THIRD EDITION

Concepts of Chemical Dependency

THIRD EDITION

Concepts of Chemical Dependency

Harold E. Doweiko

Brooks/Cole Publishing Company

I(T)P An International Thomson Publishing Company

Pacific Grove • Albany • Bonn • Boston • Cincinnati • Detroit • London • Madrid • Melbourne
Mexico City • New York • Paris • San Francisco • Singapore • Tokyo • Toronto • Washington

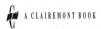 A CLAIREMONT BOOK

Sponsoring Editor: *Claire Verduin*
Marketing Team: *Nancy Kernal, Jean Thompson*
Editorial Associate: *Patsy Vienneau*
Production Editor: *Kirk Bomont*
Manuscript Editor: *Barbara Kimmel*
Interior Design: *Laurie Albrecht*

Interior Illustration: *Graphic Arts*
Cover Design: *Roy R. Neuhaus*
Cover Photo: *Dennis O'Clair/Tony Stone Images*
Art Editor: *Kathy Joneson*
Typesetting: *Kachina Typesetting, Inc.*
Printing and Binding: *Malloy Lithographing, Inc.*

For more information, contact:

BROOKS/COLE PUBLISHING COMPANY
511 Forest Lodge Road
Pacific Grove, CA 93950
USA

International Thomson Publishing Europe
Berkshire House 168-173
High Holborn
London WC1V 7AA
England

Thomas Nelson Australia
102 Dodds Street
South Melbourne, 3205
Victoria, Australia

Nelson Canada
1120 Birchmount Road
Scarborough, Ontario
Canada M1K 5G4

International Thomson Editores
Campos Eliseos 385, Piso 7
Col. Polanco
11560 México D. F. México

International Thomson Publishing GmbH
Königswinterer Strasse 418
53227 Bonn
Germany

International Thomson Publishing Asia
221 Henderson Road
#05-10 Henderson Building
Singapore 0315

International Thomson Publishing Japan
Hirakawacho Kyowa Building, 3F
2-2-1 Hirakawacho
Chiyoda-ku, Tokyo 102
Japan

Printed in the United States of America

10 9 8 7 6 5 4 3 2 1

Library of Congress Cataloging-in-Publication Data
Doweiko, Harold E., [date]
    Concepts of chemical dependency / Harold E. Doweiko. — 3rd ed.
       p.   cm.
    Includes bibliographical references and index.
    ISBM 0–534–33904-2 (paperback : alk. paper)
    1. Substance abuse.   I. Title.
RC564.D68 1996
362.29—dc20   95–19833
                                                    CIP

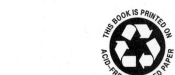

To Jan

Contents

12 Over-the-Counter Analgesics   148

13 The Hallucinogens   163

14 Inhalants and Aerosols   175

15 Anabolic Steroid Abuse   182

Preface

There have been a number of major advances in our understanding of the addictive disorders since the second edition of *Concepts of Chemical Dependency* was published in 1993. For example, much of what we thought we knew about the impact of maternal cocaine use on the developing fetus has since been proven to be based on mistaken assumptions. Once-promising theories, such as the TIQ hypothesis of alcohol's effects, have been disproven and for the most part abandoned. At the same time, new discoveries in neurology and neuropsychology promise fresh insights into the effects of the drugs of abuse on the user's brain and consciousness.

This new edition of *Concepts of Chemical Dependency* includes a number of significant changes from the second edition. Each chapter has been revised to include the latest research. For example, the section on the effects of maternal cocaine use during pregnancy has been revised and updated. The chapter on OTC analgesics has also been revised, not only to include the latest information on aspirin, ibuprofen, and acetaminophen but also to include information on the latest OTC analgesic drug: naproxen.

Another significant change is the addition of a chapter on basic pharmacology to help the reader understand *why* the drugs of abuse work the way they do. The chapter on cocaine use and abuse has been revised to include the latest information on cocaine's effects on the body, and

the chapter on narcotic analgesics has also been updated. The chapter on adolescent drug use now includes the latest information on chemical use by adolescents as revealed by the ongoing National Institute on Drug Abuse surveys. Furthermore, the chapters on treatment formats and intervention have been extensively rewritten, both to make the material more enjoyable to read and to reflect the latest findings in the ongoing debate over which forms of treatment are best. Also in this edition of *Concepts of Chemical Dependency* is information on new self-help groups, such as Rational Recovery, that are emerging as alternatives to the traditional Alcoholics Anonymous.

When the second edition of this text was being published, the chemical LAAM was hardly known outside of research circles. Chapter 31 describes how this chemical is increasingly being viewed as an acceptable alternative to methadone maintenance programs for the treatment of narcotics addiction. Similarly, the ongoing debate over whether drugs should be legalized has made an extensive revision of the chapter on Drugs and Crime necessary.

Several reviewers have inquired why this text does not address caffeine addiction. There are several reasons for the decision not to include caffeine in the current edition of *Concepts*. First, the current evidence seems to suggest that, as addictions go, the addiction to caffeine is relatively benign. Second, the chemical structure of caffeine is so different from the other drugs of abuse that it falls into a class of its own. Third, the pattern of use of caffeine is somewhat different than those of the other drugs of abuse. Finally, for sociological and political reasons, the use of caffeine is not viewed as a serious problem in the United States at this time. Rather than cross this boundary in terms of social perception, a discussion on caffeine addiction was not included in this edition.

The accumulation of all the discoveries in the field of substance abuse over the past 3 years requires a new text edition to keep this text current. Although every effort has been made to include the latest information, there is always a lag between when discoveries are announced in the press or professional journals and when the research can be incorporated into a new edition of *Concepts*. This is one reason the field of addictive medicine is so exciting: it is constantly changing. There are few generally accepted answers, a multitude of unanswered questions, and, as compared to the other branches of science, few interdisciplinary boundaries to limit one's exploration of the field.

This text was written to share the knowledge and experience of the author with others interested in the field of substance abuse. Although every effort has been made to ensure that the information reviewed in this text is accurate, this book is *not* designed, nor should it be used, as a guide to patient care.

This text provides a great deal of information about the current drugs of abuse, their dosage levels, and their effects. This information is provided not to advocate or encourage the use of chemicals but to inform the reader of current trends in the field of drug addiction. This text is not intended as a guide to self-medication, and neither the author nor publisher assumes any responsibility for individuals who attempt to use this text either as a guide for the administration of drugs to themselves or to others or as a guide to treatment.

Acknowledgments

It would not be possible to mention every person who has helped make this book a reality. However, I would like to thank Mr. Jim Plantikow for his continued feedback and support. Certainly, I must mention the library staff at Lutheran Hospital-La Crosse for their assistance in tracking down many obscure references; Ann Emmel, Marilyn Paulson, Kitty Meyer, Kay Wagner, and Sally Harvey have provided an invaluable service as part of their everyday routine, and they deserve my warmest thanks. I would also like to thank the reviewers who read the manuscript, offering valuable suggestions and insights: Iris Heckman, Washburn University; Ron Jackson, University of Washington; and Charles Kutscher, Syracuse University. My sincere thanks also to sponsoring editor Claire Verduin and the rest of the staff at Brooks/Cole.

Finally, I would like to thank my wife, Jan, for all her support. She read each chapter of the first edition—several times over—and still volunteered to help review material for the third edition. She corrected my spelling (many, many times) and encouraged me when I was up against the brick wall of writer's block. At first, her feedback was received with the same openness that any author receives "constructive criticism." But she persisted, and more often than not she was right. She is indeed my best friend and my "editor in chief." Thanks, Jan!

Harold E. Doweiko

THIRD EDITION

Concepts of Chemical Dependency

Foundations

It is difficult to look at a newspaper or listen to a news broadcast without seeing or hearing at least one reference to drug abuse, drug-related crime, or a celebrity who has checked into a treatment center. In a very real sense, drugs have become the center of modern life, either because we are using them, fighting against them, or are afraid of the actions of those who might be using them.

Although drugs seem to be so much a part of our lives, it is difficult to write a book about substance abuse because readers have such diverse backgrounds. Some readers know a great deal about one or more drugs of abuse from their own experience. Others may be curious about recreational chemicals but have limited experience with various drugs of abuse. Still other readers have virtually no information about the drugs of abuse. This immediately poses a dilemma: where to begin?

Substance Abuse—A New Phenomenon?

Although politicians speak of the problem of recreational chemical use as if it were an invention of the post–World War II era, people have struggled with the problem of chemical use and abuse for hundreds, if not thousands, of years. For example, in the United States, one of the first problems that President Washington had to face was how to deal with the so-called Whiskey Rebellion of 1790. But English Royal decrees attempting to control or regulate recreational chemical use in one form or another date back to hundreds of years before President Washington assumed office.

Indeed, historical evidence suggests that for thousands of years, people have attempted to find ways to alter their normal state of consciousness. In the past, people have accomplished this by such methods as ingesting naturally occurring hallucinogenics, employing techniques to induce oxygen deprivation, using opioids, and consuming alcohol. The "pharmacological revolution" of the 1940s and 1950s did not create the problem of recreational chemical use. However, with the advance of pharmacology after World War II, biochemists began to develop new chemicals that held the potential for abuse.

The use of mood-altering agents appears to be a common characteristic among the many diverse human cultures that have evolved over time. Indeed, so common is the problem of recreational chemical use that every known society has been forced to develop rules that govern the time and manner in which its members can use mood-altering chemicals (*Health News*, 1990). The rules that have evolved in different societies vary significantly. For example, in the Middle East, hashish use is tolerated, but strong religious sanctions exist against the use of alcohol. In the United States, just the reverse is true: there are strong social sanctions against hashish use, but the use of alcohol is not only accepted, it is even supported by government subsidies! Perhaps more than any other form of behavior, recreational chemical use defines human culture. As we will see in Chapter 4, some evidence suggests that the very roots of civilization might be traced to early humans' need for a home base to produce beer and wine!

Surprisingly, the drive to alter consciousness by chemical means is also found in many different animal species, including elephants, bighorn sheep, and primates. Research suggests that a number of different animal species go out of their way to ingest plants "whose only attraction is a fast-acting buzz" (Engelman, 1989, p. 12 E). The animals' tendency to seek out substances that have psychoactive properties suggests a possible biological basis for the use of chemicals that alter the state of consciousness.

This behavior in animals would also explain how prehistoric humans learned which plants could be used for mood-altering purposes. Scientists believe that prehistoric humans observed which plants the animals around them ingested to learn which were dangerous and which were safe to eat. Through observation and experimentation, prehistoric observers learned which plants could be used for food, which plants might have pleasurable psychoactive effects, and which plants were harmful if ingested and were to be avoided.

Thus, there appears to be a long tradition of recreational chemical use among humans. But this is a text about *current* drug use trends and the problems of recreational chemical use in the present age. How has this society responded to the challenge of drug use and abuse?

Society's Current Drug-Use Standards: An Exercise in Schizophrenia?

At first glance, the rules that govern the use of mood-altering chemicals within U.S. society might seem rather confusing. The drug-use standards of this society—like those of all societies—have evolved over time as a result of a complex mixture of different social, historical, religious, and legal forces. Because of the different factors that help shape the evolution of social standards, the rules of behavior for any given society often contain bits and pieces that seem somewhat irrational. Social rules also constantly evolve, as societies change. For example, the change in social attitude in the United States toward marijuana use between 1950 and the 1990s illustrates how the social rules of behavior can change over time.

Alcohol occupies a special place in many cultures. In spite of the fact that, pharmacologically, alcohol is as much a "drug" as any other chemical substance (Weil, 1986), most people have stopped thinking of it as a drug. Even among those who admit that alcohol is a drug, many claim that "at least it is not one of those bad drugs" (Weil, 1986, p. 18) like heroin or cocaine. Unfortunately, the role alcohol plays in U.S. society illustrates a social paradox. Since 1970, the United States has spent a great deal of time, energy, and money, attempting to understand the reasons people use drugs. But, in reality, all the time, energy, and money was invested to understand not why people use chemicals but simply "why some people are taking some drugs that we disapprove of" (Weil, 1986, p. 18). Consider that, in the United States

> alcohol is legal, but it is not legal to drive under the influence of alcohol or to sell it to children. Conversely, we speak about cocaine and the opiates as *il*legal, but in fact doctors can prescribe these drugs. (Nadelmann, Kleiman, & Earls, 1990, p. 44)

There are other examples of how unrealistic U.S. society's standards have become. In certain parts of the United States, the sale, possession, or use of alcohol might be legal on Saturday and illegal on Sunday; but, with the proper prescription signed by a physician, a person can purchase narcotics or cocaine for medicinal use any day of the week. The church minister might denounce the use of alcohol, yet wine is a central component to the celebration of communion in many sects. Health problems associated with cigarette smoking are well known, but the "tobacco industry" spent "millions of dollars in communities throughout California" (Traynor, Begay, & Glantz, 1993, p. 479) fighting anti-smoking laws under consideration, in spite of the fact that there is a known association between "second-hand smoke" and illness (a topic discussed further in Chapter 16). Is it any wonder that the whole subject of substance use, abuse, and addiction is rather confusing?

Definitions of Substance Abuse Terms

To understand the phenomenon of substance abuse, we need to develop a common language so individuals who study this problem can understand each other when discussing their work. Unfortunately, the world of substance abuse seems to have a language all its own, which makes drug abuse terminology rather confusing to the newcomer to the field.

Occasionally, addicts themselves use the ambiguity of this terminology as a defense. An example is a man who hotly denies being alcoholic, although the opinion of numerous human service professionals, as well as a judge, is somewhat different. This man defines himself as simply a "problem drinker." This statement is a classic example of a defense often used by people addicted to chemicals: rationalization. In this man's perception, he is not *alcoholic*, only a *problem drinker*. As long as he clings to this belief, he does not have to accept the fact that he is indeed addicted to alcohol.

To avoid as many misunderstandings as possible, here are definitions of some basic terms that will be used throughout this text.

Substance Abuse

An individual who is using a drug when there is no legitimate medical need to do so or who is drinking in excess of accepted social standards is said to be abusing that chemical (Schuckit, 1989). Thus, current social standards or accepted medical practice are used to classify the individual's chemical use as either appropriate or abusive.

Social Use

The "social use" of a substance is defined by traditional social standards. When we use the term *social use*, we usually mean the rare or infrequent use of a drug in a social setting. Furthermore, the drug is not used in such a manner as to cause employment, physical, family or marital, or legal problems. The use of the chemical is confined to a social setting, where its use is governed by social rules and regulations. Currently, alcohol is the chemical most frequently used in a social context, often in religious or family functions. In some circles, marijuana is also used in a social context, although its use is less acceptable than alcohol's.

Drug of Choice

At one time, clinicians spoke about an individual's *drug of choice* as an important component of the addictive process. In theory, it was assumed that the drug(s) a person would use if he or she had the choice was considered an important clue to the nature of his or her addiction. However, clinicians no longer put much emphasis on the individual's drug of choice (Walters, 1994).

The reason for this change is that the nature of addiction itself is changing. In this era of polypharmacology, it is rare for an addicted person to use just one chemical. Many cocaine addicts supplement their cocaine or amphetamine use with alcohol or minor tranquilizers to take the edge off the side effects of cocaine, commonly known as the "coke jitters." Furthermore, the chemical(s) a person uses at any point in time is frequently influenced by its availability and price. Thus, clinicians no longer focus on the concept of drug of choice.

Addiction

Morse and Flavin (1992) offer an updated definition of alcoholism that might be viewed as a model for all forms of addiction. In their opinion, alcoholism is:

> a primary, chronic disease with genetic, psychosocial and environmental factors influencing its development and manifestations. The disease is often progressive and fatal. It is characterized by impaired control over drinking, preoccupation with the drug alcohol, use of alcohol despite adverse consequences, and distortions in thinking. (p. 1013)

In this definition, one finds all the core concepts used to define drug addiction. Each form of drug addiction is viewed as follows:

1. It is a primary disease.
2. There are multiple manifestations in the person's social, psychological, spiritual, and economic life.
3. It is often progressive.
4. It is potentially fatal.
5. It is marked by an inability to control the use of that drug(s).
6. The individual is preoccupied with chemical use.
7. The individual develops a distorted way of looking at the world that supports his or her continued use of the chemical despite the many consequences inherent in its use.

In addition, addiction to a chemical is marked by the development of *tolerance* to the chemical's effects, and a *withdrawal syndrome* when the drug is discontinued (Schuckit, 1989).

Tolerance develops over time, as the body struggles to maintain normal function in spite of the presence of one or more foreign chemicals. Technically, there are several different forms of tolerance. For the sake of this text, we will limit our discussion to just two forms of tolerance: (1) metabolic tolerance and (2) pharmacodynamic tolerance.

Metabolic tolerance takes place when, after being exposed to a drug for a period of time, the body becomes more effective in biotransforming that chemical into a form that can be easily eliminated from the body. (The process of biotransformation will be discussed in more detail in Chapter 3). The liver is the main organ in which the process of biotransformation is carried out. In some cases, the constant exposure to a chemical causes the liver to become more efficient at breaking down the foreign chemical.

Pharmacodynamic tolerance is a term applied to the central nervous system's increasing insensitivity to the drug's effects. When the cells of the central nervous system are continuously exposed to a chemical, they often try to maintain normal function by making minute changes in their cell structure to compensate for the drug's effects. The cells of the central nervous system then become less sensitive to the effects of that chemical, and the person must use more of the drug to achieve the initial effect.

Each drug of abuse will, if used for a long enough period of time, bring about a characteristic *withdrawal syndrome*. The exact nature of the withdrawal syndrome will vary, depending on such factors as the class of drug, the period of time it has been used, and the individual's state of health. But each group of drugs will produce certain physical symptoms when the person stops taking the drug.

The existence of a withdrawal syndrome is evidence that pharmacodynamic tolerance has developed. In a very real sense, the withdrawal syndrome is caused by the absence of the chemical the central nervous system had previously adapted to. When the drug is discontinued, the central nervous system goes through a period of readaptation as it learns to function normally again. It is during this period of time that the individual experiences the physical signs of withdrawal.

Consider the case of alcohol, which is a central nervous system depressant. Alcohol functions very much as a chemical "brake" on the cells of the central nervous system, similar to the brakes on a car. If you attempt to drive while the brakes are engaged, it might be possible to eventually force the car to go fast enough to meet the posted speed limits. But if you then suddenly release the pressure on the brakes, the car will suddenly leap ahead because the brakes are no longer fighting the forward motion of the car. You would need to ease up on the gas pedal to slow the engine down enough to keep you within the posted speed limit.

During that period of readjustment, the car is, in a sense, going through a withdrawal phase. Much the same thing happens in the body when the individual stops using drugs. The body must adjust to the absence of a chemical that it had previously learned would always be there. This withdrawal syndrome, like the presence of tolerance to the drug's effects, provides strong evidence that the individual is addicted to one or more chemicals.

How Serious *Is* the Problem of Illicit Drug Use?

We have been waging a "war on drugs" in the United States for several generations. For many years, a basic strategy of this "war" has been to exaggerate the dangers associated with chemical use (Musto, 1991). Indeed, there seemed to be an unwritten law that one had to present drugs in such a negative light that "anyone reading or hearing of them would not be tempted to experiment with the substances" (Musto, 1991, p. 46). It is almost as if disinformation became the government's unofficial policy against chemical use. An excellent example of this "disinformation policy" is a statement by an antidrug speaker claiming that 1 ounce of heroin could make 2000 people addicts (Musto, 1991).

As a result of this process of disinformation, a certain degree of hysteria surrounding chemical abuse has become part of the social structure. People have lost sight of the fact that even the use of such chemicals as cocaine or heroin does not *automatically* bring about the more advanced, destructive forms of compulsive drug use usually associated with these substances. Indeed, in spite of the popular image associated with various drugs of abuse, research

suggests that, although many people might abuse drugs on occasion, addiction to a drug is a problem for only a small percentage of the population. This is not to deny that substance abuse and addiction has not extracted a terrible cost from those who are within its grasp. However, an open, honest examination of the research data shows that only a small percentage of the population is actually addicted to chemicals.

Holloway (1991), for example, reported that only 5.5 million people (or, about 2% of the current U.S. population of approximately 260 million) are addicted to illegal drugs. This estimate does not include people addicted to alcohol. Gazzaniga (1988) arrived at a different estimate, stating that perhaps 26 million, or 10% of the U.S. population, "falls into addictive patterns with drugs" (p. 143). Although it is not the goal of this text to advocate substance use, one must wonder how serious the problem of drug use and abuse actually is if it affects only a minority of the population.

The Growth of New "Addictions"

In addition to the media's tendency to exaggerate the dangers associated with chemical abuse, there is a disturbing trend to refer to larger and larger numbers of people as addicts. Many substance abuse professionals now speak of "addiction" to food, sex, gambling, men, women, play, television, shopping, credit cards, making money, carbohydrates, shoplifting, unhappy relationships, and a multitude of other nondrug behaviors and substances (Peele, 1989; Peele, Brodsky, & Arnold, 1991). This expansion of the definition of the term *addiction*, unfortunately, does not appear to have an end in sight.

In this text, we will limit the term *addiction* to references to the various drugs of abuse, and we will use the criterion of a demonstrated withdrawal syndrome to identify whether an individual is actually addicted. As we will discuss in the next chapter, substance abuse often blends into an addiction to the chemical. In this text, we will often use the terms *substance use, chemical dependency, substance abuse,* and *addiction* interchangeably, but these terms apply only to the problem of drug abuse and addiction.

The Neurological Foundation and Unity of Addictions

Many years ago, professionals would speak of alcoholism, or heroin addiction, or addiction to barbiturates as if they were separate disorders. Yet, in the past generation, neuropsychological researchers have uncovered evidence suggesting that, in spite of superficial differences among the various drugs of abuse, they all seem to activate a "pleasure center" of the brain (Restak, 1994). Indeed, neuropharmacological researchers have concluded that the pleasure center is within a region of the brain known as the *limbic system.* Currently, it is suspected that the various drugs of abuse cause their pleasurable effects by altering the normal chemical interactions within this region of the brain (Miller & Gold, 1993).

Unfortunately, researchers have yet to agree on the exact subunits of the limbic system where the drugs of abuse have their main effects. Some researchers believe that the various drugs of abuse alter the normal function of the *nucleus accumbens,* a subunit of the region of the brain known as the *basal ganglia* (Restak, 1994; Fischbach, 1992). Other researchers believe that the various drugs of abuse alter the function of the median forebrain bundle of the brain (Miller & Gold, 1993). In contrast, Beitner-Johnson and Nestler (1992) identified the meso-limbic dopamine system as the region of the brain where the CNS stimulants, CNS depressants, nicotine, and marijuana all seem to produce their euphoric effects. So although there is still considerable disagreement over which specific sections of the limbic system are involved, researchers now believe that it is in this region of the brain that drug-induced euphoria is generated.

The discovery that, ultimately, the various drugs of abuse impact on the same nerve pathways within the brain is consistent with clinical observations made by mental health professionals over the years. Substance abuse professionals have long known that polydrug addiction is the norm rather than the exception (Miller & Gold, 1993; Miller & Gold, 1991a). For example, 90% of adult alcoholics also smoke cigarettes (Myers & Brown, 1994). (The properties of nicotine are discussed in Chapter 14.) Research also suggests that 80% of cocaine addicts and up to 75% of opiate addicts are also addicted to alcohol (Miller & Gold, 1991a). Perhaps the reason addicts find it so easy to switch from one drug to another is because they all work through the limbic system of the brain.

Further evidence of the unitary nature of addictive disorders can be found in the observation that, as a general rule, addicts all use the same psychological defense mechanisms. Regardless of the exact nature of their specific addiction, all addicts struggle to defend, as well as to control, their individual addiction. They engage in many of the same behaviors while addicted and often utilize many of the same drugs. The alcoholic, for example, might use amphetamines or cocaine to help fight off the sedating effects of alcohol so that he or she could drink more. The concept of a common pleasure center also might explain why such a large percentage of alcoholics smoke cigarettes; nicotine is a powerful CNS stimulant.[1]

Another reflection of the common nature of addictions is the similarities found among the self-help programs of Alcoholics Anonymous (AA), Narcotics Anonymous (NA), and Cocaine Anonymous (CA). With few exceptions, all three programs utilize the same language and concepts to help addicts come to terms with their addiction. The fact that it is possible

[1]The reverse is also true: Individuals who abuse CNS stimulants like cocaine or the amphetamines often try to control the harsh, abrasive side effects of the drug through the use of CNS depressants like alcohol, the benzodiazepines, or similar agents.

to adapt the AA philosophy for NA and CA again demonstrates the unitary nature of addictive disorders.

Social Differences Within Unity

Thus, all forms of drug addiction might be viewed as different forms of a single disease. One hallmark of this disease is the compulsive use of any number of different chemicals (Miller & Gold, 1993; Franklin, 1987). But whereas neuropharmacologists identified the common specific neural pathways associated with the addictive disorders, sociologists discovered that the face of addiction is quite different in different social groups.

Franklin (1987) noted that, historically, different social groups have tended to gravitate toward different chemicals. Indeed, there appeared to be a social stratification process at work in the field of chemical abuse and dependency. To "many inner-city blacks . . . heroin was their history, their balm . . . and their master" (Franklin, 1987, p. 58). However, middle-class whites tended to use one of the barbiturates or the barbituratelike drugs. This pattern of chemical use remained true in the United States for the white middle class until Valium replaced the barbiturates as the "opiate of the suburbs" (p. 57) in the mid-1960s. Even today, researchers find that "crack" cocaine is more common in the inner-city areas, whereas powdered cocaine is more common in the suburbs. Thus, even as neuropharmacologists have laid the groundwork for viewing the various forms of drug abuse and addiction as different manifestations of one basic disorder, sociologists have found clear-cut class differences in the United States in how individuals have come to use recreational chemicals.

Chemical Dependency: A "Disease" with Nobody Trained to Diagnose It

The confusion surrounding substance use and abuse is not limited to the general public. Within the medical community, there are those who argue that drug addiction is a "disease" and those who argue just as strongly that it is not a true "disease." No matter which position one adopts, modern medicine's response to the problem of substance use, abuse, and addiction is no less confusing than society's.

Consider the following facts in the United States.

- At any given time, up to one-half of the patients in the hospital emergency room are there either directly or indirectly because of chemical abuse (Evans & Sullivan, 1990).
- Either directly or indirectly, chemical abuse plays a role in between one-third and one-half of those individuals seen for psychiatric emergencies (Evans & Sullivan, 1990; Galanter, Castaneda, & Ferman, 1988).
- The medical treatment of alcoholism and drug addiction, combined with the various psychiatric consequences of these disorders, accounts for up to 60% of hospital usage in this country (Ciraulo, Shader, Ciraulo, Greenblatt, & von Moltke, 1994a).
- The economic cost of chemical abuse *alone* is more than two and a half times that of all other forms of mental illness combined (Group for the Advancement of Psychiatry, 1990).
- Either directly or indirectly, substance abuse is the most common "disease" the modern physician encounters (American Medical Association, 1993a).

Even though these statistics suggest that substance abuse is a major contributing factor to illness and disease, *less than 1% of the typical medical school curriculum addresses alcohol or drug abuse* (Selwyn, 1993). It is only recently that psychiatric residency programs have even started to focus on the issue of alcohol or drug addiction. And even these psychiatric residency programs tend to focus more on the mechanics of detoxification, without addressing the subject of substance abuse rehabilitation (Galanter, 1993).

The situation is even worse for the typical general practice physician. In his or her medical training, the general practice physician is exposed to information on many rare and infrequently encountered diseases (Twerski, 1989). But when it comes to the identification or treatment of substance abuse, "medical education and training remain seriously inadequate in preparing physicians to identify and to treat substance abuse" (Selwyn, 1993, p. 1045).

Unfortunately, one result of this oversight in physicians' training is that most doctors are not able to recognize the early signs of addictive disorders such as alcoholism. For example, Rydon, Redman, Sanson-Fisher, and Reid (1992) examined the primary care physicians' ability to detect alcohol-related problems in more than 300 patients. The patients who took part in this study had completed either a modified form of the Michigan Alcoholism Screening Test (MAST) or a standard assessment tool for alcoholism known as the CAGE. The authors found that the primary care physicians failed to identify alcoholism in 65% of those patients classified as alcoholic by the CAGE, and in 82% of the alcoholics classified as such on the modified form of the MAST. In other words, the primary care physicians failed to identify the majority of the individuals who, on the basis of either the MAST or CAGE, were classified as alcoholic. This diagnostic failure might reflect the fact that many physicians consider alcoholism "untreatable" (Rains, 1990, p. 40). At best, physicians are "often pessimistic about the efficacy of treatment" for substance abuse or addiction (Group for the Advancement of Psychiatry, 1990, p. 1295).

Diagnostic blindness is not limited to physicians, however; psychologists can be affected, too. Although substance abuse is not the only reason families become troubled, it does play a role in up to 50% of the cases presented for family or marital counseling (Treadway, 1987), yet the chemical abuse within the family is often not diagnosed. Family/marital therapists only

rarely ask the proper questions to identify addicted individuals within the marital or family unit, according to Treadway. When the addiction is not uncovered, therapy proceeds in a haphazard fashion and vital clues to a very real illness within the family are missed. The attempt at family or marital therapy is often ineffective because the addictive disorder is not identified and addressed.

In spite of the obvious relationship between substance abuse and the various forms of psychopathology, Youngstrom (1991) reported that of the approximately 68,000 psychologists who are members of the American Psychological Association (APA), "only 504 identified substance abuse as their primary specialty, and 789 list it as their secondary specialty" (p. 14). Obviously, the professional response to the problem of substance abuse has been far short of the need. In a very real sense, despite whether or not substance abuse and addiction is a true "disease" (a matter that is still disputed), the health care and mental health professions have not responded to the problem by training practitioners to recognize and treat this disorder.

Summary

Historical evidence suggests that, for thousands of years, people have attempted to find ways to alter their normal state of consciousness. In this sense, recreational drug use might be said to be a defining characteristic of human culture. But the recreational chemical use standards of U.S. society are often unrealistic and seemingly contradictory, as with sanctions against alcohol use only on Sunday.

It has been estimated that 2–10% of adults in the United States either abuse or are addicted to illegal drugs. Although this percentage suggests that large numbers of people are using illicit chemicals in this society, it also suggests that the drugs of abuse are not universally addictive. The reality is that only a small percentage of the total population of this country becomes addicted. In this chapter, we introduced and defined key concepts such as substance abuse, social use, addiction, and the individual's drug of choice. We also proposed that the various forms of chemical abuse and addiction may reflect different manifestations of a single disorder: chemical abuse/addiction. Finally, although drug addiction is classified as a "disease," we noted that most physicians are ill-prepared to treat substance abusing patients.

The Scope of Chemical Abuse and Addiction

In the last chapter, we introduced the basic terminology of the field of substance abuse. In this chapter, we will explore the scope of the problem of drug abuse and addiction within the United States. We will also briefly discuss some issues the professional faces in accurately diagnosing chemical dependency.

The Continuum of Addiction

It is not uncommon these days to hear health care and mental health professionals speak about substance *use, abuse,* and *dependency* as if these terms were synonymous. In reality, there are subtle but very real differences between the use of a recreational chemical, the abuse of that substance, and dependency on that drug. Because a person uses a certain chemical does not automatically mean he or she is addicted to it. Unfortunately, even today there are those who continue to confuse the abuse of a chemical with the more serious problem of drug addiction.

This is not to deny that substance abuse is a serious problem or that there is a great potential for harm in the misuse of chemicals for personal pleasure. Rather, the point is that chemical addiction is not simply an either/or condition. There are a variety of different chemical use patterns, of which the addict's habitual, compulsive use of a drug is an extreme.

Unfortunately, because of society's attitudes and prejudices, there are few clear-cut lines between experimental chemical use, the "social" use of a substance, drug abuse, and chemical dependency (*Health News*, 1990). Even in the case of alcohol, humankind's oldest drug, professionals often disagree over what constitutes alcohol abuse and the more serious condition of alcoholism (Washton, 1990).

One reason for this disagreement is that substance abuse can follow one of many different patterns. Addiction "is not an all-or-nothing thing, but a continuum from moderate excess to severe compulsion" (Peele, Brodsky, & Arnold, 1991, p. 133). Thus the severity of a given individual's substance use must be considered along a continuum that ranges from total abstinence from all chemical use, through rare (or, for want of a better word, "social") use, to heavy use, and ultimately to addiction to chemicals (Sellers, Ciraulo, DuPont, Griffiths, Kosten, Romach, & Woody, 1993; Brower, Blow, Young, & Hill, 1991). Thus, at any given time, an individual might be (1) abstaining from all recreational chemical use, (2) using one or more chemicals on a social basis, (3) abusing one or more chemicals on an episodic basis, (4) abusing one or more drugs on a continual basis, or (5) addicted to a drug or drugs. Admittedly, there are no firm boundaries between these points on the continuum (Sellers et al., 1993). For the purpose of this text, we will use a similar continuum, as illustrated in Figure 2.1.

The Scope of Chemical Abuse and Addiction

0	1	2	3	4
Total abstinence from drug use	Rare social use of drugs	Heavy social use/early problem use of drugs	Heavy problem use/early addiction to drugs	Clear-cut addiction to drugs

FIGURE 2.1 The continuum of chemical use

As with any continuum, movement back and forth from one stage to another is possible. For example, alcoholism is not simply the result of a progression from occasional social drinking to alcohol addiction. Rather, as Vaillant (1983) discovered in his research, there is a great deal of variation in any given individual's pattern of alcohol use over a lifetime. Vaillant found that movement back and forth from more serious to less offensive drinking, or the opposite, is actually the rule rather than the exception. For example, a rare social drinker might abuse alcohol for a period of several months following the break up of a relationship, after which he or she might return to the occasional social use of alcohol.

The advantage of viewing drug use on a continuum such as the one in Figure 2.1 is that it allows us to classify various intensities and patterns of chemical use. Drug use, abuse, or addiction thus becomes a behavior, not a condition that either is or is not present. The different stages of chemical use on the continuum are as follows.

Level 0: Total abstinence The individual abstains from all recreational alcohol or chemical use.

Level 1: Rare social use The individual rarely uses alcohol or chemicals for recreational purposes but is able to drink or use chemicals without social, financial, interpersonal, or legal problems associated with more serious levels of alcohol or drug use.

Level 2: Heavy social use/early problem drug use A person at this point in the continuum (1) uses chemicals in a manner that is clearly above the norm for his or her social group, or (2) begins to experience various combinations of legal, social, financial, occupational, and personal problems associated with chemical use. For example, 30% to 45% of all adults in the United States will experience at least one episode of transient alcohol-related problems (such as blackouts) (Kaplan, Sadock, & Grebb, 1994). The individual in this category might try to hide or deny the problems that arise from his or her chemical use. But many will learn from their experience and alter their chemical use so that they are unlikely to encounter future problems.

Level 3: Heavy problem use/early addiction This person's alcohol or chemical use has reached the point where there clearly is a problem. Indeed, this person may have become addicted to chemicals, although he or she may argue the point. For some drugs of abuse, medical complications associated with addiction become apparent. Also at this phase, the individual demonstrates classic withdrawal symptoms when unable to continue the use of drugs or alcohol. The early addict also experiences various combinations of ongoing legal, financial, social, occupational, and personal problems either directly or indirectly caused by his or her chemical use.

Level 4: Clear-cut addiction to drugs At this point on the continuum, the person demonstrates the classic addiction syndrome in combination with multiple social, legal, financial, occupational, and personal problems. The person also demonstrates various medical complications associated with chemical abuse and may be near death as a result of chronic addiction. This individual is clearly addicted beyond any shadow of a doubt in an observer's mind. However, even at this level of substance use, the addicted individual might try to rationalize away or deny problems associated with his or her alcohol or drug use. More than one elderly alcoholic, for example, has tried to explain away an abnormal liver function as the aftermath of a childhood illness. However, to an impartial outside observer, the person at this level is clearly addicted to alcohol or drugs.

Admittedly, this classification system, like all others, is imperfect. The criteria used to determine the different levels are arbitrary and subject to debate. As Vaillant (1983) observed, it is often "the variety of alcohol related problems, not any unique criterion, that captures what clinicians really mean when they label a person alcoholic" (p. 42). That is, it is a constellation of various symptoms, rather than the existence of any single symptom, that identifies alcoholism or any other drug dependency.

However, as outlined in the next section, even with such drugs of abuse as narcotics or cocaine, significant percentages of those who use these drugs—even if they do so on a regular basis—are not necessarily *addicted*. Physical addiction to a chemical is just one point on the continuum of drug use styles.

The Extent of Chemical Dependency[1]

Over the years, various estimates of the scope of the problem of drug abuse and addiction in the

United States have been offered. Franklin (1987), for example, concluded that, when drug rehabilitation professionals examined the statistics on alcoholism, illegal drug abuse, and the abuse of prescription drugs, it appeared "that perhaps one in every five Americans (is) hopelessly addicted to something—and another one or two (are) steady users (p. 59). If we accept Franklin's estimate that 20% of the U.S. population is addicted, then (assuming a national population of 260 million) approximately 52 million people are addicted to chemicals, and another 52 million are steady users. These figures are indeed quite alarming. Fortunately, other estimates do not suggest a problem of this magnitude.

The study that came closest to supporting Franklin's estimate was the study by Kessler, McGonagle, Zhao, Nelson, Hughes, Eshleman, Hans-Ulrich, and Kendler (1994). These authors based their conclusions on the responses of a sample of 8,098 individuals, selected to approximate the characteristics of the population of the United States as a whole. This sample represented the percentage of the population that would meet diagnostic criteria for one of 14 psychiatric conditions, both in the preceeding 12 months and during their lifetime. On the basis of their research, the authors concluded that more than 14% of their respondents had a lifetime history of alcohol dependence; more than 7% of their sample were dependent on alcohol in the past 12 months; more than 4% of their sample had used a drug for recreational purposes at some point in their lives but were not dependent on chemicals; and more than 7% of their sample would meet the diagnostic criteria for drug dependence at some point in their lives.

These results, while suggestive, failed to answer some significant questions. For example, the study did not identify the degree of overlap that might have existed between those who were found to be alcohol dependent and those who were judged to be drug dependent. Individuals who are addicted to chemicals rarely limit themselves just to alcohol or to a single drug. Thus, it is possible that Kessler et al.

[1]Although this section explains that not everyone who uses a given chemical will become addicted, this is not to be interpreted as an endorsement of experimentation with, or use of, chemicals. If only because it is not possible to predict in advance who will ultimately become addicted, recreational drug use is not encouraged.

counted some of their respondents in *both* the alcohol and drug dependent samples. Furthermore, the authors failed to identify whether tobacco was defined as a drug of abuse. These methodological flaws in the research may have resulted in inaccurate conclusions.

Certainly, the results obtained by Kessler et al. (1994) were significantly different from those obtained by Regier, Farmer, Rae, Locke, Keith, Judd, and Goodwin (1990). These researchers also examined the lifetime prevalence rates of various forms of mental illness—including alcohol and substance abuse disorders—in the United States. Regier et al. (1990) used a different methodology, and their results suggest that, at any given point in time, only 2.8% of the population meet the criteria for a diagnosis of either alcohol abuse or dependence. Another 1.3 % of the population meet the diagnostic criteria for a drug abuse or dependence problem. The authors also concluded that, over the course of their lives, approximately 13.5% of the population would meet the criteria for either alcohol abuse or dependence. Another 6.1% would meet the criteria for a diagnosis of substance abuse or dependence.

Again, if we assume that the population of the United States is approximately 260 million people and apply the figures suggested by these two studies, we reach some interesting conclusions. On the basis of the study by Regier et al. (1990), at any given time about 7.3 million people in the United States meet the diagnostic criteria for alcohol abuse or dependence; another 3.4 million qualify for a diagnosis of drug abuse or dependence. In contrast, Kessler et al.'s (1994) conclusions suggest that 18.2 million people in the United States were physically dependent on alcohol at some point in the preceding 12 months, and 10.4 million had used a recreational chemical other than alcohol in the same 12-month period. The data also suggests that, at some point in their lives, approximately 36.4 million people would be physically dependent on alcohol, and 18.2 million would be dependent on a recreational drug.

Galanter and Frances (1992) estimated that a slightly higher percentage, 15% of the U.S. population, will meet the diagnostic criteria for alcohol abuse at some point in their lives, and they predicted a lifetime prevalence rate of 6% for drug abuse. Again, if we assume that the population of the United States is approximately 260 million people and apply the lifetime prevalence figures suggested by Galanter and Frances (1992), the authors postulate that 39 million people in the United States will meet the diagnostic criteria for a formal diagnosis of alcohol abuse at some point in their lives, and, sooner or later, another 15.6 million will meet the diagnostic criteria for drug abuse.

Now we can compare the preceding estimates with what researchers have found out about the drug abuse problem in the United States. Approximately 12.9 million people in the United States used an illicit substance at least once in 1991 (*Playboy*, 1992), a number that was down from the estimated 23 million who used an illegal drug in 1985. If we use a population estimate of 260 million Americans, we calculate that about 5% of the population used one or more illicit drugs at least once in 1991. White (1993) suggests that only 12 million Americans might be classified as "frequent users" of illicit chemicals (p. 26A). Overall, there are an estimated 1.1 to 1.8 million intravenous drug users in the United States. This estimate includes both those who are addicted and those who are abusing intravenous drugs but who are not addicted to chemicals (Selwyn, 1993).

These estimates and the predictions reviewed earlier in this chapter are significantly lower than Franklin's (1987) estimated 20% of the population (or 52 million people) who were presumed to be addicted to chemicals, and 20% of the population who were abusing chemicals. The reader might consider Franklin's figures a "worst case" estimate that has not been supported by the research data.

However, the wide differences among the various estimates of the scope of substance abuse and addiction in the United States underscore a serious shortcoming in the field of substance abuse rehabilitation: the lack of clear data. Depending on who you talk to, substance abuse is or is not a serious problem, is or is not getting worse (or, better), will or will not be resolved in the next decade, and is or is not something that parents should worry about. The truth is that large numbers of people use one or more recreational chemicals, but only a small percentage of people who use them will ultimately become addicted (Peele, Brodsky, & Arnold, 1991). In the next section, we will provide an overview of the problem of substance abuse in this country.

Estimates of Substance Use, Abuse, and Addiction

Alcohol

Only a small minority of those who drink are actually addicted to alcohol. The American Psychiatric Association (1994) estimated that, in the United States, 90% of adults have used alcohol at least once. However, alcohol abuse or addiction are a problem only for a minority of those who drink, according to the American Psychiatric Association.

Unfortunately, even after many decades of study, researchers still disagree as to the exact scope of the problem of alcohol addiction in the United States. Various estimates have been offered, suggesting that 6 million (Ellis, McInerney, DiGiuseppe, & Yeager, 1988) to 10 million (Bays, 1990) to 12 million (L. Siegel, 1989) to perhaps as many as 18 million (McMicken, 1990) adults in the United States are addicted to alcohol. This number does not include another estimated 1 million (Ellis, McInerney, DiGiuseppe, & Yeager, 1988) to 3 million children and adolescents (Turbo, 1989) thought to be addicted to alcohol.

Researchers do agree that, to a very large degree, alcohol abuse and addiction could be called a "male disease." The majority of those who abuse or who are addicted to alcohol are male. But this does not mean that alcohol abuse and addiction is *exclusively* a male problem. The ratio of male to female alcohol abusers and

addicts is thought to fall between 2:1 and 3:1 (Blume, 1994; Cyr & Moulton, 1993). These figures suggest that significant numbers of women are also abusing or are addicted to alcohol.

Because alcohol can be legally purchased, many people forget that it is also a drug. However, the grim reality is that this legal chemical makes up the greatest part of the drug abuse and addiction problem in the United States. Franklin (1987) stated that alcoholism alone accounts for 85% of the problem of drug addiction.

Narcotics

When many people hear the term *drugs of abuse*, they think of narcotics, especially heroin. Although narcotic analgesics have the reputation of being quite addictive, significant evidence suggests that a large number of people abuse the narcotic analgesics without ever becoming addicted to them. Jenike (1991) estimates that only half of those who abuse narcotics go on to become addicted to them.

In contrast, the American Academy of Family Physicians (1989) estimated that 2 million Americans use narcotics occasionally, in addition to the 500,000 who are addicted. This gives a ratio of 4 abusers to every 1 addict. Kaufman and McNaul (1992) reported that 1 million Americans use heroin at least once a week but did not estimate how many were addicted to the drug or how many were casual users.

Obviously, not every person who abuses narcotics will become addicted.[2] Of those who *are* addicted to narcotics, the greatest number are addicted to heroin. However, as we will discuss later in this book, there are individuals who are addicted to various prescription narcotic analgesics who never use heroin.

It should not be surprising to learn that the estimates of the number of active heroin addicts

[2]Unfortunately, it is not possible to determine in advance who will or will not become addicted to narcotics. Thus, if only for this reason, narcotics abuse should be discouraged.

vary. Because heroin is illegal in the United States, individuals who are addicted are unlikely to volunteer that information. Furthermore, it is natural to assume that these individuals will go to great lengths to hide their addiction. It has been estimated, however, that there are between 500,000 (Kaplan, Sadock, & Grebb, 1994; Kanof, Aronson, & Ness, 1992) and 600,000 (Witkin & Griffin, 1994) heroin addicts in the United States; it is believed that about half of them live in New York City (Kaplan, Sadock, & Grebb, 1994; Witkin & Griffin, 1994).

A significant percentage of those addicted to heroin are women. Peluso and Peluso (1988) estimate that perhaps as many as 100,000 of the known heroin addicts are women, whereas Kaplan and Sadock (1990) give a ratio of three male heroin addicts to every female. Given the estimates of 400,000 to 600,000 heroin addicts, this means that there are between 100,000 and 150,000 women addicted to heroin in the United States.

Unfortunately, estimates of the scope of narcotics addiction are, for the most part, based on data drawn from public treatment programs and social service agency reports (Eisenhandler & Drucker, 1993). Individuals who utilize these services are largely indigent and dependent on public services. But, in spite of the popular stereotype of the narcotics addict, many individuals who are addicted to narcotic analgesics have regular jobs and private health care insurance. Unfortunately, when these individuals enter the health care system, they do so at a private health care facility, so their addiction to narcotic analgesics is unlikely to be included in a database drawn from public treatment programs or social service agency reports. Their addiction would be hidden from most researchers in the field of substance abuse.

This is exactly the population that Eisenhandler and Drucker (1993) discovered in their study. In their exploration of treatment histories of individuals covered by a major private health care insurance agency, the authors identified a subgroup of opiate addicts about whom little is known: the employed, financially stable addict

with private health care insurance. Because virtually nothing is known about this population, the authors' research was significant. This study helped identify a new subgroup of narcotics addicts different from those who are addicted to heroin and who live "on the street."

The truth is that there are many "hidden" narcotics addicts in the population about whom health care professionals have virtually no information. For example, it *is* known that some pharmaceutical narcotic analgesics are diverted to the illicit drug market; however, there is virtually no information available on the person addicted to pharmaceutical narcotics. Thus, the estimated 400,000 to 600,000 intravenous heroin addicts must be accepted as only a minimal estimate of the problem of narcotics addiction in the United States.

Cocaine

Although evidence suggests that cocaine abuse peaked in the mid-1980s, it still remains a popular drug of abuse. Angell and Kassifer (1994) estimate that, in the United States, 1.6 million people use cocaine on a regular basis. However, the authors do not differentiate between those who were addicted to the drug and those who used cocaine infrequently. In a report issued by the RAND Corporation on the subject of the U.S. drug policy, it was estimated that there are currently 7 million cocaine users in the United States (*Alcoholism & Drug Abuse Week*, 1994b). Of this number, 1.7 million are thought to consume cocaine at least once a week, using 8 times as much cocaine as the other 5.3 million combined.

Surprisingly, in spite of its reputation for causing addiction, only a small percentage of those who use cocaine ever become addicted to this or any other drug. Musto (1991), for example, estimated that between 3 and 20% of those who use cocaine go on to become addicted. In support of this estimate, consider that, between 1 cocaine user in 6 (Peele, Brodsky & Arnold, 1991) to 1 in 12 (Peluso & Peluso, 1988) is actually addicted to the drug. The rest are cocaine abusers but not addicts.

Marijuana

Researchers have only recently concluded that it is possible to become addicted, in the traditional sense of the word, to marijuana. The possibility of an individual going through withdrawal symptoms as a result of chronic marijuana use will be discussed in more detail in Chapter 10.

Marijuana is currently the most commonly abused illegal drug in the United States (Kaufman & McNaul, 1992) and Canada (Russell, Newman, & Bland, 1994). It is estimated that 68 million (Kaufman & McNaul, 1992), or approximately 25% of the entire U.S. population, has used marijuana at least once.

Angell and Kassifer (1994, p. 537) estimate that there are presently 9 million "regular" users of marijuana in the United States; however, the authors do not identify what they mean by "regular" users of this substance. Apparently, only a fraction of those who use marijuana do so daily.

Hallucinogenics

There are questions as to whether one can become addicted to hallucinogenics. For this reason, we speak of the "problem of hallucinogenic abuse" rather than addiction. Perhaps as many as one-fifth of the U.S. population under the age of 25 have used hallucinogenics at one time or another (Kaplan & Sadock, 1990), but hallucinogenic use is actually quite rare. Of those young adults who have used hallucinogenic drugs, only 1 or 2% will have done so in the past 30 days, according to Kaplan and Sadock. This data suggests that the problem of *addiction* to hallucinogenics is exceedingly rare.

Tobacco

Tobacco is a special drug; like alcohol, it is legally sold to adults. Unfortunately, tobacco products are also readily obtained by adolescents, who make up a significant proportion of tobacco users in the United States. Traditionally, it has been quite difficult to obtain accurate estimates

of how many people smoke, but current estimates are that approximately 46 million people in the United States smoke cigarettes (Brownlee, Roberts, Cooper, Goode, Hetter, & Wright, 1994). Of this number, an estimated 24 million smokers are male and 22.3 million are female.

Future Trends in Substance Use and Abuse

As stated earlier, there is strong evidence (*Mayo Clinic Health Letter*, 1989; Gold, 1990a) that casual drug use in the United States peaked in the early to mid-1980s. Official estimates provided by the U.S. government suggest a 45% drop in the number of illicit drug users between 1985 and 1991 (*Playboy*, 1992). But no one *really* knows what is going on in the world of illicit drug use.

The Limitations of Current Research

If you were to watch the television talk shows or read a small sample of the multitude of self-help books currently on the market, you would be left with the impression that researchers fully understand the causes and treatment of drug abuse. Nothing could be further from the truth. Much of what we think we know about addiction is based on mistaken assumptions or, at best, incomplete data. Furthermore, because of the illicit nature of recreational chemical use, many drug-use trends remain hidden or only poorly understood.

Much of the research on substance abuse is flawed for several reasons. For example, a great deal of research is based on a distorted sample of people: those who are in treatment for substance abuse problems (Gazzaniga, 1988). Virtually nothing is known about those people who use chemicals on a social basis, never become addicted, and never enter treatment programs for their drug use. These people, who are known as "chippers," make up a subpopulation of drug users about which virtually nothing is known. Researchers are not even able to make an educated guess as to their number, but it is known that there are "chippers" for virtually every recreational drug currently in use.

Second, much of the research on substance abuse is based on the assumption that all chemical abuse is the same. Thus, much of the research done in this field is carried out either in Veteran's Administration hospitals or public facilities such as state hospitals. However, the simple fact that an individual was able to complete a term of military service (required for admission into a Veteran's Administration facility) or is employed and able to afford treatment in a private treatment center means that he or she is far different from the indigent alcoholic who must be treated in a publicly funded treatment program.

Third, although many in the treatment industry will not admit it, the majority of those who abuse chemicals either stop or significantly reduce their chemical use without professional intervention (Gazzaniga, 1988; *Mayo Clinic Health Letter*, 1989; Peele, 1985, 1989; Tucker & Sobell, 1992; Carroll & Rounsaville, 1992). Indeed, the *Mayo Clinic Health Letter* (1989) concluded that "despite the widespread availability of drugs and their addictive qualities, millions of Americans who once used them regularly appear now to have given them up" (p. 2).

This phenomenon can be seen clearly in the histories of soldiers who used chemicals while serving in Vietnam. Although many U.S. military personnel used drugs in Vietnam and many were addicted, the majority apparently stopped using chemicals without professional intervention. Of 1,400 U.S. soldiers who tested positive for drugs on their return from Vietnam in 1971, only one-third, or 495 men, were still using chemicals eight months later (Gazzaniga, 1988). Jenike (1991) pointed out that up to 40% of the enlisted men who served in Vietnam had abused heroin at one time or another, but only 5% of the men continued to abuse narcotics after their return to the United States.

Fourth, as stated earlier, much of what we think we know about substance abuse is based on research carried out on those in treatment for drug addiction. Unfortunately, much of this research has failed to differentiate between abusers of a chemical and those who are ad-

dicted (Peele, 1985). Rather, it is assumed that if the person is in treatment, he or she is by definition an addict. But people enter "treatment" for a number of reasons, not just because they are addicted to chemicals. Consider the (all too common) case of a drug "pusher" who enters treatment to impress the court with his or her desire for sobriety, while holding the sincere desire to continue to sell drugs after release from "treatment."

It is also important to keep in mind that those who seek treatment for their substance abuse problem are not representative of all substance abusers. Addicts who seek treatment are quite different from those addicts who do not (Carroll & Rounsaville, 1992). Indeed, as a group, addicts who do not seek treatment seem to be better able to control their substance use and have shorter drug use histories than do addicts who seek treatment.

The available literature on the subject of drug addiction is extremely limited in other ways as well. Only a small portion of the current literature addresses forms of addiction other than alcoholism. An even smaller proportion addresses the impact of chemicals on women (Griffin, Weiss, Mirin, & Lang, 1989). Much of the research conducted to date has simply failed to differentiate between male and female drug addicts. Virtually no research has been done on the subject of drug abuse and addiction in children or adolescents (Newcomb & Bentler, 1989). Yet, as will be discussed in Chapter 23, the problem of child and adolescent drug and alcohol abuse is a serious one. Children and adolescents who abuse chemicals are not simply small adults. It is thus not possible to automatically generalize from research done on adults to the effects of substance abuse on children or adolescents.

Thus, much of what we think we know about addiction is based on research that is quite limited at best, seriously flawed in many cases, and, all too often, simply nonexistent. Yet this is the foundation on which an entire "industry" of treatment has evolved. It is not the purpose of this text to deny that large numbers of people abuse drugs or that such drug abuse carries with it a terrible cost in personal suffering. It is also not the purpose of this text to deny that many people are harmed by drug abuse; admittedly, people become addicted to chemicals. The purpose of this section is to make the reader aware of the shortcomings of the current body of research on substance abuse.

The Cost of Chemical Abuse and Addiction

It is difficult to estimate the total financial cost of drug abuse and addiction, if only because there are so many "hidden" aspects of the problem of substance abuse. For example, McGinnis and Foege (1993) noted that, in 1990, only 9,000 deaths in the United States were directly attributed to chemical abuse. However, when one considers the impact of drug-related infant deaths, overdose, suicide, homicide, motor vehicle deaths, and the various forms of drug-abuse related disease (such as hepatitis, HIV infection, pneumonia, endocarditis, and so on), the true cost of drug abuse and addiction is closer to 20,000 premature deaths a year (Paulos, 1994; McGinnis & Foege, 1993). And these figures do not reflect the estimated 200,000 people who die each year from alcohol use (Kaplan, Sadock, & Grebb, 1994) or the 500,000 who die each year from tobacco-related illness.

Thus, the information available at this time suggests that chemical use or abuse is a significant factor in premature death, illness, loss of productivity, and medical expenses. However, because chemical abuse and addiction has so many hidden facets, we have only rough estimates of what the various forms of substance abuse cost society each year.

The Cost of Alcohol Abuse

Kaplan, Sadock, and Grebb (1994) place cost of alcohol use and abuse at $600 for every man, woman, and child in the United States, but they do not specify what factors they considered in

reaching this estimate. A number of factors must be considered in calculating the annual financial cost of alcohol abuse and addiction in the United States. Included in this list are direct and indirect costs, such as the cost of alcohol-related criminal activity, motor vehicle accidents, destruction of property, social welfare programs, private and public hospitalization for alcohol-related illness, and public and private treatment programs. When all these costs are computed, it appears that the total financial loss for alcohol abuse and addiction in the United States is from just over $90 billion (National Foundation for Brain Research, 1992) to $98.6 billion (Rice, 1993) a year. Angell and Kassifer (1994) give an even higher estimate of the cost of alcohol use and abuse in the United States, stating that when all the various expenses are added together, alcohol use and abuse costs between $100 and $130 billion each year.

Alcohol abuse and addiction are significant factors in the growing health care financial crisis. The American Medical Association (1993b) estimated that between 25 and 40% of the people hospitalized in the United States are there for treatment of some complication of alcoholism. Between 15 and 30% of the nursing home beds in this country are occupied by individuals whose alcohol use has contributed at least in some measure for their need for placement in a nursing home (Schuckit, 1989). Many of these nursing homes are supported at least in part by public funds, making chronic alcohol abuse a major factor in the growing cost of nursing home care for the elderly.

In addition, approximately 540,000 people in the United States are injured in alcohol-related automobile accidents each year (Massing, 1992), and alcohol use was a factor in approximately 46% of motor vehicle deaths in 1992 (American Medical Association, 1993b). Whether they ultimately survive their injuries or not, individuals involved in alcohol-related motor vehicle accidents often require emergency medical treatment, which is ultimately paid for by the public through higher insurance costs and higher taxes.

It has been reported that between 30 and 40% of the homeless in the United States are alcohol abusers, and 10% to 15% abuse drugs (McCarty, Argeriou, Huebner, & Lubran, 1991; Calsyn & Morse, 1991). Some estimates of the yearly cost of providing social service support (housing, medical treatment, food, and so on) to this population are as high as $23,000 per client (Whitman, Friedman, & Thomas, 1990). When one considers the number of homeless in this country, these figures amount to a massive investment of social support dollars that must also be included in the cost that addiction extracts from U.S. resources.

The Cost of Substance Abuse

Various estimates of the financial cost of drug abuse and dependence in this country have been advanced. The American Medical Association (AMA) (1992) suggests that drug abuse costs $76 billion each year. Angell and Kassifer (1994) estimate that the annual cost of illicit drug use in this country is between $76 and $150 billion. These figures represent the estimated financial impact of premature death or illness caused by substance abuse, lost wages from those who lose their jobs because of substance abuse, financial losses incurred by victims of drug-related crimes, and expected costs of drug-related law-enforcement activities. White (1993), on the other hand, suggests that, when measured in terms of law enforcement, treatment, medical care, insurance costs, and the financial impact of crime, the cost of substance abuse is close to $300 billion each year. No matter which of these estimates you believe, it is clear that drug abuse is an expensive luxury.

Drug Use as a Way of Life

In a very real sense, the drugs of abuse are luxury items. It is estimated that between $40 billion (Scheer, 1994b) and perhaps as much as $150 billion (Collier, 1989) is spent on illicit recreational chemicals each year in the United States. A large part of this money is spent by casual, recreational drug users, not hardened addicts. This expenditure represents a sum greater than *the total combined income* of the 80 poorest Third World countries (Corwin, 1994).

Substance Abuse and Victimization

There is a known relationship between chemical abuse in one form or another and various forms of victimization. It has been reported, for example, that alcohol is implicated in one way or another in 50% of all homicides (National Foundation for Brain Research, 1992).

There appears to be a relationship between being a victim of sexual assault and subsequent substance abuse, at least for women (Burnam, Stein, Golding, Siegel, Sorensen, Forsythe, & Telles, 1989). There also appears to be a relationship between being a victim of a violent assault and subsequent alcohol or drug abuse. Kilpatrick (1990) estimated that women who were victims of some form of violent crime were three to six times as likely to have alcohol or drug problems as were those women who were never victimized.

Walker, Bonner, and Kaufman (1988) observed that both alcohol and drug addiction are "frequently associated with physical abuse" (p. 45) of children. Chemical use is also frequently associated with spouse abuse. The research team of Gondalf and Foster (1991) found that 39% of their sample of 218 male veterans in an alcohol treatment program "reported assaulting their wives or partners at least once during the past year" (p. 76). Of this number, one-fifth of the men reported that the assault might be classified as "severe" (p. 76).

Collins and Messerschmidt (1993) suggested an even stronger relationship between alcohol use and domestic violence, stating that alcohol abuse is involved in approximately 60% to 70% of spouse abuse cases. Alcohol use is also thought to be a factor in 38% of the cases of child abuse (Beasley, 1987). Chasnoff (1988) noted that alcohol and/or drug abuse was involved in 64% of all child abuse cases in New York City, and Bays (1990) concluded that "at least 675,000 children each year are seriously mistreated by an alcoholic or drug abusing caretaker" (p. 881). Although these estimates disagree as to the exact nature of the relationship between alcohol and/or drug abuse and family violence, they all point to a strong connection between these two social problems.

This is not to say that alcohol or drug use *caused* the child or spouse abuse. The relationship between chemical use and physical abuse is a complex one. However, as Gelles and Straus (1988) discovered, alcohol or drug use is more likely to be present in a home where physical abuse takes place because such families tend to demonstrate a number of antisocial behaviors. In other words, such families suffer from multiple problems, of which chemical use and physical abuse are only two of the more visible examples.

Substance Abuse and Suicide

There is a known association between suicide and alcohol and drug abuse. Approximately one-fourth of the successful suicides in any given year are alcoholics (National Foundation for Brain Research, 1992), and as much as 60% of suicide attempts can be traced either directly or indirectly to alcoholism (Beasley, 1987).

There is no way to determine the ultimate role of drug abuse and addiction in suicide, but certain classes of drugs—specifically the amphetamines and cocaine—are known to cause suicidal depression following prolonged use. Indeed, as will be discussed in Chapter 9, some researchers have found that cocaine has been involved in a significant percentage of the successful suicides in at least some regions of the United States.

Substance Abuse and Intimacy Dysfunctions

Chemical abuse may result in various forms of sexual dysfunction, including changes in the individual's ability to achieve a stage of sexual excitement, orgasm, and resolution following sexuality activity. Furthermore, drug abuse could lead to various forms of performance dysfunction as well as interfere with the individual's ability to enjoy sexual relations (Gold, 1988).

In conclusion, there is no way to fully estimate the personal, economic, or social impact that various forms of chemical addiction have had on society. When one considers the possible economic impact of medical costs incurred, lost productivity, or other indirect costs from hidden drug abuse and addiction, one can begin to appreciate just how chemical abuse and addiction affects society.

The State of the Art: Unanswered Questions, Uncertain Answers

It is clear that there is much confusion in the professional community over the problems of substance abuse and addiction. Even in the case of alcoholism, which is perhaps the most common of the drug addictions, there is an element of confusion or uncertainty over its essential features. For example, 30% to 45% of all adults will have at least one transient alcohol-related problem (such as a blackout or legal problem) (Kaplan, Sadock, & Grebb, 1994), yet this does not mean that 30% to 45% of the adult population is alcoholic! Rather, this fact underscores the need for researchers to more clearly identify the features that might identify the potential alcoholic.

What Constitutes a Valid Diagnosis of Chemical Dependency?

Another unanswered question is where one might draw the line between casual use, problem use, and addiction to one or more drugs. Ultimately, there are no clear guidelines. Rather, as Vaillant (1983) suggests, "it is not who is drinking but *who is watching*" (p. 22, italics added) that defines whether alcoholism is present. Peele (1985) agrees, noting that what we define as alcoholism actually is "a social convention" (p. 35).

Are there valid diagnostic signs of drug addiction that are not simply matters of social convention? At present, the diagnosis of chemical dependency remains difficult (Lewis, Dana, & Blevens, 1988), and in the final analysis it may be considered a value judgment. Criteria such as the American Psychiatric Association's DSM-IV may make such judgment easier, but even in rather advanced cases of drug dependency, the issue of whether or not the individual is addicted is not always clear-cut.

For the moment, we will focus on the problem of alcoholism and its diagnosis. Although the work of Greenblatt and Shader (1975) is more than a generation old, it still is of value to illustrate the problems of diagnosing alcohol addiction (alcoholism). According to the authors, three elements are necessary to diagnose alcoholism: (1) a deterioration in the person's work performance, family relationships, and social behavior, termed a *pathological psychosocial behavior pattern*; (2) a classic drug addiction process, including withdrawal symptoms following abstinence from alcohol severe enough for the person to try to avoid them by continued use of alcohol; and (3) a medical disease, such as cirrhosis of the liver, certain nutritional disorders, and/or certain forms of neurological damage, considered a complication of alcoholism.

It is certainly easy to recognize alcoholism when all three elements are present (Greenblatt & Shader, 1975). However, as the authors observed, many "skid row" alcoholics may be hospitalized many times for alcohol withdrawal symptoms but never develop any of the diseases associated with chronic alcoholism. Thus, Conditions 1 and 2 are satisfied, but not Condition 3. Similarly, a heavy-drinking business executive whose drinking pattern never interferes with family or occupational performance may develop withdrawal symptoms when hospitalized for elective surgery (say for a hernia repair). In this case, Condition 2 is satisfied, but Conditions 1 and 3 are not. Finally, many "binge" drinkers never become addicted to alcohol and never develop any of the physical complications associated with al-

coholism, yet these individuals still have a problem with alcohol (Greenblatt & Shader, 1975). The binge drinker meets Conditions 1 and 3, but not Condition 2; still, many will ultimately suffer broken families and loss of employment as a result of their drinking.

Thus, as Greenblatt and Shader (1975) point out, even alcoholism, perhaps our best understood form of addiction, is not easy to diagnose. In the final analysis, the diagnosis of chemical dependency is still an opinion made by a professional about another person's chemical use. The issue of assessing another individual's substance use pattern will be discussed in a later chapter. The point being made here is that there is still much to be learned, about how best to assess a person's chemical use pattern and provide an accurate diagnosis.

What Is the Role of News Media in Chemical Use Trends?

One of the most serious of the unanswered questions facing mental health or substance abuse professionals is whether the media have been a positive or negative influence on those who have not yet experimented with alcohol or drugs. Because it is illegal to use or import a variety of drugs, activities surrounding these drugs become "newsworthy."

It has been suggested that media reports of the dangers inherent in the use of certain drugs have actually contributed to the aura surrounding inhalant abuse (Brecher, 1972) and use of a new form of amphetamine known as "ice" (Cotton, 1990). Media reports often describe how to use the drug in question, the profits earned by those who sell drugs, and what effects certain chemicals will produce. The media have been charged with actually making these drugs appear more attractive to many who might otherwise have not been motivated to try them.

The Dutch experiment in dealing with their drug problem (see Chapter 33) supports the theory that, when legal sanctions against drug use are removed, drugs actually become *less* attractive to the average individual, and casual drug use declines. For a number of years, substance abuse in Holland has been viewed from a public health perspective, not a legal one. It was only after large number of foreign chemical users moved to Holland to take advantage of this permissiveness that Dutch authorities began to utilize law enforcement as a means of controlling substance use.

The point to remember is that there is a great deal of evidence suggesting that media reports have actually contributed to the problem of substance abuse in this country by adding to the aura of mystery and "charm" that surrounds the street drug world. The question to be asked is, Whose side is the media on?

Summary

In this chapter, we introduced the concept of a continuum of drug use and reviewed research studies outlining the extent of substance abuse and addiction. We also explored the issues of actual and hidden costs of chemical use and abuse, which are often reflected solely in financial or economic terms. However, it is important that society not lose sight of the "hidden" impact substance abuse has on the individual's spouse, family members, and the entire community. We also raised some unanswered questions about chemical abuse and concluded with a look at the media's role in the evolution of the problem of substance abuse.

CHAPTER THREE

An Introduction to Pharmacology

It is virtually impossible to discuss the effects of the various drugs of abuse without touching on a number of basic pharmacological concepts. In this chapter, we will review some of the basic principles of pharmacology to help you better understand the impact different drugs of abuse may have on the user's body.

A good starting point is to clear up two common misconceptions about recreational chemicals. First, recreational chemicals work in the same manner that other pharmaceuticals do: they modify (strengthen or weaken) a potential that already exists in the cells of the body (Williams & Baer, 1994; Ciancio & Bourgault, 1989). The drugs of abuse, all of which exert their desired effects in the brain, modify the normal function of the neurons of the brain.

The second misconception is that drugs of abuse are somehow different than legitimate pharmaceuticals; this is simply not true. Many drugs of abuse are, or were once, legitimate pharmaceuticals used by physicians to treat disease and control human suffering. Drugs of abuse must obey the same laws and mechanisms of pharmacology that apply to other medications in use today.

This chapter is designed to provide a brief overview of some important principles of pharmacology. It is not intended to serve as, nor should it be used for, a guide to patient care. Those interested in reading more on pharmacology can find several good selections in any medical or nursing school bookstore.

The Site of Action

We begin our overview of pharmacology by examining the concept of the *site of action*. Consider a person with an "athlete's foot" infection; this condition is caused by a fungus that attacks the skin. Obviously, the individual who has such an infection will want to have it cured, and there are several excellent over-the-counter antifungal compounds available. In most cases, the individual need select only one and apply it to the proper area to be cured of the infection.

Although antifungal compounds have little to do with drug abuse, the example of the athlete's foot infection helps illustrate the concept of the *site of action*. Put simply, the site of action is where the drug being used will have its prime effect. In the case of the antifungal compound, the site of action is the infected skin on the person's foot. For most drugs of abuse, the central nervous system (CNS) is the site of action.

The Prime Effect and Side Effects of Chemicals

One rule of pharmacology is that there is an element of risk whenever a chemical is introduced into the body (Laurence & Bennett, 1992). *Every* chemical agent presents the potential to harm the individual, although the degree of risk varies depending on a number of factors, such as the specific chemical being used, the individual's state of health and so on.

The localized infection on the surface of the skin caused by a fungus presents both a localized site of action and one that is on the surface of the body. This makes it easy to limit the impact that a medication used to treat the infection might have on the rest of the body. The patient is unlikely to need more than a topical medication that can be applied directly to the necessary region of the body.

But consider the drugs of abuse. As mentioned before, the site of action for each recreational chemical lies deep within the CNS. And, we discussed in Chapter 2, there is increasing evidence that each of the various drugs of abuse ultimately will impact on the limbic system of the brain. However, the drugs of abuse are very much like a blast of shotgun pellets spewing from the end of a "scattergun": they will have an impact not only on the brain but also on many other organ systems in the body.

For example, cocaine causes the user to experience a sense of well-being or euphoria (see Chapter 9). The euphoria and sense of well-being that result can be called the *primary effects*[1] of cocaine use. But the chemical has a number of other effects, including constriction of the coronary arteries of the user's heart. Causing coronary artery constriction is hardly a desired effect, and it may be a factor in the development of heart attacks in cocaine users. Such unwanted effects of a chemical are often called *secondary effects,* or *side effects.* A chemicals' side effects may make the patient feel uncomfortable at times and, in more extreme cases, could actually threaten the user's life.

A second example is aspirin's ability to inhibit the production of chemicals known as prostaglandins at the site of an injury. This

action helps reduce the individual's discomfort if he or she suffered an injury. But, the body also produces prostaglandins in the kidneys and stomach, where the chemical helps modify the function of these organs. Unfortunately, an unwanted side effect is that aspirin tends to block prostaglandin production nonselectively *throughout* the body—including the stomach and kidneys—which could put the individual's life at risk.

Similarly, when a person with a bacterial infection of the middle ear (a condition known as *otitis media*) takes an antibiotic such as penicillin, the desired outcome is for the antibiotic to destroy the bacteria causing the infection. However, a side effect might be a case of drug-induced diarrhea, because the antibiotic interferes with normal bacteria growth patterns in the intestines. Thus, one needs to keep in mind that all pharmaceuticals, and the drugs of abuse, have both desired effects, and numerous side effects.

Drug Forms and Their Administration

Essentially, a drug is a foreign chemical introduced into the individual's body to bring about a specific, desired response. Antihypertensive medications are used to control excessively high blood pressure; antibiotics are used to eliminate unwanted bacteria. Recreational drugs are introduced into the body, as a general rule, to bring about feelings of euphoria, relaxation, and relief from stress.

The specific *form* in which a drug is administered will have a major effect on the speed with which that chemical is able to work, and the way the chemical is distributed throughout the body. In general, the drugs of abuse are administered by either the *enteral* or *parenteral* route.

Enteral Drug Administration

Medications administered by the enteral route are administered *orally, sublingually, or rectally* (Williams & Baer, 1994; Ciancio & Bourgault,

---

[1]Shannon, Wilson, and Stang (1992) refer to a chemical's *primary effects* by the term *therapeutic effects* (p. 21). However, their text is devoted to medications and their uses, not to the drugs of abuse. To keep the differentiation between the use of a medication in the treatment of disease and the abuse of chemicals for recreational purposes, I will use the term *primary effects.*

1989). The most common means by which a medication is administered orally is the tablet. Essentially, a tablet is "a compounded form in which the drug is mixed with a binding agent to hold the tablet together before administration. . . . Most tablets are designed to be swallowed whole" (Shannon, Wilson, & Stang, 1992, p. 8). A number of the drugs of abuse are often administered in tablet form, including aspirin, the hallucinogens LSD and MDMA, and the amphetamines. Sometimes amphetamine tablets are made in illicit laboratories and are known on the street by a variety of names (such as "white cross" or "cartwheels").

A second common form that oral medication might take is the *capsule*. Essentially, capsules are modified tablets with the inside medication surrounded by a gelatin capsule. The capsule is designed to be swallowed whole; once it reaches the stomach, the gelatin capsule breaks down, allowing the medication to be released into the gastrointestinal tract (Shannon, Wilson, & Stang, 1992).

There are many other forms that medication might take. For example, some medications intended for oral use are administered in liquid form. Antibiotics and some over-the-counter analgesics often are administered in liquid form, especially when the patient is a very young child. Liquid forms make it possible to tailor each dose to the patient's weight, and they are ideal for patients who have trouble taking pills or capsules by mouth. Of the drugs of abuse, alcohol is perhaps the best example of a chemical administered in liquid form.

Some medications, and a small number of the drugs of abuse, can be absorbed through the blood-rich tissues under the tongue. A chemical that enters the body by this method is said to be administered *sublingually*. The sublingual method of drug administration is a variation of the oral form of drug administration. Certain drugs, like nitroglycerin, and fentanyl (discussed in Chapter 11) are well absorbed by the sublingual method. However, for the most part, the drugs of abuse are not administered through sublingual means, and we will not discuss this method of introducing chemicals into the body any further.

Parenteral Forms of Drug Administration

The parenteral method of drug administration essentially involves injecting the medication directly into the body. Several forms of parenteral administration are commonly used in both the world of medicine and the world of drug abuse. First is the *subcutaneous* method of drug administration. In this process, a chemical is injected just under the skin, which allows the drug to avoid the dangers of passing through the stomach and gastrointestinal tracts. However, drugs administered in a subcutaneous injection are absorbed more slowly than are chemicals injected either into muscle tissue or into a vein. As we will see in Chapter 11, heroin addicts often use subcutaneous injections, a process that they call "skin popping."

A second method of parenteral administration involves the *intramuscular* injection of a medication. Muscle tissues have a good supply of blood, and medications injected into muscle tissue are absorbed into the general circulation more rapidly than when injected just under the skin. Individuals abusing anabolic steroids commonly inject the chemical(s) into the muscle tissue (see Chapter 15).

The third method of parenteral administration is the *intravenous* (I.V.) injection, whereby the chemical is injected directly into a vein. When a chemical is injected into a vein, it is deposited directly into the general circulation (Schwertz, 1991). Heroin, cocaine, and the amphetamines are all examples of drugs of abuse administered by intravenous injection.

Unfortunately, because of the speed with which the chemical reaches the general circulation when administered by intravenous injection, there is a very real potential for undesirable reactions. The very nature of intravenously administered drugs provides the body very little time to adapt to the arrival of the foreign chemical (Ciancio & Bourgault, 1989). This is one reason users of intravenously administered chemicals, such as heroin, frequently experience a wide range of adverse effects in addition to the desired euphoria caused by the chemical being abused.

The reader should keep in mind that, just because a parenteral method of drug administration is utilized, the chemical in question does not necessarily have an instantaneous effect. The speed at which all forms of drugs administered by parenteral administration begin to work is influenced by a number of factors, which will be discussed in the section on drug distribution in this chapter.

Other Forms of Drug Administration

A number of additional methods of drug administration need to be identified briefly. Some chemicals can be absorbed through the skin, a *transdermal* method of drug administration. Chemicals absorbed transdermally eventually reach the general circulation and are then distributed throughout the body.

Physicians often take advantage of the potential to provide the patient with a low, steady blood level of a chemical that transdermal drug administration offers. A drawback of this method is that it is a very slow way to introduce a drug into the body. But, for certain agents, it is a very useful method. For example, a "skin patch" is used to administer nicotine transdermally to patients who want to quit smoking. Some antihistamines are administered transdermally, especially those used for motion sickness. There also is a transdermal "patch" available for the narcotic analgesic fentanyl, although its success as a means of providing analgesia has been quite limited.

Occasionally, chemicals are administered *intranasally*. The intranasal administration of a chemical involves nasal inhalation so the material in question is deposited on the blood-rich tissues of the sinuses. From that point, many chemicals can be absorbed into the general circulation. For example, both cocaine and heroin powders are frequently "snorted."

The process of *inhalation* is used by both physicians and illicit drug users. Depending on the characteristics of the chemical(s) being inhaled, one of two different processes takes place. In the first case, the molecules of the chemical being inhaled are small enough to pass through the lungs into the general circulation, as with surgical anesthetics and some drugs of abuse. In the second form of inhalation, the particles being inhaled are suspended in smoke. These particles are small enough to reach the deep tissues of the lungs, where they are deposited. In a short time, the particles are broken down into smaller and smaller units, until they are small enough to pass through the walls of the lungs and reach the general circulation. This is the process that takes place when tobacco products are smoked. Each subform of inhalation takes advantage of the fact that the lungs offer a blood-rich, extremely large surface area through which chemical agents can be absorbed (Benet, Mitchell, & Sheiner, 1991). Depending on how quickly the chemical being inhaled can cross over into the general circulation, this method introduces chemicals into the body relatively quickly.

However, researchers have found that, for a number of reasons, the actual amount of a chemical absorbed through inhalation varies. First, the individual must inhale at just the right time to allow the chemical to reach the desired region of the lungs. Second, some chemicals pass through the tissues of the lung only very poorly and are not well absorbed by inhalation. For example, smoking a marijuana cigarette involves a different technique than smoking a tobacco cigarette to get the maximum effect (see also Chapter 10). The variability in the amount of chemical absorbed through the lungs limits the utility of inhalation as a means of administering medications. However, for some drugs of abuse, inhalation is the preferred method of administration.

There are a number of other methods for introducing pharmaceuticals into the body, such as rectally or through enteral tubes. However, because the drugs of abuse are generally introduced into the body by injection, by mouth, or through smoking, we will not discuss the more obscure methods of drug administration.

Bioavailability

To produce the desired effect, the drug(s) being abused must enter the body in sufficient strength. Pharmacists refer to this as the chemical's *bioavailability: the concentration of the unchanged chemical at the site of action* (Loebl, Spratto, & Woods, 1994; Sands, Knapp, & Ciraulo, 1993). The bioavailability of a chemical in the body is influenced, in turn, by four factors (Sands, Knapp, & Ciraulo, 1993; Benet, Mitchell, & Sheiner, 1991): absorption, distribution, metabolism (or "biotransformation"), and elimination. To better understand the process of bioavailability, we will consider each of these factors in more detail.

Absorption

Except for topical agents, which are deposited directly on the site of action, chemicals must be absorbed into the body. Ultimately, the concentration of a chemical in the serum and at the site of action is influenced by the process of *absorption* (Loebl, Spratto, & Woods, 1994). The process of absorption involves the movement of drug molecules from the site of entry, through various cell boundaries, to the site of action.

The human body is composed of layers of specialized cells, organized in specific patterns to carry out certain functions. For example, the cells of the bladder are organized to form a muscular reservoir in which to store waste products and from which to allow excretion. The cells of the circulatory system are organized to form tubes (blood vessels), which contain the cells and fluids of the circulatory system.

As a general rule, each layer of cells that the drug must pass through to reach the general circulation slows the absorption rate. For exam-ple, just one layer of cells separates the air in our lungs from the general circulation. Drugs that are able to pass this boundary may reach the circulation in just a few seconds. In contrast, a drug ingested orally must pass from the gastrointestinal tract through several layers of cells before reaching the general circulation, as shown in Figure 3.1. Thus, the oral method is generally recognized as one of the slowest methods of drug administration.

Drug molecules can take advantage of a number of specialized *cellular transport mechanisms* to pass through the walls of the cells. These cellular transport mechanisms are quite complex and function at the molecular level. Some drug molecules simply diffuse across the cell membrane, a process known as *passive diffusion*, or *passive transport*. This is the most common method of drug transport across cell boundaries, and it operates on the principle that chemicals tend to diffuse from areas of high concentration to areas of lower concentration. Other drug molecules utilize *molecular* transport mechanisms, which move various essential molecules into (and out of) cells. Collectively, these molecular transport mechanisms provide a system of *active transport* across cell boundaries and into the interior of the body.

Several specialized absorption-modification variables influence the speed at which a drug is absorbed from the site of entry. For example, there is the *rate of blood flow* at the site of entry and the *molecular characteristics of the drug molecule* being admitted to the body. However, for the sake of this text, it is important to remember simply that the process of absorption refers to the movement of drug molecules from the site of entry to the site of action. In the next section, we will discuss the second factor that influences how a chemical acts in the body, its distribution.

Distribution

The process of *distribution* refers to how the chemical molecules are moved about in the body. This movement includes both the process

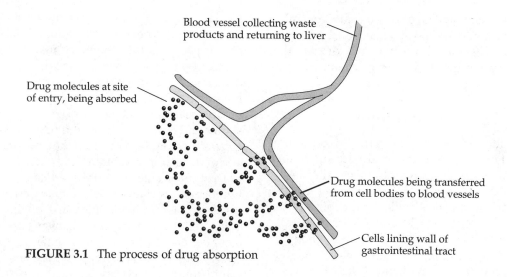

Blood vessel collecting waste products and returning to liver

Drug molecules at site of entry, being absorbed

Drug molecules being transferred from cell bodies to blood vessels

Cells lining wall of gastrointestinal tract

FIGURE 3.1 The process of drug absorption

of drug transport and the pattern of drug accumulation within the body. For example, PCP tends to accumulate within both the brain and the adipose (fat) tissues in the body (see Chapter 13).

Drug Transport

Once a chemical has reached the general circulation, that substance can then be transported to the site of action. The main purpose of the circulatory system, however, is not to provide a distribution system for drugs! A drug molecule is a foreign substance in the circulatory system that takes advantage of the body's own chemical distribution system to move from the point of entry to the site of action.

A chemical can use the circulatory system to reach the site of action in several different ways. Some chemicals are able to mix freely with the blood plasma; they are classified as water-soluble drugs. Because water is such a large part of the human body, the drug molecules from water-soluble chemicals are rapidly and easily distributed throughout the fluid in the body. Alcohol is an excellent example of a water-soluble chemical. Shortly after gaining admission into the body, alcohol is rapidly distributed throughout

the body to *all* blood-rich organs, including the brain.

Other drugs utilize a different approach. Their chemical structure allows them to "bind" to fat molecules in the blood known as *lipids;* these chemicals are often called *lipid soluble.* Because fat molecules are used to build cell walls within the body, lipids have the ability to move rapidly out of the circulatory system into the body tissues. Indeed, one characteristic of blood lipids is that they are constantly passing out of the circulatory system and into the body tissues.

Thus, chemicals that are lipid soluble will be distributed throughout the body, concentrating in organs with a high percentage of lipids. In comparison to other organ systems in the body, which are composed of between 6 and 20% lipid molecules, fully 50% of the weight of the brain is made up of lipids (Cooper, Bloom, & Roth, 1986). Thus, lipid-soluble chemicals will tend to concentrate in the tissues of the brain.

Some ultrashort- and short-acting barbiturates are good examples of lipid-soluble drugs. Although all the barbiturates are lipid soluble, there is a great deal of variability in the speed with which various barbiturates can bind to lipids. How quickly a given barbiturate will begin to have an effect will depend, in part, on its ability to form bonds with lipid molecules. For the ultrashort-acting barbiturates, which are extremely lipid soluble, the effects might be felt within seconds of the time they are injected into a vein. This is one reason the ultrashort-duration barbiturates are so useful as surgical anesthetics.

Because drug molecules are foreign substances in the body, their presence might be tolerated, but only until the body's natural defenses against chemical intruders are able to eliminate the foreign substance. The body will thus be working to detoxify (biotransform) or eliminate the foreign chemical molecules in the body almost from the moment they arrive.

Some drugs avoid being metabolized or eliminated before they have an effect by joining with protein molecules in the blood. The chemical structures of many drugs allow the individual molecules to bind with protein molecules in the general circulation, especially with the one known as *albumin*. For this reason, such chemicals are said to become "protein bound" (or, if they bind to albumin, might be said to be "albumin bound").[2] The advantage of protein binding is that it makes the drug difficult for the body to either metabolize or excrete. Some drugs form stronger chemical bonds with protein molecules than do others. The bond strength determines how long the drug will remain in the body before elimination.

However, while they are protein bound, drug molecules have no biological effect. To have an effect, the molecules must be free of chemical bonds (*unbound*). Fortunately, although a chemical might be strongly protein bound, a certain percentage of the drug molecules will always be unbound. It is this unbound fraction that produces an effect on the bodily function, or is biologically active. Because the protein-bound molecules have no effect at the site of action, they are biologically inactive while bound (Shannon, Wilson, & Stang, 1992; Rasymas, 1992).

Thus, for largely protein-bound chemicals, the unbound drug molecules must be extremely potent. The antidepressant amitriptyline is 95% protein bound. This means that only 5% of a given dose of this drug is actually biologically active at any time (Ciraulo, Shader, Greenblatt, & Barnhill, 1989). Diazepam is another strongly protein-bound drug. Over 99% of the diazepam molecules that reach the general circulation will become protein bound. Thus, the sedative effect of diazepam (see Chapter 7) is actually caused by the small fraction (approximately 1%) of the diazepam molecules that remain unbound.

As noted earlier, unbound drug molecules are easily metabolized or excreted (the process of metabolism and excretion of chemicals will be discussed in a later section of this chapter). Thus, one advantage of protein binding is that the protein-bound drug molecules form a "reservoir" of unmetabolized drug molecules. These unmetabolized drug molecules are gradually released back into the general circulation as the chemical bond between the drug and the protein molecules weakens. The drug molecules gradually released back into the general circulation then replace those molecules that have been metabolized or excreted. The *proportion* of unbound to bound molecules, however, remains approximately the same. For a drug that is 75% protein bound and 25% unbound when at its greatest concentration in the blood, as it is eliminated, the proportion of bound to unbound drug continues to be approximately 75 : 25. That is, as the drug is being removed from the general circulation, some of the protein-bound molecules are also breaking the chemical bonds that held them to the protein molecule, becoming unbound once again. Thus, although the amount of chemical in the general circulation gradually diminishes as the body biotransforms or elim-

[2]In general, acidic drugs tend to bind to albumin, whereas basic drugs tend to bind to alpha$_1$-acid glycoprotein (Ciancio & Bourgault, 1989).

inates the unbound drug molecules, the proportion of bound to unbound drug molecules remains essentially unchanged.

The characteristic of protein binding actually is related to another trait of a drug: its biological half-life. This topic will be discussed in more detail later in this chapter. However, protein binding allows the drug in question to have a longer duration of effect. Because the protein-bound molecules are gradually released back into the general circulation over an extended period of time, the total period of time in which that drug is present in sufficient quantities to remain biologically active is extended.

Metabolism or Biotransformation

Because drugs are foreign substances, the body's natural defenses try to eliminate the drug almost immediately. In some cases, the body is able to eliminate the drug without modifying its chemical structure. Penicillin is an example of a drug that is excreted unchanged from the body.

However, as a general rule, the chemical structure of most chemicals must be modified before they can be eliminated from the body. This is accomplished through what was once called *detoxification*. As researchers have come to understand how the body prepares a drug molecule for elimination, the term *detoxification* has been replaced by the term drug *metabolism* or the more accurate term *biotransformation*.

The process of biotransformation takes place mainly in the liver, usually through enzymes produced by the region of the liver known as the *microsomal endoplasmic reticulum*. Technically, the new compound that emerges from each step of the process of biotransformation is known as a *metabolite* of the chemical that was admitted to the body. The original chemical is occasionally called the metabolite's *parent compound*.

In general, metabolites are less biologically active than the parent compound, but there are exceptions to this rule. Depending on the substance being biotransformed, the metabolite might have a psychoactive effect of its own. On rare occasions, a drug has a metabolite that is more biologically active than the parent compound. It is for this reason that pharmacologists have abandoned the term *detoxification*. It became rather confusing to think of a metabolite more active than its parent compound as being the end product of a process of "detoxification." Thus, we now speak of the process of biotransformation, or metabolism, of chemicals.

Although the liver is the organ in which drug metabolism is performed, some biotransformation can also be carried out by other organs. For example, as we will discuss in Chapter 4, at least some alcohol is metabolized in the stomach, even before it is absorbed into the circulation and brought to the liver for metabolism.

Although we speak of drug metabolism as if it were a single process, there are four subforms of metabolism (Ciraulo, Shader, Greenblatt, & Barnhill, 1989): oxidation, reduction, hydrolysis, and conjugation. The specifics of each form of drug metabolism are quite complex and are best reserved for pharmacology texts. For our purposes, it is enough to know that there are four different processes collectively called drug metabolism, or biotransformation. Many chemicals must go through more than one step in the biotransformation process before that agent is ready for the next step: *elimination*.

One major goal of the process of metabolism is to transform the foreign chemical into a form that can be rapidly eliminated from the body (Clark, Bratler, & Johnson, 1991), but this process does not take place instantly. Because the process of biotransformation involves chemical reactions with enzymes, it is carried out over a period of time. Thus, depending on the drug involved, there are often a number of intermediate steps to the process of biotransformation.

The general goal of the process of biotransformation, however, is to change the chemical structure of the foreign substance to make it less lipid soluble and thus more easily eliminated from the body. There are two major subtypes of drug metabolism. In the first subtype, a constant fraction of the drug is biotransformed each hour; this is called a *first order biotransformation* process. Certain antibiotics are metabolized in this manner, with a set percentage of the medication in the body being biotransformed each hour. Other chemicals are eliminated from the body by what is known as a *zero order biotransformation* process. These drugs are metabolized at a set rate no matter how high the concentration of that chemical in the blood.

Alcohol is a good example of a chemical biotransformed through a zero order biotransformation process (see also Chapter 4). Alcohol is biotransformed at the rate of about one regular mixed drink or one can of beer per hour. Whether a person ingests just one beer or one mixed drink or twenty beers or mixed drinks in an hour, his or her body still biotransforms the equivalent of only one beer or mixed drink per hour.

As stated in the section on absorption, most of the chemicals administered orally must pass through the stomach to the small intestine before they can be absorbed. However, the human circulatory system is designed so that chemicals absorbed through the gastrointestinal system are carried first to the liver, which has the task of protecting the body from toxins. By taking chemicals absorbed from the gastrointestinal tract directly to the liver, the body is able to begin to break down any toxins in the substance before they damage other organs in the body.

Unfortunately, one effect of this process is that the liver is often able to break down a beneficent chemical before it has a chance to reach the site of action. This is called *first pass metabolism*, and it is one reason it is difficult to control pain through the use of orally administered narcotic analgesic medications. When taken by mouth, a significant part of the dose of an analgesic such as morphine is metabolized by the liver into inactive forms, *before* it reaches the site of action.

Elimination

In the human body, biotransformation and elimination are closely intertwined. Indeed, some authorities on the subject of pharmacology consider these to be a single process, given that one goal of the process of drug metabolism is to change the foreign chemical into a water-soluble metabolite that can then be removed easily from the circulation (Clark, Bratler, & Johnson, 1991).

The most common method of drug elimination is through the kidneys (Benet, Mitchell, & Sheiner, 1991). However, the biliary tract, lungs, and sweat glands may also play a role in drug elimination (Shannon, Wilson, & Stang, 1992). For example, a small percentage of alcohol ingested is excreted through the breath; a small percentage is also eliminated through the sweat glands. These characteristics of alcohol contribute to the characteristic smell of the intoxicated individual.

As discussed earlier in this chapter, some drugs are eliminated from the body virtually unchanged. These chemicals are introduced into the body in a form that is easily removed from the general circulation without biotransformation. Penicillin is rapidly removed from the blood by the kidneys and is excreted in its active form through urine. As we will discuss in Chapter 13, many of the inhalants, as well as many of the surgical anesthetics, are also eliminated from the body without being metabolized to any significant degree.

Chemical Dosage and Drug Effects

The Drug Half-Life

The speed at which the body is able to metabolize or eliminate a drug illustrates a helpful concept that physicians use to estimate the period of time during which a chemical might remain biologically active. This is the *biological half-life* (or simply *half-life*) of that chemical. Sometimes, the half-life is abbreviated by the

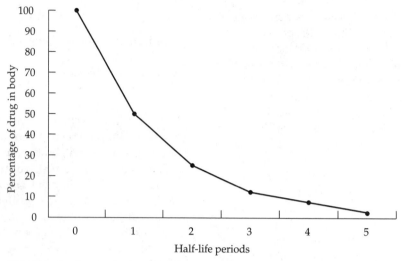

FIGURE 3.2 Drug elimination in half-life stages

symbol $t_{1/2}$. Essentially, the half-life of a chemical is the period of time needed for the individual's body to reduce the amount of active drug in the circulation by one-half (Benet, Mitchell, & Sheiner, 1991). The concept of $t_{1/2}$ is based on the assumption that the individual ingested only one dose of the drug. Although the $t_{1/2}$ concept is often a source of confusion, even among health professionals, it does allow health care workers to estimate roughly how long a drug's effects will last when that chemical is used at normal dosage levels.

One popular misconception is that it takes two half-lives for the body to totally eliminate a drug. In reality, 25% of the original dose remains at the end of the second half-life period, and 12% of the original dose still is in the body at the end of three half-life periods. As a general rule, it takes five half-life periods before the body is able to eliminate virtually all of a single dose of a chemical (Williams & Baer, 1994), as illustrated in Figure 3.2.

Generally, drugs with long half-life periods tend to remain biologically active for long periods of time. The reverse is also true: chemicals with a short biological half-life tend to be active for short periods of time. This is where the process of protein binding comes into play:

drugs with long half-lives tend to become protein bound. As stated earlier, the process of protein binding allows a "reservoir" of unmetabolized drug to be released gradually back into the general circulation as the drug molecules become unbound. This allows a chemical to remain in the circulation at a sufficient concentration to have an effect for an extended period of time.

The Effective Dose

The concept of the effective dose (ED) is based on dose-response calculations, in which pharmacologists calculate the percentage of a population that will respond to a given dose of a chemical. Scientists usually estimate the percentage of the population that is expected to experience an effect by a chemical at different dosage levels. For example, at dosage level ED_{10}, 10% of the population will achieve the desired effects from the ingested chemical; ED_{50} is the dosage level at which 50% of the population is expected to respond. Obviously, for medications, the goal is to find a dosage level where the largest percentage of the population will respond to the medication. However, you cannot keep increasing the dose of a medication forever. Sooner or later the dosage level will reach the point of toxicity and people will become ill and possibly die from the chemical's effects.

The Lethal Dose Index

Because chemicals are foreign to the human body, when introduced they will disrupt the body's function one way or another. Indeed, a common purpose of administering pharmaceuticals and the drugs of abuse is to alter the body's function in a desired direction. But chemicals also hold the potential to disrupt the function of one or more organ systems beyond the point of normal functioning. At the extreme, chemicals may so disrupt the body's activities that the individual's life is in danger.

Scientists express this continuum as a modified dose-response curve. In the typical dose-response curve, scientists calculate the percentage of the population expected to benefit from a certain dose of a chemical; the calculation for a fatal exposure level is slightly different. In such a dose-response curve, scientists calculate the percentage of the general population expected to die as a result of being exposed to a certain dose of a chemical or toxin.

This figure is then expressed in terms of a *lethal dose* (or LD) ratio. The percentage of the population that would die as a result of exposure to that chemical or toxin is identified as a subscript to the LD heading. Thus, if a certain level of exposure to a chemical or toxin resulted in a 25% death rate, this would be abbreviated as the LD_{25} for that chemical or toxin. A level of exposure that resulted in a 50% death rate would be abbreviated as the LD_{50} for that substance.[3]

For example, as we will discuss in the next chapter, a person with a blood alcohol level of 0.35 mg/mL would stand a 1% chance of death without medical intervention. Thus a blood alcohol level of 0.35 mg/mL is the LD_{01} for alcohol. It is possible to calculate the potential lethal exposure level for virtually every chemical. These figures provide scientists with a way to calculate the relative safety of different levels of exposure to chemicals or radiation and a way to determine when medical intervention is necessary.

The Therapeutic Index

Scientists have devised the *therapeutic index* (TI) to measure the relative safety of a chemical. Essentially, the TI is the ratio between the ED_{50} and the LD_{50}, or between a chemical's effectiveness and its potential for harm. A smaller TI means that there is only a small margin between a therapeutic dosage level and a toxic dosage level. A large TI suggests that a great deal of latitude exists between the normal therapeutic dosage range and the toxic dosage range.

Unfortunately, as we will see in the next few chapters, many of the drugs of abuse have a small TI; they are potentially quite toxic to the user. For example, the ratio between the normal dosage range and the toxic dosage range for the barbiturates is only about 3:1. In contrast, the ratio between the normal dosage range and the toxic dosage level for the benzodiazepines is estimated to be about 200:1. Thus, relatively speaking, the benzodiazepines are much safer than the barbiturates.

Peak Effects

The effects of a chemical develop in the body over a period of time until the drug reaches the *therapeutic threshold*. The therapeutic threshold is the point at which the concentration of a specific chemical in the body begins to have a therapeutic effect. The chemical's effects continue to build until the strongest possible effects are reached. This is the period of *peak effects*.

After the peak is reached, the impact of the drug gradually becomes less and less pro-

---

[3]Occasionally, scientists will calculate the dose-response curves for radiation exposure levels as well as for chemicals. For example, the LD_{50} for radiation exposure would be the level of radiation exposure at which 50% of the population would be expected to die.

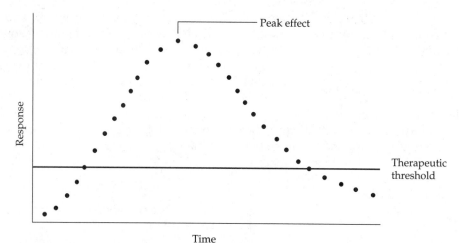

FIGURE 3.3 Hypothetical dose-response curve

nounced as the chemical is eliminated or bio-transformed over a period of time. Eventually, the concentration of the chemical in the body falls below the therapeutic level. Dose-response curves estimate a chemical's potential effect at any given point in time after administration. Figure 3.3 illustrates a hypothetical dose-response curve.

The period of peak effects following a single dose of a drug varies from one chemical to another. For example, the peak effects of an ultrashort-acting barbiturate might be achieved in a matter of seconds following a single dose, whereas the long-term barbiturate phenobarbital might take hours to achieve its strongest effects. Thus, clinicians must remember that the period of peak effects is not the same for every chemical.

Receptor Sites

The receptor site is the exact spot where the chemical carries out its main effects (Olson, 1992). Most drugs bind to specific receptor sites either on the cell wall or on one of various proteins within the cell itself. For example, forms of bacteria susceptible to the antibiotic penicillin have a characteristic receptor site, the enzyme transpeptidase, which carries out essential work

building the germ's cell wall. If the bacteria lacks the appropriate receptor site, penicillin will not be effective.

Cells usually have a number of the same kind of receptor sites. When enough of one kind of receptor site is occupied at once, the normal function of the cell is either enhanced or inhibited. The recreational drugs simply modify an existing potential within the cells of the central nervous system (CNS) in some way (Ciancio & Bourgault, 1989). In other words, when a sufficient number of drug molecules reach receptor sites either on or within the cell, they either facilitate or inhibit a potential that already exists within that neuron.

To understand how the drugs of abuse work, it is necessary to introduce the twin concepts of a drug *agonist* and *antagonist*. These may be difficult concepts for students of drug abuse to understand. Essentially, a drug agonist mimics the effect(s) of a chemical that is naturally found in the body (Shannon, Wilson, & Stang, 1992). The agonist either tricks the body into reacting as if the endogenous chemical were present, or it enhances the effect(s) of the naturally occurring chemical.

For example, morphinelike chemicals in the human brain help control the level of pain that the individual is experiencing (see Chapter 11).

Heroin, morphine, and the other narcotic analgesics mimic the actions of these chemicals and so could be classified as agonists of the naturally occurring painkilling chemicals.

The antagonist essentially blocks the effects of a chemical within the body. In a sense, aspirin is a prostaglandin antagonist because it blocks the normal actions of the prostaglandins. Antagonists may also block the effects of certain chemicals introduced into the body. For example, the drug Narcan blocks the receptor sites in the CNS that opiates normally bind to in order to have their effect. Narcan thus is an antagonist for opiates and is of value in reversing the effects of an opiate overdose.

The Blood-Brain Barrier

The blood-brain barrier (BBB) is a unique structure in the human body. Its role is to function as a "gateway" to the brain. In this role, the BBB allows only certain molecules needed by the brain to pass through. For example, oxygen and glucose, both essential to life, will pass easily through the BBB (Angier, 1990). But the BBB exists to protect the brain from toxins or infectious organisms. To this end, endothelial cells that form the lining of the BBB have established tight seals, with overlapping cells.

Initially, students of neuroanatomy may be confused by the term *blood-brain barrier*, because the word "barrier" seems to imply the existence of a single structure. Actually, the BBB is the result of a unique feature of the cells that form the capillaries through which cerebral blood flows. Unlike capillary walls in the rest of the body, those in the cerebral circulatory system are joined tightly together: each endothelial cell is joined tightly to its neighbors, forming a tight tube-like structure that protects the brain from direct contact with the general circulation.

Thus many chemicals in the general circulation are blocked from entering the CNS. However, the individual cells of the brain require nutritional support, and some of the very substances needed by the brain are those blocked by the endothelial cell boundary. Thus, water-soluble substances needed by the neurons of the brain for proper function—like glucose and iron—are blocked by the lining of the endothelial cells.

To overcome this problem, specialized transport systems, have evolved in the endothelial cells in the cerebral circulatory system. These transport systems selectively allow needed nutrients to pass through the BBB, to reach the brain (Angier, 1990). Each of these transport systems will selectively allow one specific type of water-soluble molecule, such as a glucose, to pass through the lining of the endothelial cell to reach the brain.

But lipids also pass through the lining of the endothelial cells and are able to reach the central nervous system beyond. Lipids are essentially molecules of fat and are necessary elements of cell walls, which are composed of lipids, carbohydrates, and protein molecules arranged in a specific order. As the lipid molecule reaches the endothelial cell wall, it gradually merges with the molecules of the cell wall and passes through to the interior of the endothelial cell. Later, it also passes through the lining of the far side of the endothelial cell to reach the neurons beyond the lining of the BBB.

Summary

In this chapter, we examined some of the basic components of pharmacology. Students in the field of substance abuse do not need to have the same depth of knowledge pharmacists possess in order to begin to understand how the recreational chemicals achieve their effects. However, it is important for the reader to understand at least some of the basic concepts of pharmacology, to understand the ways that the drugs of abuse achieve their primary and secondary effects.

Basic information regarding drug forms,

methods of drug administration, and biotransformation and elimination were discussed in
this chapter. Other concepts discussed were a
drug's bioavailability, the therapeutic half-life
of a chemical, the effective dose and lethal
dose ratios, the therapeutic dose ratio, and
receptor sites. The student should have at least
a basic understanding of these concepts before
starting to review the different drugs of abuse
discussed in the next chapters.

An Introduction to Alcohol Use

Historians now believe that, thousands of years ago, early man learned about intoxication by watching animals eat fermented fruits from the forest floor. One or two brave souls probably tried some of the fermented fruit, became intoxicated themselves, and promptly spread the good word to their friends (R. Siegel, 1986). Over time, prehistoric humans tried to reproduce the effect and eventually discovered how to produce alcoholic beverages.

The regular use of alcohol, also known as *ethanol* or *ethyl alcohol*,[1] thus became commonplace well before the advent of written history. Indeed, the use of alcohol is a form of a "yardstick" by which cultural development may be measured. As Beasley (1987) suggested, "virtually all cultures in time and place— whether hunter-gatherers or farmers; whether technologically advanced or primitive—share two universals: the development of a noodle and the discovery and use of the natural fermentation process" (p. 17). It has even been suggested that early civilization came about in response to the need for a stable home base from which to ferment a form of beer known as *mead* (Stone, 1991). If this theory is correct, then human civilization owes much to alcohol.

<hr>

[1]Other forms of alcohol also exist, but these are not normally used for human consumption and will not be discussed further. It is enough to understand that ethyl alcohol has been with us for a long, long time.

A Brief History of Alcohol

Mead, an early form of beer, was brewed from fermented honey. The earliest written records describing how beer is made date back only 4,000 years, to approximately 1800 B.C. (Stone, 1991). However, historical evidence suggests that a form of beer was in common use around the year 8000 B.C. (Ray & Ksir, 1993), nearly 10,000 years ago. Unlike modern beers its thick liquid was quite nutritious, and it provided necessary vitamins and amino acids to the drinker's diet. Modern beer is very thin and almost anemic in comparison.

Although no one knows how the practice of drinking wine first began, Youcha (1978) relates a 4,000-year-old Persian legend about the discovery of wine. According to this legend, a mythical Persian king, Jamshid, had vats of grapes stored in the basement of the palace. Jamshid loved grapes, and apparently wanted to store some away to enjoy during the cold winter months when grapes were out of season. However, as time passed, he discovered that some of the vats developed a sour liquid at the bottom, and, and, thinking that this liquid was poison, he set the sour fluid aside for future use against political rivals.

According to the legend, a lady of his court was subject to such severe headaches that she decided to end her life. She opened the jar marked "poison" and, expecting death, drank some of the fluid. Instead of death, she found relief from her headaches and began to sneak into the storeroom from time to time to drink some of the mystical fluid. When the supply of the fluid was exhausted, our nameless heroine confessed her discovery to the king, who ordered that grapes be fermented and that the secret of wine be made known to his countrymen.

This, admittedly, is only a legend. But there is a great deal of evidence to suggest that alcohol use was common in the developing civilizations of the Mediterranean basin. Indeed, more than 5,000 years ago, Osiris was worshiped as both the Egyptian god of wine and the ruler of the dead (Bohn, 1993). Beer and wine are also mentioned several times in Homer's *Iliad* and *Odyssey*, legends that date back thousands of years. Historical evidence suggests that humans had discovered how to ferment berries to make wine by around 6400 B.C. (Ray & Ksir, 1993); by about 3500 B.C., they had discovered how to make wine from grapes (Patrick McGovern, quoted in Wilford, 1991). Thus, a significant body of evidence suggests that humans have known how to produce alcoholic beverages, and have known something of their effects on the user, for thousands of years.

How Alcohol Is Produced

By whatever means, humans somehow discovered that if you crush certain forms of fruit and allow it to stand for a period of time in a container, alcohol is produced. We now know that unseen microorganisms called yeast float in the air, settle on the crushed fruit, multiply, and begin to digest the sugars in the fruit through a chemical process called *fermentation*. The yeast breaks down the carbon, hydrogen, and oxygen atoms in the sugar for food, and in the process recombines these atoms into ethyl alcohol and carbon dioxide.

Alcohol is actually a waste product of the process of fermentation. As with other waste products, it is a poison. When the concentration

of alcohol reaches about 15%, it becomes toxic to the yeast and fermentation stops. Thus, people were able to produce alcoholic beverages whose highest concentration of alcohol was about 15% since before the time of Babylon.

However, to obtain alcohol concentrations above 15% took several thousand years more. The process of *distillation* did not appear until around the year 800 A.D., or just over 1,100 years ago. In the distillation process, the wine obtained from fermentation is heated, causing some of the alcohol content to boil off as a vapor, or steam. Alcohol boils at a much lower temperature than water does, so the steam that forms when wine is boiled contains more alcohol than water vapor.

The steam is then collected in a special cooling coil and allowed to cool down, forming a liquid again. This liquid contains a higher concentration of alcohol and a lower concentration of water than the original mixture. The liquid, with its higher alcohol content, then drips from the end of the coil into a container of some kind. This device is the famous "still" of lore and legend.

For thousands of years, wine was considered a necessary part of any meal; in Homer's *Iliad* and *Odyssey*, people drank wine with meals. In some parts of the world today, people drink wine with meals on a regular basis, sometimes because the local water supply cannot be trusted as fit to drink. Wine may also supply valuable vitamins and minerals to the consumer's diet.

Unfortunately, many vitamins and minerals in the original wine are lost in the process of distillation. Furthermore, when the body breaks down alcohol, it finds "empty calories." When the body metabolizes alcohol, the alcohol is eventually transformed into a form of carbohydrates and carbon dioxide but without the protein, vitamins, and minerals the body needs. Over time, this may contribute to a state of vitamin depletion called *avitaminosis*, which will be discussed in the next chapter.

The process of distillation was developed in Arabia, and within two centuries of its discovery, it had spread to Europe. It is reported that by the year 1000 A.D., Italian wine growers were distilling wine to produce various drinks with higher concentrations of alcohol, mixing the distilled "spirits" with various herbs and spices. This mixture was then used for medicinal purposes. Indeed, distilled spirits were viewed as the ultimate in medicines in Europe, where they were called the *aqua vitae*, or the "water of life" (Ray & Ksir, 1993).

The history of alcohol in Western society is marked by increasing use over time. Over the years, efforts made to control or regulate alcohol use have been almost uniformly unsuccessful.[2]

Alcohol Today

Over the last 1200 years since the development of the distillation process, various forms of fermented wines using various ingredients, different forms of beer, and distilled spirits combined with various flavorings have emerged. With the march of civilization, some degree of standardization has resulted in uniform definitions of various classes of alcohol, although there still exists some regional variation.

Today, most American beer has an alcohol content of between 3.5 and 5% (Herman, 1993). As a class, wine continues to be made by allowing fermentation to take place in vats containing various grapes or other fruits. Occasionally, the fermentation involves other products than grapes, such as the famous "rice wine" from Japan called sake. Wine usually has an alcohol content of approximately 8% to 17% (Herman, 1993), and there are only minor variations in how different wines are made.

Another class of wines is "fortified" wines. They are produced by adding distilled wine to fermented wine, raising the total alcohol content to about 20%. This class contains the various brands of sherry, and port (Herman, 1993). Finally, the "hard liquors" are distilled spirits whose alcohol content may range from 20% to

95% (in the case of "Everclear" and similar distilled spirits).

Beverages that contain alcohol are moderately popular drinks. In the United States, it has been estimated that 103 million people over the age of 12 (or 41% of the population) consumed alcohol at least once in the preceding year. Of this number, 61 million drank less than once a week on average, and the remainder consumed at least one alcoholic beverage per week.

Many people are surprised to learn that alcohol consumption in the United States peaked around the year 1830, when the annual per capita consumption of alcohol was an estimated 7.1 gallons of pure alcohol (Heerema, 1990). In contrast, the per capita consumption of alcohol in the United States for the year 1989 was estimated at only about one-third of the 1830 figure, or about 2.43 gallons of pure alcohol per person (*Hospital and Community Psychiatry*, 1994), or 576 cans of beer per person.

Because the majority of those who do consume alcohol do so less than once a week, it is apparent that a minority of those who use alcohol consume a disproportionate amount. Ten percent of those who drink consume fifty percent of the alcohol used in the United States (Kaplan, Sadock, & Grebb, 1994). These are the individuals whose alcohol use will interfere with their physical health and their social well being. The impact of excess alcohol use will be discussed in more detail in the next chapter. In this chapter, we will focus on the casual drinker.

The Pharmacology of Alcohol

Alcohol is usually introduced into the body in a liquid form consumed orally. Alcohol can also be introduced into the body intravenously or as a vapor, however these methods are very dangerous and are used by physicians only rarely.

The alcohol molecule is quite small, and it is soluble in both water and lipids. Therefore, alcohol molecules are rapidly distributed to all blood-rich tissues throughout the body, includ-

[2]The text by Ray and Ksir (1993) is an excellent source for more information about the various attempts at the regulation of alcohol use throughout history.

ing the brain. Because alcohol is so easily soluble in lipids, high concentrations of alcohol in the brain are achieved very rapidly.

When a person drinks on an empty stomach, about 10% (Kaplan, Sadock, & Grebb, 1994) to 20% (Julien, 1992) of the alcohol is immediately absorbed through the stomach lining. The remainder is absorbed through the small intestine. When a person drinks on an empty stomach, alcohol first appears in the bloodstream in as little as one minute (Rose, 1988).

The concentration of alcohol in any individual's blood may be influenced by a number of factors. When alcohol is mixed with food, only about 20% of the alcohol is absorbed immediately. It was once thought that the speed at which the remaining 80% of the alcohol enters the bloodstream and is detoxified by the liver was determined by how quickly the stomach empties into the small intestine. Therefore, it was once thought that, sooner or later, all the alcohol ingested would be absorbed (Julien, 1992).

However, recent research (Frezza, Di Padova, Pozzato, Terpin, Baraona, & Lieber, 1990) suggests that, for some drinkers, the process of alcohol metabolism begins in the gastrointestinal tract. In other words, the body begins to break down the alcohol even before it reaches the general circulation—at least for some drinkers. Frezza et al. found that people produce an enzyme in the gastrointestinal tract known as *gastric alcohol dehydrogenase.* This enzyme begins to break down alcohol in the stomach, even before it reaches the bloodstream.

Measured levels of gastric alcohol dehydrogenase were highest in rare social drinkers and significantly lower in regular drinkers. It was also found that men produced more of this enzyme than did women, a discovery that the authors concluded might explain why women often have higher blood alcohol levels than men after drinking a similar amount of alcohol.

A popular method for avoiding a hangover is to ingest aspirin before drinking, so that the aspirin is already in the system for the morning after. Surprisingly, research suggests that taking aspirin an hour before drinking alcohol will *decrease* the effectiveness of gastric alcohol dehydrogenase. This will result in a higher blood alcohol level for the rare social drinker than had been intended (Roine, Gentry, Hernandez-Munoz, Baraona, and Lieber, 1990).

The exact mechanism through which alcohol is able to alter the function of the brain remains unknown (Nace & Isbell, 1991). But it is known that alcohol has a number of effects on the cellular and regional levels of the brain. There are a number of theories on how alcohol is able to alter the normal activity of the neurons, but scientists are still not sure which theory best explains alcohol's effects.

At one time, it was thought that alcohol's effects were caused by its ability to disrupt the structure and the function of the lipids in the walls of the neurons. Along with protein molecules, lipid molecules help to form the cell walls of the neurons in the brain. This theory dates back to the turn of the century (Tabakoff & Hoffman, 1992) and is known as the *membrane fluidization theory,* or the *membrane hypothesis.* In the late 1970s, researchers developed techniques to measure actual alcohol-induced changes in the membranes of neurons. They discovered that alcohol is able to disrupt the structure of lipids, making it more difficult for the neurons to maintain normal functioning. However, researchers are still not sure which lipids are affected by alcohol or which components within the neuron are most sensitive to alcohol's effects. Indeed, there are strong reasons to question whether the membrane hypothesis can account for alcohol's effects.

Another theory suggests that, on the cellular level, alcohol disrupts the normal function of neurons in the brain by interacting with protein molecules within those neurons (Tabakoff & Hoffman, 1992). These protein molecules help form the ion channels and neurotransmitter receptor sites in the walls of neurons. Other protein molecules help to form some of the enzymes found in the brain, according to Tabakoff and Hoffman. It is thought that alcohol is able to interfere with the normal function of individual neurons through the interaction with these protein molecules.

The neurons of the brain are actually microscopic chemical-electrical generators, which produce a small electrical "message" by actively moving sodium and calcium ions back and forth across the cell wall. The sodium and calcium ions pass through the cell wall through special "channels," which are formed by protein molecules. Currently, it is thought that at least some of alcohol's effects might be caused by this chemical's ability to interact with the protein molecules that form the sodium/calcium ion channels. For example, alcohol inhibits the action of the amino acid N-methyl-D-aspartate (NMDA), which functions as an excitatory amino acid within the brain. Alcohol blocks the influx of calcium atoms through the ion channels normally activated when NMDA binds at those sites.

At the same time, alcohol enhances the influx of chloride atoms through an ion channel normally utilized by gamma-amino-butyric acid (GABA) (Marshall, 1994). GABA is the main inhibitory neurotransmitter in the brain (Tabakoff & Hoffman, 1992). This allows alcohol to block the effects of the excitatory amino acid NMDA while facilitating the inhibitory neurotransmitter GABA. This is one mechanism through which alcohol is thought to depress the action of the central nervous system.

It is clear that scientists still do not understand how alcohol is able to affect the function of the brain on the cellular level. However, it is known that, on the regional level, alcohol stimulates the release of the neurotransmitter dopamine, especially in the nucleus accumbens region of the brain. This is a region of the brain thought to be the "pleasure center." It is thought that, by causing the brain to release dopamine in this region, alcohol causes a sense of pleasure, or euphoria, for the drinker. Alcohol also causes an increase in serotonin levels in many parts of the brain. However, the exact importance of this increase in serotonin is not known at this time.

The Metabolism of Alcohol

Once in the blood, alcohol passes into all body tissues rapidly, including those of the brain. Because alcohol may diffuse into muscle and fat tissue, an obese or muscular person would normally have a slightly lower blood alcohol level than a leaner person would after a given dose. About 95% of the alcohol that reaches the blood is metabolized by the liver before it is excreted, at about the rate of one-third of an ounce (1/3 oz) of pure alcohol per hour in the normal, healthy individual. The other 5% of the alcohol in the bloodstream is excreted unchanged through the lungs, skin, and urine (Ashton, 1992).

The body biotransforms alcohol in two steps. First, the liver produces the enzyme *alcohol dehydrogenase* (or ADH), which breaks the alcohol down into acetaldehyde. Unlike many enzymes produced in the body, which play multiple roles in different organs, ADH has no known function other than to metabolize alcohol (Goodwin, 1989). The exact reason for this specialization is not known.

The second enzyme required to metabolize alcohol is *aldehyde dehydrogenase*, an enzyme produced in many different parts of the body. This enzyme breaks down the acetaldehyde into acetic acid.[3] Ultimately, alcohol is biotransformed into carbon dioxide, water, and fatty acids (carbohydrates). The latter are the source of the "empty calories" obtained by ingesting alcohol (Goodwin, 1989). As will be discussed in the next chapter, chronic alcoholics may obtain a significant portion of their daily energy requirements from the empty calories obtained from alcohol.

The Alcohol-Flush Reaction

After drinking even a small amount of alcohol, a small group of people in the United States, and perhaps 50% of the Asian population, experience

---

[3]The medication Antabuse (disulfiram), used to help people stop drinking, works by blocking the enzyme aldehyde dehydrogenase. This allows acetaldehyde to build up in the individual's blood, causing the individual to become ill from the toxic effects of the acetaldehyde.

what is known as the *alcohol-flush reaction*. The alcohol-flush reaction is caused by a genetic mutation found predominantly in persons of Asian descent. Because of this genetic mutation, the liver is unable to manufacture sufficient aldehyde dehydrogenase to metabolize the acetaldehyde manufactured in the first stage of alcohol biotransformation.

Persons with the alcohol-flush syndrome experience facial flushing, heart palpitations, dizziness, and nausea as the blood levels of acetaldehyde climb to 20 times the level seen in unaffected individuals consuming the same amount of alcohol. Acetaldehyde is a toxin, and anyone with a significant amount of this chemical in his or her blood will become quite ill. This phenomenon is thought to be one reason heavy drinking is so rare in persons of Asian descent.

The Speed of Alcohol Biotransformation

Maguire (1990) offers this rule of thumb for estimating the rate at which the body might metabolize alcohol: the liver may biotransform about one mixed drink of 80-proof alcohol or one can of beer per hour. Unfortunately, as we discussed in the last chapter, alcohol is biotransformed through a zero order biotransformation process. In other words, the rate at which alcohol is metabolized by the liver is "independent of the concentration of alcohol in the blood" (Julien, 1992, p. 72).

If a person drinks at the rate of about one ounce of whiskey (or one 5-ounce glass of wine or one 12-ounce can of beer) per hour, the body metabolizes the alcohol at a rate fairly close to the speed at which the alcohol is consumed. If you were to measure the level of alcohol in the blood, you would find that it stayed relatively constant until the person stopped drinking. At that point, the body would be able to finish metabolizing the ingested alcohol. If, as is often the case, more than one ounce of whiskey or one can of beer per hour is consumed, the amount of alcohol in the bloodstream increases, possibly to the point of intoxication. One rough measure

of the level of intoxication is the blood alcohol level.

The Blood Alcohol Level

Because it is not possible to measure the alcohol level in the brain of a living person, physicians have developed an indirect measure of the amount of alcohol in a person's body. This is accomplished through a measurement known as the blood alcohol level (BAL). The BAL is, essentially, a measure of the level of alcohol actually in a given person's bloodstream. It is reported in terms of milligrams of alcohol per 100 milliliters of blood, or, mg/mL. A BAL of 0.10 is thus one-tenth of a milligram of alcohol per 100 milliliters of blood.

Surprisingly, researchers have also discovered that there is only a mild relationship between the BAL and the individual's *subjective* level of intoxication. For reasons that are still not clear, the individual's subjective level of intoxication is highest when the BAL is still rising, a phenomenon known as the *Mellanby effect* (Lehman, Pilich, & Andrews, 1994). As we will discuss further in the next chapter, chronic drinkers become somewhat tolerant to alcohol's intoxicating effects. Thus, someone who has developed some tolerance to alcohol might have a rather high BAL while appearing relatively normal.

Although the BAL does provide a *crude* estimate of the individual's level of intoxication, it is far from perfect. The BAL achieved by two people who consume a similar amount of alcohol will vary as a result of a number of different factors. For example, the drinker's body size (or volume) influences the BAL. Remember, once it is in the body, the alcohol molecule rapidly diffuses into *all* body tissues; because larger individuals have a greater body mass, the alcohol has a greater body volume to diffuse into.

To illustrate this confusing characteristic of alcohol, consider the hypothetical example of a person weighing 100 pounds who consumes

	Weight (pounds)						
Number of drinks in one hour	100	120	140	160	180	200	220
2	.07	.06	.05	.05 *	.04	.04 *	.03
3	.10	.09	.07	.07 *	.06	.05	.05 *
4	.14	.11	.10	.08	.08*	.07	.06
5	.18	.14	.12	.11	.10	.08	.08*
6	.20	.18	.14	.12	.12*	.10	.09
7	.25	.20	.18	.16	.12	.12*	.11
8	.30	.25	.20	.18	.16	.14	.12

*Rounded off

Level of legal intoxication
(0.10 blood alcohol level)

FIGURE 4.1 Estimated blood alcohol levels

two regular drinks in one hour. Blood tests would reveal that this individual has a BAL of 0.09 mg/mL, slightly below legal intoxication in most states (Maguire, 1990). But, an individual who weighs 200 pounds would have a measured BAL of only 0.04 mg/mL after consuming the same amount of alcohol. Although each person consumed the same amount of alcohol, it would be more concentrated in the smaller individual, resulting in a higher BAL.

A variety of other factors influence both the speed with which alcohol enters the blood and the individual's blood alcohol level. However, Figure 4.1 provides a rough estimate of the blood alcohol levels that might be achieved through the consumption of different amounts of alcohol.[4] This chart is based on the assumption that one "drink" is either one standard can of beer or one regular mixed drink.

[4]This chart is provided as an illustration only and is not sufficiently accurate to be used as legal evidence or as a guide to "safe" drinking. Individual blood alcohol levels from the same dose of alcohol vary widely, and these figures provide only an average blood alcohol level for an individual of a given body weight.

Subjective Effects of Alcohol

Normal Doses for the Average Drinker

For the sake of discussion, we will define a normal dose of alcohol as less than the amount necessary to produce a BAL of 0.10 mg/mL. The definition of legal intoxication is 0.10 mg/mL in most states, and the typical 160-pound person would reach this BAL after drinking 3 to 4 drinks in an hour.

After 2 to 3 drinks, which would result in a BAL of 0.05 for the typical 160-pound drinker, the individual usually reports a sense of relaxation and possibly a sense of confidence or even euphoria (McGuire, 1990). A person with a BAL of 0.05 mg/mL also experiences lowered alertness, a loss of inhibitions, and impaired judgment (Kaminski, 1992; Ray & Ksir, 1993).

After a couple of drinks, the average drinker also experiences some degree of respiratory stimulation. The heart rate increases briefly, and the blood vessels on the surface of the skin dilate, often causing the person to feel warm. But, although the person feels warmer, the dilation of the blood vessels in the skin actually causes the body to lose heat more rapidly.

Years ago, people interpreted the initial increase in respiration and heart rate as evidence that alcohol was a stimulant. Actually, alcohol functions as a pseudostimulant (Lingeman, 1974). Alcohol is a CNS depressant every bit as potent as the barbiturates, and it is not a stimulant. Eventually, the depressant effect of alcohol asserts itself, and the individual experiences some degree of respiratory and cardiovascular depression. In the normal drinker, these effects are minimal and are not normally a cause for alarm.

Surprisingly, at low to moderate dosage levels, the individual's expectations play a role in how a person interprets the effects of alcohol (Brown, 1990). Drawing on her previous research into the role of expectancies and alcohol use, Brown noted that "expectancies are closely linked to actual drinking practices of both adolescents and adults" (p. 17). Individuals who drink will have their alcohol experience shaped not only by the actual pharmacological effects of alcohol but also by their expectations for its effects.

According to Brown (1990), males are most likely to expect that alcohol will make them less anxious, enhance their sexual arousal, and make them more aggressive. Females are more likely to anticipate more pleasurable changes from moderate drinking (Brown, 1990). Such expectations are common, and these beliefs tend to reinforce the use of alcohol (Brown, 1990).

Brown, Creamer, and Stetson (1987) explored the expectations of adolescents who did and did not abuse alcohol. Adolescents who abused alcohol were more likely to anticipate a positive experience when they drank than did adolescents who did not abuse alcohol. This finding was attributed to the adolescents' home environment: adolescents who abused alcohol were more likely to come from a home where alcohol use was viewed favorably than were nonabusing adolescents.

Thus, at low to moderate dosage levels, one

factor that influences alcohol's effect is the expectation the person has for alcohol. Indeed, Brown (1990) suggested that at low to moderate dosage levels, the individual's expectations and subjective interpretation of alcohol's effects may be at least as important as the pharmacological effects of the alcohol consumed, if not more so.

After one or two drinks, alcohol causes a second effect, known as the *disinhibition effect*. The disinhibition effect comes about as the alcohol starts to interfere with the normal function of the nerve cells in the cortex. This is the part of the brain most responsible for "higher" functions, such as abstract thinking and speech. The cortex is also the part of the brain where much of our voluntary behavior is planned.

As the alcohol interferes with cortical nerve function, one tends to temporarily "forget" social inhibitions (Elliott, 1992; Julien, 1992). During periods of alcohol-induced disinhibition, the individual may engage in some behavior that, under normal conditions, he or she would never carry out. It is this disinhibition effect that may contribute to the relationship between alcohol use and aggressive behavior.

Alcohol is also able to interfere with the function of a neurotransmitter in the brain known as *serotonin* (Pihl & Peterson, 1993). Neuroscientists suspect that, when the serotonin level in the brain drops, the person is more likely to act in a violent manner. Although it is not clear whether alcohol contributes to violence by lowering brain serotonin levels or through the disinhibition effect, it is known that there is a strong relationship between alcohol use and violence. For example, researchers have long been aware that between 40 and 50% of those who commit homicide had used alcohol prior to committing the murder (Parker, 1993).

Individuals with either developmental or acquired brain damage are especially at risk for the disinhibition effects of alcohol (Elliott, 1992). This is not to say that the disinhibition effect is seen *only* in individuals with some form of neurological trauma; they are just more susceptible. Individuals without any known form of brain damage may also experience alcohol-induced disinhibition.

Above-Normal Doses for the Average Drinker

The definition of legal intoxication is usually 0.10 mg/mL for the "normal" drinker. A 160-pound person who consumed just *two* drinks in 1 hour would have a BAL of about 0.03 mg/mL. Although this is far below the level of legal intoxication in most states, even this modest BAL would still result in some degree of impairment in hand-eye coordination (*Alcohol Alert*, 1994).

For a 160-pound person, four drinks in an hour would result in a BAL of 0.10 mg/mL or higher (Maguire, 1990). At this level of intoxication, the individual would demonstrate slower than normal reaction times and an impaired ability to coordinate muscle actions (a condition called *ataxia*). A person with a BAL of 0.15 mg/mL would be above the level of legal intoxication in every state, and would definitely be experiencing some alcohol-induced physical problems. This individual would have serious difficulty reacting in time to avoid an accident while driving (Lingeman, 1974).

The person with a BAL of 0.20 mg/mL is definitely intoxicated, with a marked ataxia (P. R. Matuschka, 1985). The person with a BAL of 0.25 mg/mL would stagger and have difficulty making sense of sensory data (Kaminski, 1992; Ray & Ksir, 1993). The person with a BAL of 0.30 mg/mL would be stuporous, and although conscious, would likely be unable to remember what happened while intoxicated (P. R. Matuschka, 1985).

With a BAL of 0.35 mg/mL, the stage of surgical anesthesia is achieved (P. R. Matuschka, 1985). At high dosage levels, alcohol's effects are analogous to those of the anesthetic ether (Maguire, 1990). Unfortunately, the amount of alcohol in the blood necessary to bring about a state of unconsciousness is only a little less than the level necessary to bring about a fatal overdose of alcohol. Thus, when a person drinks to the point of losing consciousness, he or she might be dangerously close to overdosing on alcohol. Although many people do not understand that it is possible to *die* from an alcohol overdose, this occasionally does actually happen.

About 1% of the people whose BAL is 0.35 mg/mL will die without medical treatment (Ray & Ksir, 1993); this is the LD_{01} dosage level for alcohol. At this concentration, alcohol is thought to interfere with the activity of the nerves that control respiration (Lehman, Pilich, & Andrews, 1994). A BAL of 0.40 mg/mL will result in about a 50% death rate from alcohol overdose without medical intervention (Bohn, 1993); the LD_{50} is thus around 0.40 mg/mL. However, there are cases on record in which people tolerant to the effects of alcohol were still conscious and able to talk with a BAL as high as 0.78 mg/mL (Bohn, 1993; Schuckit, 1989).

Segal and Sisson (1985) reported that the approximate lethal BAL in human beings is 0.5 mg/mL, whereas Lingeman (1974) places the fatal concentration of alcohol in the blood somewhere between 0.5 and 0.8 mg/mL. Thus, in theory, the LD_{100} is reached when the drinker has a BAL between 0.5 and 0.8 mg/mL. However, since a BAL of 0.35 mg/mL or above may result in death, *all cases of known or suspected alcohol overdose should immediately be treated by a physician.*

The effects of alcohol on the rare drinker are summarized in Table 4.1.

Remember that alcohol is a toxin, or poison. When a great deal of alcohol has been consumed, the body calls on several defense mechanisms to limit its exposure to this chemical. When the level of alcohol in the stomach rises to extremely high levels, the stomach excretes higher levels of mucus than is normal, and the pyloric valve between the stomach and the small intestine closes (Kaplan, Sadock, & Grebb, 1994). These actions slow down the absorption of the alcohol that remains in the stomach,

TABLE 4.1 Effects of Alcohol on the Rare Drinker

Blood alcohol level (BAL)	Behavior and physical effects
0.05–0.09	Euphoria, mild ataxia
0.10–0.19	Slurred speech, severe ataxia, mood instability, drowsiness, nausea
0.20–0.29	Lethargy, combativeness, stupor, incoherent speech, vomiting
0.30–0.39	Coma, respiratory depression
Above 0.40	Death

Source: Based on material provided by Lehman, L. B., Pilich, A., & Andrews, N. (1994). Neurological disorders resulting from alcoholism. *Alcohol Health & Research World, 17*, 306–309.

giving the body more time to metabolize the alcohol in the blood.

These actions will also contribute to feelings of nausea and may cause the drinker to vomit, allowing the body to rid itself of the alcohol. If this happens when the individual is unconscious, some of the material being regurgitated might be aspirated, which could precipitate a condition known as aspirative pneumonia. This is a very real, if rarely discussed, danger of drinking.

Medical Complications of Alcohol Use for the Average Drinker

The Hangover

The exact mechanism by which alcohol causes a "hangover" is not well understood (Ray & Ksir, 1993). We do know that both the stomach and the brain react to alcohol's toxic effects. If the drinker has ingested enough alcohol, he or she will experience a hangover the next day. Some symptoms of the hangover include malaise, headache, tremor, and nausea (Kaminski, 1992). Although a severe hangover may make the victim wish for death (O'Donnell, 1986), in general, the alcoholic hangover is self-limiting.

A hangover is not generally considered a medical emergency. The victim of an alcoholic hangover may treat his or her suffering with antacids, bed rest, solid foods, fruit juice, and aspirin (Kaminski, 1992). Surprisingly, some experts believe that the hangover is a symptom of an early alcohol withdrawal syndrome (Ray & Ksir, 1993). Thus, the individual suffering from a hangover, be it after a single night of drinking or a more protracted period, may be going through a mild alcohol withdrawal process.

Sleep Disorders

Although it is a CNS depressant, alcohol interferes with the normal sleep cycle. Like other CNS depressants, alcohol may initially induce sleep, but it does not allow a normal dream cycle. This effect is not noted for the person who drinks only on a social basis. But for the chronic alcoholic, the cumulative effects might be quite disruptive. The impact of chronic alcohol use on the normal sleep cycle will be discussed in the next chapter.

Even the occasional drinker should be aware, however, that alcohol can impair an individual's ability to breathe during sleep. Even moderate amounts of alcohol ingested within two hours of going to sleep could contribute to *sleep apnea* (*Science Digest*, 1989). Sleep apnea is a disorder in which the individual's ability to breathe is disrupted during sleep. Other complications caused by sleep apnea include high blood pressure, abnormal heart rate, and possibly death. Individuals who consumed even moderate amounts of alcohol before sleeping experienced twice as many apnea episodes as they did when abstaining from alcohol use. Anyone with a respiratory disorder, especially sleep apnea, should not drink, especially during the hours prior to going to sleep.

Adverse Drug Interactions

When a person combines alcohol with a drug that has a sedating effect, the two chemicals are said to *potentiate* each other. The sedating effects of alcohol combine with the sedating effects of such drugs as antihistamines, tranquilizers, and many antidepressants. This potentiation effect may become so powerful that it interferes with the normal functioning of the body, and may even result in the person's death.

Alcohol interacts with a wide range of medications in addition to the drugs that have a sedating effect.[5] For example, individuals who drink while taking nitroglycerin, a medication often used to treat heart conditions, frequently develop significantly reduced blood pressure levels, possibly to the point of dizziness and loss of consciousness (Pappas, 1990).

Alcohol combined with aspirin may contribute to bleeding in the stomach, because both alcohol and aspirin irritate the stomach lining (Sands, Knapp, & Ciraulo, 1993). Although acetaminophen does not irritate the stomach lining, the chronic use of alcohol causes the liver to release enzymes that transform acetaminophen into a poison, even when the drug is used at recommended dosage levels. Thus, active alcoholics are advised not to use acetaminophen for the relief of pain.

Oral medications for diabetes may negate the body's ability to metabolize alcohol, possibly resulting in acute alcohol poisoning from even moderate amounts of alcohol. Furthermore, because the antidiabetic medication prevents the body from biotransforming alcohol, the individual will remain intoxicated far longer than he or she would normally. In such a case, the individual might underestimate the time before which it would be safe for him or her to drive a motor vehicle.

Patients on the antidepressant medications known as *monoamine oxidase inhibitors* (or MAO inhibitors) should not consume alcohol. The fermentation process produces tyramine along with the alcohol. Tyramine is normally used by the body to produce an important amino acid, but tyramine interacts with the MAO inhibitors, causing dangerously high, and possibly fatal, blood pressure levels.

Alcohol also interacts with the tricyclic antidepressants, such as amitriptyline, doxepin, and their related agents. This interaction results in an increase in sedation and difficulty in muscle movement coordination (ataxia) (Sands, Knapp, & Ciraulo, 1993). Sands et al. also note that the chronic use of alcohol causes the liver to metabolize the tricyclic antidepressants more quickly, limiting their effectiveness.

The effects of alcohol are similar to other CNS depressant drugs. This class of drugs includes narcotic analgesics, the barbiturates and barbituratelike drugs, the benzodiazepines, and a number of other chemicals. So similar are the effects of the various CNS depressants to alcohol that one class of drug potentiates the effects of the other. The interaction between alcohol and the CNS depressants is quite serious and potentially fatal, because the different chemicals combine to produce a greater degree of CNS depression than either one could achieve individually.

At one time, patients who were using the antiulcer medications Zantac (ranitidine)[6] and Tagamet (cimetidine) were advised not to drink while taking these drugs. Sicherman (1992) warned that patients who drink alcohol while taking prescribed doses of these medications experience a faster-than-normal rise in blood alcohol levels. Patients who drank while on Tagamet (cimetidine) experienced a 92% increase in measured blood alcohol levels as compared with nonmedicated drinkers. Sicherman warned that patients on these drugs might find themselves over the legal limit for intoxication after only two or three drinks.

However, Wormsley (1993) challenged this

---

[5]The list of potential alcohol/drug interactions is quite extensive. Patients taking *any* medication should refrain from consuming alcohol without first checking with a physician or pharmacist.

[6]The most common brand name is given first, with the generic name in parenthesis.

conclusion, noting that earlier studies of the effects of alcohol and ranitidine were flawed. Wormsley noted that earlier research studies into the interaction between alcohol and ranitidine used either fasting subjects or atypical dosing schedules that did not reflect how the medication would be used in real life by patients. When these variables were controlled for, Wormsley concluded that there was no evidence to suggest that ranitidineuse resulted in higher blood alcohol levels. Still, considering the damage alcohol can cause to the user's gastrointestinal tract (which will be discussed in more detail in the next chapter), ranitidine users are wise to avoid drinking alcohol, even if there is no evidence of a significant clinical interaction between alcohol and ranitidine at this time.

Patients taking the antibiotic medications chloramphenicol, furazolidone, or metronidazole should also avoid alcohol. The combination of these antibiotics with alcohol may produce a reaction very similar to that with disulfiram (discussed in Chapter 31) (Meyers, 1992). The combination of alcohol and the antitubercular drug isoniazid (or INH, as it is often called) reduces isoniazid's effectiveness and may increase the individual's chances of developing hepatitis.

Because of the potentiation effect between narcotic analgesics and alcohol, both of which are CNS depressants, patients who are using narcotics should not drink. And alcohol combined with the analgesic propoxyphene (Darvon) can cause potentially dangerous levels of CNS depression or even death (Sands, Knapp, & Ciraulo, 1993).

Alcohol Use and Accidental Injury or Death

Alcohol is quite popular as a recreational beverage. Media advertisements proclaim the benefits of recreational alcohol use at parties, social encounters, or as a way to celebrate good news.

Unfortunately, media advertisements often fail to mention that recreational alcohol is associated with an increased risk of accidental injury, or even premature death.

The relationship between motor vehicle accidents and alcohol use is well known. Yet, in spite of a protracted campaign to reduce "drunk driving" in the United States, significant numbers of people still attempt to drive motor vehicles while under the influence of alcohol. Between 40 and 50% of motor vehicle fatalities are alcohol related (McGinnis & Foege, 1993). In 1992 alone, approximately 46% of all motor vehicle fatalities (or 18,032 individual deaths) were alcohol related (Skolnick, 1993).[7]

However, some forms of motor vehicle transportation are more dangerous than others. It has been estimated that 60% of all boating fatalities are alcohol related (*Alcohol Alert*, 1994), and an estimated 70% of the motorcycle drivers killed in accidents are thought to have been drinking prior to the accident (Colburn, Meyer, Wrigley, & Bradley, 1993). These figures indicate that alcohol-related motor vehicle accidents remain a significant cause of premature death in the United States.

Alcohol use is a factor in 41% of all fatalities due to falling and 42% of all fatalities associated with fires (Rice, 1993). Furthermore, approximately 30,000 individuals lose their lives each year because of alcohol-related accidental injuries[8] (drownings, injuries in the home, and so on) (McGinnis & Foege, 1993). Researchers have found that 42% of those individuals treated at one major trauma center had alcohol in their blood at the time of admission (Milzman & Soderstrom, 1994). No matter how you look at it, even casual alcohol use carries with it a significantly increased risk of accidental injury, or death.

[7]In one study, it was found that 59% of those reckless drivers who were not under the influence of alcohol were later found to have been under the influence of marijuana or cocaine (Brookoff, Cook, Williams, & Mann, 1994).

[8]This number is part of the 200,000 alcohol-related deaths that will be discussed in the next chapter.

Summary

This chapter briefly explored the history of alcohol, including its early history as man's first recreational chemical. We discussed the process of distillation and the manner in which wine is obtained from fruit. We reviewed the use of distillation to achieve concentrations of alcohol above 15% and questions surrounding the use of alcohol. Finally, we briefly reviewed the history of alcohol consumption and the present pattern of alcohol use in the United States.

CHAPTER FIVE

Chronic Alcohol Addiction

The focus of Chapter 4 was the acute effects of alcohol on the "average" drinker, one who consumes alcohol on a social basis. However, alcohol is also capable of causing the user to become both psychologically and physically dependent on its effects. Individuals who are dependent on alcohol often ingest it on a regular basis, thus chronically exposing their bodies to the chemical. In such cases, the chronic effects of alcohol are quite different from those seen in the social drinker. In this chapter, we will explore some of the consequences of chronic alcohol use.

The Scope of the Problem

Alcohol is a popular recreational chemical. It is also by far the most popular drug of abuse, accounting for an astounding 85% of the drug addiction problem in the United States (Franklin, 1987). However, only a small proportion of alcohol users will experience problems as a result of their drinking. Regier, Farmer, Rae, Locke, Keith, Judd, and Goodwin (1990) conclude that approximately 13.5% of the population, at some time over the course of their lives, will meet the criteria for either alcohol abuse or dependence.

Although this estimate is useful, it does little to shed light on the question of how many people are using alcohol to excess *at this point in time*. Furthermore, the estimate provided by Regier et al. does not identify how many of those individuals will experience only isolated periods of alcohol abuse, and how many will become alcoholics. Remember, 30 to 45% of those who drink alcohol will experience one sign of alcohol abuse for a short period of time without going on to become alcoholic (Kaplan, Sadock, & Grebb, 1994).

Estimates of the scope of the problem of alcoholism vary. Bays (1990) suggests that there are about 10 million adult alcoholics in the United States. A decade ago, Beasley (1987) presented a higher figure, reporting that between 10 and 15 million people were alcoholic, with an additional 10 million "on the cusp of alcoholism" (p. 21). Nor is the problem of alcohol abuse and addiction limited to adults. It is estimated that between 1 million (Ellis, McInerney, DiGiuseppe, & Yeager, 1988) and 3 million (Turbo, 1989) children and adolescents are also addicted to alcohol.

Alcoholism is predominately a male disease, in the sense that male alcoholics outnumber female alcoholics by a ratio of about 2:1 (Blume, 1994). However, if it is assumed that there are about 10 to 15 million individuals in this country whose alcohol use is beyond the range of just social drinking, then 6 to 10 million men and 3 to 5 million women either abuse alcohol or are addicted to it.

Clinicians who specialize in substance abuse often hear clients deny that they are alcoholic, insisting that they are "only problem drinkers." Schuckit, Zisook, and Mortola (1985) explored whether there are significant differences between those who are physically addicted to alcohol and those who might be said to be "abusive drinkers." The authors found that a group of men identified as abusers was virtually identical to a group of men diagnosed as alcohol dependent. The major difference between these two groups was that men in the latter group drank more when they did drink and were more likely to have had alcohol-related medical problems.

On the basis of their research, the authors conclude it is "not clear whether the distinction between alcohol abuse and alcohol dependence carries any important prognostic or treatment implications" (p. 1403). When alcohol use has reached the point where the drinker is experiencing various physical, legal, social, financial, and legal problems, the distinction between *abuse* and *dependence* becomes virtually meaningless.

What the research *does* suggest is that it usually takes about 10 years of heavy drinking before the typical person becomes dependent on alcohol (Meyer, 1994). However, once a person *does* become dependent on alcohol, even if that person stops drinking for a period of time, he or she will again become dependent "in a matter of days to weeks" (Meyer, 1994, p. 165). Thus, once an individual becomes dependent on alcohol, it is unlikely that he or she can return to nonabusive drinking.

Alcohol Tolerance, Dependence, and "Craving": Signposts of Addiction

Chronic alcohol use can result in psychological or physical dependence. Specific signs indicate that a given individual has moved past the point of simple social drinking to the point of alcoholism. We will briefly discuss each of these warning signs of alcoholism in turn.

Alcohol Tolerance

If an individual repeatedly consumes alcohol, over time his or her body will make certain adaptations to try to maintain normal function in the presence of the foreign chemical. First, the individual's liver becomes more efficient at metabolizing alcohol, at least in the earlier stages of his or her drinking career. This is known as *metabolic tolerance* to alcohol.

For example, during clinical interviews, it is not uncommon for alcoholics to admit that they need to drink far more alcohol to become intoxicated than they did 5 or 10 years ago. Drinkers might admit, for example, that they could become intoxicated on "just" a 6-pack of beer when they were 21, but that it now takes 12 to 18 cans of beer to reach the same level of intoxication, a reflection of a growing tolerance to alcohol's effects. Compare the effects of alcohol for the chronic drinker in Table 5.1 with those of the social drinker (Table 4.1).

Another expression of alcohol tolerance is known as *behavioral tolerance*. Whereas a novice drinker might appear quite intoxicated after 5 or 6 beers, the chronic drinker might appear quite sober even when legally intoxicated. If judged on the basis of physical appearance alone, many chronic alcoholics appear relatively sober, at least to the untrained observer, even when blood tests reveal significant amounts of alcohol in their blood.

TABLE 5.1 Effects of Alcohol on the Chronic Drinker

Blood alcohol level (BAL)	Behavior and physical effects
0.05–0.09	None to minimal effect
0.10–0.19	Mild ataxia, euphoria
0.20–0.29	Mild emotional changes, ataxia
0.30–0.39	Drowsiness, lethargy, stupor
Above 0.40	Coma

Source: Based on material provided by Lehman, L.B., Pilich, A., & Andrews, N. (1994). Neurological disorders resulting from alcoholism. *Alcohol Health & Research World, 17*, 306–309.

Pharmacodynamic tolerance is another form of tolerance. In pharmacodynamic tolerance, the cells of the central nervous system attempt to carry out their normal function in spite of the continual presence of a toxin, such as alcohol. The cells of the brain become less and less sensitive to the chemical's effects, and the individual has to use more of the substance to achieve the same effect.

In general, clinicians simply say that the individual is "tolerant" to the effects of alcohol. Each form of tolerance discussed is actually a part of the overall process of tolerance to the effects of a chemical. There are several points to keep in mind about tolerance to alcohol's effects. First, in spite of the development of tolerance, the lethal dose of alcohol remains the same (P. R. Matuschka, 1985). Chronic alcohol users can overdose on alcohol, just as the novice drinker can. Thus, *any suspected alcohol overdose should immediately be evaluated and treated by a physician.*

The physical adaptations the drinker's body goes through to try to maintain normal function in spite of the continuous presence of alcohol are *not* permanent. Over time, the drinker may actually become *less* tolerant to alcohol's effects. Alcohol is a toxin, and over time the liver becomes less efficient in metabolizing the alcohol in the individual's body. When this occurs, clinicians say the individual's tolerance is "on the downswing." Lowered tolerance to alcohol's effects indicates the later stages of alcohol dependence and is a sign of serious alcoholism.

Alcohol Dependence

There are two forms of alcohol dependence; psychological and physical dependence. *Psychological dependence* refers to repeated self-administration of alcohol because the individual finds it rewarding. The individual continues to use alcohol as a "crutch," believing that he or she is unable to be sexual, sleep, or socialize without first ingesting alcohol.

Physical dependence, also referred to as "alcoholism" or the more generic term *addiction,* is characterized by a withdrawal syndrome that occurs when the alcohol supply is suddenly removed. Physical dependence automatically implies that the individual has become tolerant to a chemical's effects. In the case of alcohol dependence, there is a period of adjustment during which the body functions slowly return to normal again after a period of chronic alcohol use. There is some subjective discomfort for the individual, and, unfortunately, some physical danger as well. It is for this reason that *all cases of alcohol withdrawal should be evaluated and treated by a physician.*

The severity of the withdrawal from alcohol depends on (1) the intensity with which the individual used alcohol, (2) the duration of time over which the individual drank, and (3) the individual's state of health. Thus, the longer the period of alcohol use and the greater the amount ingested, the more severe the alcohol withdrawal syndrome. The symptoms of alcohol withdrawal for the chronic alcoholic will be discussed in more detail later in this chapter.

Alcohol Cravings

Recovering alcoholics often speak of a "craving" for alcohol that continues long after they have stopped drinking. Some alcoholics feel "thirsty" or find themselves preoccupied with the possibility of having a drink. At present, it is not known why alcoholics "crave" alcohol. However, the fact that the individual does become preoccupied with alcohol use, or craves a drink, is a sign that he or she has become dependent upon alcohol.

The TIQ Hypothesis

Trachtenberg and Blum (1987) theorize that cravings occur because chronic alcohol use significantly reduces the brain's production of opiatelike neurotransmitters known as the *endorphins,* the *enkephalins,* and the *dynorphins.* These neurotransmitters function in the brain's pleasure center to help moderate an individual's emotions and behavior.

Blum (1988) suggests that a byproduct of

alcohol metabolism combines with neurotransmitters normally found in the brain and forms *tetrahydroisoquinoline* (TIQ). TIQ is thought to be capable of binding to opiatelike receptor sites within the brain's pleasure center, causing a sense of well-being (Blum & Payne, 1991; Blum & Trachtenberg, 1988). This seems to be the mechanism through which alcohol use is rewarding to the individual. However, TIQ's effects are apparently short-lived, which forces the individual to drink more alcohol to regain or maintain the initial pleasurable feeling.

Chronic use of alcohol is thought to reduce the brain's production of enkephalins, as the ever-present TIQ is substituted for these naturally produced opiatelike neurotransmitters (Blum & Payne, 1991; Blum & Trachtenberg, 1988). When alcohol intake ceases, a neurochemical deficit results, which the individual then attempts to relieve through further chemical use (Blum & Payne, 1991; Blum & Trachtenberg, 1988). This deficit is the "craving" for alcohol recovering alcoholics commonly experience.

Although the TIQ theory had a number of strong adherents in the late 1980s and early 1990s, it has gradually fallen into disfavor. A number of research studies have failed to find evidence to support the TIQ hypothesis. At this time, few researchers in the field of alcohol addiction believe that TIQ plays a major role in the phenomenon of alcohol craving.

Complications from Chronic Alcohol Use

The chronic use of alcohol may contribute directly or indirectly to a number of health problems for the drinker. Because alcohol is a mild toxin, its effects over time often manifest themselves in damage to one or more organ systems. It is also important to recognize that chronic alcohol use includes "weekend" or "binge" drinking. Repeated episodic alcohol abuse may bring about many of the same effects that occur with chronic alcohol use.

Unfortunately, there is no simple formula by which to calculate the risk of alcohol-related organ damage or to determine which organs will be affected. As Segal and Sisson (1985) note:

> Some heavy drinkers of many years' duration appear to go relatively unscathed, while others develop complications early (e.g., after five years) in their drinking careers. Some develop brain damage; others liver disease; still others, both. The reasons for this are simply not known. (p. 145)

However, it is known that chronic alcohol use will have an impact on virtually every body system. Exactly which ones will be affected in any one person will vary from individual to individual.

Effects on the Digestive System

As we discussed in Chapter 4, many of the original vitamins and minerals in wine are lost during distillation. Furthermore, the body obtains carbohydrates from the alcohol it metabolizes without the protein, vitamins, calcium, and other minerals the body needs. This may contribute to a state of vitamin depletion, which will be discussed in more detail later in this chapter.

It has been known for many years that chronic alcoholic use increases the risk of many forms of cancer. There is a known relationship between chronic alcohol abuse and cancer of the upper digestive tract, respiratory system, mouth, pharynx, larynx, esophagus, and liver (Garro, Espina, & Lieber, 1992). Alcohol use is associated with 75% of all deaths due to cancer of the esophagus (Rice, 1993). Although the research data is not clear at this time, there is also evidence suggesting a link between chronic alcohol use and both cancer of the large bowel and cancer of the breast (Garro, Espina, & Lieber, 1992).

The combination of cigarettes and alcohol is especially dangerous. Chronic alcoholics experience almost a 6-fold increase in their risk of developing cancer of the mouth or pharynx (Garro, Espina, & Lieber, 1992, p. 83). In comparison, cigarette smokers have slightly more than a 7-fold increased risk of developing cancer of the mouth or pharynx. However, alcoholics who also smoke have a *38-fold increased risk* of cancer in these regions, according to Garro et al.

Chronic exposure to alcohol has a profound impact on the liver. Ultimately, the liver is "the organ most commonly thought to be affected by alcohol" (Nace, 1987, p. 23). Indeed, in humans, the liver is the primary site at which alcohol is metabolized within the body (Frezza et al. 1990; Schenker & Speeg, 1990). Not surprisingly, the liver is a likely place for alcohol-related problems to develop, and alcohol addiction is the primary cause of liver disease in the United States.

The first manifestation of alcohol-related liver problems is the development of a *fatty liver*, a condition in which the liver becomes enlarged and does not function at full efficiency (Nace, 1987). This condition can usually be detected by physical examination or through various blood tests (Schuckit, 1989). A fatty liver is a common consequence of chronic alcohol use, and eventually, every heavy drinker will develop a fatty liver (*Alcohol Alert*, 1993a; Sherman, Ward, Warren-Perry, Williams, & Peters, 1993).

If alcohol consumption continues, the individual is likely to develop *alcoholic hepatitis*. For reasons that are not well understood, only between 10 and 35% of chronic drinkers develop this condition (*Alcohol Alert*, 1993a). Sherman, et al. found evidence suggesting that the individual's vulnerability to progressing from a fatty liver to alcoholic liver disease may be mediated by genetic factors. That is, by virtue of his or her genetic inheritance, a drinker is more or less likely to develop alcohol-induced liver damage.

Symptoms of alcoholic hepatitis include a low-grade fever; malaise; jaundice; an enlarged, tender liver; and dark urine (Nace, 1987). A physical examination may reveal characteristic changes in the blood chemistry (Schuckit, 1989), and the patient may complain of abdominal pain (*Alcohol Alert*, 1993a). If possible, surgery should be avoided for recovering alcoholics as

patients going through the acute states of alcohol withdrawal are poor surgical risks.

Unfortunately, if a patient with alcoholic hepatitis is examined by a physician who is not aware of the patient's history of alcoholism, the abdominal pain may be misinterpreted as a symptom of another condition, such as appendicitis, pancreatitis, or inflammation of the gall bladder. As with any medical condition, proper diagnosis is essential to provide for the appropriate care of the patient. Death is possible from alcoholic hepatitis, especially if the amount of damage to the individual's liver exceeds its ability to recover (*Alcohol Alert*, 1993a).

In spite of the best medical care, 60% of those individuals hospitalized for acute, severe alcoholic hepatitis die within 6 weeks of their admission to the hospital (Thomson, 1994). Thus, by the time the individual develops the symptoms of alcoholic hepatitis, his or her drinking has passed far beyond "problem" drinking to the point where alcohol use has become life-threatening.

Alcoholic hepatitis is "a slow, smoldering process which may proceed or coexist with cirrhosis" (Nace, 1987, p. 25). Although some researchers believe that alcoholic hepatitis precedes the development of cirrhosis of the liver, this has not been proved. Indeed, "alcoholics may progress to cirrhosis without passing through any visible stage resembling hepatitis" (*Alcohol Alert*, 1993a, p. 1). Thus, many chronic alcoholics never develop alcoholic hepatitis, and the first outward sign of serious liver disease is the development of cirrhosis of the liver.

Statistically, *cirrhosis of the liver* is the sixth leading cause of death in the United States (Nace, 1987). For reasons that are not fully understood, less than 20% of alcoholics ultimately develop cirrhosis of the liver (*Alcohol Alert*, 1993a). But the 20% of alcoholics who do develop liver disease comprise between 60 and 90% of all serious cases of liver disease seen in the United States (American Medical Association, 1993a).

Repeated episodes of abusive drinking result in what are known as physical "insults," or injury, to the liver. As the tissue of the liver is damaged, scar tissue develops, and large areas of the liver may become permanently damaged over time. In general, cirrhosis of the liver does not develop until after 10 to 20 years of heavy drinking (*Alcohol Alert*, 1993a). A physical examination often reveals a hard, nodular liver as well as an enlarged spleen, "spider" angiomas on the skin, tremors, jaundice, mental confusion, and a number of other possible symptoms including testicular atrophy in males (Nace, 1987).

Cirrhosis itself can bring about severe complications, including liver cancer and sodium and water retention (Nace, 1987; Schuckit, 1989). Furthermore, the scar tissue and fat deposits prevent the liver from filtering the blood as efficiently as before, causing toxins to build up in the blood and adding to the damage being done to the brain by the alcohol (Willoughby, 1984). At the same time, the now-enlarged liver puts a greater work load on the heart, as it causes the pressure to build up within the vessels. This condition is known as *portal hypertension*, which in turn may contribute to a swelling of the blood vessels in the esophagus. When the blood vessels in the esophagus swell, weak spots form on their walls, much as weak spots form on an inner tube of a tire. These weak spots may rupture, leading to massive bleeding (Willoughby, 1984; Schuckit, 1989). Esophageal bleeding is a medical emergency which, even with the most advanced forms of medical treatment, may result in the patient's death (Ciraulo, Shader, Ciraulo, Greenblatt, & von Moltke, 1994b).

As if that were not enough, alcohol has been implicated as one cause of a painful inflammation of the pancreas known as *pancreatitis*. Approximately 35% of all known cases of pancreatitis are thought to be brought on by chronic alcohol use, and some research centers have found that alcoholism is the major cause of between 66 and 75% of the cases of pancreatitis treated at those facilities (Steinberg & Tenner, 1994). Pancreatitis develops slowly and usually requires a history of "10 to 15 years of heavy drinking" (Nace, 1987, p. 26) before it can

develop. Although pancreatitis can be caused by a number of toxic agents, such as the venom of scorpions or exposure to certain insecticides, ethyl alcohol is the leading cause of toxin-induced pancreatitis (Steinberg & Tenner, 1994).

Alcohol is also quite irritating to the stomach lining. Chronic alcohol use has been shown to cause *gastritis*, an inflammation of the stomach lining that may cause it to bleed or that may contribute to the formation of ulcers (Willoughby, 1984). It has been estimated that about 30% of heavy drinkers will suffer from chronic gastritis (P. R. Matuschka, 1985). If an ulcer forms over a major blood vessel, the individual may experience a "bleeding ulcer" as the stomach acid eats through the stomach lining and blood vessel walls. This is a severe medical emergency that frequently results in death. Sometimes part of the stomach is removed to control the bleeding, which makes it difficult for the body to find and absorb suitable amounts of vitamins from the food ingested (Willoughby, 1984). Either alone or in combination with further alcohol use, this impairment may lead to a chronic state of malnutrition, which in turn makes the individual a prime candidate for the developing of tuberculosis (TB) (Willoughby, 1984).

The treatment of TB is rather slow and difficult, sometimes requiring that medication be taken on a regular basis for up to 18 months. Sometimes, surgery is necessary to remove the infected tissues, a process both painful and life-threatening, and there are a number of treatment-resistant strains of TB. Willoughby (1984) estimates that at least 95% of those alcoholics who had a portion of their stomach removed secondary to bleeding ulcers and who continue to drink will ultimately develop TB.

However, even with the stomach intact, chronic alcohol ingestion contributes to a number of *malabsorption syndromes*, in which the individual's body is no longer able to absorb needed vitamins or minerals from food (Marsano, 1994). Beasley (1987) termed this condition a "leaky gut," a common problem for chronic alcoholics. Some minerals that might not be absorbed include zinc (Marsano, 1994), sodium, calcium, phosphorus, and magnesium (Lehman, Pilich, & Andrews, 1994). Chronic alcohol use will also interfere with the body's ability to absorb or properly utilize Vitamin A, Vitamin D, Vitamin B-6, thiamine, and folic acid (Marsano, 1994).

In some cases, the chronic use of alcohol contributes to *glossitis,* a very painful inflammation of the tongue (Marsano, 1994). Marsano also targets alcoholism as one factor that may cause stricture of the esophagus, making it harder for the individual to absorb adequate levels of food.

When the body metabolizes alcohol, one of the eventual by-products is a form of carbohydrate, which the body then burns in the place of normal food (Charness, Simon, & Greenberg, 1989). This results in a form of anorexia, as the body replaces the normal calorie intake with "empty" calories obtained from alcohol. Many chronic alcoholics obtain up to half of their daily caloric intake from alcohol, rather than from more traditional food sources (Suter, Schultz, & Jequier, 1992). Alcoholics' tendency to substitute calories obtained from alcohol for those normally obtained from food contributes to the decline in the effectiveness of the immune system, making the individual vulnerable to infectious diseases such as pneumonia and TB.

However, there are other consequences of heavy alcohol use for both the alcoholic and the heavy social drinker, such as the development of a number of metabolic disorders. For example, chronic alcohol use interferes with the body's ability to adequately control blood glucose levels (*Alcohol Alert,* 1993c). Heavy drinkers may experience episodes of either abnormally high or abnormally low blood sugar levels as the body struggles to adjust to alcohol's effects. These conditions are known as *hyperglycemia* and *hypoglycemia,* respectively, and reflect alcohol's ability to interfere with the secretion of digestive enzymes from the pancreas (*Alcohol Alert,* 1993c).

Chronic alcohol use may also interfere with the way the drinker's body metabolizes fats.

When the individual reaches the point where 10% or more of his or her daily energy requirements are obtained from alcohol rather than from more traditional foods, the individual's body goes through a series of alcohol-induced changes (Suter, Schultz, & Jequier, 1992). First, the body's energy expenditure (metabolism) slows down, which in turn, causes the body to store the unused lipids as fatty tissue. This is the mechanism by which the so-called "beer belly" commonly seen in the heavy drinker is formed.

Effects on the Cardiopulmonary System

Surprisingly, researchers have discovered that the moderate daily use of alcohol (that is, 1 or 2 drinks), especially wine, has been found to have a beneficial effect on the cardiovascular system. The consumption of *no more than* 2½ drinks per day seems to be associated with a significant reduction in the risk of heart attack in both men (Klatsky, 1990) and women (Doria, 1990). Kemm measures alcohol in "units," a unit being ½-pint of beer, 1 glass of wine, or 1 standard drink. Although Kemm (1993) suggests that the safe limit is 21 units (p. 1373) of alcohol per week for males and 14 units per week for females, the 2-drinks-a-day average still appears valid.

Wine's ability to reduce the risk of heart attack seems to be the result of alcohol's ability to inhibit blood platelets' "binding" together (Renaud & DeLorgeril, 1992). By reducing the ability of blood platelets to start the clotting process, the moderate use of alcohol may result in a lower risk of heart attack. This should not be surprising, given that wine contains salicylic acid, the active ingredient of aspirin (*Discover,* 1994). As will be discussed in Chapter 12, aspirin has been found to inhibit the ability of blood platelets to form clots.

However, there is a fine line between "just enough" alcohol and too much (Herman, 1993). For women, consuming even 1 drink a day significantly increases the risk of breast cancer (Brody, 1993). Thus, the role of alcohol in reducing the risk of heart attack is limited, at best, and carries with it other forms of health risks.

When an individual drinks more than 2½ drinks (or 12 ounces of beer or 5 ounces of wine) on a daily basis, alcohol not only loses its protective action but actually harms the cardiovascular system. The excessive, chronic use of alcohol suppresses normal red blood cell formation, and both blood clotting problems and anemia are common results (Nace, 1987).

For a number of reasons, bacterial pneumonia is at least twice as common in alcoholics as in nonalcoholics (Nace, 1987). First, chronic alcohol use lowers resistance to disease by lowering the immune system's effectiveness. This increases the chances that the alcoholic will experience infectious diseases. On occasion, a drinker might aspirate (inhale) some of the material vomited during and after periods of drinking which may result in a condition we referred to earlier as *aspirative pneumonia*. As mentioned in Chapter 4, if the individual is unconscious when he or she vomits, there is a very real danger that the drinker will suffocate.

Alcohol is also implicated in damage to the cardiovascular system itself. In large amounts (defined as more than 1 to 2 drinks per day), alcohol is known to be *cardiotoxic*, or toxic to the muscle tissue of the heart. Indeed, chronic alcohol use is considered the most common cause of heart muscle disease (Rubin & Doria, 1990). Prolonged exposure to alcohol may result in permanent damage to the heart muscle tissue, resulting in hypertension (or high blood pressure) and inflammation and weakening of the heart muscle (a condition known as *alcoholic cardiomyopathy*).

Alcoholic cardiomyopathy actually appears to be a special example of a more generalized process in which chronic alcohol use results in damage to *all* striated muscle tissues, not just those in the heart muscle. Fernandez-Sola, Estruch, Grau, Pare, Rubin, and Urbano-Marquez (1994) examined a number of men, both alcoholics and nonalcoholics. They found that alcoholic men in general had less muscle strength and greater levels of muscle tissue damage than did the nonalcoholics in this study. The authors concluded that alcohol is toxic to muscle tissue

and that chronic alcohol use will result in a loss of muscle tissue throughout the body.

Cardiomyopathy itself develops in between 25% (Schuckit, 1989) and 36% of chronic alcoholics (Fernandez-Sola et al., 1994). But even this figure may not reflect the true scope of alcohol-induced heart disease. Rubin and Doria (1990) suggest that "the majority of alcoholics" (p. 279), whom they define as those individuals who obtain between 30 and 50% of their daily caloric requirement through alcohol, will ultimately develop "pre-clinical heart disease" (p. 279). But, because of the body's compensatory mechanisms, many chronic alcoholics will not show gross evidence of heart disease.

Although many individuals take comfort in the fact that they drink to excess only occasionally, even "binge" drinking is not without its dangers. Binge drinking may result in a condition known as the "holiday heart syndrome" (Lange, White, & Robinson, 1992). Episodic drinkers, such as those who go on binges only around the holidays, are prone to develop an irregular heartbeat known as *atrial fibrillation*. Atrial fibrillation may be fatal, if not diagnosed and treated before the body suffers permanent physical damage. Thus, even episodic alcohol use is not without some degree of risk.

Effects on the Central Nervous System (CNS)

Alcohol is toxic to the cells of the central nervous system and will prevent the CNS from working properly. One example of the toxic effects of alcohol is the way alcohol interferes with memory formation. Neuropsychological testing has revealed that alcohol may begin to affect memory trace formation after as little as one drink. Fortunately, one normally needs to consume more than five drinks in an hour's time, before alcohol is able to significantly impact on the process of memory formation (Browning, Hoffer, & Dunwiddie, 1993). One thus does not normally see significant memory problems in the casual or social drinker.

But memory disturbance is one of the most frequent symptoms experienced by the heavy drinker. The individual may find it impossible to remember events that took place while intoxicated, a condition commonly known as a *blackout*. These periods of alcohol-induced amnesia may last several days, although for the most part they involve shorter periods of time (Segal & Sisson, 1985; Willoughby, 1984).[1] During a blackout, the individual may *appear* conscious and be able to carry out many complex tasks. However, the drinker will not have any memory of having performed those tasks. In a sense, the alcohol-induced blackout is similar to another condition, known as *transient global amnesia* (Kaplan, Sadock, & Grebb, 1994; Rubino, 1992). Scientists do not understand the mechanism behind either the episode of transient global amnesia or the alcoholic blackout. However, it is generally believed that alcohol prevents the individual from being able to form (encode) memories during the period of acute intoxication (Browning, Hoffer, & Dunwiddie, 1993).

The alcoholic blackout is "an early and serious indicator of the development of alcoholism" (Rubino, 1992, p. 360). Although not every alcoholic will experience blackouts, the majority of chronic alcoholics admit they have had them. For example, of the 636 male alcoholics in their sample, Schuckit, Smith, Anthenelli, and Irwin (1993) found that 521 men, or 82% of their sample, admitted to having experienced alcohol-related blackouts at some point in their drinking history.

Chronic alcohol use may result in more serious forms of neurological dysfunction than blackouts. It was once thought that alcohol-induced central nervous system damage did not appear until after relatively late in the individual's drinking career, but recent research sug-

gests that this may not be true. Indeed, it is possible that alcohol-induced brain damage can be detected even before the development of alcohol-related liver damage (Berg, Franzen, & Wedding, 1994).

Volkow, Hitzemann, Wang, Fowler, Burr, Pascani, Dewey, and Wolf (1992) used the recently developed technique of *positron emission tomography*, or the PET scan, to measure the metabolism of different regions of the brain of both normal and alcoholic males. The alcoholic male subjects used in this study had at least a 15-year history of alcohol abuse and had only recently completed alcohol withdrawal. The men in both groups were free from major illness, and there was no evidence of major neurological impairment on standard neuropsychological tests for any of the men in the study.

The PET scan results demonstrated significantly reduced levels of brain metabolism in the left parietal and right frontal cortex regions of the alcoholic volunteers, areas of the brain known to be affected by chronic alcohol use. On the basis of their research, the authors concluded that the effects of alcohol on the brain last well beyond the stage of acute withdrawal. Furthermore, the authors found that the PET scan identified evidence of alcohol-induced neurological dysfunction at a stage before the brain damage was severe enough to be measured using standard neuropsychological tests. These findings point the way for further research and suggest that the PET scan might be used to identify individuals who are at risk for alcohol-induced brain damage if they continue to abuse alcohol.

Certainly, the problem of alcohol-induced brain damage is a serious one. Between 15 and 30% of all nursing home patients are there because of permanent alcohol-induced brain damage (Schuckit, 1989). And it has been estimated that alcohol-induced dementia is the "second most common adult dementia after Alzheimer's disease" (Nace & Isbell, 1991, p. 56). Tarter, Ott, and Mezzich (1991) conclude that 75% of chronic alcohol users demonstrate some evidence of CNS dysfunction on standard

---

[1]Individuals who suffer from *multiple personality disorder* (MPD) might attribute the loss of memory experienced by the main personality when another personality emerges to alcohol or drug use, rather than to the psychiatric disorder. This is because an alcohol- or drug-induced memory blackout is less threatening to the core personality. Because nonalcoholic blackouts may reflect serious psychiatric disease, the clinician must carefully determine whether the client has been using alcohol or chemicals and make the appropriate referrals.

neuropsychological tests. Chronic alcohol use has been called the single most preventable cause of dementia in this country (Beasley, 1987).

Not every case of alcohol-related brain damage will require that the individual be institutionalized. Grant (1987), however, questions whether such brain damage is permanent or whether some limited degree of recovery is possible for the chronic alcoholic. At this time, it seems that a limited degree of improvement in cognitive function is possible in alcoholics who remain abstinent from alcohol for extended periods of time (Grant, 1987; Løberg, 1986). But this does not mean that every alcoholic who abstains from alcohol will achieve a complete recovery. Following a protracted period of abstinence, only 20% of chronic alcoholics can return to their previous level of intellectual function (Nace & Isbell, 1991). Some limited degree of recovery is possible in perhaps 60% of the cases, and virtually no recovery of lost intellectual function is seen in 20% of the cases.

It is not known how chronic alcohol use contributes to the death of nerve cells, but one theory suggests that it causes vitamin deficiencies in the body, or *avitaminosis* (Willoughby, 1984). As we discussed earlier, avitaminosis is caused by either a lack of adequate vitamin intake or the body's inability to use available vitamins effectively (Beasley, 1987). This process slowly depletes the body's reserves of many vitamins, some of which are needed for the proper functioning of the nervous system.

One outcome of avitaminosis is the gradual deterioration of the peripheral nerves in the hands and feet, a condition known as *peripheral neuropathy*. This condition is found in 5% to 15% of the chronic alcoholics, but it is also found in some diabetics and, rarely, as a complication to other medical conditions. Some of the symptoms of peripheral neuropathy include feelings of weakness, pain, and a burning sensation in the afflicted region of the body (Lehman, Pilich, & Andrews, 1994). Peripheral neuropathy is thought to be caused by a deficiency of the B

family of vitamins in the body. The vitamin deficiency itself is caused by either the poor eating habits commonly found in chronic alcohol use, the vitamin malabsorption syndrome that is a common complication of alcoholism, or a combination of these two factors (Charness, Simon, & Greenberg, 1989; Nace, 1987; Beasley, 1987).

Another CNS complication of chronic alcohol abuse is *vitamin deficiency amblyopia*. This condition causes blurred vision, a loss of visual perception in the center of the visual field known as central scotomata, and, in extreme cases, atrophy of the optic nerve (Mirin, Weiss, & Greenfield, 1991). Alcohol-induced damage to the visual system may be permanent.

Wernicke–Korsakoff's Syndrome

Perhaps the most serious complication of chronic alcohol use is a form of brain damage known as *Wernicke's encephalopathy* (Charness, Simon, & Greenberg, 1989), which is caused by alcohol-related avitaminosis. Inadequate vitamin intake leads to a gradual depletion of the body's reserves of thiamine, one of the B family of vitamins. Chronic thiamine deficiency results in characteristic patterns of brain damage, with a 15% to 20% mortality rate (Ciraulo et al., 1994b).

The patient suffering from Wernicke's encephalopathy often appears confused, possibly to the point of being delirious and disoriented. He or she is also apathetic and unable to sustain physical or mental activities (Victor, 1993). Symptoms include a characteristic pattern of abnormal eye movements known as *nystagmus* and such signs of brain damage as gait disturbances and ataxia (Lehman, Pilich, & Andrews, 1994).

Of those who survive this condition without treatment, up to 80% will go on to develop a condition known as *Korsakoff's psychosis*, or *Korsakoff's syndrome* (also called the *alcohol amnesic disorder*) (Victor, 1993; Charness, Simon, & Greenberg, 1989). Even when Wernicke's encephalopathy is properly treated through aggressive thiamine replacement procedures, fully

25% of the patients who develop Wernicke's disease go on to develop Korsakoff's syndrome (Sagar, 1991).

Some suggest that Korsakoff's syndrome is the psychological manifestation of Wernicke's disease (Lehman, Pilich, & Andrews, 1994). One of the most prominent symptoms of Korsakoff's syndrome is a memory disturbance, making the patient unable to remember the past accurately. The afflicted individual also has difficulty learning new information. Surprisingly, the patient appears indifferent to his or her memory loss (Ciraulo et al., 1994b).

Over time, the face of Korsakoff's syndrome changes as the individual's central nervous system adapts to the alcohol-induced damage. In the early stages, the person is confused by the inability to remember the past clearly and often "fills in" these memory gaps by making up answers to questions. This process is called *confabulation*. Confabulation is not always found in cases of Korsakoff's syndrome, but when it is found it is most common in the earlier stages (Victor, 1993; Parsons & Nixon, 1993). As the individual adjusts to the memory loss, he or she is not as likely to use confabulation to cover up memory problems (Blansjaar & Zwinderman, 1992; Brandt & Butters, 1986).

In rare cases the individual loses virtually all memories after a certain period of their lives and is almost "frozen in time" (Sacks, 1970). For example, Sacks (1970) offered an example of a man examined in the 1960s, who was unable to recall anything that happened after the late 1940s. This example of confabulation, while extremely rare, can result from chronic alcoholism. More frequent are the less pronounced cases, in which significant portions of the memory are lost but the individual retains some ability to recall the past.

Unfortunately, the exact mechanism of Korsakoff's syndrome is unknown at this time. The characteristic nystagmus seems to reflect a vitamin malabsorption syndrome, which may respond to massive doses of thiamine, or Vitamin B-1. It is possible that victims of Korsakoff's syndrome possess a genetic susceptibility to the effects of the alcohol-induced thiamine deficiency (Parsons & Nixon, 1993). In other words, some individuals may be more likely to develop thiamine deficiency when they use alcohol on a chronic basis. Although this is an attractive theory, it remains just a theory.

Other researchers have theorized that the intellectual decline noted in Korsakoff's syndrome is caused by a mechanism other than the characteristic ocular nystagmus of this disorder. It has been suggested that the person with Korsakoff's syndrome is suffering from the neurotoxic effects of his or her long-term exposure to alcohol (Brandt & Butters, 1986). Brandt and Butters point out that alcohol is a known neurotoxin, and the chronic alcoholic may experience a gradual loss of the neurons necessary for intellectual performance.

Jensen and Pakkenberg (1993) offer a unique theory about the effects of alcohol on the physical structure of the brain. The authors examined the brains of 55 individuals who were active alcoholics before they died. They found that, rather than cause the *death* of neurons, chronic alcohol use caused them to become *disconnected* from their neighbors. The authors found evidence of degeneration *in specific regions of the nerve cells*, the axons and dendrites, rather than evidence that the entire nerve cells died as a result of chronic alcohol exposure. Jensen and Pakkenberg suggest that the loss of intellectual function seen in chronic alcohol use may reflect the disruption of established nerve pathways caused by the degeneration of the axons and dendrites of some brain cells.

These are only theories, which remain to be proved. It is known that, once Korsakoff's syndrome has developed, only a minority of its victims escape without lifelong neurological damage. It is estimated that even with the most aggressive vitamin replacement therapy, only 20% (Nace & Isbell, 1991) to 25% (Brandt & Butters, 1986) of its victims will return to their previous level of intellectual function. The remaining 75% to 80% will experience greater or lesser degrees of neurological damage. In addition, very little is known about the process of rehabilitation for the victim of Korsakoff's syndrome or whether rehabilitation is even possible (Parsons & Nixon, 1993; Blansjaar & Zwinderman, 1992).

Wernicke's disease (or Wernicke's encephalopathy) was once thought to be a separate disorder from Korsakoff's syndrome. Now, both Wernicke's encephalopathy and Korsakoff's syndrome are understood to be different stages of the same disease. This disorder is now frequently referred to as the *Wernicke–Korsakoff's syndrome.*

Alcohol's Effects on the Sleep Cycle

In Chapter 4, we discussed how alcohol interferes with the normal sleep pattern. Clinicians often encounter patients who complain of sleep problems without revealing their alcohol abuse. For example, the staff of one sleep disorders clinic found that 12% of the patients who were seen for insomnia were found to have a history of alcohol abuse or alcohol dependence (Frederickson, Richardson, Esther, & Lin, 1990).

Alcohol, like the other CNS depressants, may bring about a state of sleep, but it does not allow for a normal dream cycle. As a result of chronic alcohol use, the individual may experience a decrease in dream time, which takes place during the rapid eye movement (or REM) phase of sleep. When the individual stops drinking, he or she enters a period of abnormal sleep known as "REM rebound."

During REM rebound sleep, the person dreams more intensely and more vividly, often to the point of frequent nightmares. These "rebound" dreams may be so frightening that the individual returns to using alcohol just to get a decent night's sleep. REM rebound can last up to 6 months after the person has stopped drinking. In rare cases, the effects of alcohol can interfere with the normal sleep cycle for 1 to 2 years after detoxification (Satel, Kosten, Schuckit, & Fischman, 1993; Frederickson et al., 1990).

Effects on the Emotional State

As stated many times earlier, alcohol is a CNS depressant. Willoughby (1984) notes that the depressant effects from one drink may last as long as 96 hours. The effects of an alcohol binge of even 1 or 2 days may last for several weeks after abstinence (Segal & Sisson, 1985).

Chronic alcohol use often results in a range of symptoms similar to those seen in neurotic and psychotic conditions. These symptoms are thought to be secondary to the individual's malnutrition and the toxic effects of chronic alcohol use (Beasley, 1987). Symptoms may include depressive reactions (Schuckit, 1989), generalized anxiety disorders, and panic attacks (Beasley, 1987). This is not to say that all anxiety episodes or panic attacks in an alcoholic are alcohol-induced. But the relationship between alcohol use and the anxiety disorders in alcoholics is quite complex.

Toneatto, Sobell, Sobell, and Leo (1991) suggest that anxiety disorders are "more prevalent in alcohol abusers" (p. 91) than in the general population. However, of those patients who are diagnosed as having a generalized anxiety disorder, more than 20% are alcoholics whose "anxiety" was actually an early symptom of alcohol withdrawal (Beasley, 1987). Decker and Ries (1993) estimate that between 10 and 28% of patients who report anxiety symptoms also have an alcohol use disorder. Stockwell and Town (1989) agree, warning that "many" (p. 223) who seek help for anxiety attacks are experiencing withdrawal-related "rebound anxiety" episodes. They suggest that this rebound anxiety would clear up after alcohol use is discontinued.

The differentiation between "true" anxiety disorders and alcohol-related anxiety-like disorders is thus quite complex. Kushner, Sher, and Beitman (1990) conclude that alcohol withdrawal symptoms may be "indistinguishable" (p. 692) from the symptoms of panic attacks and generalized anxiety disorder. They also conclude that agoraphobia and social phobias usually predate alcohol use. Victims of these disorders often attempt self-medication using alcohol and then develop problems associated with alcohol abuse. Still, Kushner, Sher, and Beitman conclude that symptoms of simple panic attacks and generalized anxiety disorder are more likely to reflect the effects of alcohol withdrawal than a psychiatric disorder.

Another form of phobia that frequently coexists with alcoholism is *social phobia* (Marshall, 1994). Individuals with social phobias, who fear situations in which they are exposed to other people, are twice as likely as the general population to have alcohol-use problems.

Unfortunately, many patients who drink complain of anxietylike symptoms and are treated with benzodiazepines. As we discussed in the last chapter, alcohol tends to bind at some of the same receptor sites in the brain that the benzodiazepines utilize (Marshall, 1994). This characteristic allows the benzodiazepines to mask the symptoms of alcohol withdrawal, which makes them so effective in treating alcohol withdrawal. Thus, the chronic alcoholic can control his or her withdrawal symptoms by using benzodiazepines during the day without having the smell of alcohol on the breath. (One alcoholic explained that the effects of diazepam were similar to the effects of having had 3 to 4 quick drinks). However, benzodiazepines are themselves potentially addictive. Research suggests that 25% to 50% of alcoholics are also addicted to benzodiazepines (Miller & Gold, 1991b).

If the physician fails to obtain an adequate history or physical exam, or if the patient lies about his or her alcohol use, there is also a risk that the alcoholic might combine the use of antianxiety medication with alcohol. The potential for an overdose exists when two different classes of CNS depressants are combined. Also, as Beasley (1987) notes, the benzodiazepines may bring about a *paradoxical rage reaction* when combined with alcohol. In this condition, a drug that is normally a depressant brings about an unexpected period of rage in the individual, who may become self-destructive or harm oth-

ers. The individual may have no conscious memory of what he or she did during the paradoxical rage reaction (Lehman, Pilich, & Andrews, 1994). The concept of the paradoxical rage reaction, or *pathological intoxication* as it is also called, has been challenged, according to Lehman et al. (1994). The symptoms are very similar to those in certain forms of epilepsy, brain trauma, hysteria, and some psychotic disorders.

Because alcohol's effects are very similar to those of the barbiturates, it should not be surprising that alcohol has a fair antianxiety effect in the short run. Unfortunately, many of those who suffer from anxiety, whether alcohol induced or not, will further use alcohol as a way to deal with the rebound anxiety experienced when the alcohol wears off. The chronic use of alcohol causes a paradoxical stimulation of the autonomic nervous system, which the drinker interprets as additional anxiety. A cycle is then started where the chronic use of alcohol actually sets the stage for further anxiety, resulting in the need for more alcohol. Stockwell and Town (1989) conclude that "Many clients who drink heavily or abuse other anixolytic drugs will experience substantial or complete recovery from extreme anxiety following successful detoxification" (p. 223). Stockwell and Town recommend a drug-free period of *at least 2 weeks* in which to assess the need for pharmacological intervention for anxiety. Although the topic of the pharmacological treatment of anxiety lies outside of the scope of this text, the reader should keep in mind the need for a drug-free period of at least 2 weeks in which to assess whether further treatment is needed.

As noted before, alcohol has been implicated in depressive reactions for chronic alcoholics. Surprisingly, many people who are clinically depressed will use alcohol to "numb" their depressive feelings. This form of self-medication adds to the individual's feelings of depression over time. Many people are unaware of this fact, thus setting up a vicious cycle where the individual feels depressed, turns to alcohol to deal with the feelings of depression, then ends up feeling even more depressed because of the additional use of alcohol.

It has been suggested that during the first 2 weeks of treatment, most alcoholics will meet the diagnostic criteria for major depression (Wolf-Reeve, 1990). However, in the vast majority of these cases, the individual will be found to suffer from an alcohol-induced depression, which usually clears after 2 to 5 weeks of abstinence (Decker & Ries, 1993; Clark, Gibbons, Haviland, & Hendryx, 1993; Satel, Kosten, Schuckit, & Fischman, 1993). Experts in the field of alcoholism still do not agree as to the minimum length of time necessary to wait for an alcohol-induced depressive reaction to clear. Decker and Ries (1993) note that various experts in psychiatry suggest that waiting periods of between 4 weeks and "several months" (p. 704) after the person stops drinking are necessary for the alcohol-induced depression to resolve itself.

Primary depression, in which the depression predates the alcohol use, was once considered rare in chronic alcoholics. It was estimated that only from 2% to 3% (Powell, Read, Penick, Miller, & Bingham, 1987) to perhaps as many as 5% (Schuckit, 1989) of the cases of depression seen in alcoholics are actually primary depression. However, Blume (1994) issues a note of caution. She warns that because most research into the effects of alcohol has been conducted using male subjects, there is little understanding of the effects of alcohol on women. Blume (1994) suggests that in 60% to 65% of the cases where an alcoholic woman is depressed, the woman is experiencing a major depression that should be treated.

There is a strong relationship between depression and suicide (Hirschfield & Davidson, 1988). Because alcoholics experience depressive symptoms either as a consequence of their drinking or because of a coexisting major depression, they are a high-risk group for suicide. The lifetime risk for suicide among alcoholics, whether the depression is primary or secondary to drinking, is almost 15% (Hirschfield & Davidson, 1988; Schuckit, 1986). Brent, Kupfer, Bromet, and Dew (1988) suggest that suicide is most likely to occur late in the course of alcoholism, when the individual first begins to experience such medical complications as cirrhosis of the liver.

Murphy, Wetzel, Robins, and McEvoy (1992) attempted to isolate the factors that may predict suicide in the chronic male alcoholic. On the basis of their research, the authors identified the following seven factors that appear to suggest a possible suicide risk in the chronic male alcoholic.

1. The victim was drinking heavily in the days and weeks just prior to the act of suicide.
2. The victim had talked about the possibility of committing suicide prior to the act.
3. The victim had little social support.
4. The victim suffered from a major depressive disorder.
5. The victim was unemployed at the time of the suicide.
6. The victim was living alone.
7. The victim was suffering from a major medical problem at the time of the act of suicide.

Although the authors failed to find any single factor that seemed to predict a possible suicide, they did conclude that "as the number of risk factors increases, the likelihood of a suicidal outcome does likewise" (p. 461).

Roy (1993) also identified several factors that seemed to be associated with an increased risk of suicide for adult alcoholics. Like Murphy et al. (1992), Roy failed to find a single factor that seemed to predict the possibility of suicide for the adult alcoholic. However, he did suggest that the following factors were potential indicators for an increased risk of suicide for the adult alcoholic.

1. *Gender:* Men tend to commit suicide more often than women, and the ratio of male to female suicides for alcoholics may be about 4:1.
2. *Marital status:* Single, divorced, or widowed adults are significantly more likely to attempt suicide than are married adults.

3. *Co-existing depressive disorder*: Depression is associated with an increased risk of suicide.
4. *Adverse life events*: The individual who has suffered an adverse life event such as the loss of a loved one, a major illness, or legal problems, is at increased risk for suicide.
5. *Recent discharge from treatment for alcoholism*: The first 4 years following treatment are associated with a significantly higher risk for suicide, although the reason for this is not clear.
6. *A history of previous suicide attempts*: Approximately one-third of alcoholic suicide victims had attempted suicide at some point in the past.
7. *Biological factors*: Such factors as decreased levels of serotonin in the brain are thought to be associated with increased risk for violent behavior, including suicide.

Although mental health professionals know that it is impossible to identify every potential suicide victim, some factors are associated with an increased risk for suicide. Thus, substance abuse professionals should have a working knowledge of the risk factors that may alert health care providers to the possibility that a specific individual is at high risk for suicide in the near future.

Alcohol Withdrawal for the Chronic Alcoholic

Unlike the social drinker, who may recover from a night's heavy drinking with little more than a hangover, chronic alcoholic may experience an alcohol withdrawal syndrome when they attempt to stop drinking. This is an acute brain syndrome that develops within 24 to 96 hours after the last drink in 90% of the cases (Lehman, Pilich, & Andrews, 1994; Weiss & Mirin, 1988). However, there are cases of an alcohol withdrawal syndrome occurring up to 10 days after the last drink (Slaby, Lieb, & Tancredi, 1981).

As noted before, the severity of the alcohol withdrawal symptoms experienced depends on (1) the intensity with which the individual used alcohol, (2) the duration of time over which the individual drank, and (3) the individual's state of health. Approximately 6 to 8 hours after the last drink, the individual may begin to experience any or all of the following symptoms: agitation, anxiety, diarrhea, hyperactivity, exaggerated reflexes, insomnia, nausea, restlessness, sweating, tachycardia, vomiting, and vertigo (Lehman, Pilich, & Andrews, 1994; Lieveld & Aruna, 1991).

In mild withdrawal cases, the patient may experience only a few of these symptoms and may not progress on to the next level of withdrawal. However, in more advanced cases, the symptoms may become more intense over the first 6 to 24 hours following the last use of alcohol. The patient may also begin to experience *alcoholic hallucinosis*, or hallucinations (both visual and auditory) brought on by the withdrawal process. These hallucinations are different than those seen in disorders such as schizophrenia, and although they usually do not indicate the onset of a schizophrenic disorder, they still may be quite frightening to the individual.

In extreme cases of alcohol withdrawal, the symptoms will continue to become more intense over the next 24 to 48 hours, and by the third day following the last drink, the patient will start to experience fever, incontinence, and/or tremors in addition to the other symptoms. In approximately 16% of the cases, the withdrawal syndrome will also result in alcohol-related seizures (Lehman, Pilich, & Andrews, 1994; Nace & Isbell, 1991).

A further complication of chronic alcohol use in extreme cases is a condition known as the *delirium tremens* (DTs). It has been estimated that only about 5% (Lieveld & Aruna, 1991) to 10% (Weiss & Mirin, 1988) of alcoholics will develop the DTs, but they are certainly to be feared. The DTs involve a period of delirium, hallucinations, delusional beliefs that one is being followed, fever, tachycardia (Lieveld & Aruna, 1991), and, in some cases, a disruption of normal fluid levels in the brain (Trabert, Caspari, Bernhard, & Biro, 1992).

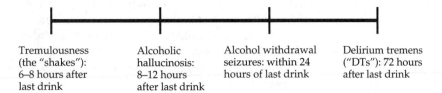

Tremulousness   Alcoholic   Alcohol withdrawal   Delirium tremens
(the "shakes"):   hallucinosis: seizures: within 24   ("DTs"): 72 hours
6–8 hours after   8–12 hours   hours of last drink   after last drink
last drink   after last drink

FIGURE 5.1 Continuum of alcohol withdrawal symptoms. (Chart suggested by Rubino, F.A. (1992). Neurologic complications of alcoholism. *Psychiatric Clinics of North America, 15,* 359–372.)

The latter condition results when the mechanism that regulates normal fluid levels in the drinker's body is disrupted. During withdrawal, the bodies of at least some alcoholics become hypersensitive to the antidiuretic hormone (ADH) that is normally secreted to slow the rate of fluid loss through the kidneys. Whereas traditional medical theory holds that the alcoholic in withdrawal is dehydrated, research has shown that some individuals retain too much fluid within their bodies. This excess fluid may contribute to the damage alcohol has caused the brain, possibly by bringing about a state of cerebral edema (Trabert et al., 1992). Trabert et al. found, surprisingly, that only patients going through the DTs were found to have higher levels of ADH in spite of low body fluid levels, suggesting that a body fluid dysregulation process might be involved in the development of the DTs.

Rubino (1992) suggests viewing the alcohol withdrawal syndrome on a continuum, as illustrated in Figure 5.1. The least severe symptoms of alcohol withdrawal would be the tremulousness ("shakes") experienced as the central nervous system tries to adjust to the sudden absence of the long-present alcohol. The syndrome of alcoholic hallucinosis might be viewed as a more severe manifestation of the alcohol withdrawal syndrome than the "shakes" but less severe than withdrawal seizures. Finally, the most severe symptom of alcohol withdrawal would be the delirium tremens.

As useful as this continuum might be as a guide for judging the severity of the alcohol withdrawal syndrome, Rubino (1992) warns

that "The syndrome may stop at any point spontaneously, however, or skip any part of the continuum for unknown reasons" (p. 360). Furthermore, there is some variation among individuals who go through the alcohol withdrawal syndrome. For example, as mentioned earlier, there are cases on record of a person going into an alcohol withdrawal syndrome up to 10 days after the last drink (Slaby, Lieb, & Tancredi, 1981). Thus, this continuum must be viewed as only a rough guide to the severity of the alcohol withdrawal syndrome.

In the past, death from exhaustion resulted in between 5 and 25% of the cases of the most severe form of the alcohol withdrawal syndrome, the DTs (Lehman, Pilich, & Andrews, 1994; Schuckit, 1989). However, improved medical care has decreased the mortality from the DTs to about 1% (Milzman & Soderstrom, 1994). The main causes of death from the DTs include sepsis, cardiac and/or respiratory arrest, or cardiac and/or circulatory collapse (Lieveld & Aruna, 1991). People going through the DTs are also a high-risk group for suicide as they struggle to come to terms with the emotional pain and terror associated with this condition (Hirschfield & Davidson, 1988; Weiss & Mirin, 1988).

Although a number of different chemicals may be of value in controlling the symptoms of alcohol withdrawal, the current medical practice is to use one of the benzodiazepines, usually chlordiazepoxide or diazepam. The judicious use of either drug has been found to control the tremor, hyperactivity, convulsions, and anxiety associated with alcohol withdrawal (Milhorn,

1992; Miller, Frances, & Holmes, 1989). However, not every alcoholic going through withdrawal will automatically require benzodiazepines (Saitz, Mayo-Smith, Roberts, Redmond, Bernard, & Calkins, 1994).

Indeed, evidence suggests that categorically administering benzodiazepines whenever a patient goes into alcohol withdrawal may actually contribute to excessive hospital stays, according to Saitz et al. (1994). Instead, Saitz et al. (1994) recommend a "symptom-triggered" (p. 519) approach, in which chlordiazepoxide is administered only if the patient's physical status suggests that he or she is going into acute alcohol withdrawal. The authors found that this method results in fewer doses of medication being administered and a shorter hospital stay than the standard approach, which places each patient on a rigid dosing schedule of benzodiazepines, followed by a gradual reduction in the daily dosage.

Thus, the approach suggested by Saitz, et al. (1994) is an alternative to the "standard" withdrawal schedule, which suggests that after the withdrawal symptoms have been controlled, the daily dosage level of benzodiazepines should be reduced by 10–20 percent each day until finally the drug is discontinued (Miller, Frances, & Holmes, 1989).

If a patient is going through alcohol hallucinosis, Milhorn (1992) advocates administering low doses of the antipsychotic medication haloperidol in conjunction with benzodiazepines to control the withdrawal symptoms. Usually 1 to 2 mg of haloperidol every 4 hours, in addition to the benzodiazepines, will control the symptoms of alcohol hallucinosis.

Other Complications from Chronic Alcohol Use

Either directly or indirectly, alcohol contributes to a large number of head injuries (Anderson, 1991; Sparadeo & Gill, 1989). It is not uncommon for an intoxicated individual to fall and strike his or her head on coffee tables, magazine stands, or whatever happens to be in the way. Unfortunately, the chronic use of alcohol also contributes to the development of three different bone disorders (Griffiths, Parantainen, & Olson, 1994): (1) *osteoporosis* (loss of bone mass); (2) *osteomalacia* (a condition in which new bone tissue fails to absorb minerals appropriately); and, (3) *secondary hyperparathyroidism* (a hormonal disorder that develops when alcohol interferes with the body's ability to regulate calcium levels in the blood; the calcium in the bones is reabsorbed into the blood, and the bones become weakened through calcium loss). These bone disorders in turn contribute to the higher-than-expected level of injury and death when alcoholics fall or are involved in automobile accidents.

Alcohol is also a factor in traumatic brain injury. Researchers believe that approximately 50% of the estimated 1 million people who suffer a traumatic head injury each year have alcohol in their blood at the time of the injury (Anderson, 1991; Sparadeo & Gill, 1989).

Schuckit (1989) warns that chronic alcohol use may reduce the individual's life expectancy by 15 years, with the leading causes of death being (in decreasing order of frequency) heart disease, cancer, accidents, and suicide. In the United States, between 90,000 (Paulos, 1994) and 200,000 (Kaplan, Sadock, & Grebb, 1994) people die each year from alcohol-related diseases or accidents, in addition to those who commit suicide as a result of their alcohol use.

Women who drink while pregnant run the risk of causing alcohol-induced birth defects, a condition known as the *fetal alcohol syndrome*. This condition will be discussed in detail in Chapter 20, "Chemicals and the Neonate."

Chronic alcoholism has also been associated with a premature aging syndrome, in which individuals appear much older than they actually are (Brandt & Butters, 1986). In many cases, the overall physical and intellectual condition of the individual corresponds to that of a person between 15 and 20 years older than the actual chronological age. One alcoholic, a man in his 50s, was told by his physician that he was in good health—for a man about to turn 70!

Admittedly, every alcoholic will not suffer from every consequence we have reviewed. Some alcoholics will never suffer from stomach problems, for example, but may suffer from advanced heart disease. However, Schuckit (1989) notes that in one research study, 93% of those alcoholics admitted to treatment had at least one important medical problem in addition to their alcoholism.

Research has demonstrated that, in most cases, the first alcohol-related problems are experienced during a person's late 20s or early 30s. Schuckit, Smith, Anthenelli, and Irwin (1993) outlined a progressive course for alcoholism, based on their study of 636 male alcoholics. The authors admitted that their subjects experienced wide differences in the specific problems caused by their drinking, but as a group the alcoholics began to experience severe alcohol-related problems in their late 20s. By their mid-30s, alcoholics are likely to recognize that they have a drinking problem and begin to experience more severe problems as a result of continued drinking. However, as the authors point out, there is a wide variation in this pattern, and some subgroups of alcoholics fail to follow this pattern.

The issue of whether an "addictive personality" exists will be discussed in a later chapter. Essentially, the only generalization that can be made about the risk factors for alcoholism at this time is that the children of alcoholics appear to be between 3 and 4 times as likely as children of nonalcoholics to become alcoholics as well (Schuckit, 1987; Ackerman, 1983; Vaillant, 1983). Researchers interpret this tendency as reflecting a genetic predisposition toward alcoholism that is thought to be passed from one generation to another, especially in males. Evidence suggests that this genetic predisposition also requires certain environmental factors to trigger the development of alcoholism. However, if the individual has *ever* had an addiction disorder, then this person should certainly be considered at risk for alcoholism.

Summary

In this chapter we explored the many facets of alcoholism. We reviewed the scope of alcohol abuse and addiction in the United States, noting that alcoholism accounts for approximately 85% of the drug addiction problem in the United States.

We discussed the different forms of tolerance and the ways that the chronic use of alcohol can affect the body, including the central nervous system, the cardiopulmonary system, the digestive system, and the skeletal bone structure. We examined the process of alcohol withdrawal and explored the relationship between chronic alcohol use and physical injuries. Finally, we saw how chronic alcohol use can lead to a decreased lifespan and premature aging.

Barbiturates and Similar Drugs

Throughout much of recorded history, mankind has struggled against the twin demons of anxiety and insomnia. Even today, in spite of all that is known about the unconscious sources of emotional distress, anxiety disorders remain the most common form of psychiatric disorder found in the United States (Cohn, Wilcox, Bowden, Fisher, & Rodos, 1992). The prevalence of anxiety is reflected in the fact that 11% of the adults in the United States use an antianxiety[1] agent at least once a year (Sussman, 1988). Furthermore, at least 35% of U.S. adults suffer each year from at least a transient sleep disturbance (Lacks & Morin, 1992).

For thousands of years, alcohol was the only agent available to reduce anxiety or help induce sleep. However, as we discussed in Chapter 5, the effectiveness of alcohol as an antianxiety agent (often called a "sedative") is quite limited. Thus, there has been a demand for effective antianxiety or hypnotic[2] medications for a very long time. In this chapter, we will review the various medications used to control anxiety or promote sleep before the benzodiazepines were introduced in the early 1960s. In Chapter 7, we will focus on the benzodiazepine family of drugs

and on medications introduced after the benzodiazepines first appeared.

Early Pharmacological Therapy for Anxiety Disorders and Insomnia

It was not until 1870 that *chloral hydrate* was introduced as a hypnotic. Researchers discovered that chloral hydrate was rapidly absorbed from the digestive tract, and an oral dose of 1 to 2 grams would cause the typical person to fall asleep in less than an hour. The effects usually lasted 8 to 11 hours, which appeared to make it ideal for use as a hypnotic.

However, physicians quickly discovered that chloral hydrate had several major drawbacks. Most important, researchers soon found that chloral hydrate was quite irritating to the stomach lining, and when used for extended periods of time, it caused extensive damage. Furthermore, patients who used chloral hydrate for extended periods often became physically dependent on the drug. Withdrawal from chloral hydrate was quite dangerous, and many patients developed life-threatening withdrawal seizures.

Since the time of its introduction, pharmacologists have discovered a great deal about chloral hydrate. After it is ingested, chloral hydrate is rapidly biotransformed into *trichloroethanol*. It is

---

[1]Occasionally, mental health professionals will use the term *anxiolytic* rather than *antianxiety*. For the purpose of this text, we will use the term *antianxiety*.

[2]A "hypnotic" is a medication designed to help the user fall asleep.

this metabolite of chloral hydrate that makes the drug an effective hypnotic. Surprisingly, in spite of its known dangers, chloral hydrate's relatively short biological half-life makes it of value in treating some elderly patients who suffer from insomnia. Thus, even with all the newer medications available to physicians, some patients still receive chloral hydrate to help them sleep.

Paraldehyde was first used as a hypnotic in 1882, although it was first isolated in 1829. As a hypnotic, paraldehyde is quite effective. It produces little respiratory or cardiac depression, making it a relatively safe drug to use with patients who have some forms of pulmonary or cardiac disease. However, it tends to produce a very noxious taste and odor. After the barbiturates were introduced, paraldehyde gradually fell into disfavor, although it does have a very limited role in medicine even today.

The *bromide salts* were first used for the treatment of insomnia in the mid-1800s. Although bromides are indeed capable of inducing sleep, it was soon discovered that they tend to accumulate in the chronic user's body, causing a drug-induced depression after as little as just a few days of continuous use. The bromide salts have been totally replaced by newer drugs, such as the barbiturates.

Despite superficial differences in their chemical structure, all these chemicals are central nervous system depressants, and they share many common characteristics. To a significant degree, the CNS depressants potentiate the effects of other CNS depressants. And, as a group, the CNS depressants all have a potential for abuse. In spite of these shortcomings, these agents were the treatment of choice for anxiety and insomnia until the barbiturate family of chemicals was introduced.

The History and Current Medical Uses of the Barbiturates

Chemists discovered the barbiturates in the late 19th century. Experimentation quickly revealed that, depending on the dose, the barbiturates act either as a sedative or as a hypnotic. The barbiturates were also safer and less noxious than either the bromides, chloral hydrate, or paraldehyde (Greenberg, 1993). In 1903, the first barbiturate—Veronal—was introduced for human use (Peluso & Peluso, 1988).

Since the time of their introduction, some 2,500 different barbiturates have been isolated in laboratories. Most of these barbiturates were never marketed, and they have remained only laboratory curiosities. Indeed, after the introduction of the benzodiazepines in the 1960s, many of the barbiturates previously in use gradually fell into disfavor. Only about a dozen forms of barbiturate are used in the United States today (Kaminski, 1992).

In spite of the introduction of new pharmaceuticals, however, there are still some areas of medicine—for certain surgical procedures and the control of epilepsy, for example—where barbiturates remain the pharmaceutical of choice. Surprisingly, in light of the fact that newer drugs have all but replaced the barbiturates in modern medicine, controversy still rages around the appropriate use of many of these chemicals.

In some states, one form of barbiturate is used to execute criminals by "lethal injection" (Truog, Berde, Mitchell, & Grier, 1992). Another, equally controversial, use of the barbiturates is in the sedation of terminally ill cancer patients who are in extreme pain (Truog et al., 1992). Truog et al. advocate using extremely large doses of select barbiturates to sedate patients in extreme pain from the terminal stages of cancer. Although extremely large doses of barbiturates may hasten the patient's death through respiratory depression, Truog et al. argue that by allowing some freedom from extreme pain, the barbiturates are an attractive adjunct to the treatment for at least some terminal cancer patients.

The Abuse Potential of Barbiturates

The barbiturates have considerable abuse potential. In the past, as much as one-half of the 300 tons of barbiturates manufactured in the United States each year was diverted to the black market

(P. R. Matuschka, 1985). It is not known what quantity of barbiturates are being diverted to the black market today. At one time, heroin addicts routinely used barbiturates to "boost" the effects of low-potency heroin by mixing the barbiturate with the heroin (Kaminski, 1992). However, in this era of high-potency heroin (see Chapter 11), it is not known whether heroin addicts still add barbiturates to their heroin to increase the drug's effects.

There are a number of older people, usually over the age of 40, who became addicted to pre-scribed barbiturates when they were younger. For people of this generation, the barbiturates were the most effective treatment for anxiety and insomnia, and many users became—and re-main—addicted (Kaplan, Sadock, & Grebb, 1994). Thus, in spite of their limited role in modern medicine, the barbiturates continue to represent a significant part of the drug abuse problem.

Over the past 30 years, the benzodiazepines have replaced the barbiturates as the primary family of antianxiety drugs (Gillin, 1991). As the benzodiazepines became more popular, the use and abuse of the barbiturates declined for a num-ber of years. However, evidence now indicates that, with the increasing restrictions on physi-cians for prescribing benzodiazepines in many states, the number of prescriptions for barbitu-rates may even be on the increase (American Society of Hospital Pharmacists, 1994).

The Pharmacology of the Barbiturates

Even now, more than a century after their intro-duction, the exact mechanism by which the barbi-turates work is still not entirely known (American Society of Hospital Pharmacists, 1994). The barbi-turates are all remarkably similar; the only major difference between the various members of the barbiturate family of drugs is the length of time it takes the individual's body to absorb, metabolize (or break down), and then excrete the specific bar-biturate.

This difference arises because the different forms of barbiturates on the market differ in terms of lipid solubility and their degree of pro-tein binding. Those barbiturates that are easily soluble in lipids are rapidly distributed to all blood-rich tissues, including the brain. Thus, pentobarbital, which is very lipid soluble, may begin to have an effect in 10 to 15 minutes. In contrast, phenobarbital is poorly lipid soluble and does not begin to have an effect until 60 minutes or more after ingestion.

Although neuropharmacologists understand why different forms of barbiturates have a dif-ferent duration of effect and speed of action, they still do not know how the barbiturates work. However, the barbiturates can be grouped into four different classes,[3] using the *duration of action* as the criterion for classification.

1. The effects of the *ultrashort-acting* barbitu-rates begin in a matter of seconds and last for less than 1 hour. Examples of ultrashort barbiturates are Pentothal and Brevital. The ultrashort barbi-turates are highly lipid soluble and thus reach the brain in just a few seconds. These medica-tions are often utilized in surgical procedures where a short duration of action is desirable (Snyder, 1986).

2. The effects of the *short-acting* barbiturates begin in a matter of minutes and last for 4 to 8 hours. Nembutal is one example of short-acting barbiturates. (Kaplan, Sadock, & Grebb, 1994). In terms of lipid solubility, the short-acting barbi-turates fall between the ultrashort-acting barbi-turates and the intermediate-acting barbiturates.

3. The effects of the *intermediate-acting* barbi-turates begin within an hour, and last 6 to 8 hours. Included in this group are such drugs as Amytal (Schuckit, 1989).

4. The effects of the *long-acting* barbiturates begin as long as an hour after ingestion and last for 10 to 12 hours (Snyder, 1986). Phenobarbital is perhaps the most common drug in this class.

[3]Other researchers may use classification systems other than the one presented here. For example, some researchers use the chemical structure of the different forms of barbiturate as the defining criterion for classification. In this text, we will follow the classification system suggested by Snyder (1986).

TABLE 6.1 Drug Equivalency Table

Generic name	Dose equivalent to 600 mg of secobarbital
Barbiturates	
Amobarbital	600 mg
Butabarbital	600 mg
Butabital	600 mg
Pentobarbital	600 mg
Secobarbital	600 mg
Phenobarbital	180 mg
Barbituratelike drugs	
Meprobamate	2,400 mg
Glutethimide	1,500 mg
Methaqualone	1,800 mg

Source: Based on Miller, N. S., & Gold, M. S. (1989). Identification and treatment of benzodiazepine abuse. *American Family Physician, 40* (4), 175–183.

Overall, the chemical structure of the various forms of barbiturates are quite similar and tend to have similar effects on the user. Table 6.1 provides an overview of the relative potency of some of the commonly used barbiturates and barbituratelike drugs, using a standard dose of 600 mg of secobarbital as the reference dose.

In reviewing Table 6.1, it is obvious that there are few significant differences in relative potency among various barbiturates. Indeed, as a group, the barbiturates' effects are remarkably similar. However, there are a number of interesting differences between the various forms. First, as a general rule, the short-term barbiturates are metabolized by the liver before being excreted. In contrast, a significant proportion of the long-term barbiturates are eliminated from the body essentially unchanged. Phenobarbital has a half-life of 2 to 6 days, and between 25 and 50% of the drug is excreted by the kidneys virtually unchanged. However, the barbiturate methohexital has a half-life of only 3 to 6 hours, and virtually all of it is metabolized by the liver before it is excreted from the body (American Society of

Hospital Pharmacists, 1994). Another difference among the various barbiturates is the degree to which the drug molecules become protein-bound. As a general rule, the longer the drug's half-life, the stronger its degree of protein binding.

When used on outpatients, the barbiturates are typically administered orally. On occasion, especially when used as a surgical anesthetic, ultrashort-acting barbiturates may be administered intravenously. On rare occasions, the barbiturates are administered rectally through suppositories.

When taken orally, the barbiturate molecule is rapidly and completely absorbed from the small intestine (Julien, 1992; Winchester, 1990). Once it reaches the blood, the barbiturate is distributed throughout the body, but concentration will be highest in the liver and the brain (American Society of Hospital Pharmacists, 1994). The barbiturates are all lipid soluble, but they vary in their ability to form bonds with blood lipids. As a general rule, the more lipid soluble a barbiturate is, the more highly protein-bound that chemical will also be (Winchester, 1990).

The behavioral effects of the barbiturates are very similar to those of alcohol (*Harvard Medical School Mental Health Letter*, 1988). Thus, like alcohol, once the barbiturate reaches the bloodstream, it is distributed throughout the body and will affect all body tissues to some degree. At normal dosage levels, the barbiturates depress not only the activity of the brain but also, to a lesser degree, the activity of the muscle tissues, the heart, and the respiratory system (P. R. Matuschka, 1985). However, it is within the central nervous system that the barbiturates have their strongest effect (Rall, 1990).

Within the brain, the barbiturates are thought to have the greatest impact on the cortex and the reticular activating system (or RAS, which is responsible for awareness) as well as on the medulla oblongata (which controls respiration) (American Society of Hospital Pharmacists, 1994; P. R. Matuschka, 1985). At low dosage levels, the barbiturates reduce the function of the nerve cells in these regions of the brain, bringing on a state of relaxation; at slightly higher doses, they produce a drug-induced sleep. At extremely high dosage levels, the barbiturates interfere with the normal function of the neurons of the central nervous system to such a degree that death is possible.

The therapeutic dose of the typical barbiturate is relatively close to the level necessary to bring about an overdose. Indeed, some of the barbiturates have a therapeutic dosage to lethal dosage level ratio of only 1:3, suggesting that they have little safety margin. This low safety margin, and the significantly higher safety margin offered by the benzodiazepines, is one reason the barbiturates have largely been replaced by the benzodiazepines.

Effects of the Barbiturates at Normal Dosage Levels

At low doses for the occasional user, the barbiturates reduce feelings of anxiety, and possibly bring on a sense of euphoria. The individual may also report a feeling of sedation or fatigue, possibly to the point of drowsiness. At low dosage levels, the barbiturates may also bring about a decrease in motor activity. Thus, the individual's reaction time will increase, and he or she may have trouble coordinating muscle movements.

The physical sensations brought about by low doses of barbiturates are very similar to those of alcohol, and the subjective effects are "practically indistinguishable from alcohol's" (Peluso & Peluso, 1988, p. 54; *Harvard Medical School Mental Health Letter*, 1988). This is to be expected, because both alcohol and the barbiturates affect the cortex of the brain through a similar pharmacological mechanism. Thus, on occasion, the disinhibition effects of the barbiturates, like alcohol's, may cause a state of "paradoxical" excitement.

Complications from Barbiturate Use at Normal Dosage Levels

For almost 60 years, the barbiturates were the treatment of choice for insomnia. Given the fact that the barbiturates were so extensively prescribed, it is surprising to learn that research has shown that tolerance to the hypnotic effects of barbiturates develops rapidly. Indeed, research suggests that barbiturates are not effective as hypnotics after just a few days of regular use (Ray & Ksir, 1993; Rall, 1990).

In spite of barbiturates' traditional use as a treatment for insomnia, the sleep achieved is not a normal state of sleep. Scientists believe that people need to experience REM sleep for their emotional well-being. Normally, about 25% of a young adult's total sleep time is spent in REM sleep (Kaplan, Sadock, & Grebb, 1994). But the barbiturates suppress a portion of the REM stage (Peluso & Peluso, 1988), reducing the total amount of time spent in REM sleep (Rall, 1990). Thus, by disrupting the normal sleep pattern, barbiturate-induced sleep may adversely affect the individual's emotional and physical health.

When the barbiturates are used as a sleep aid for a long period of time and then discontinued, the person enters a state of REM rebound. As previously mentioned, in this state, a person will dream more intensely and more vividly for a period of time as the body tries to catch up on lost REM sleep time. These dreams have been described as nightmares strong enough to tempt the individual to return to the use of drugs to get a good night's sleep again. This rebound effect may last for 1 to 3 weeks, although in rare cases it has been known to last for up to 2 months (Tyrer, 1993).

Another drawback of the barbiturates is the possibility of experiencing a drug "hangover" (Shannon, Wilson, & Stang, 1992). The physical experience of the barbiturate hangover is similar to that of an alcohol hangover; the individual simply feels that he or she is "unable to get going" the next day. This feeling derives from the extended period of time often needed for the body to completely metabolize and excrete the drug.

It generally takes 5 half-life periods to completely eliminate a single dose of a chemical from the blood. Because many of the barbiturates have extended biological half-lives, some small amounts of a barbiturate may remain in the person's bloodstream for hours or days. Thus, in some cases, the effects of the barbiturates on judgment, motor skills, and behavior might last for several days after a single dose of the drug (Kaminski, 1992).

If a person continually adds to this reservoir of unmetabolized drug by ingesting additional doses of the barbiturate, there is a greater chance that he or she will experience a drug hangover. However, whether the result of a single dose or repeated doses, the drug "hangover" is caused by traces of unmetabolized barbiturates remaining in the bloodstream when the medication is discontinued.

The elderly, or those with impaired liver function, are especially likely to have difficulty with the barbiturates because the liver's ability to metabolize many drugs declines with age. Sheridan, Patterson, and Gustafson (1982) advise starting older individuals at half the usual adult dosage of the barbiturate, gradually increasing the dose until the desired effect is achieved.

Children suffering from attention deficit-hyperactivity disorder (ADHD) (what was once called "hyperactivity") who receive phenobarbital are likely to experience a resurgence of their ADHD symptoms. This effect reflects the barbiturates' ability to suppress the action of the reticular activating system (RAS) in the brain. The current belief is that the RAS of children with ADHD is underactive, so any medication that further reduces its effectiveness will contribute to the development of ADHD symptoms.

Hypersensitivity reactions have also been reported with the barbiturates, most commonly in (but not limited to) individuals with asthma. Other complications occasionally seen at normal dosage levels include nausea, vomiting, diarrhea, and constipation. Some patients develop skin rashes while receiving barbiturates, although the reason for this is not clear. Finally, patients who are prescribed barbiturates often develop an extreme sensitivity to sunlight known as *photosensitivity*. Thus, patients who receive barbiturates must take special precautions to avoid sunburn, even after limited exposure to the sun's rays.

Because of these problems and because medications are now available that do not share the dangers associated with barbiturate use, barbiturates are no longer considered appropriate in the treatment of anxiety or insomnia (Tyrer, 1993).

Drug Interactions with Other Medications

Research has found that the barbiturates are capable of interacting with numerous other chemicals, increasing or decreasing the amount of these drugs in the blood through various mechanisms. The mixture of alcohol with barbiturates is especially dangerous and may result in death (Barnhill, Ciraulo, & Ciraulo, 1989). Each drug potentiates the effects of the other by interfering with the metabolism of the other chemical in the liver. This allows the toxic effects of both drugs to continue with greater intensity than one would expect from either chemical alone. In extreme cases, death can result.

The barbiturates should not be mixed with drugs classified as CNS depressants, except under a physician's supervision. The barbiturates will often potentiate the depressant effect of another CNS depressant, with possibly serious or even fatal consequences. Examples of CNS depressants include the benzodiazepines, sleep medications, some forms of pain medication, many antidepressants, alcohol, and the phenothiazines. Antihistamines are another class of CNS depressants that might cause a potentiation effect in combination with a barbiturate (Rall, 1990). Because many antihistamines are available without a prescription, there is a very real danger of unintentional potentiation effects.

Patients using barbiturates should also avoid

the antibiotic doxycycline, except under a physician's supervision. The barbiturates reduce the effectiveness of this antibiotic, which may have serious consequences for the patient (Meyers, 1992). If a patient is using barbiturates and trycyclic antidepressants concurrently, the barbiturate will cause the blood plasma levels of the tricyclic antidepressant to drop by as much as 60% (Barnhill, Ciraulo, & Ciraulo, 1989). The barbiturates increase the speed with which the antidepressants are metabolized by activating the liver's microsomal enzymes. This is the same process through which the barbiturates speed up the metabolism of many oral contraceptives, corticosteroids, and the antibiotic Flagyl (metronidazole) (Kaminski, 1992), thus reducing their effectiveness. Women who are taking both oral contraceptives and barbiturates should be aware of the potential for barbiturates to reduce the effectiveness of oral contraceptives.

It is obvious from this list of potential interactions that the barbiturates are a powerful family of drugs. A physician should always be consulted before combining different medications.

Complications from Barbiturate Use at Above-Normal Dosage Levels

When used at above-normal dosage levels, barbiturates may cause a state of intoxication similar to alcohol intoxication. Patients intoxicated by barbiturates demonstrate such behaviors as slurred speech and unsteady gait but without the characteristic smell of alcohol (Jenike, 1991). These individuals will not test positive for alcohol on blood or urine toxicology tests (unless they also have alcohol in their systems). Specific blood or urine toxicology screens must be carried out to detect barbiturate intoxication.

If the dosage level is increased beyond that normally necessary to induce sleep, or if the individual has used more than one CNS depressant, several things may occur. As the increasing blood levels of barbiturate interfere with the nor-

mal function of the medulla oblongata (the part of the brain that maintains respiration), there is a reduction in respiratory response. There is also a progressive loss of reflex activity, which may then progress to coma and ultimately, death (Jenike, 1991).

Before the introduction of the benzodiazepines, the barbiturates accounted for as much as 75% of all drug-related deaths in the United States (Peluso & Peluso, 1988). Even now, intentional or unintentional barbiturate overdose is one of the most common causes of drug-related deaths. For example, the estimated death rate in England and Wales for barbiturates is calculated at 69 to 176 deaths for each 1 million prescriptions written (Serfaty & Masterson, 1993). In their study of successful suicides in the San Diego, California, area, Mendelson and Rich (1993) found that approximately 10% of those individuals who committed suicide via a drug overdose used barbiturates, either exclusively or in combination with other chemicals.

Fortunately, the barbiturates do not directly cause any damage to the central nervous system. If an overdose victim reaches medical support before he or she develops shock or hypoxia, a complete recovery is likely (Sagar, 1991). For this reason, *any suspected barbiturate overdose should be treated by a physician immediately.*

Barbiturate Tolerance and Addiction

The primary use for barbiturates today is quite limited, as newer, more effective drugs have replaced this family of pharmaceutical agents. But barbiturates continue to have limited medical applications, including the control of epilepsy and the treatment of some forms of severe head injury (Julien, 1992).

Tolerance to the Barbiturates

Tolerance to many of the effects of the barbiturates will develop quite rapidly with regular use. When the barbiturates are used for medical reasons, the development of tolerance may not be a significant problem. For example, a patient who is taking phenobarbital for the control of seizures will eventually become somewhat tolerant to the sedative effect of the medication, although he or she will not become tolerant to its anticonvulsant effect.

Unfortunately, tolerance also may develop to the barbiturate's *desired* effect. For example, when used for extended periods of time to control anxiety or help the individual sleep, the barbiturates may become less and less effective. One characteristic of the barbiturates is that tolerance to the drug's effects does not develop at a uniform rate. One patient may go for years without adjusting the daily dosage level, whereas another patient may need to increase the dosage in a matter of months.

Barbiturate users have been known to try to overcome their tolerance to the drug by increasing their dosage of the drug without consulting their physician. These attempts at self-medication have resulted in a large number of unintentional barbiturate overdoses, some of which have been fatal. When the barbiturates are being abused for an extended period of time and the individual begins to become tolerant to the effects of the drug, he or she may be tempted to increase the dose to maintain the drug-induced euphoria. However, although tolerance to the euphoric effects of the barbiturates may develop, there is no concomitant increase in the lethal dose (Jenike, 1991). Thus, as the person abusing the barbiturates increases the dosage levels to achieve the same effect, he or she will come closer and closer to the lethal dose.

Cross-tolerance is also possible between barbiturates and other similar chemical agents. Cross-tolerance occurs when a person who has become tolerant to certain chemicals becomes tolerant to the effects of other similar drugs, even if the person has never used them. Cross-tolerance between alcohol and the barbiturates is common, as is some degree of cross-tolerance between the barbiturates and the opiates and between the barbiturates and the hallucinogen PCP (Kaplan, Sadock, & Grebb, 1994).

Addiction to the Barbiturates

The United States experienced a wave of barbiturate abuse and addiction in the 1950s. Thus, physicians have long been aware that *once the person is addicted, withdrawal from barbiturates is potentially life-threatening and should be attempted only under the supervision of a physician* (Jenike, 1991). The barbiturates should never be abruptly withdrawn, as to do so might bring about an organic brain syndrome that can include such symptoms as confusion, seizures, possible brain damage, and even death. According to Jenike (1991), approximately 80% of barbiturate addicts who abruptly discontinue the drug will experience withdrawal seizures.

Unfortunately, there is no set formula to estimate the danger period for barbiturate withdrawal problems. Indeed, the exact period during withdrawal when the barbiturate addict is most "at risk" for problems such as seizures depends on the specific barbiturate being abused (Jenike, 1991). As a general rule, the longer-lasting forms of barbiturates tend to have longer withdrawal periods. For short-acting to intermediate-acting barbiturates, one can normally expect withdrawal seizures to begin after 2 or 3 days, and they rarely occur after 12 days. For the longer-acting barbiturates, withdrawal seizures may not occur until as late as 7 days after the last dose of the drug (Tyrer, 1993).

A number of symptoms accompany the withdrawal process. Virtually every barbiturate-dependent patient will experience a feeling of apprehension, which will last for the first 3 to 14 days of withdrawal (Shader, Greenblatt, & Ciraulo, 1994). Other symptoms include muscle weakness, tremors, anorexia, muscle twitches, and possibly delirium. All these symptoms will pass after 3 to 14 days, depending on the individual. Although physicians can minimize these withdrawal symptoms through other medications, there is no such thing as a symptom-free withdrawal.

Barbituratelike Drugs

Because of the many adverse side effects of the barbiturates, pharmaceutical companies have long searched for substitutes that are as effective but safe to use. During the 1950s, a number of new drugs were introduced to treat anxiety and insomnia, including Miltown (meprobamate), Quaalude and Sopor (both brand names of methaqualone), Doriden (glutethimide), Placidyl (ethchlorvynol), and Noludar (methyprylon). Table 6.2 lists the equivalent dosage levels for some of these barbituratelike drugs.

Although these drugs were thought to be non-addicting when first introduced, research has shown that barbituratelike drugs have an abuse potential very similar to that of the barbiturates. This should not be surprising, because many have a chemical structure similar to that of the barbiturates (Julien, 1992). For example, like the barbiturates, glutethimide and methyprylon are metabolized mainly in the liver.

Both Placidyl (ethchlorvynol) and Doriden (glutethimide) are considered especially danger-ous and should not be used for a number of reasons (Schuckit, 1989). For example, the pro-longed use of ethchlorvynol may result in a drug-induced loss of vision known as *amblyopia*. Fortunately, this drug-induced condition is not permanent, and it will gradually clear when

TABLE 6.2 Dosage Equivalency Table for Barbituratelike Drugs

Generic name	Dose equivalent to 30 mg of phenobarbital
Chloral hydrate	500 mg
Ethchlorvynol	350 mg
Meprobamate	400 mg
Methyprylon	300 mg
Glutethimide	250 mg

the drug is discontinued (Michelson, Carroll, McLane, & Robin, 1988). Since its introduction, glutethimide has become "notorious for its high mortality associated with overdose" (Sagar, 1991, p. 304). The high mortality is a result of the drug's narrow therapeutic range. The lethal dose of glutethimide is only 10 grams, a dose only slightly above the normal dosage level (Sagar, 1991).

Meprobamate was a popular sedative in the 1950s, when it was sold under at least 32 different brand names, including Miltown or Equanil (Lingeman, 1974). However, it is considered "ob-solete" by current standards (Rosenthal, 1992). Surprisingly, this medication is still quite popu-lar with older patients, and older physicians often continue to prescribe it. Meprobamate is quite addictive, although its addictive potential was not clearly recognized when it was first introduced. Some older patients have been using this medication for 30 years or more, and quite a few have been addicted to it for much of this period (Rosenthal, 1992).

Methaqualone achieved significant popular-ity in the drug world, especially in the late 1960s and early 1970s. It was originally introduced as a nonaddicting substitute for the barbiturates and, depending on the dosage level, was sold both as a sedative and as a hypnotic (Lingeman, 1974). Taken orally, methaqualone is rapidly ab-sorbed from the gastrointestinal tract, and its effects are felt in 15 to 20 minutes. Methaqualone was purported to have aphrodisiac properties (which was never proved) and was said to pro-vide a mild sense of euphoria (Mirin, Weiss, & Greenfield, 1991). People who used methaqua-lone reported feelings of euphoria, well-being, and behavioral disinhibition.

Shortly after methaqualone was introduced, reports of its abuse surfaced. The usual dose for methaqualone as a sedative was 75 mg, and the hypnotic dose was between 150 and 300 mg. Because tolerance to methaqualone developed rapidly, many abusers gradually increased their daily dosage levels in an attempt to re-create the initial effect. Some individuals who abused methaqualone were known to use as much as

2,000 mg in a single day (Mirin, Weiss, & Green-field, 1991), a very dangerous dosage level. The lethal dose of methaqualone is estimated as approximately 8,000 mg for a typical 150-pound user (Lingeman, 1974). As with the barbiturates, although tolerance to the drug's effects develops quickly, the lethal dosage of methaqualone remains the same. Death from methaqualone overdose was common, especially when the drug was taken with alcohol. The typical cause of death was heart failure (Lingeman, 1974).

In the United States, methaqualone was withdrawn from the market in the mid-1980s, although it is still manufactured by pharmaceutical companies in other countries. It is often smuggled into the United States or manufactured in illicit laboratories and sold on the street. Thus, the substance abuse counselor must have a working knowledge of methaqualone and its effects.

Summary

For thousands of years, alcohol was the only chemical that was even marginally effective as an antianxiety or hypnotic agent. Although a number of chemicals with hypnotic action were introduced in the mid-1800s, each was of limited value in the fight against anxiety or insomnia. Then, in the early 1900s, the barbiturates were introduced and rapidly became popular. The barbiturates have a mechanism of action very similar to that of alcohol and were found to have both an antianxiety and a hypnotic effect.

However, like alcohol, the barbiturates were also found to have a significant potential for addiction. This resulted in a search for non-addictive medications that could replace the barbiturates. In the post–World War II era, a number of synthetic drugs with chemical structures very similar to the barbiturates were introduced, often with the claim that these drugs were nonaddicting. However, these drugs were ultimately found to have an addiction potential similar to that of the barbiturates. Since the introduction of the benzodiazepines (to be discussed in the next chapter), the barbiturates and similar drugs have fallen into disfavor. However, there is evidence to suggest that they might be making a comeback.

Benzodiazepines and Beyond

In 1960, the first of a new class of antianxiety drugs, chlordiazepoxide, was introduced in the United States. Chlordiazepoxide is a member of a family of chemicals known as the *benzodiazepines*. The benzodiazepines were found to be effective in the treatment of a wide range of disorders to control such symptoms as anxiety, insomnia, muscle strains, and seizures. This is one reason the benzodiazepines have become *the* most frequently prescribed psychotropic medication in the United States (Gonzales, Stern, Emmerich, & Rauch, 1992). Currently, more than 20 different benzodiazepines are in use in different countries around the world, 14 of which are in use in the United States (Bohn, 1993).

The benzodiazepines were initially viewed as nonaddicting substitutes for the barbiturates or barbituratelike drugs. However, in the 35 years since their introduction, serious questions have been raised about the abuse potential of the benzodiazepines. In this chapter, we will look at the history of the benzodiazepines, their medical applications, and their role in the drug abuse problem in the United States.

Medical Uses of the Benzodiazepines

The benzodiazepines were initially introduced as antianxiety agents, and this remains a major use for this group of medications. But several benzodiazepines have been found to be of value in treating other medical problems as well, such as seizure disorders and muscle strains (Shader & Greenblatt, 1993). Because the effects of the benzodiazepines are more selective than those of the barbiturates, they are able to reduce anxiety without causing the same degree of sedation and fatigue barbiturates do. This is the main reason the benzodiazepines have become the drug of choice for treating anxiety, specifically Valium (diazepam), Librium (chlordiazepoxide), Tranxene (clorazepate), Xanax (alprazolam), and Ativan (lorazepam).

At least one benzodiazepine, Valium (diazepam), is quite useful in treating many forms of human suffering. It is an antianxiety medication that can be used to control seizures and to help damaged muscles recover (American Psychiatric Association, 1990). Another benzodiazepine, Clonopin[1] (clonazepam), is also effective in the long-term control of seizures, and as an antianxiety agent (Shader & Greenblatt, 1993). Other benzodiazepines are used as a short-term treatment for insomnia: Restoril (temazepam), Halcion (triazolam), Dalmane (flurazepam), and the recently introduced Doral (quazepam) (Gillin, 1991; Hussar, 1990).

Two different benzodiazepines, Xanax (alprazolam) and Deracyn (adinazolam), are reportedly of value in the treatment of depression.

[1]This is sometimes spelled "Klonopin."

Alprazolam has been used to treat the anxiety that often accompanies depression, thus indirectly helping the patient feel better. However, Deracyn (adinazolam) appears to have a direct antidepressant effect, a feature that makes it unique among the benzodiazepines. Researchers believe that Deracyn (adinazolam) works by increasing the sensitivity of certain neurons within the brain to serotonin (Cardoni, 1990). Serotonin deficit or insensitivity is thought to be the cause of at least some forms of depression. Thus, by increasing the neurons' sensitivity to serotonin, Deracyn (adinazolam) seems to have a direct antidepressant effect that is lacking in most benzodiazepines.

The possibility of suicide through a drug overdose is a very real concern for the physician, especially when the patient is depressed. Since the time of their introduction, the benzodiazepines have had a reputation as being "safe" drugs to use with patients who are potentially suicidal because the benzodiazepines have a high therapeutic index (discussed in Chapter 3). Unlike the low safety factor of barbiturates (see Chapter 6), the benzodiazepines have a therapeutic index of 1:200 (Kaplan & Sadock, 1990).

Animal research suggests, for example, that the LD_{50} for diazepam is around 720 mg per kilogram of body weight for mice and 1,240 mg/kg for rats (Medical Economics Company, 1993). Although the LD_{50} for humans is not known, these figures suggest that an exceptionally large dose of diazepam can be tolerated with minimal risk of death from overdose.[2]

However, this is not to say that the benzodiazepines are *totally* safe. In the last decade, approximately 5.9 deaths were recorded for each million prescriptions written for a benzodiazepine in England and Wales (Serfaty & Masterton, 1993). Although this is a significant improvement over the death rate per million prescriptions of barbiturates (discussed in the last chapter), these statistics illustrate that the benzodiazepines still retain a potential for harm. Furthermore, the safety margin for the benzo-

diazepines is drastically reduced, when these medications are mixed with other CNS depressants, such as alcohol.

To treat an overdose, physicians can use a medication that blocks the receptor site within the brain utilized by benzodiazepines. This medication, Mazicon (flumazenil), occupies the benzodiazepine receptor site without causing any sedation, thus protecting the individual from the effects of a benzodiazepine overdose. However, physicians must administer flumazenil in a hospital setting. Because multiple agents are often ingested in suicide attempts and because flumazenil is effective in blocking only the effects of benzodiazepines, *any suspected drug overdose should be treated by a physician.*

Pharmacology of the Benzodiazepines

The benzodiazepines are all very similar in their effects, differing mainly in their duration of action (*Harvard Medical School Mental Health Letter,* 1988). Table 7.1 reviews the relative potency and biological half-lives of some of the benzodiazepines currently in use in the United States.

Like many pharmaceuticals, the benzodiazepines can be classified on the basis of their pharmacological characteristics. Tyrer (1993), for example, adopted a classification system based not on the duration of the effects of the benzodiazepines but on their biological half-lives. Tyrer separated the benzodiazepines into four groups: those with (1) *very short half-lives* (4 hours or less), (2) *short half-lives* (4 to 12 hours), (3) *intermediate half-lives* (12 to 20 hours), and (4) *long half-lives* (20 or more hours).

The various benzodiazepines currently in use range from moderately to highly lipid soluble (Ayd, 1994). The more lipid soluble a benzodiazepine is, the faster it is absorbed through the small intestine after being taken by mouth (Roberts & Tafure, 1990).

Once in the general circulation, the benzodiazepines are all protein-bound. However, there is some degree of variation in what percentage of each medication will be protein-

---

[2] *All* suspected overdoses should be treated by a physician.

TABLE 7.1 Selected Pharmacological
Characteristics of Some Benzodiazepines

Generic name	Equivalent dose	Half-life
Alprazolam	0.5 mg	6–20 hours
Chlordiazepoxide	25 mg	30–100 hours
Clonazepam	0.25 mg	20–40 hours
Clorazepate	7.5 mg	30–100 hours
Diazepam	5 mg	30–100 hours
Flurazepam	30 mg	50–100 hours
Halazepam	20 mg	30–100 hours
Lorazepam	1 mg	10–20 hours
Oxazepam	15 mg	5–21 hours
Prazepam	10 mg	30–100 hours
Temazepam	30 mg	9.5–12.4 hours
Triazolam	0.25 mg	1.7–3.0 hours

Source: Based on Hyman, S. E. (1988). *Manual of Psychiatric Emergencies* (2nd ed). Boston: Little, Brown.

bound. Diazepam, for example, is more than 99% protein-bound (American Psychiatric Association, 1990), whereas alprazolam is about 80% protein-bound (Medical Economics Company, 1993).

As a general rule, the benzodiazepines are poorly absorbed from intramuscular or subcutaneous injection sites. It is thus difficult to predict in advance the degree of bioavailability when benzodiazepines are injected. Except for rare situations, such as for uncontrolled seizures, the benzodiazepines are usually administered orally. This allows the prescribing physician a greater degree of control over the drug's effects, because it is easier to predict the bioavailability of orally administered benzodiazepines than it is of injected forms.

Most members of the benzodiazepine family of chemicals must be biotransformed before elimination can proceed. This task is mainly carried out in the liver. In the process of biotransformation, metabolites that have biological effects of their own are produced. These biologically active metabolites may contribute to the drug's effects and may require extended periods of time before they are eliminated from the body. For example, the benzodiazepine chlordiazepoxide produces a total of four different metabolites before it is finally eliminated from the body.

The exceptions to this rule are lorazepam, oxazepam, and temazepam. These benzodiazepines either are eliminated without biotransformation or produce metabolites that have minimal physical effects on the patient. As we will discuss later in this chapter, these benzodiazepines are often preferred for older patients, who may become oversedated as a result of the long half-lives of some benzodiazepine metabolites.

Although the benzodiazepines are often compared with the barbiturates, they are very different in the way they function in the brain. The barbiturates nonselectively depress the *entire* range of activity of neurons in many different parts of the brain, including the cortex. This results in significant degrees of sedation along with the desired effect of a reduction in anxiety levels.

The benzodiazepines, on the other hand, are more selective in their action. Clinical research suggests that the benzodiazepines affect the action of only a single neurotransmitter, known as *gamma aminobutyric acid* (or GABA). Scientists believe that GABA is the most important "inhibitory" neurotransmitter in the brain (Bohn, 1993; Tabakoff & Hoffman, 1992).

The benzodiazepines are thought to facilitate the action of GABA by binding to the GABA receptor site and a chloride channel on the neuron surface. This, in turn, makes the receptor more sensitive to GABA, reducing the level of neurological activity. Neurons that utilize GABA are found throughout the brain, especially in a specific portion of the brain known as the *locus ceruleus* (Cardoni, 1990; Upjohn Company, 1989). Nerve fibers from the locus ceruleus connect with other parts of the brain believed to be involved in fear and panic reactions. Thus, by reducing the level of activity of the neurons in the locus ceruleus, the benzodiazepines are thought to reduce the individual's anxiety level.

Unlike the barbiturates, excessive sedation at normal dosage levels of the benzodiazepines is rare. It is for this reason that benzodiazepines are often called "tranquilizers" but not "sedatives." When excessive sedation *is* observed with a benzodiazepine, it is usually a result of too large a dose being used for that particular person (Rickels, Schweizer, & Lucki, 1987).

Advanced age is one factor that may make an individual more susceptible to benzodiazepine-induced oversedation (Ayd, 1994). There are two reasons for this. First, with advancing age, the individual's liver becomes less efficient at metabolizing many drugs, including the benzodiazepines. Second, there is an age-related decline in blood flow to the liver and kidneys, which adds to the difficulty of metabolizing or excreting many drugs (Bleidt & Moss, 1989). The result of the combination of these two forces is that many older patients become oversedated or experience a paradoxical excitement as their bodies struggle to adjust to the effects of the benzodiazepines. One exception to this rule is Deracyn (adinazolam). It is not uncommon for patients of any age to experience sedation from adinazolam. As many as two-thirds of those who receive Deracyn may experience some degree of drowsiness, at least until their bodies adapt to the drug's effects (Cardoni, 1990).

To put the impact of these age-related changes on benzodiazepine metabolism in some perspective, consider that the elderly may require *three times as long* to fully metabolize diazepam and chlordiazepoxide as would a young adult (Cohen, 1989). If benzodiazepines are to be used in older patients, lorazepam or oxazepam might be better than long-acting benzodiazepines such as diazepam (Graedon & Graedon, 1991; Bleidt & Moss, 1989). Lorazepam and oxazepam have a shorter half-life and are more easily metabolized than diazepam and similar benzodiazepines.

In Chapter 6, we discussed the phenomenon of a barbiturate hangover. It is also possible for the benzodiazepine user to experience a drug hangover, especially when using some of the longer-lasting benzodiazepines (Ashton, 1992).

From Table 7.1, we see that for some individuals the half-life of some benzodiazepines may be as long as 100 hours. If such a patient were to take a second, or even a third dose of the medication before the first dose was fully metabolized, he or she would begin to accumulate unmetabolized medication in body tissues. The unmetabolized medication would continue to have an effect on the individual's function well past the time that he or she thought the drug's effects had ended.

Although the benzodiazepines are most often prescribed as antianxiety agents, there is actually a great deal of controversy as to how effective they are in this capacity. Indeed, Ayd (1994) notes that although the benzodiazepines are of value in the short-term treatment of anxiety, "There is a paucity of research studies that have investigated the therapeutic efficacy of a benzodiazepine anxiolytic after six months to a year" (p. 92). Thus, in Ayd's opinion, the long-term effectiveness of benzodiazepines in the treatment of anxiety has not been adequately studied.

Schuckit (1989) suggests that, because the antianxiety effects of the benzodiazepines last about 1 to 2 months, these drugs are not useful for continuously treating anxiety over a long period of time. The *Harvard Medical School Mental Health Letter* (1988) does support this conclusion, however, stating that although patients may develop some tolerance to the sedative effects of benzodiazepines, they do not become tolerant to the antianxiety effects.

Benzodiazepine Tolerance, Abuse, and Addiction

Benzodiazepine Tolerance and Dependence

After taking a benzodiazepine for an extended period of time, users go through a process of "neuroadaptation" (Sellers, Ciraulo, DuPont, Griffiths, Kosten, Romach, & Woody, 1993, p. 65), in which the central nervous system becomes tolerant to the drug's effects. The *discontinuance syndrome* is the outcome of a state of pharmacological dependence, or pharmacological tolerance, that develops after using benzodiazepines on a daily basis for several months. As a result of this pharmacological dependence, users experience "rebound" or "discontinuance" symptoms when they stop taking the benzodiazepine, even if they had been taking the recommended dosage.

Some researchers believe that this state of pharmacological dependence is evidence that the patient has become addicted to the benzodiazepine. Remember that two signs of addiction are a state of physical dependence and tolerance to the drug's effects. Some physicians believe that the discontinuance syndrome is clear evidence that the user becomes both tolerant to benzodiazepines and physically dependent on them "within a few weeks, perhaps days" (Miller & Gold, 1991b, p. 28).

Other researchers view the rebound or discontinuance symptoms as a natural consequence of benzodiazepine use. Sellers et al. (1993) argued, for example, that evidence "of neuroadaptation is not sufficient to define drug-taking behavior as dependent" (p. 65). Thus, although the patient may experience a discontinuance syndrome if the medication is discontinued, this is seen as a natural process. Advocates of this position argue that the body must go through a period of adjustment whenever *any* medication is discontinued.

Researchers disagree as to how long a patient must use the benzodiazepines at normal dosage levels before he or she might experience a discontinuance syndrome. Some believe that in rare cases pharmacological dependence on the benzodiazepines may develop in just days or weeks (Miller & Gold, 1991b; American Psychiatric Association, 1990; *Harvard Medical School Mental Health Letter,* 1988). Others believe that it takes several weeks of continual use before the patient runs any risk of significant discontinuance distress (Graedon & Graedon, 1991).

In most cases in which the benzodiazepines are used at normal dosage levels, 4 to 6 months of daily use would be required for patients to become physically dependent on these drugs (*Harvard Medical School Mental Health Letter,*

1988). According to the *Harvard Medical School Mental Health Letter* (1988), "most" (p. 3) patients would experience withdrawal symptoms after 8 months of daily benzodiazepine use at normal dosage levels, and "after a year almost all" (p. 3) patients would experience some symptoms during withdrawal. Some of the factors that influence the development of pharmacological dependence on the benzodiazepines include (1) the frequency with which the individual has used a benzodiazepine, (2) the total period of time during which the individual was using benzodiazepines, (3) the individual's unique biochemistry, (4) the individual's history of prior addiction to chemicals, and (5) the pharmacological characteristics (the potency, biological halflife, and so on) of the specific benzodiazepine being used.

Benzodiazepine Abuse

Until now, we have been talking about the discontinuance syndrome that develops after a patient has been using a benzodiazepine daily at recommended dosage levels. What about the actual abuse potential of these drugs? Researchers disagree as to the abuse potential of the benzodiazepines. Some researchers have concluded that the benzodiazepines have a rather low "reward potential"; that is, in contrast to heroin, cocaine, or the other drugs of abuse, the benzodiazepines do not provide a "buzz" or a "high." These findings mirror clinical research evidence, which suggests that most people do not find benzodiazepine use pharmacologically rewarding. For this reason, the abuse potential of the benzodiazepines is said to be quite low, and so there is little incentive for most people to increase the daily dosage level above what was prescribed.[3] On the other hand, many who work in the field of substance abuse believe that the benzodiazepines have a significant potential for abuse. These individuals point to the clinical

[3]Yet Graedon and Graedon (1991) conclude that one reason BuSpar (discussed later in this chapter) has not won wide acceptance as an antianxiety medication is that, unlike the benzodiazepines, it does not produce a "buzz" for the user.

cases of benzodiazepine dependence that are occasionally reported in the literature to support their belief that the abuse potential of this family of drugs is underrated.

To explain this apparent contradiction, Cole and Kando (1993) suggest that the vast majority of those who abuse benzodiazepines do so as part of a pattern of polydrug abuse: "Patients taking only benzodiazepine in large doses to get 'high' are quite rare" (p. 58). Cole and Kando also acknowledge that an exception to this rule might be the medical patient who increases his or her daily dosage level in an attempt to come to terms with chronic feelings of dysphoria. However, overall, they believe it is rare for a patient to be abusing only benzodiazepines.

This conclusion seems difficult to defend in light of the results of clinical research conducted in the field. Substance abuse workers have long been aware that at least some drug users find the benzodiazepines attractive as recreational drugs. The pharmacological characteristics of alprazolam, for example, might make it a prime drug of abuse (Sellers et al., 1993; Juergens & Morse, 1988). Alprazolam reaches peak blood levels in 1 to 2 hours, and in the healthy individual it is fully metabolized in 6 to 16 hours. These characteristics allow the abuser to experience an intense "high," followed by a rapid drop in the drug's effects.

It is quite difficult to reconcile the conclusions of Cole and Kando (1993) with those of Robertson and Ronald (1992), who called the benzodiazepines "the single most misused category of drug in Scotland" (p. 1169). It is also difficult to reconcile the work of Cole and Kando (1993) with the observation that there are an estimated 500,000 benzodiazepine addicts in England alone (Ashton, 1992). And the American Psychiatric Association (1990) concluded that perhaps 2% of the adults in the United States have abused benzodiazepines on at least one occasion in their lives.

There is thus some disagreement as to the extent of benzodiazepine abuse in the United States. Some researchers maintain that in the vast majority of cases the benzodiazepines *are* both

appropriately prescribed and properly used (Appelbaum, 1992; Woods, Katz, & Winger, 1988). Other researchers maintain that the benzodiazepines present the user with a very real potential for abuse.

Benzodiazepine Withdrawal

In any case, once a person is addicted to benzodiazepines, withdrawal from these drugs can be quite difficult. For example, Schweizer, Rickels, Case, and Greenblatt (1990) worked with a group of 63 benzodiazepine-dependent individuals and attempted to implement a 25% per week reduction in their dosage benzodiazepine levels. In spite of this slow withdrawal schedule, the authors found that only one-third of those individuals addicted to benzodiazepines with long half-lives and 42% of those addicted to benzodiazepines with short half-lives were able to complete the withdrawal program. The authors attribute their findings to individual personality structures, suggesting that some patients may have greater difficulty during withdrawal than others.

Rickels, Schweizer, Case, and Greenblatt (1990) studied benzodiazepine withdrawal to try to identify factors that might influence the withdrawal process. They conclude that the severity of benzodiazepine withdrawal is dependent on five different "drug treatment" factors and several "patient factors." The drug treatment factors are (1) the total daily dose of benzodiazepines being used, (2) the total time over which benzodiazepines have been used, (3) the half-life of the benzodiazepine being used (short half-life benzodiazepines tend to produce more withdrawal symptoms than do long half-life benzodiazepines) (4) the potency of the benzodiazepine being used, and (5) the rate of withdrawal (gradual, tapered, or abrupt withdrawal). The patient factors include the patient's premorbid personality structure, his or her expectations for the withdrawal process, and individual differences in the neurobiological structures in the brain thought to be involved in the withdrawal process. Rickels et al. believe that interactions between these two sets of factors determine the severity of withdrawal, which can be a complex and difficult process.

Complications from Benzodiazepine Use at Normal Dosage Levels

The benzodiazepines are not perfect drugs. As a group, the benzodiazepines have a number of drawbacks. For example, because tolerance to the anticonvulsant effects of benzodiazepines can develop over time, they are of only limited value in the long-term control of epilepsy (Morton & Santos, 1989). Also, although benzodiazepines are not general neuronal depressants as are the barbiturates, excessive sedation still occasionally occurs, even at normal dosage levels. As we noted earlier, this effect is most prevalent in the older patient or in the patient with significant levels of liver damage. The fact that the elderly are most likely to experience excessive sedation is unfortunate, as evidence suggests that two-thirds of the prescriptions for benzodiazepines are for people over the age of 60 (Ayd, 1994).

Different benzodiazepines will have slightly different side-effect profiles, depending on their chemical structure. The side effects of Halcion (triazolam) have received a great deal of media attention. When used at low doses, triazolam may cause the user to experience periods of confusion and disorientation (Gillin, 1991; Salzman, 1990). Other possible side effects of triazolam are behavioral disinhibition, hyperexcitability, daytime anxiety, and amnesia (O'Donovan & McGuffin, 1993; Gillin, 1991). These side effects have been observed both in the elderly and in younger adults and will be discussed in more detail in the section "The Trials of Halcion."

Another benzodiazepine, flurazepam (sold under the brand name of Dalmane), also tends to cause confusion and oversedation, especially in the elderly. This medication is often used as a treatment for insomnia. When introduced into the body, flurazepam is biotransformed into the metabolite desalkylflurazepam. Unfortunately, desalkylflurazepam has a half-life of between 40 and 280 hours (Gillin, 1991), which means that the effects of a single dose might last for *up to 12 days* in some patients. If a person should ingest alcohol or an over-the-counter cold remedy before the flurazepam is fully metabolized, the unmetabolized drug could combine with the depressant effects of the alcohol or cold remedy to produce serious levels of CNS depression.

Cross-tolerance between the benzodiazepines, alcohol, the barbiturates, and meprobamate is also possible (Snyder, 1986; Barnhill, Ciraulo, & Ciraulo, 1989). The benzodiazepines may also potentiate the effects of other CNS depressants such as antihistamines, alcohol, or narcotics, presenting a danger of oversedation or even death.[4] Thus, if there is any doubt about whether two or more medications should be used together, one should *always* consult a physician, pharmacist, or the local poison control center.

Another problem associated with the long-term use of benzodiazepines, even at normal dosage levels, is that, when the medication is discontinued, the withdrawal symptoms may mimic the symptoms of anxiety and sleep disorders (Miller & Gold, 1991b). Miller and Gold state that the benzodiazepine withdrawal symptoms are "virtually indistinguishable from" (p. 34) the symptoms of anxiety and sleep disorders for which the medication was first prescribed. The danger is that the patient may begin to take benzodiazepines again, in the mistaken belief that the withdrawal symptoms indicate that the original problem still exists.

Occasionally, normal doses of the benzodiazepines bring about a degree of irritability, hostility, rage, or outright aggression (Juergens, 1993; Cole & Kando, 1993). This *paradoxical rage reaction* is thought to be the result of the disinhibition effects of the benzodiazepines. Because the benzodiazepines lower social inhibitions, the person is more likely to engage in

---

[4]For example, the movie star Judy Garland reportedly died as a result of the combined effects of alcohol and the benzodiazepine diazepam (Snyder, 1986).

behavior that was previously controlled successfully. A similar effect is often seen in persons who drink alcohol. The disinhibition effect of alcohol is thought to be the reason the combination of alcohol and benzodiazepines sometimes precipitates a paradoxical rage reaction (Beasley, 1987).

Another complication of benzodiazepines is that they may interfere with the formation of memory patterns (Ayd, 1994; Plasky, Marcus, & Salzman, 1988). Although often the memory disturbance is so subtle it escapes notice (O'Donovan & McGuffin, 1993; Juergens, 1993), every benzodiazepine can cause some degree of memory loss. Although Halcion (triazolam) in particular has acquired a reputation for causing memory disturbance when used at therapeutic dosage levels, this effect is a characteristic common to *all* the benzodiazepines (O'Donovan & McGuffin, 1993; Juergens, 1993). This kind of memory disturbance is termed *anterograde amnesia,* a form of amnesia that involves the formation of memories after a specific event (Plasky, Marcus, & Salzman, 1988). A person with anterograde amnesia might be unable to remember information presented to them after ingesting the drug, a process similar to the alcohol-induced "blackout" (Juergens, 1993).

At normal dosage levels, the benzodiazepines may also disrupt the normal psychomotor skills necessary to drive an automobile or work with dangerous power tools. This effect is not as apparent in situations in which the individual is "allowed to compensate on a difficult task by performing it more slowly" (Rickels, Schweizer, & Lucki, 1987, p. 784). However, tasks that require vigilance or speed of motor performance might be adversely affected by benzodiazepine use. Rickels, Schweizer, and Lucki (1987) warn that "caution should be exercised" (p. 785) by patients who use benzodiazepines and who also drive. Problems with psychomotor coordination may persist for several days following the initial use of benzodiazepines (Woods, Katz, & Winger, 1988).

The benzodiazepine family of drugs occasionally will produce mild respiratory depression, even at normal therapeutic dosage levels. This is especially true for people with pulmonary disease. However, the use of the benzodiazepines should also be avoided by patients who suffer from sleep apnea, chronic lung disease, or other sleep-related breathing disorders (Rickels, Schweizer, & Lucki, 1987). Doghramji (1989) warns against using CNS depressants for patients who suffer from Alzheimer's disease, as such medications might potentiate preexisting sleep apnea problems.

In addition to their other side effects, the benzodiazepines occasionally interfere with normal sexual functioning. Although clinical depression is not a commonly encountered side effect of benzodiazepine use, rare cases of drug-induced depression have been reported (Cole & Kando, 1993; Juergens, 1993; Ashton, 1992; Smith & Salzman, 1991). The exact mechanism by which the benzodiazepines might cause or contribute to depressive episodes is not clear at this time. Unfortunately, suicide is a possible outcome of the benzodiazepine-induced depressive episode, and there is evidence to suggest that benzodiazepine use might contribute to thoughts of suicide (Juergens, 1993; Ashton, 1992).

The Trials of Halcion

Since the benzodiazepine Halcion (triazolam) was first introduced, it has been a controversial drug. Intended as a hypnotic, Halcion has been the subject of at least 100 lawsuits against the manufacturer by various individuals who believe they have been harmed by their own or another person's use of this drug (Dyer, 1992). Furthermore, in the United States alone, at least 2,300 adverse reactions have been reported to the manufacturer, Upjohn Pharmaceuticals (Hand, 1989). At least 1,100 reports of adverse reactions were filed by physicians in Holland before the drug was banned in that country ("60 Minutes," 1994).

Simply put, Halcion (triazolam) has been

called "a very, very dangerous drug" (Kayles, quoted in "60 Minutes," 1994, p. 2). It has been suggested that

> compared with other benzodiazepines, triazolam causes more agitation, confusion, amnesia, hallucinations, and bizarre or abnormal behavior. Suicides, attempted suicides, deaths, and violent crimes have been associated with triazolam administration. In most of the adverse reaction reports, the drug was taken as recommended. (Hand, 1989, p. 3)

Recent evidence has come to light suggesting that, for reasons that are still unclear, the manufacturer *under*reported some of the side effects associated with Halcion during at least one early study of the drug's safety ("60 Minutes," 1994; Cowley, 1992). In the United States and in a number of other countries, government agencies have reviewed the side effects of triazolam and reconsidered whether this drug meets their safety standards. As a result of their review, the British government banned the sale of Halcion (triazolam) in England as of October, 1991 (Dyer, 1992). Since then, triazolam has also been banned in 12 other countries, including Norway, Finland, Brazil, and Jamaica (Dyer, 1993).

In the United States, the Food and Drug Administration (FDA) set up a special review panel to determine whether the drug was safe. After a year-long study, the FDA panel concluded that Halcion was safe but recommended that the manufacturer issue stronger warnings about potential side effects (Dyer, 1992). However, there are questions as to how objective the FDA review panel might have been and whether the manufacturer presented *all* the facts to the panel for its consideration.

For example, when they met with the FDA review panel, Upjohn Pharmaceutical's representatives claimed that there were no studies to substantiate the reports of adverse Halcion-induced effects. Indeed, they presented the results of one study, known as "Protocol 321," as evidence that the drug was safe ("60 Minutes," 1994). However, the true findings of this study

were apparently not provided to the FDA review panel. The study actually found that 70% of the subjects experienced major side effects from the drug ("60 Minutes," 1994). But this information was "either missing or minimized when Upjohn sent this official summary of the test to the FDA" ("60 Minutes," 1994, p. 3).

Thus, serious questions about the safety of the drug Halcion (triazolam) have been raised, and it will take many years for the lawsuits against the manufacturer to be settled. Halcion will probably remain a controversial drug for some time to come.

Drug Interactions Involving the Benzodiazepines

Creelman, Ciraulo, and Shader (1989) observe that there are a "few anecdotal case reports" (p. 144) of patients who have suffered adverse effects from the use of benzodiazepines while on lithium carbonate. The authors reviewed a single case report of "profound hypothermia resulting from the combined use of lithium and diazepam" (p. 144). In this case, lithium was implicated as the agent that caused the individual to suffer a progressive loss of body temperature. The authors further note that the sedative effects of diazepam appear to be potentiated by lithium in rats, although the implications of this research on human subjects is not clear at this time.

Patients on Antabuse (disulfiram) should use benzodiazepines with caution, because disulfiram reduces the speed at which the body can metabolize benzodiazepines such as diazepam and chlordiazepoxide (Zito, 1994). Zito recommends that, when a patient must use both medications concurrently, a benzodiazepine such as oxazepam or lorazepam, which does not have any biologically active metabolites, should be used.

Patients who are taking a benzodiazepine should avoid the antipsychotic medication clozapine (Zito, 1994). There have been reports of severe respiratory depression caused by the combination of these two medications, possibly resulting in several deaths.

Women who are using oral contraceptives should discuss the use of benzodiazepines with a physician before combining these medications. According to Zito (1994), oral contraceptives reduce the rate at which the body metabolizes some benzodiazepines. Thus it may be necessary to reduce the dose of the benzodiazepine. Patients who are taking antitubercular medications such as isoniazid may also need to adjust their benzodiazepine dosage (Zito, 1994). Because isoniazid also reduces the rate at which the body metabolizes some benzodiazepines, it may be necessary to reduce the dosage level of the benzodiazepine to avoid oversedation.

Benzodiazepines should *never* be intermixed with medications that are classified as CNS depressants, except under the supervision of a physician. Some examples of such medications are alcohol, narcotic analgesics, and the antihistamines. The combined effects of the two classes of medications may result in excessive, if not dangerous, levels of sedation.

Although this list is not exhaustive, it does illustrate that there is potential for interaction between the benzodiazepines and a number of other medications. Again, a physician or pharmacist should always be consulted before taking any two medications at the same time.

Subjective Experience of Benzodiazepine Use

As antianxiety agents, the benzodiazepines have very similar effects on the user. At normal dosage levels, the person experiences a state of gentle relaxation. When used in the treatment of insomnia, the benzodiazepines initially reduce the sleep latency period, the period of time between going to bed and falling asleep. At first, those who use benzodiazepines to help them sleep often report a sense of deep and refreshing sleep.

However, the benzodiazepines also interfere with the normal sleep cycle, reducing the amount of REM sleep. It is during the REM phase of sleep that we dream, and experimental research suggests that dreaming is necessary for mental health (Hobson, 1989). Alcohol, the barbiturates, and the benzodiazepines have all been noted to interfere with REM sleep.

As we noted earlier, when a person discontinues the use of a CNS depressant such as alcohol, the barbiturates, or the benzodiazepines, he or she will experience REM rebound (Woods, Katz, & Winger, 1988), a phenomenon in which the individual experiences an *increase* in the amount of sleep time spent in REM sleep. During this period, he or she will have vivid dreams, which may be quite frightening. After protracted periods of benzodiazepine use, the individual may experience a significant REM rebound effect. But the term *protracted* is a relative term. There have been cases involving individuals who had used a benzodiazepine as a hypnotic for only 1 or 2 weeks who still experienced significant "rebound" symptoms (Tyrer, 1993; *Harvard Medical School Mental Health Letter*, 1988).

REM rebound is not the only rebound effect that may occur. Patients who have used a benzodiazepine for daytime relief from anxiety have reported symptoms such as anxiety, agitation, tremor, fatigue, difficulty concentrating, headache, nausea, gastrointestinal upset, a sense of paranoia, depersonalization, impaired memory, and insomnia (Graedon & Graedon, 1991). Rebound insomnia may last from 3 to 21 days after the last benzodiazepine use. Nor are prolonged episodes of benzodiazepine use required for rebound symptoms to develop.

The benzodiazepines with short half-lives are most likely to cause rebound symptoms (Ayd, 1994; O'Donovan & McGuffin, 1993; Rosenbaum, 1990). Such rebound symptoms may be precipitated by an abrupt drop in medication blood levels. For example, alprazolam has a short half-life, and the blood levels drop rather rapidly just before it is time for the next dose. It is during this period that the individual is most likely to experience an increase in anxiety levels.

This process results in a phenomenon known as "clock watching" (Rosenbaum, 1990, p. 1302), as the patient waits with increasing anxiety until it is time for the next dose.

In withdrawing patients from benzodiazepines with short half-lives, Rosenbaum (1990) recommends gradually switching to clonazepam, a long-acting medication. Clonazepam is about twice as potent as alprazolam but has a longer half-life. The transition between alprazolam and clonazepam takes about 1 week, after which time the patient should be taking only clonazepam. This medication can then be gradually withdrawn, resulting in a slower decline in blood levels. However, the patient still should be warned that there will be some rebound anxiety symptoms. Although the patient might believe otherwise, these rebound symptoms are not a sign that the original anxiety is still present; rather, they are simply a sign that the body is adjusting to the gradual reduction in clonazepam blood levels.

Complications from Chronic Benzodiazepine Use

Although introduced as safe and nonaddicting substitutes for the barbiturates, the benzodiazepines do indeed have a significant abuse potential. Dietch (1983) explored the nature of benzodiazepine abuse and outlined several criteria by which to identify benzodiazepine abuse. These criteria include (1) use of the drug after the medical or psychiatric need for its use has passed, (2) symptoms of physical or psychological dependence on one of the benzodiazepines, (3) use of the drug in amounts greater than the prescribed amount, (4) use of the drug to obtain an euphoriant effect, and (5) use of the drug to decrease self-awareness, or the possibility of change.

Benzodiazepine withdrawal symptoms include anxiety, insomnia, dizziness, nausea and vomiting, muscle weakness, tremor, confusion, convulsions (seizures), irritability, sweating, and a drug-induced withdrawal psychosis (Juergens,

1993). There have also been rare reports of depression, manic reactions, and obsessive-compulsive symptoms as a result of benzodiazepine withdrawal (Juergens, 1993).

In addition to the problems of physical dependence, Dietch (1983) notes that it is possible to become *psychologically* dependent on benzodiazepines. Indeed, according to Dietch (1983), "Psychological dependence on benzodiazepines appears to be more common than physical dependence" (p. 1140). Psychologically dependent users may take the drug either continuously or intermittently because they *believe* they need benzodiazepines. Their actual medical requirements may be quite different.

For example, research shows that tolerance to the sleep-inducing (or hypnotic) effect of the benzodiazepines develops in 2 to 4 weeks (Ayd, 1994; American Psychiatric Association, 1990). Yet many people continue to take benzodiazepines as a sleep aid for much longer periods of time, believing that the medication is still helping them get a good night's sleep.

Some benzodiazepine users increase their dosage levels above that prescribed by their physician. Why they do so is not well understood. Although tolerance to benzodiazepines does develop (Snyder, 1986), "the magnitude of such increases appears to be small" (Dietch, 1983, p. 1141), and, in general, "subjects [tend] to titrate their dose according to the level of environmental stress." The limited information we have on this phenomenon is based on patients who were prescribed one of the benzodiazepines for medical or psychiatric reasons. There is virtually no information on how drug abusers utilize this class of drugs or what dosage level they prefer. Woods, Katz, and Winger (1988) postulate that the person most likely to abuse benzodiazepines is one with a history of polydrug abuse.

As is true for all CNS depressants, the benzodiazepines are capable of producing a *toxic psychosis,* especially in overdose situations. This condition is also referred to as *organic brain syndrome* by some professionals. Some of the symptoms of a benzodiazepine-related toxic psychosis are visual and auditory hallucinations and/or paranoid delusions. This drug-induced psychosis usually clears after 2 to 14 days (Miller & Gold, 1991b; Schuckit, 1989).

As with the barbiturates, *withdrawal from benzodiazepines should be attempted only under the supervision of a physician.* Severe withdrawal symptoms may include hyperthermia, delirium, convulsions, a drug-induced psychosis, and possible death (Jenike, 1991). Detoxification may be necessary on an inpatient basis in some cases. Although most patients can be slowly withdrawn from benzodiazepines with few or no side effects (Woods, Katz, & Winger, 1988), some patients will experience some degree of discomfort during withdrawal.

Benzodiazepines as Substitutes for Other Drugs of Abuse

Juergens (1993) reports that many individuals who abuse the amphetamines and cocaine often also abuse benzodiazepines. Such polydrug abuse is done either to control some of the side effects of the stimulant use or to "come down" from the stimulants in order to sleep.

Alcoholics who do not have access to alcohol during the day have been known to substitute benzodiazepines. Some recovering alcoholics have likened the effects of 10 mg of diazepam to the effects of 3 to 4 "stiff" drinks. Furthermore, diazepam's long half-life is often sufficient to allow the individual to work the entire day without going into alcohol withdrawal.

Finally, opiate addicts in methadone maintenance programs often take a single, massive dose of a benzodiazepine (the equivalent of 100 to 300 mg of diazepam) to "boost" the effect of their daily methadone dose (Juergens, 1993; American Psychiatric Association, 1990). There is also evidence to suggest that the experimental narcotic buprenorphine may, when mixed with benzodiazepines, offer the narcotics user a lesser "high," thus reducing the incentive for mixing medications (Sellers et al., 1993). However, at present, buprenorphine has still not been approved for use as a substitute for methadone in the United States.

Buspirone: The First Decade

In 1986, a new medication by the name of BuSpar (buspirone) was introduced. Buspirone is a member of a new class of medications known as the *azapirones,* which are chemically different from the benzodiazepine family of drugs. Buspirone was found as a result of a search by pharmaceutical companies for antipsychotic drugs that did not have the harsh side effects of the phenothiazines or similar chemicals (Sussman, 1994).

Buspirone has an antianxiety effect, "comparable with that of both diazepam and clorazepate" in terms of its ultimate effectiveness, but with fewer side effects than the benzodiazepines (Feighner, 1987, p. 15; Manfredi, Kales, Vgontzas, Bixler, Isaac, & Falcone, 1991). Buspirone only infrequently causes sedation or fatigue (Sussman, 1994; Rosenbaum & Gelenberg, 1991). Furthermore, no evidence has been found of potentiation between buspirone and select benzodiazepines or between buspirone and alcohol (Feighner, 1987; Manfredi et al., 1991).[5]

However, clinical trials of buspirone *do* suggest that some patients may experience gastrointestinal problems, drowsiness, decreased concentration, dizziness, headache, feelings of lightheadedness, nervousness, diarrhea, excitement, sweating/clamminess, nausea, depression, and some feelings of fatigue (Manfredi et al., 1991; Graedon & Graedon, 1991; Feighner, 1987; Newton, Marunycz, Alderdice, & Napoliello (1986).

Unlike the benzodiazepine family of drugs, buspirone has no anticonvulsant action and no muscle-relaxant effect (Eison & Temple, 1987). It has been found to be of value in controlling the anxiety of general anxiety disorder but not the anxiety of panic attacks. Indeed, buspirone has been found to be of little value in anxiety cases that involve insomnia, which is a significant

---

[5]This is not, however, a suggestion that the user try to use alcohol and buspirone at the same time. The author does *not* recommend the use of alcohol with any prescription medication.

proportion of anxiety cases (Manfredi et al., 1991).

However, buspirone has been effective in the treatment of anxiety disorders with a depressive component (Cohn, Wilcox, Bowden, Fisher, & Rodos, 1992). Indeed, evidence suggests that buspirone might be of value in the treatment of some forms of depression, both as the primary form of treatment and as an agent to potentiate the effects of other antidepressants (Sussman, 1994). In addition, buspirone has been found to be of value in the treatment of obsessive-compulsive disorder, social phobias, posttraumatic stress disorder, and possibly alcohol withdrawal (Sussman, 1994; Schweizer & Rickels, 1994). Finally, there is some evidence to suggest that buspirone might be able to control the "craving" that many cigarette smokers report when they try to stop smoking (Schweizer & Rickels, 1994).

The Pharmacology of Buspirone

The mechanism of action for buspirone is different from that of the benzodiazepines (Eison & Temple, 1987). For example, whereas the benzodiazepines are effective almost immediately, buspirone must be used for up to 2 to 4 weeks before its maximum effects are evident (Sussman, 1994; Graedon & Graedon, 1991; Thornton, 1990). Furthermore, the short half-life of buspirone requires that the individual take the drug in 3 to 4 divided doses, whereas the half-life of the benzodiazepine diazepam makes it possible for the drug to be used 1 to 2 times a day (Schweizer & Rickels, 1994). Finally, unlike many other sedating chemicals, there does not appear to be any degree of cross-tolerance between buspirone and either the benzodiazepines, alcohol, the barbiturates, or meprobamate (Sussman, 1994).

As we discussed earlier in this chapter, the benzodiazepines tend to bind to receptor sites that utilize the neurotransmitter GABA. However, buspirone tends to bind to one of the many serotonin receptor sites known as the 5-HT_{1A} sites (Sussman, 1994). There are several subforms of serotonin receptors, each of which

appears to be involved in a different neurobehavioral function, according to Sussman. Depending on the dosage level being used, the individual differences in the distribution of 5-HT_{1A} receptor sites in the brain, and the individual's normal level of serotonin in the brain, buspirone might either enhance or decrease the effects of serotonin as a neurotransmitter. Another difference between buspirone and the benzodiazepines is that BuSpar binds to dopamine and serotonin type 1 receptors in the hippocampus, a different portion of the brain than where the benzodiazepines exert their effect (Manfredi et al., 1991).

Research into the abuse potential of buspirone is mixed at this time. Lader (1987) concludes that buspirone has "failed to demonstrate any abuse liability in either animal or human studies" (p. 25), a conclusion supported by Thornton (1990) and Rosenbaum and Gelenberg (1991). Sussman (1994) found no evidence of a withdrawal syndrome from buspirone such as that seen in chronic benzodiazepine abuse. Indeed, "recreational users (of chemicals) rated buspirone as no more attractive than placebo with regard to 'stimulant/euphoria' (potential) and buspirone was not sought in self-administration studies" (Sussman, 1994, p. 14). However, in an earlier study, Murphy, Owen, and Tyrer (1989) found both an addictive effect and a characteristic withdrawal syndrome from buspirone. Thus, at this point, the potential for buspirone abuse and addiction remains unclear.

As you will recall, one of the side effects of benzodiazepine use is occasional memory problems. Rickels, Giesecke, and Geller (1987) found that buspirone failed to demonstrate any impact on memory in a sample of 39 subjects suffering from generalized anxiety disorder, as measured by psychological tests. These results suggest that buspirone does not cause the amnesia that many benzodiazepines do.

Rickels, Schweizer, Csanalosi, Case, and Chung (1988) note that buspirone has not been shown to lessen the intensity of withdrawal symptoms experienced by patients addicted to benzodiazepines. They attempted to identify the long-term effects of buspirone and found no evidence of tolerance over a 6-month period. They also failed to uncover any evidence of a physical dependence or withdrawal syndrome from buspirone in that time frame.

Unfortunately, the manufacturer's claim that buspirone offers many advantages over the benzodiazepines in the treatment of anxiety states has not yet been totally fulfilled. Indeed, Rosenbaum and Gelenberg (1991) caution that "many clinicians and patients have found buspirone to be a generally disappointing alternative to benzodiazepines" (p. 200). In spite of this note, however, they recommend a trial of buspirone for "persistently anxious patients" (p. 200). At present, buspirone seems to be the drug of choice in the treatment of anxiety states in the addiction-prone individual.

Zolpidem: The Next Generation's Hypnotic?

Zolpidem has been used as a sleep-inducing drug in Europe for a number of years and was recently introduced to the United States. It is administered orally, and it is marketed as a hypnotic in both the United States and Europe.

Pharmacologically, zolpidem is not a member of the benzodiazepine family of drugs. Rather, it is the first of a new family of sleep-inducing chemicals that binds to just one of the receptor sites in the brain used by the benzodiazepines. Zolpidem thus is more selective than the benzodiazepines, which use a number of receptor sites in the brain. Unlike the benzodiazepines, zolpidem has only a minor anticonvulsant effect. The biological half-life of zolpidem is about 1.5 to 2.4 hours (Kryger, Steljes, Pouliot, Neufeld, & Odynski, 1991; Merlotti, Roehrs, Koshorek, Zorick, Lamphere, & Roth, 1989).

Unlike earlier hypnotics, at therapeutic dosage levels zolpidem causes only a minor reduction in REM sleep (Merlotti et al., 1989). There is a dose-related progression in the side effects, however, with the most serious side effects occurring at the highest dosage levels. As dosage levels approach or exceed 20 mg per day, zolpidem significantly reduces REM sleep. Also, at dosage levels of 20 mg per day or more, zolpidem causes rebound insomnia when the drug is discontinued.

As the dosage levels approached 50 mg per day, volunteers who received zolpidem reported visual perceptual disturbances, ataxia, dizziness, nausea and/or vomiting. Because most serious side effects are encountered at higher dosage levels, the recommended dosage level should not exceed 10 mg per day (Evans, Funderburk, & Griffiths, 1990; Merlotti et al., 1989).

Zolpidem "may have some abuse potential in people with histories of sedative-hypnotic abuse" (Evans, Funderburk, & Griffiths, 1990, p. 1254). However, the authors suggest that the abuse potential of zolpidem is less than that of a commonly prescribed benzodiazepine, triazolam. Thus, the prescribing physician must balance the potential for abuse against the potential benefit that this medication would bring to the patient.

There are also rare reports of patients who have developed some degree of tolerance to the hypnotic effects of zolpidem, as well as very rare reports of drug-induced psychotic reactions (Ayd, 1994). Thus, although this medication has some promise as a clinical hypnotic, it is not without side effects.

Summary

Since their introduction in the 1960s, the benzodiazepines have become one of the most frequently prescribed medications. As a class, the benzodiazepines are the treatment of choice for the control of anxiety, insomnia, and many other conditions. They have also become a significant part of the drug abuse problem. Although many of the benzodiazepines were first introduced as "nonaddicting and safe" substitutes for the barbiturates, there is evidence to suggest that they have an abuse potential similar to that of the barbiturate family of drugs.

In the past decade a new series of pharmaceuticals has been introduced, including buspirone, sold under the brand name BuSpar, and zolpidem. Buspirone is the first of a new class of antianxiety agents that works through a different mechanism than the benzodiazepines. Although buspirone was introduced as nonaddicting, this claim has been challenged by at least one team of researchers. Zolpidem has an admitted potential for abuse; however, current research suggests that this abuse potential is less than that of the benzodiazepine triazolam, commonly used as a hypnotic. Researchers are presently actively discussing the potential benefits and liabilities of these new medications.

Amphetamines and CNS Stimulants

Students in the field of substance abuse are often surprised to learn that the use of CNS stimulants dates back several thousand years. Indeed, historical evidence suggests that gladiators in ancient Rome used CNS stimulants to overcome the effects of fatigue (Wadler, 1994). Not surprisingly, people *still* use CNS stimulants to fight off fatigue. Thus, at first glance, stimulant use patterns seem to have changed very little in the last two thousand years or so.

There are currently several different families of chemicals that can be classified as CNS stimulants. CNS stimulant drugs in use today include cocaine, the amphetamines, amphetaminelike drugs such as Ritalin, and over-the-counter agents such as ephedrine. Because all these agents act as CNS stimulants, the behavioral effects of many of these drugs are remarkably similar (Gawin & Ellinwood, 1988). We will discuss cocaine in Chapter 9. In this chapter, we will review amphetamines and amphetamine-like drugs.

History of the Amphetamines

The amphetamine family of chemicals was first discovered in 1887 (Lingeman, 1974; Kaplan & Sadock, 1990), but it was not until 1927 that these drugs were found to be useful to medicine. In that year, Benzedrine was introduced for use in the treatment of asthma and rhinitis (Derlet &

Heischober, 1990). The drug, which could be purchased over the counter,[1] was contained in a cloth-covered ampoule. When broken, the ampoule released the concentrated amphetamine liquid into the surrounding cloth, to be held under the nose and inhaled, much as "smelling salts" are.

It was not long, however, before it was discovered that these ampoules of Benzedrine could be unwrapped, carefully broken open, and the concentrated Benzedrine used for injection. Street drug users quickly discovered that the effects of the amphetamines were quite similar to those of cocaine. Indeed, the amphetamines were introduced in an era when the dangers of cocaine were well known, and they came to be viewed by many as a "safe" substitute for cocaine.

During World War II, the amphetamines were used by American, British, German, and Japanese armed forces to counteract fatigue and heighten endurance (Brecher, 1972). The Army Air Corp crew members stationed in England in World War II alone took 180,000,000 benzedrine pills to help them stay awake and work longer (Lovett, 1994). Immediately following World War II, for reasons that are still not well understood, there was a wave of amphetamine abuse in Sweden (Snyder, 1986) and Japan.

---

[1]Needless to say, the amphetamines are no longer sold without a prescription. In some regions of the country, ephedrine can be purchased without a prescription for use in the treatment of asthma, narcolepsy and some forms of heart disease.

In the late 1960s and early 1970s, the amphetamines had become popular medications, and U.S. physicians routinely prescribed them for depression and weight loss. Indeed, so popular were the amphetamines that, by the early 1970s, some *10 billion* 5-mg tablets of amphetamine were legally produced in the United States alone (Kaplan & Sadock, 1990). And, because the amphetamines were also a popular drug of abuse, an unknown quantity was also produced in various illegal laboratories.

Amphetamine use in the United States reached "epidemic proportions" (Kaplan & Sadock, 1990, p. 305) during the late 1960s and early 1970s. It is ironic that, just a generation later, the amphetamines were no longer used in weight loss programs, and their role in the treatment of depression has been filled by the newer, more effective antidepressant medications. Yet even then, drug addicts had discovered that with chronic use the amphetamines would ultimately dominate the user's life. At high doses, the amphetamines caused agitation and, when discontinued, frequently caused a severe, drug-induced depression that could last for days or weeks.

By the early 1970s, people began to understand that "speed kills," either directly (through its impact on the heart and vascular system) or indirectly (by causing a deterioration in the person's self-care activities, a drug-induced psychosis, or a drug-induced depressive state that could reach suicidal proportions). Amphetamine use died out during the late 1970s and early 1980s as cocaine became the preferred stimulant of abuse.

The Scope of the Problem of Stimulant Abuse and Addiction

Now, with the trend moving away from cocaine, a new generation of drug abusers are exploring the amphetamines. Methamphetamine abuse has been a problem in Japan since the drug was first developed more than 50 years ago (*Forensic Drug Abuse Advisor*, 1994d). Although we have not returned to the levels of amphetamine use in the United States that characterized the late 1960s, there *is* evidence that the amphetamines are becoming increasingly popular as drugs of abuse. Illicit drug laboratories in California and Mexico supply large amounts of relatively pure amphetamine to users in the United States (Lovett, 1994). It is estimated that 7% of the adults in the United States used a CNS stimulant at least once in 1991 (Kaplan, Sadock, & Grebb, 1994).

Medical Uses of Amphetamines and CNS Stimulants

The amphetamine family of drugs is one of the more powerful groups of CNS stimulants (Jaffe, 1990). In addition to acting on the brain, the CNS stimulants affect a number of other body systems. The amphetamines and similar drugs (Ritalin, for example) improve the action of the smooth muscles of the body (Weiner, 1985). Because these drugs thus have some potential for improving athletic performance, at least to some degree, they are often abused for this purpose. However, these effects are not uniform, and overuse of the CNS stimulants can actually bring about a *decrease* in athletic abilities (Weiner, 1985).

The amphetamines have an *anorexic* side effect, causing a loss of appetite. This side effect was once thought to be useful in controlling weight. Subsequent research, however, has demonstrated that the amphetamines are only minimally effective as a weight control agent. Tolerance to the appetite-suppressing side effect of the amphetamines develops in only 4 weeks (Snyder, 1986), and physicians discovered that, after tolerance to the anorexic effect of amphetamines develops, many people regain the weight lost on amphetamines. For these reasons, the amphetamines are no longer utilized in weight control programs (Weiner, 1985).

Although the amphetamines were once thought to be antidepressants, they are now only rarely used in the treatment of depression (Potter, Rudorfer, & Goodwin, 1987). The amphetamines and related compounds do have a limited medical value, however. First, in a limited number of cases, these drugs have been found to be useful in controlling the symptoms of hyperactivity in children (Kaplan & Sadock, 1990). Surprisingly, although the amphetamines are CNS *stimulants,* they have a calming effect on children whose hyperactivity is a result of a condition known as *minimal brain damage,* which is also referred to as "hyperactivity" or "attention deficit syndrome."

The amphetamines are thought to be able to achieve this calming effect by enhancing the function of the reticular activating system (RAS) of the brain, the portion of the brain thought to be involved in focusing attention (Gold & Verebey, 1984). The RAS is believed to "screen out" extraneous stimuli to allow concentration on one specific task. Children who suffer from hyperactivity are believed to have an underactive RAS and so are easily distracted. The amphetamines are thought to stimulate the RAS to the point where the child is able to function more effectively.

The amphetamines have also been found to be the treatment of choice for a rare condition known as *narcolepsy.* Narcolepsy is a lifelong neurological condition in which the person is subject to sudden spells of falling asleep during waking hours (*Harvard Medical School Mental Health Letter,* 1990; Mirin, Weiss, & Greenfield, 1991). Doghramji (1989) describes narcolepsy as an incurable disorder thought to reflect a chemical imbalance within the brain. One of the chemicals involved, dopamine, is the neurotransmitter that the amphetamines cause to be released from neurons in the brain. Current thinking is that the amphetamines may at least partially correct the dopamine imbalance that causes narcolepsy.

Pharmacology of Amphetamines and Similar Drugs

The amphetamines can be administered in a number of ways. The drug molecule tends to be basic and when taken orally is easily absorbed through the small intestine (Laurence & Bennett, 1992). Amphetamine powder is also absorbed through the tissues of the nasopharynx when the person "snorts" amphetamine powder, and the drug is absorbed through the lungs when the amphetamines are smoked (Shields, 1990).

Once in the circulation, the amphetamine molecule is highly lipid soluble. When ingested orally, the amphetamines begin to have an effect on the user within 20 (Siegel, 1991) to 30 minutes (Mirin, Weiss, & Greenfield, 1991). When smoked, the amphetamines reach the brain in just a matter of seconds.

The chemical structure of the amphetamines closely resembles that of two different neurotransmitters, norepinephrine and dopamine. Because of this similarity, they are thought to impact on many different parts of the central nervous system as well as the muscles of the body. The exact mechanism through which the amphetamines stimulate the brain and central nervous system is still not entirely known, although evidence suggests that the amphetamines facilitate the selective release of norepinephrine and dopamine within the brain (King & Ellinwood, 1992; Mirin, Weiss, & Greenfield, 1991).

Once in the brain, the amphetamines stimulate the medulla (which is involved in the control of respiration), causing the individual to breathe more deeply and more rapidly. At normal dosage levels, the cortex is also stimulated, resulting in reduced feelings of fatigue and possibly increased concentration (Kaplan & Sadock, 1990). Many amphetamine users also report a feeling of euphoria or well-being, which may be quite intense. If the amphetamine is injected or smoked, the user may experience an intense "rush," once described as "instant euphoria" by the late Truman Capote (quoted in Siegel, 1991, p. 72).

In the average patient, the peak plasma levels of amphetamines are achieved in 1 to 3 hours after a single dose is ingested. The biological half-life of the amphetamines varies, depending on the chemical structure of the various forms of amphetamines available for use. For example, the biological half-life of dextroamphetamine is 10.25 hours, whereas the half-life of methamphetamine is only 4 to 5 hours (Medical Economics Company, 1993; Shannon, Wilson, & Stang, 1992; Derlet & Heischober, 1990).

There is considerable variation in the level of individual sensitivity to the effects of the amphetamines. For example, some users have been known to develop toxic reactions to amphetamines at dosage levels as low as 20 to 30 mg (or 0.3 mg/kg for a 160-pound person), which is within, or just above, the normal therapeutic dosage range. The estimated lethal dose of amphetamines for a nontolerant individual is 20 to 25 mg/kg (Chan, Chen, Lee, & Deng, 1994). However, there is one clinical report of a case where a person ingested 1.5 mg/kg of amphetamine, with fatal results. There are also case reports of amphetamine-naive individuals (individuals who have not developed tolerance to the amphetamines) surviving a total single dose of 400 to 500 mg (or 7.5 mg/kg body weight for a 160-pound person), although they required medical support to overcome the toxic effects of the amphetamines.

Some amphetamines in the body are metabolized by the liver. During the process of amphetamine biotransformation, which involves several steps, a number of metabolites are formed. The exact number of metabolites varies, depending on the specific amphetamine being used. For example, during the process of methamphetamine biotransformation, seven different metabolites are formed.

Although *some* amphetamines are biotransformed by the liver, a significant percentage of the amphetamines are excreted from the body essentially unchanged. Some researchers believe that at least 50% of the drug is excreted unchanged by the kidneys (Mirin, Weiss, & Greenfield, 1991). However, the percentage of amphetamine molecules that will be excreted unchanged depends on how acidic the individual's circulatory fluids are at the time the drug molecules pass through the kidneys. If the individual's urine is quite acidic, up to 60% of a dose of amphetamine will be filtered from the blood and excreted unchanged (Shields, 1990). However, if the individual's urine is extremely alkaline, perhaps as little as 5% of a dose of amphetamine will be filtered out by the kidneys, because the kidneys tend to reabsorb the drug molecules when the urine is highly alkaline. Thus, the speed at which a dose of amphetamines is excreted from the body varies in response to how acidic the individual's urine is when the drug passes through the kidneys.

When used on a regular basis, the amphetamines are able to bring about an incomplete state of tolerance. The chronic user becomes tolerant to *some* effects of the amphetamines but not to all of them. For example, when an amphetamine is used in the treatment of narcolepsy, it is possible for a person to be maintained on a specific dosage level for years without developing tolerance (Weiner, 1985; Brecher, 1972).

But, the chronic user *will* become tolerant to the euphoric effects of the amphetamines. There are three ways that amphetamine abusers try to overcome their tolerance to the effects of these drugs. First, the person uses higher and higher dosage levels of amphetamines over time (Peluso & Peluso, 1988) in an attempt to re-achieve the sense of euphoria once felt during the initial period of amphetamine use. Second, chronic amphetamine users may use 5,000 to 15,000 mg in a day, repeatedly ingesting small doses of amphetamines over the course of the day to try to overcome their tolerance to the effects of smaller doses (Chan, Chen, Lee, & Deng, 1994). Finally, chronic users substitute intravenously administered amphetamines for the initial oral or intranasal forms of the drug. Thus, the individual "graduates" to the intravenous use of amphetamines when he or she is no longer able to achieve the desired effects through oral or intranasal use of the drug.

As noted earlier in this chapter, the chronic user will eventually become tolerant to the anorexic effects of the amphetamines. This is one major reason these drugs are no longer used in weight control programs.

Methods of Amphetamine Use

Because of the ease with which they can be manufactured, amphetamines—especially the form of amphetamine known as *methamphetamine*—are often produced in illicit laboratories. Sometimes, illicit methamphetamine tablets are sold in homemade tablet form for oral use. These tablets are often white with crossed score lines on one side. Some amphetamines are also diverted from legitimate sources, and such "pharmaceutical" amphetamines come in a variety of capsules or tablets. In the past decade, methamphetamine crystals known as "ice" have also become available in many parts of the United States.

The tablets (or powder) can be crushed and prepared for intravenous use, as is done with heroin. Methamphetamine is especially potent and so is favored by amphetamine users. Amphetamine powder may be "snorted," similar to the way in which cocaine is used. When used in this manner, it takes only about 3 minutes for the drug to be absorbed and reach the brain (Siegel, 1991). Amphetamines are also smoked, especially the ice form. The user feels the effects of ice in only 6 seconds (Siegel, 1991).

Effects of the Amphetamines

The effects of amphetamines are, to a large degree, very similar to those of cocaine or adrenaline (Kaminski, 1992). However, there are some major differences: (1) whereas the effects of cocaine might last from a few minutes to an hour at most, the effects of the amphetamines last many hours (Schuckit, 1989); (2) unlike cocaine, the amphetamines are effective when used orally; and, (3) unlike cocaine, the amphetamines have only a very small anesthetic effect (Weiner, 1985).

The effects of the amphetamines on any given individual will depend on that individual's mental state, the dosage level, the relative potency of the specific form of amphetamine, and the manner in which the drug is used. The usual oral dosage level is between 15 to 30 mg per day (Lingeman, 1974), although this depends on the potency of the particular drug being used (Julien, 1992).

At low to moderate oral dosage levels, the individual experiences feelings of increased alertness, an elevation of mood, a feeling of mild euphoria, less mental fatigue, and an improved level of concentration (Kaplan & Sadock, 1990; Weiner, 1985). Like many drugs of abuse, the amphetamines stimulate the "pleasure center" in the brain. Thus, both the amphetamines and cocaine initially produce "a neurochemical magnification of the pleasure experienced in most activities" (Gawin & Ellinwood, 1988; p. 1174). Gawin and Ellinwood also note that the initial use of amphetamines or cocaine will

> produce alertness and a sense of well-being . . . lower anxiety and social inhibitions, and heighten energy, self-esteem, and the emotions aroused by interpersonal experiences. Although they magnify pleasure, they do not distort it; hallucinations are usually absent. (p. 1174)

Some of the side effects of the amphetamines include insomnia and anxiety, as well as irritability and hostility (Derlet & Heischober, 1990). It is not uncommon for illicit drug users to try to counteract these side effects through the use of alcohol, or benzodiazepines. Indeed, Peluso and Peluso (1988) estimate that *half* of all regular users of amphetamines can also be classified as heavy drinkers. These individuals attempt to control the side effects of the amphetamines through the use of alcohol, a CNS depressant. Because of their stimulant effect, it is not uncommon for alcoholics to use amphetamines to allow them to counteract the sedating effects of the alcohol. Thus, cross-abuse is a common characteristic of both amphetamine abusers and alcoholics.

When amphetamines are injected or smoked, users have reported an almost orgasmic experience. However, as the individual begins to develop tolerance to the effects of the drug, this euphoria becomes less and less pronounced. As the individual experiments with the drug, she or he will initially discover that higher doses also intensify the euphoria experienced (Gawin & Ellinwood, 1988). There is thus a tendency for intravenous amphetamine users to increase their daily dosage level over time to recapture the euphoria that they experienced when they first started using the drug.

Chronic users of amphetamines will often embark on "speed runs," repeatedly using amphetamines to recapture and maintain the elusive euphoria initially experienced. During such speed runs, the user must inject larger and larger doses of the drug to overcome the tolerance for the drug's effects. Indeed, as noted earlier in this chapter, long-term users of amphetamines have been known to inject as much as 5,000 to 15,000 mg/day in divided doses, gradually building up to this total daily dosage level as their tolerance for the drug increases (Derlet & Heischober, 1990). These dosage levels would be fatal to the inexperienced user.

Amphetamine Abuse

Patterns of Amphetamine Abuse

In certain circles, the amphetamines are popular drugs of abuse. One study showed that methamphetamine was the preferred CNS stimulant for 80% of the adolescents in treatment (Derlet & Heischober, 1990). Not infrequently, the amphetamines have been known to have been abused by college students, especially around the final examination period. Long-distance truck drivers have been known to use illicit amphetamines to enable them to drive for longer periods of time and with fewer rest stops than they could normally accomplish on their own.

The abuse of amphetamines even extends to medical schools, although this fact is not advertised by the faculty. Conrad, Hughes, Baldwin, Achenback, and Sheehan (1989) conclude that approximately 50% of the medical students in the 1960s used amphetamines to remain awake at some point in their medical school or internship. However, with increasing restrictions on the manufacture of amphetamines, Conrad et al. conclude that medical students might be turning to the use of cocaine to help them meet the demands of their training in the 1980s and 1990s.

At present, evidence suggests that the amphetamines are becoming increasingly popular as drugs of abuse. The pendulum appears to be swinging away from cocaine, back toward the stimulant of the 1960s: the amphetamines.

Complications of Amphetamine Abuse

Effects on the Central Nervous System

As noted earlier, the amphetamines appear to have their strongest impact on the central nervous system. High dosage levels of amphetamines can result in confused behavior, irritability, fear, suspicion, drug-induced hallucinations, and delusions (Julien, 1992; King & Ellinwood, 1992). Chronic abusers of the amphetamines may also experience periods of confusion, assaultiveness, irritability, weakness, insomnia, anxiety, delirium, paranoid hallucinations, panic states, and suicidal and homicidal tendencies (Derlet & Heischober, 1990). Derlet and Heischober recommend the use of haloperidol and diazepam to control the agitation and delusions that often accompany amphetamine abuse.

The chronic use of amphetamines seems to contribute to the development of extreme sensitivity to anxiety states (Satel, Kosten, Schuckit, & Fischman, 1993). The drug-induced anxiety and panic attacks may persist for months or even years after the last actual use of amphetamines. Satel et al. propose that these drug-related anxiety and panic attacks may be intensified if the individual again abuses CNS stimulants.

Satel et al. also cite research suggesting that chronic amphetamine users may experience sleep disturbances for up to 4 weeks after the last use of the drug. They also cite evidence indicating that chronic amphetamine users may have abnormal EEG tracings (a measure of the electrical activity in the brain) for up to 3 months after their last use of the drug.

It is not uncommon for both new and chronic amphetamine abusers to experience a psychotic reaction. In its earlier stages, the amphetamine-induced psychosis is often indistinguishable from schizophrenia (Kaplan & Sadock, 1990). This drug-induced state often includes confusion, suspiciousness, hallucinations, and delusional thinking, as well as episodes of violence. In contrast to actual schizophrenia, however, the hallucinations experienced by an individual suffering from an amphetamine psychosis tend to be mainly visual (Kaplan and Sadock, 1990). Kaplan and Sadock also note that the amphetamine-induced hyperactivity and absence of a thought disorder helps distinguish an amphetamine psychosis from actual schizophrenia.

Under normal conditions, this drug-induced psychosis clears up within days after the drug is discontinued (Schuckit, 1989; Kaplan & Sadock, 1990). In some cases, however, this drug-induced psychosis may require weeks or months to clear up. On occasion, the amphetamine-induced psychosis seems to become permanent. At one time, it was thought that the amphetamines essentially brought on a latent schizophrenia in a person who was vulnerable to this condition, and that the psychosis would have manifested itself even if the person had not used amphetamines. But the amphetamines are now known to be able to cause a drug-induced psychosis even in essentially normal people.

Prolonged use of the amphetamines may also result in a condition known as *formication*, which is the sensation of having unseen insects crawling either on or just under the skin (*Harvard Medical School Mental Health Letter*, 1990; Siegel, 1991). Both amphetamine and cocaine addicts may develop this condition. Victims have been known to scratch or burn the skin in an attempt to rid themselves of these nonexistent bugs.

Fatigue and depression follow prolonged periods of amphetamine use, and the depression often reaches suicidal proportions (Slaby, Lieb, & Tancredi, 1981). Amphetamine-induced feelings of depression can last for extended periods of time, possibly for *months*, following cessation of amphetamine use.

Research evidence now exists suggesting that the chronic use of amphetamines might cause actual physical damage to the cells of the brain, which in turn affects how the brain functions. The exact mechanism by which the chronic use of amphetamines are able to cause a "sustained neurophysiologic change" (Gawin & Ellinwood, 1988, p. 1178) in the user's brain is not clear. Animal research indicates that chronic use of amphetamines changes blood flow patterns within the brain, and King and Ellinwood (1992) warn that "chronic amphetamine users are at high risk for cerebrovascular damage" (p. 255).

The exact mechanism through which the amphetamines are able to bring about changes in the blood flow pattern within the brain is not clear. However, one possibility is that, because amphetamine abuse can produce hypertensive episodes, it is possible that the rapid changes in blood pressure levels might damage the blood vessels in the brain. This is certainly the mechanism through which an individual experiences a cerebral hemorrhage (a "stroke") (Brust, 1992; King & Ellinwood, 1992); these strokes destroy some blood vessels and disrupt normal blood flow patterns in the brain.

The amphetamines are emotionally, and possibly physically, addictive. Although there *is* evidence that most amphetamine users will not become addicted (Gawin & Ellinwood, 1988), the potential is there for every person who uses amphetamines. Thus, nobody is able to predict who will become addicted to amphetamines.

A possible complication of amphetamine use is that the periods of drug-induced euphoria experienced during the amphetamine "binge" may create "vivid, long-term memories" (Gawin & Ellinwood, 1988, p. 1175). These memories, in turn, form part of the foundation of the craving that many amphetamine users report when they stop using the drug. The recovery process from prolonged amphetamine use follows the same pattern seen for cocaine, and this "euphoric recall" is a very real problem for recovering abusers.

Effects on the Digestive System

The consequences of prolonged amphetamine use include the drug-induced psychosis mentioned earlier as well as various complications that arise from neglecting dietary requirements or going for extended periods of time without adequate sleep. Vitamin deficiencies are a common consequence of chronic amphetamine abuse (Gold & Verebey, 1984). Prolonged use of the amphetamines may also result in vomiting, anorexia, and diarrhea (Kaplan & Sadock, 1990).

Effects on the Cardiovascular System

The amphetamines have the potential to cause chest pain (angina), atrial and ventricular arrhythmias, myocardial ischemia (Lange, White, & Robinson, 1992; Derlet & Heischober, 1990) and myocardial infarction (Packe, Garton, & Jennings, 1990). When abused, both the amphetamines, and cocaine (as we will discuss in the next chapter) may cause a spasm in the coronary arteries at a time when the heart's workload is increased by the drug's effects on the rest of the body (Hong, Matsuyama, & Nur, 1991; Packe, Garton, & Jennings, 1990). Often, the result is a heart attack that may prove fatal.

Other Consequences of Amphetamine Abuse

Like the narcotics addict, the intravenous user of amphetamines, if he or she fails to use proper sterile techniques, runs the risk of a number of different infections, including (but not limited to) endocarditis, hepatitis, malaria, and the virus that causes AIDS (Jenike, 1991).

When they are abused, the amphetamines have a toxic effect on the user and ultimately may prove fatal. However, as noted earlier in this

chapter, there is a wide variation in what might be considered a "toxic" dose of amphetamine (Julien, 1992). Once they have developed tolerance to the euphoric effects of the amphetamines, chronic abusers have been known to use a total of up to 15,000 mg/day in divided doses (Derlet & Heischober, 1990). Some "speed runs," or extended periods of continual amphetamine use, have been known to last for a number of days, during which time the user injects a new dose of amphetamines perhaps as often as every few minutes.

The Treatment of Amphetamine Abuse

Because the effects of the CNS stimulants are similar to the effects of cocaine in many ways, it should not be surprising that the treatment of CNS stimulant abuse is very similar to that of cocaine abuse. For this reason, the treatment of amphetamine abuse will be discussed in Chapter 9, along with treatment of CNS stimulants and cocaine.

Although the amphetamines have been abused for several generations, new forms of the drug have been introduced in an attempt to entice new users. In the next two sections, we will discuss two of the latest forms of amphetamine to be introduced into the United States; ice and cat.

"Ice"

In the late 1970s, a new form of methamphetamine known as ice was reported on the mainland United States for the first time. Ice is a colorless, odorless, form of concentrated crystal methamphetamine that resembles a chip of ice or clear rock candy. Some samples of ice sold on the street have been up to 98 to 100% pure amphetamine (Kaminski, 1992). Since its introduction, ice has become quite popular in some regions of the United States (Kaminski, 1992; *Playboy*, 1990). It is often sold on the streets as a "safe" alternative to crack cocaine (*Mayo Clinic*

Health Letter, 1989). Other names for ice include "glass," "crystal" (*The Economist*, 1989), or "batu" (Kaminski, 1992).

Apparently, ice was brought to Hawaii from Japan by Army troops just after World War II, and its use was endemic to Hawaii for many years (*Health News*, 1990). Police and drug abuse professionals now believe that ice may have reached the mainland United States in the late 1970s or early 1980s (*The Economist*, 1989). However, this form of methamphetamine did not gain much notoriety until the news media began to give the drug a certain prestige by reporting its effects and dangers.

Although it is between two and three times as expensive as crack, ice has become a popular drug of abuse both in Hawaii and on the mainland United States. Its use was once thought to be limited to the West Coast (Siegel, 1991), but there is evidence that ice has become commonly available on the streets of Texas and Florida and is spreading across the country (Gold, 1990b; *The Economist*, 1989). However, the feared "ice storm," or epidemic of ice use, predicted to take place never materialized (*Brown University Digest of Addiction Theory and Application*, 1994; *Forensic Drug Abuse Advisor*, 1994d).

How Ice Is Used

Ice is smoked in a manner similar to crack. Like crack, the drug crosses through the lungs into the blood and reaches the brain in a matter of seconds. However, whereas the "high" from crack lasts perhaps 20 minutes, the effects of ice last significantly longer. Estimates of the duration of the ice's effects range from 8 hours (*Playboy*, 1990) to 12 hours (*Minneapolis Star-Tribune*, 1989; *Health News*, 1990) to 14 hours (*The Economist*, 1989), to 18 hours (McEnroe, 1990), to 24 hours (Evanko, 1991), to as long as 30 hours (Kaminski, 1992). Although the exact duration of the effects is obviously in some dispute, their extended length is consistent with the pharmacological properties of the amphetamines. The stimulant effects of the amphetamines generally last for hours, whereas cocaine's stimulant effects usually last for a shorter period of time.

How Ice Is Produced

This form of methamphetamine is manufactured in clandestine laboratories. However, unlike crack, which must be processed from cocaine smuggled into the country, methamphetamine can be manufactured from chemicals legally purchased from any chemical supply store (Siegel, 1991).

Street addicts have found that ice has several advantages over crack cocaine. Dose for dose, ice is actually cheaper than crack cocaine and, because of its duration of effect, *seems* more potent than crack. Because ice melts at a lower temperature than crack, it does not require as much heat to use and so can be smoked without elaborate equipment. Furthermore, because it is odorless, ice can be smoked in public without alerting passersby that it is being used. Another advantage of ice is that, if the user stops smoking for a moment or two, ice will cool and reform as a crystal. This makes it highly transportable and offers an advantage over crack cocaine, in that only a piece of the drug can be used rather than having to use it all at once.

Complications of Ice Abuse

Although it is often sold as a safe alternative to crack, there have been reports of fatal overdoses of ice (*Mayo Clinic Health Letter*, 1989; *Health News*, 1990). Indeed, researchers have discovered that the complications of ice abuse parallel those of methamphetamine abuse, which is understandable given that ice is simply a form of methamphetamine. However, ice users may ultimately use dosage levels up to *150* or even *1,000 times the maximum recommended therapeutic dosage* for methamphetamine (Hong, Matsuyama, & Nur, 1991). These dosage levels are potentially toxic and may prove lethal. Some of the known consequences of methamphetamine abuse include kidney and/or lung damage, permanent damage to the structure of the brain itself (*Health*

News, 1990), pulmonary edema, vascular spasm, cardiomyopathy, drug-induced psychotic reactions, and acute myocardial infarction (heart attack) (Hong, Matsuyama, & Nur, 1991).

It now appears that the addiction potential of ice is at least as great as crack's, if not greater (*Health News*, 1990). But ice is not the last word in CNS stimulants. A new CNS stimulant has been gaining in popularity in this country even as ice spreads outward from the West Coast to the rest of the United States. This latest arrival is methcathinone.

"Cat"

The CNS stimulant known as methcathinone, or "cat," is a member of the cathinone family of chemicals, which are found naturally in several species of plants from Africa (Goldstone, 1993). The chemical structure of methcathinone is similar to that of the amphetamine family of chemicals, although drug users who have tried cat report that its effects last longer. Some addicts have reported that the effects of cat last for up to 6 days, according to Goldstone.

Cat is easily synthesized by illicit laboratories, using chemicals that can be purchased legally in the United States, including drain cleaner and epsom salts. The use of cat was limited to the former Soviet Union for many years, but in the early 1990s, the drug surfaced in parts of the United States. Illicit laboratories producing cat have been found in Michigan, Wisconsin, Illinois, Missouri, and Ohio.

Because this is a "new" drug, very little is known about cat's effects on the user. Adverse effects include drug-induced psychotic reactions, agitation, hyperactivity, a strong, offensive body odor, and depression. Death has been known to occur, although the exact mechanism of death has not been identified. In 1994, the chemical was declared a controlled substance, and its manufacture thus became illegal.

Summary

Although they had been discovered in the 1880s, the amphetamines were first introduced as a treatment for asthma some 50 years later, in the 1930s. The early forms of amphetamine were sold over the counter in cloth covered ampoules that were used in much the same way as smelling salts are used today. Within a short time, however, it was discovered that the ampoules were a source of concentrated amphetamine that could be injected. The resulting "high" was similar to that of cocaine but with the added "benefit" of lasting much longer.

The amphetamines were used extensively both during and after World War II. Following the war, U.S. physicians prescribed amphetamines for the treatment of depression and as an aid for weight loss. By 1970, amphetamines accounted for 8% of all prescriptions written. However, in the time since then, physicians have come to understand that the amphetamines present a serious potential for abuse. They have come under increasingly strict controls, limiting their manufacture and distribution.

Unfortunately, the amphetamines are easily manufactured, and there has always been an underground manufacture and distribution system for these drugs. In the late 1970s and early 1980s, street drug users drifted away from the amphetamines, to the supposedly safe stimulant of the early 1900s, cocaine. But recent evidence suggests that the pendulum has started to swing back in the opposite direction. A new generation has discovered the amphetamines, and these new users have not learned the dangers of amphetamine abuse so painfully discovered by amphetamine users of two or three decades ago: "speed" kills.

CHAPTER NINE

Cocaine

As we discussed in Chapter 8, the CNS stimulants include the amphetamines and amphetaminelike drugs, such as ephedrine and Ritalin. Although cocaine shares many characteristics of the CNS stimulants, it is also a unique drug of abuse in many ways. In this chapter, we will discuss the ways that cocaine is both similar to and different from the amphetamines.

A Brief Overview of Cocaine

Cocaine is obtained from the coca bush *Erythroxylon coca*, which grows naturally in the higher elevations of Peru, Bolivia, and Java (DiGregorio, 1990). The high mountains of South America are barely habitable, in part because the thin atmosphere makes it difficult to work for extended periods of time. However, thousands of years ago, natives learned that chewing the leaves of the coca plant reduced their feelings of fatigue, thirst, and hunger, making it possible for them to work in the high mountains (White, 1989). Cocaine use rapidly became a part of everyday life in South America.

Before the Spanish conquistadores invaded Peru in the sixteenth century, cocaine was used in religious ceremonies, as part of the burial ritual (Byck, 1987), and as a medium of exchange (Ray & Ksir, 1993). However, its use was generally reserved for the upper classes. After the Spanish conquistadores overpowered the

Incas (Mann, 1994), the practice of chewing cocaine became widespread throughout South America, especially after the Spanish landlords discovered that native workers were more productive when allowed to chew cocaine leaves.

The practice of chewing coca leaves, or drinking a form of "tea" brewed from the leaves, has continued to the present. Modern natives of the mountain regions of Peru chew the leaves mixed with lime obtained from sea shells (White, 1989). The lime works with saliva to release the cocaine from the leaves and helps reduce the bitter taste of the coca leaf. Chewing coca leaves is also thought to help the chewer absorb some of the phosphorus, vitamins, and calcium contained in the mixture (White, 1989). Thus, although its primary use is to help the natives work more efficiently at high altitudes, there may also be some small nutritional benefit obtained from the practice of chewing coca leaves.

There is some dispute as to whether the natives who chew coca leaves become addicted to the stimulant effect of the cocaine. Jaffe (1990) notes that the natives of Peru who chew cocaine on a regular basis "appear to have little difficulty in discontinuing use of the drug when they move to lower altitudes" (p. 541), perhaps because chewing the leaves is a rather inefficient method of abusing cocaine. On the other hand, Byck (1987) found that "appreciable blood levels" of cocaine can be achieved through the oral use of cocaine, concluding that "coca chewers are *de facto* users" (p. 4). Thus, the question of whether natives who chew coca leaves are addicted to cocaine has not been resolved.

What *is* clear is that the reason for growing coca plants in South America has changed in the last few decades. Since cocaine became a popular drug of abuse in the 1970s, the majority of the coca plants grown in South America have been grown expressly for the international cocaine trade (Mann, 1994). Only a small minority of the coca bushes grown are cultivated for native use or to meet the needs of medicine.

Cocaine in Recent History

Although cocaine was used in South America for thousands of years, the active agent of cocaine was isolated only in 1859[1] by Albert Neiman (Scaros, Westra, & Barone, 1990). Following the isolation of the drug, European researchers began to concentrate large amounts of relatively pure cocaine for human use. The newly developed hypodermic needle also made it possible to introduce cocaine directly into the bloodstream for the first time. The combination of the hypodermic needle and large amounts of relatively pure cocaine was to prove to be a dangerous one.

During the late 1800s, Sigmund Freud experimented with the drug, at first thinking it a cure for depression[2] (Rome, 1984). During that time, cocaine, like most medicines, was easily available without a prescription. Freud also considered cocaine a possible "cure" for the withdrawal symptoms associated with opiate addiction (Lingeman, 1974; Byck, 1987). However, when Freud discovered the drug's previously unsuspected addictive potential, he discontinued his research on cocaine.

In the late 1800s and early 1900s, cocaine found its way into a wide variety of products and medicines, often without it being listed on

the label as an active ingredient. The new drink "Coca-cola," introduced by John S. Pemberton, was one of many beverages and elixirs that contained cocaine (Mann, 1994; White, 1989). There were periodic epidemics of cocaine abuse, in Europe between 1886 and 1891, in both Europe and the United States between 1894 and 1899, and again in the United States between 1921 and 1929. The use of cocaine in so many patent medicines, combined with fears over its supposed "narcotic" qualities, prompted the passage of the Pure Food and Drug Act of 1906 (Mann, 1994), requiring that makers list the ingredients of a patent medicine or elixir on the label. As a result of this law, cocaine was removed from many patent medicines.

The Harrison Narcotics Act of 1914 prohibited nonmedical cocaine use in the United States (Derlet, 1989). This act, in combination with the isolation of the United States during World War I and World War II and the introduction of the amphetamines in the 1930s, served to virtually eliminate cocaine use in the United States. It did not surface again as a major drug of abuse in the United States until the late 1960s. By then, cocaine had the reputation of being the "champagne of drugs" (White, 1989, p. 34) for those who could afford it. Those who could not afford it were interested in learning more about this "wonder drug," and cocaine again became increasingly popular as a recreational stimulant.

There are many reasons cocaine became so popular in the late 1960s. First, the bitter lessons about the dangers of cocaine use that had been learned in the late 1800s and early 1900s were either forgotten or dismissed by physicians as "moralistic exaggerations" (Gawin & Ellinwood, 1988, p. 1173). Secondly, there was a growing disillusionment with the amphetamines as recreational drugs. The amphetamines had acquired a reputation as known killers. Also, for better or worse, cocaine had the reputation of being able to bring about many of the same sensations caused by amphetamine use. The mistaken belief that cocaine was a nonaddicting substitute for the amphetamines,

---

[1]Schuckit (1989) reports that cocaine was isolated in 1857, rather than 1859.

[2] Surprisingly, recent research (Post, Weiss, Pert, & Uhde, 1987) has cast doubt on the antidepressant properties of cocaine.

combined with its reputation as a glamorous drug and the increasing restrictions on the manufacture of amphetamines, all served to once more focus attention on cocaine as an attractive recreational drug.

As a result, cocaine became increasingly popular in different parts of the world from the 1960s to the mid-1980s. In fact, cocaine use was on the increase in other parts of the world long before it reached the United States. But drug use trends in the United States are often different from those in other parts of the world. In the 1970s, the practice of smoking coca paste popular in South America did not gain much interest in the United States. Cocaine dealers, eager to find new markets for their "product," struggled to find a form of cocaine that was easily prepared and easily smoked, without the elaborate equipment necessary to make cocaine "freebase" (*U.S. News & World Report*, 1991). The result was "crack" cocaine, which became popular in the 1980s.

The popularity of cocaine as a drug of abuse seems to have peaked sometime around 1986, and casual cocaine use continues to be on the decline at this time (Kleber, 1991). However, cocaine abuse has by no means disappeared, and a significant number of people continue to use this chemical.

Current Medical Uses of Cocaine

Cocaine is not just a drug of abuse. Although it is a potent CNS stimulant, it is also an effective local anesthetic. This property of cocaine was discovered approximately 100 years ago (Mann, 1994; Byck, 1987). Cocaine is thought to function as a local anesthetic by blocking the nerve signals, or impulses, of the peripheral nerves. Applying cocaine at the proper point will change the electrical potential of these peripheral nerves, preventing them from passing on pain impulses to the brain.

Because of its anesthetic effects, cocaine was once commonly used as a topical analgesic for medical procedures involving the ear, nose,

throat, rectum, and vagina. The onset of cocaine's analgesic action is approximately 1 minute, with a duration of effect that may last as long as 2 hours (Shannon, Wilson, & Stang, 1992). Cocaine was also included in a mixture called Brompton's cocktail, which was used to control the pain of cancer. However, this mixture has fallen out of favor and is rarely, if ever, used today (Scaros, Westra, & Barone, 1990).

As a pharmaceutical, cocaine's usefulness is limited by its often undesirable side effects. Physicians have found a number of other chemicals that offer the advantages of cocaine without its side effects or potential for abuse. Today, cocaine "has virtually no clinical use" (House, 1990, p. 41), although on rare occasions it is still used by physicians to control pain.

The Scope of the Problem of Cocaine Abuse and Addiction

The United States is still the world's largest consumer of cocaine, an "honor" this country has held for many years (Sabbag, 1994). *USA Today* (1994) estimates that 303 tons of pure cocaine are consumed annually in the United States, at an estimated expense of $18 billion (*Alcoholism & Drug Abuse Week*, 1991b) to $100 billion (Will, 1993) each year.

One would expect that, because casual cocaine abuse peaked in the mid-1980s, the total *amount* of cocaine used in the United States has declined since then. Surprisingly, the amount of cocaine consumed each year in the United States has remained at about the mid-1980 level (*Minneapolis Star-Tribune*, 1994; Gold & Palumbo, 1991). This apparent contradiction is explained by the fact that whereas there are fewer casual cocaine users, there has been an increase in the number of heavy cocaine users. If the 1994 estimate offered by *USA Today* is accurate, then cocaine users in the United States have consumed approximately 303 tons of the drug each year for about the last decade.

Estimates vary as to the scope of the problem of cocaine abuse and addiction. At least

30,000,000 Americans have at least tried cocaine at some point in their lives (DiGregorio, 1990; House, 1990), but only a small percentage of this number continue to use cocaine. Estimates of the number of current cocaine users in the United States range from 1.6 million (Angell & Kassifer, 1994) to 1.9 million (Kaplan, Sadock, & Grebb, 1994) people. This estimate is somewhat lower than the recent estimate offered by the RAND Corporation, which concludes that there are currently 1.7 million heavy users and 5.3 million light users of cocaine in the United States (*Alcoholism & Drug Abuse Week*, 1994b). "Heavy" users, defined as those who use cocaine at least once a week, are thought to consume *eight times* as much cocaine as do light users, according to the RAND Corporation. Although Gawin, Khalsa, and Ellinwood (1994) did not try to estimate the number of casual cocaine users in the United States, they did estimate that there are 1 million cocaine addicts in this country today.

Thus, there is presently no clear picture as to the number of people who are using cocaine, the way they are using cocaine, or how often they do so. About all that researchers agree on is that the casual use of cocaine in the United States seems to have peaked in the mid-1980s, and the number of casual cocaine users has been declining ever since. But, as these figures suggest, cocaine remains a significant part of the U.S. drug abuse problem.

The Pharmacology of Cocaine

Cocaine hydrochloride is a water-soluble drug, which diffuses into the general circulation after it enters the body. From there, it is rapidly transported to the brain and other blood-rich organs such as the heart. Within the brain, cocaine focuses its effects on the regions that use *dopamine* as a major neurotransmitter, including the region of the brain known as the *ventral tegmentum* (Restak, 1994). The ventral tegmentum communicates with the *nucleus accumbens*, the area of the brain known to be intimately involved in the experience of pleasure. Researchers are not exactly sure how, but apparently when cocaine reaches the ventral tegmentum, it causes a massive discharge of the neurotransmitter dopamine along the nerve pathways that communicate with the nucleus accumbens (Restak, 1994; Beitner-Johnson & Nestler, 1992).

But cocaine does not just cause the release of dopamine; it also blocks a process known as *reabsorption*. Neurotransmitter reabsorption is one method by which the individual neuron "deactivates" a neurotransmitter that has been released. Normally, the process of neurotransmitter release and reabsorption results in a pattern of "on–off" firing of the neurons along the nerve pathway. But when cocaine is present, once the dopamine supplies have been released, their reabsorption is blocked.

Thus, cocaine is able to cause a biphasic response by the neurons in the brain. First, the neurons in the ventral tegmentum region release their stores of dopamine in response to the arrival of cocaine in the brain. Then, cocaine blocks the reabsorption of the dopamine after it has been released. Through this mechanism, cocaine is thought to "flood" the nerve pathways in the nucleus accumbens with the neurotransmitters that activate the pleasure center of the brain.

The *diencephalon* is another subunit of the brain affected by cocaine. The diencephalon is responsible for temperature regulation. Cocaine use causes a higher than normal body temperature. At the same time that cocaine alters the brain's temperature regulation system, it causes the constriction of surface blood vessels. This combination of effects results in hyperthermia, or excess body heat, because the body conserves heat just when it needs to release the excess thermal energy caused by the cocaine-induced dysregulation of body temperature. This is the mechanism through which cocaine-induced hyperthermia may prove dangerous, or even fatal (Hall, Talbert, & Ereshefsky, 1990).

After periods of chronic abuse, the neurons within the brain will have released virtually all their stores of the neurotransmitter dopamine.

Unfortunately, low dopamine levels is thought to be one factor involved in the development of depressive disorders. Thus, pharmacologically, chronic cocaine use may induce a state of depression by depleting the dopamine levels in the brain.

Furthermore, tolerance to cocaine may develop within "hours or days" (Schuckit, 1989, p. 99). As tolerance develops, the individual requires more and more cocaine to achieve the same effect initially experienced at a lower dosage level. This urge to increase the dosage and continue using the drug can reach the point where it "may become a way of life and users become totally preoccupied with drug-seeking and drug-taking behaviors" (Siegel, 1982, p. 731).

Some cocaine abusers have been known to routinely administer huge amounts of cocaine in a day's time to counteract their tolerance to the drug's effects (Schuckit, 1989). Siegel (1982) reports that some cocaine users ingest as much as 30 grams (there are 1,000 mg per gram) in a day, using the cocaine as frequently as once every 5 minutes. It should be pointed out that these dosage levels are quite toxic and could be fatal to the "naive" drug user.

Cocaine's effects are very short-lived. For example, when cocaine is injected intravenously, the peak plasma levels are reached in just 5 minutes, and the effects begin to diminish in 20 to 40 minutes (Weddington, 1993). One reason the effects of intravenously administered cocaine are so short-lived is that the human body begins to metabolize cocaine quite rapidly. In the normal adult, the half-life of intravenously administered cocaine is only between 30 to 90 minutes (Julien, 1992).

About 90% of a dose of intravenously administered cocaine is biotransformed into one of two different metabolites, either *benzoylecgonine* or *ecogonine methyl ester;* only about 10% of a dose of cocaine is excreted from the body unchanged (Cone, 1993). Surprisingly, cocaine will "autometabolize"; that is, the body will continue to biotransform the cocaine in the blood even after the user has died. Thus, a postmortem blood sample may not reveal any measurable amount of cocaine in the blood, even in cases where the user was known to have used cocaine prior to his or her death.

There was a time when mental health professionals thought that cocaine was not addictive. Given the impact of the cocaine use epidemic of the 1980s, there is no question that a person can become addicted to cocaine. Gold and Verebey (1984) termed cocaine "deceptively addictive" (p. 720), and Kirsch (1986) called crack cocaine "extraordinarily addictive" (p. 47).

How Cocaine is Produced

Byrne (1989b) and White (1989) have outlined the steps involved in producing cocaine for sale on the streets in the United States. First, the cocaine leaves are harvested. In some parts of Bolivia, this may be done as often as once every 3 months, as the climate is well suited for the plant's growth. Second, the leaves are dried, usually by letting them sit in the open sunlight for a few hours or days. Byrne (1989b) reports that, although technically illegal, cocaine is openly set out to dry in some parts of Bolivia.

The third step in the production of cocaine begins when the dried leaves are put in a plastic lined pit and mixed with water and sulfuric acid (White, 1989). After the mixture is crushed by workers, who wade into the pit in their bare feet, diesel fuel and bicarbonate are added. After a period of time, during which workers reenter the pit several times to continue to stomp through the mixture, the liquids are drained off. Lime is then mixed with the residue, forming a paste (Byrne, 1989b), the cocaine base. It takes 500 kilograms of leaves to produce 1 kilogram of cocaine base (White, 1989).

The fourth step begins when water, gasoline, acid, potassium permanganate and ammonia are added to the cocaine paste. This forms a reddish brown liquid, which is then filtered. A few drops of ammonia added to the mixture produces a milky solid, which is then filtered and dried. The fifth step begins when the dried cocaine base is dissolved in a solution of hydrochloric acid and acetone. A white solid forms, which settles to the bottom of the tank (Byrne, 1989b; White, 1989). This solid material is the compound cocaine hydrochloride.

In the sixth step, the cocaine is filtered, and dried under heating lights, causing it to form a white, crystalline powder. This is gathered up, packed and shipped, usually in kilogram packages (there are 2.4 pounds in a kilogram). Before each kilogram is repackaged for sale on the street, it is diluted either with mannitol or a local anesthetic, such as lidocane (Byrne, 1989b). The cocaine is then packaged in 1-gram units and sold to individual users. For more information about how street drugs are adulterated, see Chapter 33.

How Cocaine Is Used

Cocaine may be used in a number of ways. Cocaine hydrochloride powder can be inhaled through the nose (intranasal use, or "snorting"). It can also be injected directly into a vein (intravenous injection). Cocaine hydrochloride is a water soluble form of cocaine and thus is well adapted to either intranasal or intravenous use (Sbriglio & Millman, 1987). Cocaine "base" can also be smoked or taken orally ("sublingually"). We will examine each of these methods of cocaine use in detail.

Intranasal Inhalation

When cocaine is to be snorted, the powder is diced up, usually with a razor blade, on a piece of glass or mirror. The powder is then usually arranged on the glass in thin lines, 3 to 5 cm long, each of which contains between 25 and 100 mg of cocaine (Strang, Johns, & Caan, 1993). These are the "lines" referred to by users. The powder is then inhaled through a drinking straw or rolled paper.

When it reaches the nasal passages, which are richly supplied with blood vessels, the cocaine is quickly absorbed. It gains rapid access to the bloodstream, usually in 30 to 90 seconds (House, 1990), where it is carried to the brain. Only about 5% of the available cocaine is actually absorbed when cocaine powder is snorted (Strang, Johns, & Caan, 1993). This is because cocaine's vasoconstrictive action at the site of entry reduces the blood flow to the nasal tissues, limiting the absorption of the drug.

When cocaine powder is administered intranasally, the effects gradually build for about 30 minutes, after which the effects gradually decline over the next hour or so (Strang, Johns, & Caan, 1993). As we will discuss in the section on intravenous cocaine abuse and cocaine smoking, the effects of intranasal cocaine use are quite different from these other methods of drug administration.

Intravenous Injection

Cocaine can be introduced directly into the body through intravenous injection. Cocaine hydrochloride powder is mixed with water and then injected into a vein, where it rapidly reaches the brain. Intravenous administration results in 20 times as much cocaine reaching the brain as in intranasal cocaine use (Strang, Johns, & Caan, 1993). And when injected, the cocaine reaches the brain in between 3 to 5 seconds (Restak, 1994) and 15 to 20 seconds (Jones, 1987).

Intravenous cocaine abusers have reported a rapid, intense feeling of euphoria called the "rush" or "flash," which is similar to a sexual orgasm, followed by a feeling of euphoria that lasts 10 to 15 minutes. This will be discussed in more detail in the section on the Effects of Cocaine. As we noted earlier, intravenously administered cocaine is biotransformed quite quickly, which is one reason its effects are so short-lived.

Sublingual Administration

This form of cocaine administration is becoming increasingly popular, especially when the hydrochloride salt of cocaine is utilized (Jones, 1987). The tissues in the mouth, especially under the tongue, are richly supplied with blood. Large amounts of the drug enter the bloodstream quickly and are transported to the brain, with results similar to those achieved through intranasal administration.

Cocaine Smoking

A major method of cocaine use involves inhaling the fumes, a process known as "freebasing." Actually, the practice of burning or smoking different parts of the coca plant dates back to at least 3000 B.C. Siegel (1982) reports that the Incas burned coca leaves at religious festivals. In the late 1800s, coca cigarettes were used to treat hay fever and opiate addiction and, by 1890, for the treatment of whooping cough, bronchitis, asthma, and a range of other conditions (Siegel, 1982).

However, the practice of smoking cocaine for recreational purposes is apparently a new phenomenon. Kirsch (1986) observed that, in the mid-1960s, it was discovered that it is easier to smoke freebase cocaine than cocaine hydrochloride. This is because the freebase form of cocaine is more volatile and decomposes less when heated. Unless conditions are just right, cocaine hydrochloride tends to turn into a liquid when heated (House, 1990), making it impossible to smoke.

To be smoked, cocaine must be transformed from its hydrochloride salt into freebase cocaine (or simply "base"). One method of transforming cocaine hydrochloride into freebase is to treat the cocaine hydrochloride with various solutions, such as ether (Siegel, 1982). The precipitated cocaine free base can then be filtered out and prepared for smoking. This process increases the concentration of the obtained powder but does not burn off all the impurities in the cocaine base (Siegel, 1982).

When heated, the freebase powder vaporizes and the user inhales the fumes, a process that allows the cocaine to take effect in just 7 seconds (Beebe & Walley, 1991). When cocaine is smoked, between 80 and 90% of the cocaine crosses over from the lungs into the general circulation. Thus, as with intravenously administered cocaine, a high concentration of the chemical quickly reaches the general circulation. Indeed, so potent are the effects of cocaine smoking that Gold and Verebey (1984) call it "tantamount to intravenous administration without the need for a syringe" (p. 714). The user experiences a "rush" or "flash" that lasts for a few moments, but the sense of euphoria that follows the "flash" will last for only about 10 minutes (Strang, Johns, & Caan, 1993).

The process of preparing cocaine freebase is quite long, dangerous, and complicated. The chemicals used to separate cocaine freebase from its hydrochloride salt are quite volatile, and there is a very real danger of explosion. As a result, smoking cocaine freebase has never become popular. Only a small proportion of those who abuse cocaine smoke freebase (Gawin, Allen, & Humblestone, 1989).

The drawbacks of freebase led to the development of new methods of separating cocaine from its hydrochloride salt and offered a new way of abusing cocaine. This "new" form of cocaine is known as "crack" or "rock." Essentially, crack is a solid chunk of cocaine base. When smoked, the solid crystals provide "an intense, wrenching rush in a matter of seconds" (Lamar, Riley, & Samghabadi, 1986, p. 16). The process is similar to that of freebase in that the crack is cocaine base, freed from its hydrochloride salt, and prepared for smoking.

However, there is a difference between the two compounds. With cocaine freebase, the *user* must obtain the freebase from the cocaine hydrochloride. This is a difficult and dangerous process, which involves a serious risk of explosion or fire. Crack, however, is prepared for smoking *before* it reaches the user, in what are known as illicit "factories." Breslin (1988) described how one crack "factory" worked:

> Curtis and his girlfriend dropped the cocaine and baking soda into the water, then hit the bottle with the blowtorch. The cocaine powder boiled down to its oily base. The baking soda soaked up the impurities in the cocaine. When cold water was added to the bottle, the cocaine base hardened into white balls. Curtis and Iris

spooned them out, placed them on a table covered with paper, and began to measure the hard white cocaine. (p. 212)

The crack produced in these illicit factories is sold in small, ready-to-use pellets. They are usually packaged in containers that allow the user one or two inhalations for a relatively low price (Beebe & Walley, 1991; Gawin, Allen, & Humblestone, 1989). For example, the price of one piece of crack, known as a "rock," is as low as $2 in some areas (*Forensic Drug Abuse Advisor*, 1994c). The low cost of crack is one reason it is so attractive to the under-eighteen crowd (Taylor & Gold, 1990; Bales, 1988).

The effects of crack, like the effects of freebase, are short-lived. The crack "rush" lasts only a matter of a few minutes, and the sense of euphoria is equally short-lived (Weddington, 1993). When the euphoria wears off, the person is tempted to use more crack to try to reachieve the initial "rush." Eventually, the user enters a period of severe postcocaine depression, as the brain's stores of dopamine are exhausted. This, in turn, encourages further use of cocaine to feel "normal" again.

Recent evidence indicates that many people are now smoking a combination of heroin and crack. The combination of these two drugs produces an intense initial "rush," followed by a longer period of lethargy and drowsiness as the effects of the heroin replace those of the shorter lasting cocaine.

Although accurate data is difficult to obtain—in part because so few people are willing to admit that they are using an illegal substance—some believe that a class distinction has evolved in terms of the *form* of cocaine being abused by different people. Cocaine *powder* is thought to be abused mainly by middle-class users, whereas *crack* is found most often in the ghetto areas. It is not clear at this time how accurate this observation is, but many drug rehabilitation counselors who work with inner-city clients maintain that they have seen this form-of-use class distinction evolve over the past decade.

Effects of Cocaine

As with many drugs of abuse, the individual's *expectancies* for cocaine influence both how its effects are interpreted and its patterns of use. Schafer and Brown (1991) found that experienced cocaine users anticipate both positive (euphoria) and negative (depression) effects from cocaine. Furthermore, experienced cocaine users expect a generalized feeling of arousal, some feelings of anxiety, and a sense of relaxation and reduced tension. Cocaine use may also result in a short-term indifference to pain and fatigue and a decrease in hunger.

Depending on how the cocaine is administered, some cocaine users report a feeling of "quick, intense euphoria" (Lingeman, 1974, p. 46) called the "rush" or the "flash." The "rush" experience has been described as so intense that "it alone can replace the sex partner of either sex" (Gold & Verebey, 1984, p. 719). Indeed, some male users have experienced spontaneous ejaculation without direct genital stimulation after either injecting or freebasing cocaine. Some cocaine users of both sexes speak of cocaine as they would a lover.

Within seconds, the initial "rush" is replaced by a period of excitation that lasts for several minutes (Siegel, 1982). During this period, the individual feels an increased sense of competence, energy (Gold & Verebey, 1984), or extreme self-confidence (Taylor & Gold, 1990). Some cocaine users feel powerful and "energized." Although there is no objective evidence that a person under the effects of cocaine actually is stronger, the user is likely to *feel* more powerful because of the effects of cocaine on the nervous system (Schuckit, 1989). This is one of the positive effects that experienced cocaine users anticipate.

The cocaine-induced euphoria might last from only a few minutes for the individual who smokes cocaine (Byck, 1987) to an estimated 20 minutes to an hour for the individual who "snorts" cocaine powder. However, no matter how the cocaine is administered, after a short period of time the effects begin to wear off.

One of the myths surrounding crack is that it is more pure than other forms of cocaine. Kirsch (1986) reports that, although crack contains the same adulterants and impurities found in cocaine, "it feels purer because smoking the concentrated alkaloid gives a more immediate, intensified rush. This happens because the smoke is absorbed into the bloodstream through the lung tissue—the most direct route to the brain" (p. 46). The "rush" obtained from crack begins almost instantly and subsides quickly. This makes the drug *seem* more pure than when cocaine is used intranasally. When "snorted," the cocaine must be absorbed through the mucous membranes of the nose, which is a slower process, and the "high" is less intense (Kirsch, 1986).

Psychological Effects of Cocaine

Cocaine causes the brain's reward system to function more easily, with less than normal stimulation. This is, needless to say, a very pleasurable experience. Current thought is that cocaine's psychological effects are brought about mainly through the release of the neurotransmitter dopamine (Beitner-Johnson & Nestler, 1992). Although cocaine also causes the release of norepinephrine and serotonin, it is not clear to what degree, if any, these neurotransmitters are involved in the sense of euphoria experienced.

Cocaine is self-reinforcing for humans; the person who uses cocaine is likely to experience pleasurable effects and want to repeat the experience again. As noted earlier, some methods of ingesting cocaine bring about an intense "rush" that has been described by several cocaine addicts in this manner: "If God made anything better, He kept it for Himself." Injecting cocaine intravenously, smoking crack, or "freebasing" cocaine provides a "rush" in just seven seconds, and this immediate reinforcement is quite powerful. After the initial "flash," the user experiences a feeling of confidence, power, and energy that lasts for about 20 to 30 minutes. To repeat this experience, the chronic cocaine user might begin a cycle of continuous cocaine use known

as a "coke run," repeatedly using cocaine every few minutes. The usual coke run lasts about 12 hours, although there have been cases of runs that lasted up to 7 days (Gawin, Khalsa, & Ellinwood, 1994).

A similar pattern is seen when animals are given unlimited access to cocaine. Animal research has demonstrated that rats who are given intravenous cocaine for pushing a bar set in the wall of their cage will do so repeatedly, ignoring food or even sex, until they die from convulsions or infection (Hall, Talbert, & Ereshefsky, 1990). This reflects just how rewarding the effects of cocaine can be.

Complications of Cocaine Abuse and Addiction

Cocaine is hardly a safe drug. Indeed, cocaine abuse holds the potential for a wide range of health problems, some of which can be fatal. Although this fact is not advertised by cocaine dealers, death from cocaine-related problems may be so rapid that "the victim never receives medical attention other than from the coroner" (Estroff, 1987, p. 25). It has been estimated that an average of 5 of every 1,000 deaths in hospital emergency rooms are caused either directly or indirectly by cocaine abuse (House, 1990).[3] Although death is the most extreme consequence of cocaine abuse, a number of other adverse effects are possible.

Addictive Potential

As we discussed in Chapter 2, not everyone who uses cocaine will become addicted, but cocaine does have a very real potential to cause physical and psychological addiction.

Depending on the method by which the individual uses the drug, however, there does appear to be a difference in the speed with which cocaine addiction will develop. Individ-

---

[3]This number does not include those individuals who die *before* reaching the hospital.

uals who "snort" cocaine may take as long as 3 to 4 years to become fully addicted to the drug (Lamar, Riley, & Samghabadi, 1986), whereas those who smoke crack may be fully addicted in only 6 to 10 weeks.

Respiratory System Dysfunctions

The cocaine user who smokes the drug may experience chest pain, cough, and damage to the bronchioles of the lungs (O'Connor, Chang, & Shi, 1992). In some cases, the alveloli of the user's lungs rupture, allowing the escape of air (and bacteria) into the surrounding tissues. This establishes the potential for infection to develop, and the escaping gas may inhibit the lung's ability to fully inflate (a "pneumothorax"). Other complications of cocaine smoking might include chronic bronchiolitis (also known as "crack lung"), pulmonary hemorrhage, and chronic inflammation of the throat (House, 1990; Taylor & Gold, 1990). Unfortunately, cocaine-induced lung damage may be irreversible.

The chronic intranasal use of cocaine can result in sore throats, inflamed sinuses, hoarseness, and occasionally a breakdown of the cartilage of the nose. Damage to the cartilage of the nose may develop after as little as 3 weeks of intranasal cocaine use (O'Connor, Chang, & Shi, 1992). Other medical problems that can result from intranasal cocaine use are bleeding from the nasal passages and the formation of ulcers in the nasal passages.

Cardiovascular System Damage

Although the exact mechanism by which cocaine affects the heart is not known, cocaine has a strong effect on the entire cardiovascular system. No matter how it is abused, cocaine can cause an irregular heartbeat (cardiac arrhythmia), which can ultimately be fatal. Other potential consequences of cocaine abuse may include severe hypertension, sudden aortic dissection, sudden dissection of the coronary arteries, tachycardia, and myocarditis (O'Connor, Chang, & Shi, 1992; Jaffe, 1990; Derlet, 1989; Schuckit, 1989).

Recently, Moliterno, Willard, Lange, Negus, Boehrer, Glamann, Landau, Rossen, Winniford, and Hollis (1994) measured the effects of cigarette smoking and cocaine abuse on coronary artery diameter. When the coronary artery diameter is reduced, its ability to carry adequate levels of blood to the heart is also reduced. Although it was generally known that cocaine increases the heart rate while simultaneously decreasing the blood flow through the coronary arteries, the degree to which cocaine use may interfere with blood flow through the coronary arteries was not known.

The authors first administered a 2 mg/kg intranasal dose of cocaine to volunteers who had agreed to participate in the study. Although this dosage level of cocaine is smaller than that typically used on the street, the authors found a temporary 7% decrease in coronary artery diameter for those individuals with no known coronary artery disease. For those individuals with coronary artery disease, however, the authors found that the cocaine caused a 9% reduction in coronary artery diameter for a period of time.

The authors then administered the same dose of cocaine to volunteers who were cigarette smokers and who had a known coronary artery disease. The results suggest that, for this subgroup, the combined effects of the tobacco and cocaine resulted in a 19% reduction in coronary artery diameter. This is a significant decrease, and it may be the mechanism through which cocaine is able to bring about a decrease in the supply of oxygen to the heart muscle at the very time that the cocaine is causing an increase in the performance demand on this same muscle tissue.

In theory, the outcome of this process, even for individuals with no known coronary artery disease, is potential damage to the heart muscle. This may explain how cocaine interferes with the heart's ability to regulate its own rhythm, which may prove fatal. However, O'Connor, Chang, and Shi (1992) point out that this theory has been challenged by other researchers, and the actual mechanism through which cocaine may induce heart damage has yet to be proved beyond a shadow of a doubt.

Different researchers have suggested that cocaine's cardiac complications are caused either by the cumulative effects of cocaine use or by impurities in the cocaine (Decker, Fins, & Frances, 1987; Isner & Chokshi, 1989). Another possible means by which cocaine affects cardiac function may be its ability to alter the release and utilization of the neurotransmitter norepinephrine (Beitner-Johnson & Nestler, 1992). Norepinephrine plays a significant role in normal cardiac function, and self-administered cocaine may interfere with the norepinephrine's action in the heart tissue.

Thus, although researchers are still not sure about the exact mechanism, there is little doubt that cocaine use is often associated with "profound cardiovascular effects such as sudden death from cardiac arrest, pericardial chest pain, myocardial infarction, hypertension, ventricular tachyarrhythmias, and angina pectoris" (Decker, Fins, & Frances, 1987, p. 464). In other words, cocaine can cause pain in the region over the heart and lower thorax (pericardial chest pain). The term *ventricular tachyarrhythmias* refers to a pattern of abnormally fast contractions of the ventricles of the heart, usually in excess of 150 contractions per minute (*Dorland's Illustrated Medical Dictionary*, 1988), which may rapidly prove fatal. A myocardial infarction is a technical term for a heart attack. In addition to the massive damage that results from a heart attack, cocaine use can also cause microinfarcts, or microscopic areas of damage to the heart muscle (Gawin, Khalsa, & Ellinwood, 1994). Accumulated microinfarcts ultimately reduce the heart's ability to function effectively and may lead to further heart problems later on.

As we will discuss later in this chapter, cocaine abuse often results in feelings of irritation or anxiety. Alcohol, tranquilizers, or marijuana are often used in conjunction with cocaine to control the agitation and anxiety that accompany cocaine use. Both marijuana and cocaine are capable of "significantly" (Barnhill, Ciraulo, & Ciraulo, 1989, p. 242) increasing the heart rate

above levels reached when either drug is used alone. Indeed, Barnhill et al. report a heart rate increase of almost 50 beats per minute in individuals under the influence of cocaine, a matter of some consequence for people with preexisting heart muscle damage.

There does not seem to be any pattern to cocaine-induced cardiovascular problems, and both first-time users and long-term cocaine abusers have suffered heart attacks. Unfortunately, there is a very real danger that any of these symptoms may "be misinterpreted as being of psychogenic etiology when it actually may signal cardiac damage resulting from remote or recent drug use" (Barnhill, Ciraulo, & Ciraulo, 1989, p. 465). Thus, there is a danger that the younger user will misinterpret his or her chest pain as a symptom of anxiety or some other psychological problem, rather than as a sign that the heart muscle is being destroyed by cocaine abuse.

Liver Damage

Medical research has discovered that a small percentage of the population simply cannot detoxify cocaine, no matter how small the dosage level. In these cases, the liver is unable to produce an essential enzyme necessary to break down the cocaine, a condition known as *pseudocholinesterase deficiency* (Gold, 1989). For these people, ingesting even a small amount of cocaine could result in serious, if not fatal, complications.

Central Nervous System Damage

Most of our knowledge of cocaine's effects comes from research on adults; virtually nothing is known about the effects of either intentional or accidental cocaine abuse by children (Mott, Packer, & Soldin, 1994). Mott et al. did find evidence indicating that cocaine abuse by children could cause seizures, possibly by lowering the seizure threshold for children already predisposed to seizures. The authors also found evidence suggesting actual neurological damage in almost 50% of the children studied. In fact, the authors found the relationship between cocaine abuse and seizures in children so strong that they recommended that *all* childhood or adolescent *first-time* seizure patients be tested for cocaine abuse.

For adults, research suggests that the chronic use of cocaine might result in brain damage. Cocaine is a potent vasoconstrictor, and this property is suspected to be one mechanism by which cocaine can cause brain damage. Pearlson, Jeffery, Harris, Ross, Fischman, and Camargo (1993) used the *single photon emission computed tomography* (SPECT) technique, a new scanning device that allows scientists to study blood flow patterns in living tissues, to document evidence of altered blood flow patterns within the frontal cortical and basal ganglia regions of the brains of chronic cocaine users.

To uncover this evidence, the authors administered a 48-mg intravenous dose of cocaine to eight volunteers, and then performed a SPECT analysis on each subject. They found reduced blood flow rates in the frontal and basal ganglia regions of the subjects' brains. The authors also found that the subjective experience of the "rush," or "high," was related to the degree of blood flow reduction. In other words, the greater the measured reduction in blood flow, the better the drug use experience was rated by the individual.

Pearlson et al. could not determine whether these blood-flow pattern changes reflected temporary or permanent changes in the vasculature of the brain. Nor could they determine the degree to which changes in blood flow patterns resulted in physical changes in the brain's structure. However, the possibility exists that this is one way that chronic cocaine use causes neurological dysfunctions.

A number of studies have contrasted the test performance of chronic cocaine users and normal subjects on a series of psychoneurological tests. For example, O'Malley, Adamse, Heaton, and Gawin (1992) found that 50% of regular cocaine abusers showed evidence of cognitive impairment on the test battery used in this study, as compared to only 15% of the control

subjects. The authors suggest that, when abused for long periods of time, cocaine may function as a neurotoxin. It is not clear whether the neurological impairment the authors found is permanent; however, this is the second study concluding that cocaine abuse may be the cause of neurological dysfunction.

Cocaine may cause brain damage through other methods as well. The vasoconstriction that is a side effect of cocaine use may result in elevated blood pressure levels. If the blood pressure level rises high enough, or if the person has a weak spot in the lining of a blood vessel, a "cerebrovascular accident" (CVA, or stroke) may result. It is in this manner that cocaine apparently causes strokes in both the brain and the spinal cord (Mendoza & Miller, 1992; Jaffe, 1990; Derlet, 1989). Depending on where the stroke occurs, the victim may die, become blind, or suffer permanent neurological impairment.

Unfortunately, chronic cocaine abusers are not the only ones susceptible to cocaine-induced strokes. A first-time user can also suffer from a cocaine-related stroke. Cocaine abusers may also experience transient ischemic attacks (TIAs) and seizures as unwanted side effects of the drug use (O'Connor, Chang, & Shi, 1992; Derlet, 1989). Cocaine-induced seizures can occur as late as 12 hours after the last cocaine use.

Animal research has suggested that, after repeated exposures to cocaine, it is possible to develop seizures at doses that previously had not brought on such convulsions. This process was termed a "pharmacological kindling" (Post, Weiss, Pert, & Uhde, 1987). Although cocaine itself may have a short half-life, "the sensitization effects are long lasting" (Post et al., p. 113).

Post et al. believe that the sensitizing effects of cocaine may thus lower the seizure threshold, at least in some individuals, and they went on to observe that "Repeated administration of a given dose of cocaine without resulting seizures *would in no way assure the continued safety of this drug even for that given individual* (1987, p. 159; emphasis added). Thus, although the *immediate* effects of cocaine may last only a short time, the body can become hypersensitive to cocaine after long periods of time. If this happens, the person could suffer serious—possibly fatal—side effects from a dosage level of cocaine that was once easily tolerated.

Impact on Emotional State and Perceptions

It has been suggested (Hamner, 1993) that cocaine abuse may exacerbate the symptoms of posttraumatic stress disorders (PTSD). The exact mechanism by which cocaine seems to be able to add to the emotional distress of PTSD is not clear at this time. However, there is evidence that individuals who suffer from PTSD may find that their distress is worsened by the psychobiological interaction between the effects of the drug and their traumatic experiences.

Also, after periods of extended cocaine use, some people have experienced "cocaine bugs," a hallucinatory experience of having bugs crawling on or just under their skin; the technical term is *formication* (*Harvard Medical School Mental Health Letter*, 1990). Patients who experience cocaine-induced formication sometimes burn their arms or legs with matches or cigarettes or scratch themselves repeatedly in an attempt to rid themselves of these imaginary bugs (Lingeman, 1974).

Cocaine has also been implicated as a causal factor of anxiety or panic reactions (DiGregorio, 1990). Indeed, Louie (1990) reports that 25% of the patients seen at one panic disorder clinic eventually admitted to using cocaine. Furthermore, up to 64% of cocaine users experience some degree of anxiety as a side effect. Some cocaine users try to ameliorate this side effect by using marijuana, benzodiazepines, narcotics, barbiturates, or alcohol.

Cocaine-induced anxiety and panic attacks may not stop immediately after the drug is discontinued. Indeed, these cocaine-induced panic attacks may continue for "months or years into the period of abstinence" (Satel, Kosten, Schuckit, & Fischman, 1993, p. 700). This is an apparent result of cocaine's ability to make the user sensitive to anxiety states.

Chronic cocaine use has also been implicated in the development of a drug-induced psychosis very similar in appearance to paranoid schizophrenia. However, there are often subtle differences between the symptoms of paranoid schizophrenia and those of a cocaine-induced psychosis, according to Rosse, Collins, Fay-McCarthy, Alim, Wyatt, and Deutsch (1994). They compared the symptoms of individuals with cocaine-induced psychoses with those of patients diagnosed as paranoid schizophrenics, and they found that patients with cocaine-induced psychoses were more suspicious of others and were profoundly afraid of being discovered or of being harmed while under the influence of cocaine. Furthermore, cocaine-induced psychosis was often marked by hypervigilance on the part of the individual.

Estimates of the scope of cocaine-induced psychotic reactions range from 53% (Decker & Ries, 1993) to 65% (Beebe & Walley, 1991) of cocaine users. This condition, known on the streets as "coke paranoia," usually clears within a few hours (Davis & Bresnahan, 1987) to a few days (Schuckit, 1989) after the person stops using cocaine. Gawin, Khalsa, and Ellinwood (1994) suggest that the delusions found in a cocaine-induced psychotic reaction usually clear after the individual's sleep pattern has returned to normal. However, on occasion, the cocaine-induced paranoid state apparently becomes permanent (Maranto, 1985).

It is not clear how chronic cocaine abuse may contribute to the development of this drug-induced psychosis. One possibility is that those individuals who develop a cocaine-induced paranoid state may possess a biological vulnerability for schizophrenia, which is then activated by chronic cocaine abuse (Satel & Edell, 1991). However, another possibility is that the individual's biological vulnerability is not for the development of schizophrenia but for the chronic use of cocaine to result in a short-lived paranoid state as an unwanted drug side effect (Satel, 1992).

Approximately 20% of the chronic users of crack cocaine in one study were reported to have experienced drug-induced periods of rage or outbursts of anger and violent assaultive behavior (Beebe & Walley, 1991). Finally, as noted earlier, either a few hours after snorting the drug, or within 15 minutes if the person has injected it, the person slides into a state of depression. After periods of prolonged cocaine use, the individual's postcocaine depression may reach suicidal proportions (Maranto, 1985). Cocaine-induced depression is thought to be the result of cocaine's depleting the nerve cells in the brain of the neurotransmitters norepinephrine and dopamine. After a period of abstinence, the neurotransmitter levels usually return to normal and the depressive episode gradually ends.

However, because suicide is a common consequence of depression (whether cocaine-induced or not) there is a very real danger that the cocaine user will attempt, or actually commit, suicide before recovering from the cocaine-induced depression. Indeed, one recent study in New York City found that *one-fifth* of all suicides involving a victim under the age of 60 were cocaine related (Marzuk, Tardiff, Leon, Stajic, Morgan, & Mann, 1992).

Withdrawal and Recovery from CNS Stimulant Abuse

Although the treatment process will be discussed in more detail in later chapters, brief mention of the treatment of addiction to CNS stimulants should be made here. Unfortunately, although a great deal is known about the manifestations of cocaine addiction, very little is known about the natural history of cocaine dependence (Jaffe, 1990). A great deal remains to be discovered about cocaine abuse and its effects on the user.

Although cocaine has a reputation of being exceptionally addictive, researchers disagree on exactly what percentage of those who use cocaine become addicted. The National Institute on Drug Abuse (quoted in Kotulak, 1992) suggests that only about 10% of those who use cocaine actually go on to become heavy users.

Restak (1994) gives a higher estimate of between 25 and 33%. Although not everybody who uses cocaine will become addicted to the drug, some people do become addicted to cocaine with terrible consequences for themselves and their families. There is no way of predicting in advance who will become addicted to cocaine. If for no other reason than this, cocaine use is to be discouraged.

For those who do abuse cocaine, or who might become addicted to it, hospital-based detoxification is rarely necessary (*Harvard Medical School Mental Health Letter,* 1990). However, hospital-based observation and treatment may be necessary to protect the individual who is depressed as a result of his or her cocaine abuse. Because cocaine-induced depression can reach suicidal proportions, the decision to hospitalize a cocaine abuser should be made on a case-by-case basis by qualified physicians. Some of the factors that must be considered include the abuser's current state of mind, his or her medical status, and whether he or she has adequate resources and social support to deal with the withdrawal process on an outpatient basis.

There has been very little research into the factors that bring about addiction to the CNS stimulants. In contrast to the research into the genetics of alcoholism, "research on genetic factors in stimulant abuse has not been pursued" (Gawin & Ellinwood, 1988, p. 1177). Thus, there is no information into possible genetic "markers" that may identify the person who is vulnerable to cocaine addiction.

Researchers do believe that protracted cocaine abuse may result in a withdrawal syndrome (Satel, Price, Palumbo, McDougle, Krystal, Gawin, Charney, Heninger, & Kleber, 1991; Hammer & Hazelton, 1984). Gawin and Ellinwood (1988) characterize the cocaine withdrawal syndrome as "comparable to the acute withdrawal of the alcohol hangover" (p. 1176). Although the cocaine withdrawal syndrome does not include "severe . . . symptoms such as those seen in opiate withdrawal" (Gold & Verebey, 1984, p. 720), research has shown that it is marked by such complaints as paranoia, depression, fatigue, "craving" for cocaine, agitation, chills, insomnia, nausea, changes in the individual's sleep patterns, ravenous hunger, muscle tremors, headache, and vomiting (DiGregorio, 1990). These symptoms begin within 24 to 48 hours after the last dose of cocaine and persist for 7 to 10 days.

Stages of Recovery

Gawin and colleagues have proposed the following triphasic model for the postcocaine binge recovery process (Gawin, Khalsa, & Ellinwood, 1994; Gawin & Kleber, 1986).

Stage 1. In the early part of the first stage, which lasts from 1 to 4 days, the person experiences feelings of agitation, depression, and anorexia (loss of desire to eat), as well as a strong craving for cocaine. As the person progresses through the second half of the first phase, they lose the craving for cocaine but experience insomnia and exhaustion combined with a strong desire for sleep. The second half of the first phase lasts from day 4 until day 7 of recovery.

Stage 2. The second phase of recovery begins 7 days after abstinence. The person returns to a normal sleep pattern and gradually experiences stronger cravings for cocaine and higher levels of anxiety. Conditioned cues exacerbate the individual's craving for stimulants, drawing the person back to chemical use. Those who can withstand the environmental and intrapersonal cues for further drug use move on to the extinction phase, gradually returning to a more normal level of function.

Stage 3. The third stage of recovery, the extinction phase, begins after 10 weeks of abstinence. If the person goes on another stimulant "binge," the cycle will repeat itself. If the person is able to withstand the drug craving, there is a good chance that he or she can achieve sobriety. For example, Hall, Havassy, and Wasserman (1991) found that approximately 80% of those cocaine addicts who were able to abstain from cocaine use for 12 weeks after treatment were still drug-free after 6 months.

However, successful completion of Stage 3 does not mean that the individual has fully recovered from cocaine addiction. Former cocaine and amphetamine addicts may suddenly experience craving for the drug "months or years after its last appearance" (Gawin & Ellinwood, 1988, p. 1176), and long after the last period of chemical use.

Satel et al. (1991) examined the cocaine withdrawal process and found data that failed to support the model advanced by Gawin and Kleber (1986). In Satel et al.'s sample, the cocaine withdrawal process was marked by mild withdrawal symptoms that declined over the first 3 weeks of inpatient treatment. These withdrawal symptoms were much milder than had been anticipated and failed to follow the triphasic model suggested by earlier research.

Although researchers agree that there appears to be a withdrawal syndrome following prolonged cocaine use, they do not agree on the exact nature of the post-cocaine withdrawal syndrome. Various theoretical models are still being explored to better understand what happens when a cocaine addict stops using chemicals. As part of this process, a number of pharmacological agents are being investigated in the hopes of finding a drug or combination of drugs that will control the postcocaine craving. These agents will be discussed in Chapter 31.

The treatment of stimulant addiction involves more than just helping the addict stop using the drug. One common complication of stimulant addiction is that the addict has often forgotten what a drug-free life is like (Siegel, 1982). Gold and Verebey (1984) also point out that cocaine addiction may lead to vitamin deficiencies, especially of the B complex and C vitamins. Because the stimulant effects of the amphetamines are so similar to those of cocaine, we would expect to see a pattern of vitamin deficiencies similar to that seen in chronic amphetamine abuse. Gold and Verebey found that 73% of a sample of cocaine abusers tested had at least one vitamin deficiency. They conclude that these vitamin deficiencies reflect the malnutrition that results from cocaine-induced anorexia. The authors recommend vitamin replacement therapy as part of the treatment of cocaine addiction.

Total abstinence from drugs of abuse is essential for the individual recovering from cocaine or amphetamine addiction, and follow-up treatment should include behavior modification and psychotherapy (Gold & Verebey, 1984). Indeed, Hall, Havassy, and Wasserman (1991) found that those cocaine addicts who made a commitment to full abstinence following treatment were more likely to avoid further cocaine use than were addicts who did not desire abstinence as a treatment goal. Social support and self-help group support in the form of Alcoholics Anonymous, Narcotics Anonymous, or Cocaine Anonymous is often of great help. As with the other forms of drug addiction, the recovering individual is at risk for cross-addiction to other chemicals and needs to avoid other drug use for the rest of his or her life.

Summary

Although man has used cocaine for hundreds, if not thousands, of years, the active agent of the coca bush was not isolated until 1859. About the same time, the intravenous needle was developed, which allowed users to inject large amounts of cocaine into the circulatory system, where it was rapidly transported to the brain. Users quickly discovered that intravenously administered cocaine brought on a sense of euphoria, which immediately made it a rather popular drug of abuse.

At the turn of the century, government regulations limited the availability of cocaine, which was mistakenly classified as a narcotic. The development of the amphetamine family of drugs in the 1930s, along with increasingly strict enforcement of the laws against cocaine use, allowed addicts to substitute legally purchased amphetamines for the increasingly rare cocaine. In time, the dangers of cocaine use were forgotten by all but a few medical historians.

In the late 1960s and early 1970s, government regulations began to limit the availability of amphetamines. Cocaine emerged as a substitute for the difficult-to-obtain amphetamines in the late 1970s and early 1980s. To entice users, new forms of cocaine were introduced, including concentrated "rocks" of cocaine known as crack. To the user of the 1980s, cocaine seemed to be a harmless drug, although historical evidence suggested otherwise.

In the 1980s, users rediscovered the dangers associated with cocaine abuse, and the drug gradually has fallen into disfavor. The most recent wave of cocaine addiction to date peaked around the year 1986, and fewer and fewer people are presently becoming addicted to cocaine. But a disturbing new trend is for drug abusers and addicts to smoke a combination of crack cocaine and heroin, probably in response to the growing threat of HIV infection through contaminated hypodermic needles and the growing availability of heroin.

This new method of drug abuse probably accounts for the recent increase in cocaine- and heroin-related emergency room admissions in the United States. Thus, it appears that cocaine will remain a part of the drug abuse problem well into the next century.

Marijuana

For many generations, marijuana has been a controversial substance of abuse, and misperceptions surrounding marijuana abound. For example, people talk about marijuana as if it were a chemical in its own right, but it's actually a plant. Over the years, people discovered that some of the chemicals contained in this plant seem to have beneficial properties, and if they smoke parts of the plant or, less often, consume it, some of the chemicals in the plant will enter their bodies.

Unlike recreational substances such as alcohol, cocaine, or the amphetamines, marijuana is not a recreational substance in the technical sense. Like tobacco, it is only a plant that happens to contain some chemicals that may be used for recreational purposes. The scientific name of this plant is *Cannabis sativa*. The cannabis plant, often known as "ditchweed," grows wild in the countryside of much of the United States. This "wild" marijuana is of very low potency and is rarely used as a recreational substance.

The marijuana most commonly used in the United States is the product of selective breeding programs carried out by illicit growers. As a result of such selective breeding programs, strains of marijuana have been developed that have high concentrations of the psychoactive chemicals that make it a popular recreational substance. Indeed, the marijuana most commonly sold on the streets is now *two and a half*

times as potent as the marijuana sold in the 1970s (American Academy of Family Physicians, 1990a).

A History of Marijuana Use in the United States

It has only been in the last century that marijuana has gone through a number of transformations. Before then, physicians considered marijuana a medicinal substance and used it to treat a number of different disorders. Indeed, the first historical references to marijuana date back to the reign of the Chinese Emperor Shen Nung (2737 B.C.), when it was used as a medicine (Scaros, Westra, & Barone, 1990). Thus, the medicinal use of marijuana has been documented as far back as "at least 5,000 years" (Denis Petro, quoted in *Health Facts*, 1991, p. 4).

Physicians in the United States and Europe used marijuana as an analgesic, hypnotic, and anticonvulsant as recently as the 19th century (Grinspoon & Bakalar, 1992). In an 1838 case, physicians used hashish to completely control the terror and "excitement" (Elliott, 1992, p. 600) of a patient who had contracted rabies. During the early part of the 20th century, researchers found that marijuana was either ineffective or less effective than many other pharmaceuticals being introduced to fight disease. As there did not appear to be any legitimate medical use for marijuana, it was removed from the doctor's pharmacopoeia.

The practice of smoking marijuana cigarettes for its psychoactive effects was apparently introduced to the United States by Mexican immigrants who had come north to find work in the 1920s (Mann, 1994). Recreational marijuana smoking was quickly adopted by others, especially jazz musicians (Musto, 1991). With the start of Prohibition, the working class turned to growing or importing marijuana as a substitute for alcohol (Gazzaniga, 1988). Its use declined with the end of Prohibition, when alcohol could once more be easily obtained, but a small minority of the population continued to use it as a recreational substance.

The passage of the Marijuana Tax Act of 1937 certainly drove marijuana use underground, but it did not eliminate it.[1] In the 1960s, marijuana again became popular and it has remained a popular recreational drug ever since. Currently, marijuana is "the most frequently used drug in the United States" (Nahas, 1986, p. 82), as well as the most commonly abused illicit chemical in Canada (Russell, Newman, & Bland, 1994) and the United Kingdom (Mathers & Ghodse, 1992).

In an interesting twist of events, however, physicians have once more started to explore whether some of the chemicals found in the marijuana plant can be of value in the fight against disease and suffering. Physicians are considering using the marijuana plant, or selected chemicals found in that plant, to control the nausea that often accompanies cancer chemotherapy and to control certain forms of glaucoma (Voelker, 1994; Jaffe, 1990). There is also limited evidence that suggests marijuana may be of value in the treatment of multiple sclerosis, rheumatoid arthritis, and possibly chronic pain conditions (*Health Facts*, 1991).

[1]Contrary to popular belief, the Marijuana Tax Act of 1937 did not make *possession* of marijuana illegal, but it *did* impose a small tax on it. A person who paid the tax would receive a stamp to show authorities that they had paid the tax. Obviously, illegal users of marijuana do not apply for the proper forms to pay the tax. The stamps are of interest to stamp collectors, however, and a few collectors have actually paid the tax to obtain the stamp for their collection.

The use of marijuana in the treatment of disease is not without controversy in the medical field. Some physicians point out that there is no evidence that marijuana is of value in the treatment of these or any other disorders (Dr. Janet Lapey, quoted in Voelker, 1994). On the other hand, advocates of the possible medicinal value of marijuana continue to point to anecdotal reports that marijuana seems to be effective in treating some of the disorders listed above. However, given its legal status, it is difficult to find many health care professionals who are willing to advocate its use or even to recommend that further research on its effects be carried out. Thus, marijuana will probably remain a controversial recreational substance for many years to come.

The Scope of the Problem

Marijuana currently is the most frequently abused illicit substance in the United States (Millman & Beeder, 1994; *The Addiction Letter*, 1993a; Abood & Martin, 1992). An estimated 67 million people in the United States have used marijuana at least once in their lives (Kaplan, Sadock, & Grebb, 1994), and 9 million are thought to be current users (Angell & Kassifer, 1994; *The Addiction Letter*, 1993a).

Marijuana is especially popular as a substance of abuse among the young. Perhaps 15 million young people use marijuana at least once a month, 9 million use it weekly, and 6 million use it daily (Mirin, Weiss, & Greenfield, 1991). The popularity of marijuana rests on the fact that a "few puffs on a joint is this generation's social martini" (Peluso & Peluso, 1988, p. 110). Because marijuana has become so much a part of the social scene, both the legal and the social sanctions against marijuana use have changed in the past 30 years. Indeed, in many states, possession of a small amount of marijuana has been decriminalized.

This does not mean that everyone who has used marijuana does so on a frequent basis. The majority of marijuana users experiment with the drug briefly and then discontinue its use. Only a minority of those who try marijuana go on to use the drug on a regular basis for an extended period of time.

The Pharmacology of Marijuana

The *Cannabis sativa* plant contains more than 400 different identified compounds, of which an estimated 61 have psychoactive properties (Restak, 1994; University of California, Berkeley, 1990b). Although marijuana's psychoactive effects have been known for many years, the main active ingredient of marijuana, THC,[2] was identified only in 1964 (Restak, 1994; Mirin, Weiss, & Greenfield, 1991; Schwartz, 1987; Bloodworth, 1987).

THC is found throughout the plant, but the highest concentrations of THC are found in the small upper leaves and flowering tops (Mirin, Weiss, & Greenfield, 1991). Technically, the term *marijuana* is used to identify the relatively weak preparations of the cannabis plant that are used for smoking or eating, whereas the term *hashish* is used to identify a preparation with a higher concentration of THC (Berger & Dunn, 1982). However, for the purpose of this chapter, we will use the generic term *marijuana* for any part of the plant that is to be smoked or ingested.

As with most chemicals of abuse, the primary site of THC metabolism is in the liver. The half-life of THC appears to vary depending on whether or not metabolic tolerance has developed. Research suggests that, in experienced users, marijuana has a half-life of about 3 days (Schwartz, 1987) to 1 week (Bloodworth, 1987). About 65% of the metabolites of THC are excreted in the feces, and the rest are excreted in the urine (Schwartz, 1987). However, the liver is not able to metabolize the THC in the body very quickly, and the unmetabolized THC binds to fat cells in the body. With repeated episodes of marijuana use over a short period of time, significant amounts of THC may be stored in

[2]THC is the abbreviation of delta-9-tetrahydrocannabinol.

the body's fat reserves. Between periods of active marijuana use, the fat-bound THC is slowly released back into the blood (Schwartz, 1987).

This process explains why heavy marijuana users can test positive for THC in urine toxicology screens weeks after their last use of the drug (Schwartz, 1987). However, this happens only with *very* heavy marijuana users. In the casual marijuana user, urine toxicology tests can detect evidence of THC for only about 3 days after the last use of the drug.

Tolerance to the effects of THC develop rapidly. To continue to achieve the initial effects, the chronic marijuana user must use "more potent cannabis, deeper, more sustained inhalations, or larger amounts of the crude drug" (Schwartz, 1987, p. 307).

In August of 1990, after a search that has taken more than a generation, a team of researchers from the National Institute of Mental Health discovered one receptor site within the brain that is used by the THC molecule (Matsuda, Lolait, Brownstein, Young, & Bonner, 1990). Researchers attempting to isolate certain neuropeptides that transmit pain signals between cells discovered a process through which THC inhibits the function of the enzyme *adenylate cyclase*, which is involved in the transmission of pain messages. Thus, by accident, researchers identified at least one of the sites within the brain where THC carries out its effects.

Since this initial discovery, researchers at the Hebrew University in Jerusalem identified a molecule within the brain that "binds" to the same receptor that THC does (Restak, 1993); they named this molecule *anandamide*. This research will open the door for further research into the nature of memory and pain perception. However, there is still a great deal to be discovered about how THC's effects are produced.

How Marijuana Is Used

In the United States, marijuana is usually smoked, although occasionally it is ingested by mouth (often baked in cookies, or brownies).

Sometimes marijuana is mixed with other substances, but it's usually smoked in the form of rolled marijuana cigarettes called "joints." Joints usually contain between 500 and 750 mg of marijuana and provide an effective dose of approximately 5 to 20 mg of THC per joint.

A variation on the marijuana cigarette is the "blunt." Blunts are made by removing one of the outer leaves of a cigar, unrolling it, filling it with high potency marijuana mixed with chopped cigar tobacco, and then rerolling the mixture into what is essentially a marijuana "cigar" (*The Addiction Letter*, 1993a). Users report some degree of stimulation, possibly from the nicotine in the cigar tobacco that enters the lungs along with the marijuana smoke.

The technique by which a marijuana joint is smoked is somewhat different than the smoking technique used for cigarettes or cigars (Schwartz, 1987). The user must inhale the smoke deeply into the lungs, then hold his or her breath for between 20 and 30 seconds to get as much THC into the blood as possible (Schwartz, 1987). Researchers disagree as to the amount of THC that is absorbed through the lungs into the blood. Scaros, Westra, and Barone (1990) suggest that about 18% of the available THC is absorbed by smoking. But Jaffe (1990) suggests that between 2 and 50% of the THC may be absorbed, depending on the individual and the exact method of smoking used.

When smoked, marijuana's effects begin almost immediately, usually within seconds (Weiss & Mirin, 1988) to perhaps 10 minutes (Bloodworth, 1987). It has been estimated that, to produce a sense of euphoria, the user must inhale approximately 25 to 50 micrograms per kilogram of body weight when marijuana is smoked, and between 50 to 200 micrograms per kilogram of body weight if the marijuana is ingested orally (Mann, 1994). Doses of 200 to 250 micrograms per kilogram smoked or 300 to 500 micrograms taken orally may cause the user to hallucinate, according to Mann.

As these figures suggest, it takes an extremely large dose of THC for the individual to halluci-nate. Marijuana users in some countries often have access to high potency sources of THC and thus may achieve hallucinatory doses. But, it is extremely rare for marijuana users in the United States to have access to such potent forms of the plant. In many parts of the country, marijuana is classified as a hallucinogenic by law enforcement officials, in spite of the fact that it rarely causes hallucinations at the dosage levels normally used in the United States.

The marijuana in use in the United States at present *will* produce a sense of euphoria, however. When it is smoked, the effects of marijuana reach peak intensity within 30 minutes and begin to decline in 1 hour (Weiss & Mirin, 1988). Estimates of the duration of the subjective effects of marijuana range from 2 to 3 hours (Brophy, 1993) up to 4 hours (Grinspoon & Bakalar, 1992; Bloodworth, 1987).

When ingested by mouth, the user absorbs only 4% to 12% of the available THC (Jaffe, 1990). The oral user also will not experience immediate effects, usually requiring 30 to 60 minutes (Mirin, Weiss, & Greenfield, 1991) to perhaps 2 hours (Schwartz, 1987) before feeling the euphoric effects of THC. Estimates of the duration of marijuana's effects when ingested orally range from 3 to 5 hours (Mirin, Weiss, & Greenfield, 1991; Weiss & Mirin, 1988) up to 5 to 12 hours (Kaplan, Sadock, & Grebb, 1994).

In terms of *immediate* lethality, marijuana could be called a "safe" drug. Psychiatrist Lester Grinspoon, long an advocate of further research into marijuana's potential medicinal value, rated marijuana as less harmful than alcohol or tobacco (Voelker, 1994). But, as we will discuss in the section "Complications of Chronic Marijuana Use," it is not without its dangers.

Based on animal research, the LD_{50} of THC is estimated to be about 125 mg/kg (Nahas, 1986). A 160-pound person weighs about 72.59 kilograms. If the typical marijuana cigarette contains 20 mg of THC, then the estimated LD_{50} for this person would be the equivalent of smoking 453 marijuana cigarettes at once. But we stated earlier in this chapter that only 2% to

50% of the THC in a marijuana cigarette is actually absorbed. If we take the high estimate of 50%, then the estimated number of marijuana cigarettes that a typical 160-pound person would have to smoke to reach the estimated LD_{50} is just over 900 marijuana cigarettes at once.

Thus, in terms of its immediate toxicity, marijuana appears to be "among the least toxic drugs known to modern medicine" (Weil, 1986, p. 47). The effective dose of THC is between 1/20,000 and 1/40,000 the lethal dose (Kaplan, Sadock, & Grebb, 1994; Grinspoon & Bakalar, 1992). As one would expect from these statistics, there has as yet never been a clearly documented case of a lethal overdose involving only marijuana (Nahas, 1986).

In contrast to the estimated 434,000 deaths each year from tobacco use and the total of 125,000 yearly fatalities from alcohol use, there are only an estimated 75 marijuana-related deaths in the United States each year. Indeed, in contrast to the toxic effects of alcohol and tobacco, most marijuana-related deaths occur in accidents that take place while the individual is under the influence of this substance, not as a direct result of any toxic effects of THC (Crowley, 1988).

The Subjective Effects of Marijuana

At moderate dosage levels, marijuana brings about a two-phase reaction (Brophy, 1993). The first phase begins shortly after the drug enters the bloodstream, when the individual experiences a period of mild anxiety, followed by a sense of well-being or euphoria and a sense of relaxation and friendliness (Kaplan & Sadock, 1990; Kaplan, Sadock, & Grebb, 1994). These subjective effects are consistent with the known physical effects of marijuana. Research has found that marijuana causes "a transient increase in the release of the neurotransmitter dopamine" (Friedman, 1987, p. 47), a neurochemical thought to be involved in the experience of euphoria.

As with many drugs of abuse, the individual's *expectations* will influence how he or she interprets the effects of marijuana. Marijuana users tend to anticipate that the drug will (1) impair cognitive function as well as the user's behavior, (2) help the user relax, (3) help the user interact socially and enhance sexual function, (4) enhance creative abilities and alter perception, (5) bring with it some negative effects, and (6) bring about a sense of food "craving" (Schafer & Brown, 1991).

Individuals who are intoxicated on marijuana report an altered sense of time as well as mood swings (Kaplan, Sadock, & Grebb, 1994) and feelings of well-being and happiness (Abood & Martin, 1992). Marijuana also seems to bring about a splitting of consciousness, in which users may experience the sensation of observing themselves while under the influence of the drug (Kaplan, Sadock, & Grebb, 1994; Grinspoon & Bakalar, 1992).

Marijuana users often report a sense of being on the threshold of a significant personal insight but are unable to put this insight into words. These reported drug-related insights seem to come about during the first phase of the marijuana reaction. The second phase of the marijuana experience begins when the individual becomes sleepy, which takes place following the acute intoxication phase (Brophy, 1993; Abood & Martin, 1992).

There are few immediate adverse reactions to marijuana (Mirin, Weiss, & Greenfield, 1991). One of the most common adverse reactions is drug-related anxiety or even full-blown panic reactions (Millman & Beeder, 1994; Kaplan, Sadock, & Grebb, 1994). Factors that seem to influence the development of marijuana-related panic reactions are the individual's prior experience with marijuana, expectations for the drug, the dosage level being used, and the setting in which the drug is used. Such panic reactions are most often seen in the inexperienced marijuana user (Mirin, Weiss, & Greenfield, 1991; Bloodworth, 1987) and usually respond to simple reassurance (Millman & Beeder, 1994; Kaplan, Sadock, & Grebb, 1994).

Occasionally, marijuana use is implicated as the cause of a drug-induced psychotic reaction. However, research suggests that marijuana use is unlikely to trigger a psychotic reaction unless the user either has previously suffered a psychotic episode or is predisposed to psychosis (Linszen, Dingemans, & Lenior, 1994; Mathers & Ghodse, 1992; Nahas, 1986). Researchers currently believe that marijuana-induced psychotic reactions are caused only by extremely heavy use of the drug (Kaplan, Sadock, & Grebb, 1994; Abood & Martin, 1992; Mathers & Ghodse, 1992).

A possible mechanism through which marijuana may contribute to the emergence of schizophrenia was suggested by Linszen, Dingemans, and Lenior (1994). The authors note that THC functions as a dopamine agonist in the nerve pathways of the region of the brain known as the *medial forebrain bundles* that use dopamine as the primary neurotransmitter. Dopamine is also the neurotransmitter implicated in schizophrenia, which suggests a link between marijuana use and the psychotic symptoms of schizophrenia.

Another form of marijuana-induced psychosis is the drug-induced *toxic psychosis*. The effects of a marijuana-induced toxic psychosis are usually short-lived and clear up in a few days to a few weeks (Millman & Beeder, 1994; Schuckit, 1989). Psychotic reactions that last longer are usually a reflection of an underlying psychotic condition rather than a drug-induced condition, according to Schuckit.

Finally, an extremely rare consequence of marijuana use is the development of an acute depressive reaction (Grinspoon & Bakalar, 1992). Marijuana-related depression is most common in the inexperienced user and may reflect the activation of an undetected preexisting depression. Grinspoon and Bakalar report that the depressive episode is usually mild and does not require professional intervention ex-

cept in rare cases. It usually clears up in less than 24 hours (Millman & Beeder, 1994).

Complications from Chronic Marijuana Use

The hemp plant from which marijuana is obtained contains some 400 different chemicals. More than 2,000 separate metabolites of these 400 chemicals may be found in the body after the individual has smoked marijuana (Jenike, 1991). Many of these metabolites can remain present in the body for weeks after a single episode of marijuana smoking. Unfortunately, the long-term effects of these chemicals on the human body have not been studied in detail (University of California, Berkeley, 1990b). In addition, if the marijuana used is adulterated (as it frequently is), the various adulterants will add their own contribution to the flood of chemicals being admitted to the body. Again, there is little research into the long-term effects of these adulterants or their metabolites.

The active agent of marijuana, THC, has been demonstrated to cause lung damage and reduce the effectiveness of the body's immune system. Indeed, research suggests that marijuana smokers absorb 4 *times* as much "tar" as do cigarette smokers (Tashkin, 1993). Smoking marijuana can also cause increased levels of carbon monoxide in the blood (Oliwenstein, 1988). Some reports show that the marijuana smoker absorbs 5 *times* as much carbon monoxide per joint as a cigarette smoker does after smoking a single regular cigarette (Polen, Sidney, Tekawa, Sadler, & Friedman, 1993; University of California, Berkeley, 1990b; Oliwenstein, 1988). Smoking just 4 marijuana joints appears to have the same negative impact on lung function as smoking 20 regular cigarettes (Tashkin, 1990).

Furthermore, chronic marijuana users who smoke just a few marijuana "joints" a day seemed to develop the same type of damage to the cells lining the airways as do cigarette smokers who later develop lung cancer (Tashkin,

1993; University of California, Berkeley, 1990b; Oliwenstein, 1988). Research has shown that marijuana smoke contains 5 to 15 times the amount of benzpyrene, a known carcinogen, as does tobacco smoke (Tashkin, 1993; Bloodworth, 1987). The heavy use of marijuana has been suggested as a cause of cancer of the respiratory tract and the mouth (tongue, tonsils, and so on) in a number of young individuals who would not be expected to have cancer (Tashkin, 1993).

There are several reasons for the observed relationship between heavy marijuana use and lung cancer. In terms of absolute numbers, marijuana smokers tend to smoke fewer joints than cigarette smokers do cigarettes. However, they smoke unfiltered joints, a practice that allows more of the particles of the marijuana into the lungs than is the case for cigarette smokers. Marijuana smokers also smoke more of the joint than cigarette smokers do cigarettes. This increases the individual's exposure to microscopic contaminants in the marijuana. Finally, marijuana smokers inhale more deeply than cigarette smokers do, and they retain the smoke in the lungs for a longer period of time (Polen et al., 1993). Again, this increases the individual's exposure to the potential carcinogenic agents in marijuana smoke.

Like tobacco smokers, marijuana users have an increased frequency of bronchitis and other upper respiratory infections (Mirin, Weiss, & Greenfield, 1991). The chronic use of marijuana also may contribute to the development of obstructive pulmonary diseases, similar to those seen in cigarette smokers (University of California, Berkeley, 1990b).

Another observed effect of marijuana use is drug-induced suppression of the immune system, although researchers still do not understand the mechanism through which this is accomplished. For a healthy person, this immunosuppressant effect is usually quite minor. But, unfortunately, even a weak immunosuppressant effect could have "a devastating effect on AIDS patients" (Bloodworth, 1987, p. 180) or on patients who suffer from another disorder of the immune system.

Marijuana has been implicated in a number of reproductive system dysfunctions. For example, there is evidence to suggest that marijuana is the cause of reduced sperm counts in men (Brophy, 1993). Furthermore, male chronic marijuana users have been found to have 50% lower blood testosterone levels than men who do not use marijuana (Bloodworth, 1987). Female chronic marijuana users sometimes experience abnormal menstruation or a failure to ovulate (Brophy, 1993; *Mayo Clinic Health Letter*, 1989).

Wray and Murthy (1987) conclude that chronic marijuana use can result in fertility problems in women. However, Grinspoon and Bakalar (1992) point out that research studies in this area have been flawed, as few studies have utilized proper control groups. Thus, it is not clear at this time whether the marijuana use is responsible for the changes in reproductive health for female chronic marijuana users.

Persons who have previously used hallucinogenics may also experience marijuana-related "flashback" experiences, limited to the 6-month period following the last marijuana use (Jenike, 1991). They eventually stop if the person does not use any further mood-altering chemicals (Weiss & Mirin, 1988). (The flashback experience will be discussed in more detail in Chapter 13.)

For years, researchers believed that marijuana does not cause any physical damage to the brain. But recently researchers have uncovered evidence suggesting that the chronic use of marijuana may result in physical damage to a region of the brain known as the hippocampus (Kaminski, 1992; Kaufman & McNaul, 1992; Schuster, 1990; Friedman, 1987). This is a portion of the brain that is thought to be involved in the processing of sensory information. Chronic exposure to THC "damages and destroys nerve cells and causes other pathological changes in the hippocampus" (Friedman, 1987, p. 47), suggesting that marijuana may actually be toxic to the cells in this region of the brain (Schuster, 1990).

In addition to the damage to the hippocampus, there is evidence that chronic marijuana use can cause memory problems (American Academy of Family Physicians, 1990a; Wray and Murthy, 1987), apparently because marijuana interferes with the retrieval mechanisms of memory (Wray & Murthy, 1987). This may be only a temporary effect of marijuana that clears up in a few weeks after the last marijuana use (American Academy of Family Physicians, 1990a). But there does appear to be evidence that the chronic use of marijuana can cause at least temporary brain dysfunction.

Marijuana use may also result in impaired reflexes, decreased short-term memory, and decreased attention span, at least in the period immediately after the use of the drug (Jenike, 1991). Automobile drivers under the influence of marijuana frequently misjudge the speed and length of time required for braking, factors that may contribute to accidental death while using marijuana (Mirin, Weiss, & Greenfield, 1991). Schwartz (1987) reports that marijuana use may impair coordination and reaction time for 12 to 24 hours after the euphoria from the last marijuana use ended. Schwartz also notes that teenagers who smoke marijuana as often as 6 times a month are "2.4 times more likely to be involved in traffic accidents" (p. 309) than nonusers.

Meer (1986) tested 10 private airplane pilots on a flight simulator 24 hours after they had smoked one marijuana cigarette. Although their performance had improved over their simulator performance 1 to 4 hours after smoking the marijuana cigarette, these pilots still demonstrated significant impairment on flight simulation tests; one pilot's simulation performance would have landed the plane off the runway. The exact significance of these findings are not clear at this time, but this study does suggest that marijuana's effects on coordination may be longer lasting than was once thought.

Marijuana use can cause a significant increase in heart rate, a side effect that could be of some consequence to people who suffer from heart disease (Barnhill, Ciraulo, & Ciraulo, 1989; Bloodworth, 1987). Cocaine users often smoke marijuana concurrently with cocaine use to counteract the excessive stimulation caused by the cocaine. The combination of marijuana and cocaine can increase heart rate above that seen from either drug alone, raising the heart rate an additional 50 beats per minute (Barnhill, Ciraulo, & Ciraulo, 1989).

Chronic marijuana users have been found to have changes in electrocardiographic (EKG) studies, but the exact nature of these changes is unclear. At present, the observed EKG changes do not seem to reflect marijuana-induced heart disease (Brophy, 1993; Jenike, 1991). Although marijuana use is not viewed as a *direct* cause of heart disease, the potential does exist for indirect cardiovascular problems as a result of marijuana use.

There is conflicting evidence as to whether chronic marijuana use can bring about an "amotivational syndrome." Some researchers have described a marijuana-related amotivational syndrome consisting of decreased drive and ambition, short attention span, easy distractability, and a tendency to not make plans beyond the present day (Mirin, Weiss, & Greenfield, 1991). However, many researchers do not believe that marijuana can cause this so-called amotivational syndrome (Abood & Martin, 1992). Indeed, it has been suggested that the amotivational syndrome is a research artifact. Individuals who use marijuana on a regular basis are also likely to be those individuals who are already bored, depressed, listless, alienated from society, and cynical — some of the very characteristics thought to be a result of the marijuana-induced amotivational syndrome (Grinspoon & Bakalar, 1992). Thus, it is not clear at this time whether marijuana causes observed personality characteristics, or whether people with these personality traits are most likely to use marijuana regularly. Obviously, further research is necessary to determine once and for all whether the amotivational syndrome does indeed exist and what role chronic marijuana use may play in its development (Schwartz, 1987).

More than half a century ago, it was widely believed that marijuana use was likely to induce violence. However, the sedating and euphoric effects of marijuana are more likely to *reduce* any tendency toward violence, rather than bring it about. Thus, few clinicians now believe that marijuana use is associated with increasing violent behavior.

Although marijuana is safe in terms of immediate lethality, there is significant evidence that chronic marijuana use can contribute to or is the primary cause of a number of potentially serious medical problems. Marijuana use is not as benign as advocates of this substance would have us believe.

The Addiction Potential of Marijuana

As the reader will recall from earlier chapters, two necessary conditions for addiction to any chemical are the development of tolerance to that chemical and the existence of a withdrawal syndrome when that drug is discontinued. In this sense, marijuana meets one criterion for a potential addictive substance, because smoking as few as three marijuana cigarettes a week may result in tolerance to the effects of marijuana (Bloodworth, 1987).

Chronic marijuana use may also result in a mild withdrawal syndrome. Because of its long half-life in the human body, marijuana does not cause the severity of symptoms found with narcotic or barbiturate withdrawal (Bloodworth, 1987). The withdrawal syndrome associated with heavy, chronic marijuana use has such symptoms as irritability, anxiety, insomnia, nausea, and a loss of appetite (Abood & Martin, 1992; Group for the Advancement of Psychiatry, 1990; Bloodworth, 1987). Other symptoms of withdrawal may include sweating and vomiting (Nahas, 1986). Thus, marijuana does appear to

meet the criteria necessary to classify it as an addictive drug.

The Treatment of Marijuana Abuse and Addiction

Although marijuana use has been popular in this country since the Prohibition era — and even more so after the "hippie" generation "discovered" marijuana in the 1960s — virtually nothing is known about the treatment of marijuana abuse and dependence (Stevens, Roffman, & Simpson, 1994). Researchers believe that short-term, acute reactions to marijuana do not require any special medical intervention (Brophy, 1993). Although marijuana is capable of causing transient feelings of anxiety, especially in the "naive" user, marijuana-related anxiety or panic reactions usually respond to "firm reassurance in a nonthreatening environment" (Mirin, Weiss, & Greenfield, 1991, p. 304). However, individuals with adverse reactions should be watched to ensure that no harm comes to either the marijuana user or to others.

A number of problems are associated with working with marijuana abusers. First, it is rare for a person to be abusing *only* marijuana, so treatment usually needs to focus on the abuse of a number of chemicals. Second, marijuana users usually do not seek treatment unless coerced (Bloodworth, 1987). (The use of external pressure to convince a person to enter treatment will be discussed in more detail in a later chapter.) Third, even when the marijuana user *does* enter treatment, specific therapeutic methods for working with the chronic marijuana user are not well developed (Mirin, Weiss, & Greenfield, 1991). Roffman and George (1988) suggested that this is the result of the mistaken belief that, because marijuana is not as toxic as other drugs of abuse, its use by adults is not a cause of major concern to health care providers. Thus, health care providers have not addressed the issue of how to deal with the chronic marijuana user.

As with all chemical addictions, total abstinence from *all* psychoactive drugs is required if treatment is to work (Bloodworth, 1987). The most effective treatment program is one that identifies the individual's reasons for continued drug use and helps the individual find alternatives to drugs. Supplemental groups that focus on vocational rehabilitation and socialization skills are also of value in the treatment of the chronic marijuana user (Mirin, Weiss, & Greenfield, 1991). Jenike (1991) recommends that treatment efforts focus on understanding the abuser's disturbed psychosocial relationships. Bloodworth (1987) concludes that "family therapy is almost a necessity" (p. 183). Bloodworth believes that group therapy as a means of dealing with peer pressure to use chemicals is necessary, and self-help support groups such as Alcoholics Anonymous or Narcotics Anonymous "cannot be overemphasized" (Bloodworth, 1987, p. 183).

Summary

Marijuana has been the subject of controversy for several generations. In spite of its popularity as a drug of abuse, surprisingly little is actually known about marijuana. Indeed, after a 25-year search, researchers have only recently identified what appears to be the specific receptor site where the THC molecule causes at least some of its effects on perception and memory.

In spite of the fact that very little is known about this drug, some groups have called for its complete decriminalization. Other groups maintain that marijuana is a serious drug with a high potential for abuse. Even experts differ as to the potential for marijuana to cause harm. Whereas Weil (1986) classifies marijuana as one of the safest drugs known, Oliwenstein (1988) terms marijuana a dangerous drug.

The evidence available at this time indicates that marijuana is not as benign as once thought. Marijuana, either alone or in combination with cocaine, increases the heart rate, a matter of some significance to those with cardiac disease. There is evidence that chronic use of marijuana will cause physical changes in the brain, and the smoke from marijuana cigarettes has been found to be even more harmful than tobacco smoke. In the years to come, marijuana will probably remain a most controversial drug.

Narcotic Analgesics

The existence of narcotic analgesics has been known for at least 10,000 years. Researchers have found the residue of the opium poppy plant *Papaver somniferum* in Stone Age dwellings in what is now northern Italy and Switzerland (Restak, 1994). One early reference to the medicinal uses of opium is found in the Ebers Papyri, which dates back to approximately 7000 B.C. Within this ancient record is a reference to the use of opium as a treatment for children who suffer from colic (Thomason & Dilts, 1991). Opium was known to the physicians of ancient Greece and ancient Rome, and its use was common for thousands of years.

However, the active agent of opium, morphine, was first isolated only 200 years ago (Restak, 1994). Morphine has since become both a lifesaver and an affliction. In this chapter, we will explore the history and role that narcotic analgesics play in modern medicine and as drugs of abuse.

The Classification of Analgesics

Pain is the most common complaint encountered by physicians (Fishman & Carr, 1992). Thus, there is a very real demand for medications that will control pain. To meet this demand, researchers have developed a group of medications that are known collectively as *analgesics*. An analgesic is a chemical that is able to bring about the "relief of pain without producing general anesthesia" (Abel, 1982, p. 192).

There are two groups of such drugs. The first bring about a *local anesthesia* and the second change the perception of pain—*global analgesics*. Cocaine can be used as a local anesthetic. When used properly, it blocks the transmission of nerve impulses from the site of the injury to the brain. In so doing, cocaine (or any of the other local anesthetics developed after cocaine) prevents the brain from receiving the nerve impulses that would otherwise transmit the pain message from the site of the injury.

The second group of analgesics are more global in nature and alter the individual's perception of pain. Abel (1982) further divides this group of analgesics into two subgroups. The first is the *narcotic* family of drugs, which have both a CNS depressant capability and an analgesic effect. The second subgroup are nonnarcotic analgesics such as aspirin, acetaminophen, and similar agents.

The nonnarcotic analgesics are thought to interfere with the action of chemicals released by injured tissues of the body, which reduces pain and inflammation. They are useful for controlling fever and do not have a major impact on the CNS. The nonnarcotic analgesics will be discussed in detail in another chapter; in this chapter, we will discuss only the narcotic family of drugs.

Many narcotic analgesics can be traced either

directly or indirectly to opium. The term *opiate* was once used to designate only those drugs actually derived from opium (Jaffe & Martin, 1990). Recently, a number of either synthetic or semisynthetic opiatelike painkillers have been introduced. In current terminology, the term *opioid* is used in a generic sense to refer to any drug similar to morphine in its actions. Some authors, however, utilize the terms *opiate* and *opioid* interchangeably (Jaffe & Martin, 1990). For the purpose of this text, we will use the traditional terms *opiate* or *narcotic*.

A History of Opium and Narcotic Addiction

Opium is a powder obtained by first extracting a milky sap from the plant *papaver somniferum* and then letting the juice dry. Although opium has been known for at least 10,000 years, most of its history has been lost. In the 16th and 17th centuries, opium was used for virtually every ailment that European physicians encountered (Melzack, 1990). Indeed, until recently, opium was perhaps the only medicine that physicians could use with predictable results (Ray & Ksir, 1993). Physicians used opium to control mild to severe levels of pain and (before modern sanitation) to treat dysentery.

However, no one knew what made opium able to control pain. It was not until 1803[1] that Friedrich W. A. Serturner first isolated a pure alkaloid base from opium, a chemical named *morphine* after the Greek god of dreams, Morpheus. Morphine was soon recognized as the major active ingredient in opium. With this discovery, researchers were one step closer to understanding how narcotic analgesics helped to control pain.

Chemists eventually discovered a total of 20 distinct alkaloids in addition to morphine that could be obtained from the opium poppy (Gold, 1993; Kaplan & Sadock, 1990), and medical

science found uses for many of them. Unfortunately, many of these alkaloids also have an abuse potential and are part of the narcotics abuse problem in the United States. An example is codeine, which has a modest but very real potential for abuse.

Although narcotics were abused for many years before the invention of the hypodermic needle by Alexander Wood in 1857, this invention made it possible to inject drugs into the body quickly and relatively painlessly. The introduction of the hypodermic needle, combined with the availability of relatively large amounts of pure morphine, soon resulted in a rather severe outbreak of morphine addiction (Jaffe, 1989). Furthermore, injected morphine was not thought to be addicting, at least during the early 1850s, and was freely available without a prescription (Melzack, 1990).

Morphine, or its parent compound opium, was freely utilized as a painkiller in battlefield hospitals of the American Civil War and in the later Franco-Prussian and Prussian-Austrian wars in Europe (Callahan & Pecsok, 1988). Indeed, during the Civil War, surgeons administered opium "in pill form and in a mixture with alcohol, called laudanum. . . . It also was sometimes sprinkled in powdered form directly onto a wound" (Norris, 1994, p. 53). Battlefield doctors also used morphine to treat dysentery.[2] The crowded, unsanitary army camps of the last century were prime breeding grounds for dysentery, and virtually every soldier in the American Civil War contracted dysentery at least once (Norris, 1994).

Both morphine and opium slowed down the wavelike contractions of the muscles surrounding the intestines, and so were valuable in treating dysentery. Little was known about the addictive potential of either opium or morphine at the time, and many soldiers on both sides of the Atlantic became addicted to morphine dur-

---

[1]Restak (1994) states that morphine was first isolated in 1805, not 1803.

[2]Dysentery is an infection of the lower intestinal tract that causes a great deal of pain and severe diarrhea that is often mixed with blood and mucus. It is caused by contaminated water (often found in crowded army camps) and could rapidly lead to death from dehydration.

ing the war. Indeed, by the mid-1800s, morphine addiction was known as the "soldier's disease" (Ray & Ksir, 1993, p. 304).

During the last half of the 19th century, the United States suffered from a wave of narcotics addiction. Both opium and morphine were freely available without a doctor's prescription. Indeed, as Norris (1994) notes, the vast majority of the people at the time had little faith in medical science, and it was not unusual for the patient to rely on time-honored folk remedies and the then-popular patent medicines. Unfortunately, many patent medicines contained opiates, and many users unwittingly became addicted to the narcotic contained therein. In many other cases, people who used either opium or morphine for the control of pain or diarrhea became physically dependent and continued to use the narcotic long after the need for it had passed.

By the year 1900, *more than 1% of the entire population of the United States* was addicted to opium (Restak, 1994). The practice of smoking opium was brought to the United States by Chinese immigrants, many of whom came to work on the railroad in the late 1800s. Although the practice of smoking opium never became very popular, there was still a sizable minority who engaged in this practice. By 1900, 25% of the opium imported into the United States was for smoking (Ray & Ksir, 1993).

Concern over the growing numbers of people addicted to cocaine, the opiates, or both prompted passage of the Pure Food and Drug Act of 1906. This law required that the contents of medicines be printed on the labels, so that the purchaser could know what was contained in the medicine. Eight years later, the Harrison Narcotics Act of 1914 was passed, which prohibited the use of certain drugs without a prescription. These laws were intended to help contain the growing drug addiction problem in the United States. Over the years, various other legal restrictions have been implemented, as the drug abuse problem has waxed and waned. However, the problem of narcotic abuse and addiction never entirely disappeared.

Because the synthesis of morphine in the laboratory is difficult, most morphine is still obtained from the opium poppy, and so there is a legitimate need for the continued cultivation of the opium poppy. However, experts agree that the supply of morphine obtained from poppies far exceeds the supply necessary to meet the world's needs for morphine. Unfortunately, most of the excess opium finds its way to the illicit narcotics market. Currently, virtually all the legally produced opium comes from India (Sabbag, 1994). However, illegal crops of opium poppies are raised in Southeast Asia and Afghanistan, the second-largest producer of illicit opium in the world. Other countries involved in the illicit opium trade include Iran, Pakistan, China, Burma, Laos, Thailand, Colombia, and Mexico (Sabbag, 1994).

Current Medical Uses of the Narcotic Analgesics

Since the introduction of aspirin, narcotics are no longer utilized to control mild to moderate levels of pain. An exception to this rule is codeine, which, in addition to being a useful cough suppressant (Jaffe, 1992), is occasionally used to control moderate levels of pain. However, as a general rule, the opiates are reserved for the control of acute, severe pain (Bushness & Justins, 1993). Narcotic analgesics also continue to be used to control *severe* diarrhea, by suppressing the motility of the gastrointestinal tract. This will be discussed in more detail in a later section of this chapter.

Several different forms of opiates have been developed over the years, with various potencies and various durations of effects. The generic and brand names of some of the more commonly used narcotic analgesics are listed in Table 11.1.

Codeine, first isolated from the opium poppy plant in 1832 (Melzack, 1990), has a mild analgesic effect. Once it is in the body, a small amount of codeine is biotransformed to morphine during the process of drug metabolism

TABLE 11.1 Some Commonly Utilized Narcotic Analgesics

Chemical name	Brand name
Methadone	Dolophine
Oxycodone	Percodan
Hydromorphone	Dilaudid
Pentazocine	Talwin
Codeine	—
Fentanyl	Sublimaze
Meperidine	Demerol
Oxymorphone	Numorphan
Propoxyphene	Darvon
Diphenoxylate	Lomotil
Morphine	—

(Jaffe, 1992). Like many of the narcotic analgesics, codeine is also an effective cough suppressant. As a consequence, codeine is frequently prescribed by physicians to help control coughing and moderate levels of pain.

Although a number of new analgesic medications have been developed over the years, morphine is still considered the standard against which other analgesics are measured (Bushnell & Justins, 1993). We will focus mainly on morphine in this chapter. However, no discussion of narcotic analgesic abuse would be complete without mentioning what first comes to mind when many think of narcotic abuse: heroin.

The Mystique of Heroin

Except for differences in potency, the effects of the various forms of narcotic analgesics are very similar. Researchers are thus at a loss to explain why heroin (actually, *diacetylmorphine*) is the preferred narcotic among addicts in the United States. Heroin has traditionally been viewed as the most destructive drug in the United States (Gold, 1993; Savage, 1993); now crack cocaine has that distinction.

Heroin was developed in 1898 by chemists at the Bayer pharmaceutical company in Germany. When the chemists first tried diacetylmorphine,

they reported that the drug made them feel "heroic," and thus it was given the brand name "Heroin" (Mann & Plummer, 1991, p. 26). At the time, heroin was thought to be nonaddictive and was initially sold as a cure for morphine addiction. It was not until 12 years later that the true addictive potential of heroin was finally recognized.

Heroin is more potent than morphine; a standard conversion formula is 4 milligrams of heroin is equal to 10 milligrams of morphine (Lingeman, 1974). Because of differences in its chemical structure, heroin is much more lipid soluble than morphine and is able to cross over from the bloodstream into the brain 100 times faster than morphine (Angier, 1990). Because morphine is not fully lipid soluble, it takes 20 to 30 minutes for morphine to cross over the barrier from the blood into the brain (Angier, 1990).

Thus, pharmaceutical forms of heroin offer some advantages over morphine for controlling severe pain. Heroin, however, is illegal in the United States, and the illicit sale of heroin is estimated to be a $4 billion- to $10 billion-per-year industry in this country (Witkin & Griffin, 1994). In other countries, heroin is a recognized pharmaceutical; it is utilized by physicians in Canada and England as an analgesic to control severe pain, especially the pain caused by cancer. However, even in these countries, its use is quite controversial (Parry, 1992).

As Lingeman (1974) points out, one of the factors underlying addicts' preference for heroin over morphine is their *expectation* that heroin will produce a greater degree of euphoria. Surprisingly, narcotics addicts are unable to tell the difference between morphine and heroin when equipotent doses are injected into the muscle tissue (an *intramuscular* injection). When intravenous injections are utilized, most addicts can immediately tell the difference between heroin and morphine (Lingeman, 1974).

The actions of heroin are quite similar to those of morphine. This is not surprising, since morphine is a metabolite of heroin (Jaffe, 1992; Scaros, Westra, & Barone, 1990). In other words, once heroin is injected into the body, it is transformed back into morphine by the liver. Heroin's main advantage for addicts is that it has only half the bulk of morphine, allowing for easier transportation by users and suppliers (Lingeman, 1974). The fact that it is able to pass through the blood/brain barrier so easily may also account for the intensity of the "rush" experienced when heroin is injected into a vein.

In spite of the introduction of new synthetic and semisynthetic narcotic analgesics, heroin abuse accounts for approximately 90% of the narcotics abuse problem in the United States today (Dygert & Minelli, 1993). However, the face of heroin abuse is changing, and the current methods of heroin abuse will be discussed in more detail in the section "Methods of Narcotics Abuse."

Surprisingly, in spite of the protracted U.S. "war on drugs" of the last 25 years, evidence suggests that heroin has continued to be a significant part of the drug abuse problem. Many crack cocaine addicts apparently are smoking a combination of heroin and crack called "speed ball rock," "moon rock," or "parachute rock" (Dygert & Minelli, 1993). The combination of heroin and crack cocaine reportedly produces a longer "high" and a less severe post-cocaine use depression (Levy & Rutter, 1992).

There is also evidence that heroin abuse has become more popular in the past decade (*Forensic Drug Abuse Advisor*, 1994c). The number of patients treated for heroin-related emergencies in the first 6 months of 1993 increased by 44% over the number treated in the first 6 months of 1992 (Gabriel, 1994). Furthermore, young drug users now prefer heroin over crack (Smolowe, 1993). These statistics suggest that heroin is increasing in popularity among those who are abusing chemicals.

Finally, the purity of heroin on the street is far higher than it was before the "war on drugs" began. In 1985, the average sample of heroin from the street had an average purity of about 5% to 6% (Sabbag, 1994). Researchers are currently finding samples of heroin being sold on the street with an average purity of 65% (Ga-

briel, 1994). Indeed, there is a glut of heroin on the streets at this time, and when this has happened in the past, the price of heroin on the street dropped and the purity of the drug increased. At this point, there is no end in sight to the high potency of street heroin in the United States.

The Pharmacology of the Narcotic Analgesics

Research shows that the opiates seem to mimic the actions of a family of related chemicals broadly known as the *opioid peptides*, which are found within the brain and spinal cord (Simon, 1992). The opioid peptides function as neurotransmitters and are grouped into three families: the *endorphins*, the *enkephalins*, and the *dynorphins*.

Chemically, the opioid peptides are extremely powerful. Although narcotic analgesics utilize the same receptor sites as the opioid peptides do, they are only crude copies of the naturally occurring neurotransmitters. The neurotransmitter known as *beta endorphin*, for example, is thought to be 200 times as potent an analgesic as morphine.

There are at least a dozen known opioid peptides, which are thought to carry out a number of different functions within the brain. Although researchers are still trying to understand the function of the opioid peptides, some apparently include perception of pain, moderation of emotions, perception of anxiety, sedation, appetite, suppression, anticonvulsant activity within the brain, smooth muscle motility, regulation of a number of body functions (such as temperature, heart rate, respiration, and blood pressure), and perhaps even involvement in the perception of pleasure (Restak, 1994; Hawkes, 1992; Simon, 1992).

The narcotic analgesics appear to utilize a number of the same receptor sites in the brain normally used by the opioid peptides. Researchers have identified seven different receptor sites within different regions of the brain that are utilized by the opioids (Foley, 1993). Each site is identified by a letter of the Greek alphabet. Table 11.2 summarizes what we know about the different receptor sites and the function controlled by each receptor subtype.

One of the areas in the brain where the opioids appear to work is the *medial portion of the thalamus* (Restak, 1994). It is thought that narcotic analgesics mimic the action of the opioid peptide(s) normally found in this region of the brain, thus controlling the experience of pain. The experience of euphoria often reported by narcotic abusers is thought to be caused by the effects of the opioids on the *ventral tegmental* region of the brain (Kaplan, Sadock, & Grebb, 1994). This area of the brain uses dopamine as its major neurotransmitter, and it connects the cortex of the brain with the limbic system.

Thus, morphine—and its chemical cousins—mimic the actions of naturally occurring chemicals found in the brain. But to reach the brain, morphine must first be admitted into the body. Morphine is well absorbed from injection sites and is often administered through intramuscular or intravenous injections. It is also well absorbed through the mucous membranes of the body and so is occasionally administered through rectal suppositories.

Although morphine is well absorbed through

TABLE 11.2

Opioid receptor	Biological activity associated with opioid receptor
mu	Analgesia, euphoria, respiratory depression, suppression of cough reflex
delta	Analgesia, euphoria, endocrine effects, psychomotor functions
kappa	Analgesia in spinal cord, sedation, miosis
sigma	Dysphoria, hallucinations, increased psychomotor activity, respiratory activity
epsilon	Unknown
lambda	Unknown

Source: Based on information provided in Ashton (1992) and Jaffe (1989).

the gastrointestinal tract, the effects of first-pass metabolism (discussed in Chapter 3) cause the blood levels of orally administered morphine to be quite unpredictable. The peak effects of morphine are felt about 60 minutes after an oral dose and between 30 to 60 minutes after intravenous injection (Shannon, Wilson, & Stang, 1992).

Once in the body, approximately one-third of intravenously administered morphine will become protein-bound (see Chapter 3 for a discussion of this phenomenon) (Medical Economics Company, 1993). The rest of the morphine is distributed to various blood-rich tissues, including muscle tissues, kidneys, liver, lungs, spleen, and the brain. Morphine has a biological half-life of 2 to 3 hours. It is metabolized mainly in the liver, and about 90% of the drug metabolites are eliminated by the kidneys (Shannon, Wilson, & Stang, 1992).

Morphine and other opiates produce a state of relative analgesia, reducing the recipient's experience of pain. A further advantage is that analgesia is achieved without a significant loss of consciousness, an important factor in many cases (Jaffe, 1992; Jaffe & Martin, 1990). The opiates also appear to be able to reduce the individual's anxiety level, promote drowsiness, and allow the individual to sleep in spite of severe pain (Restak, 1994; Shannon, Wilson, & Stang, 1992).

These latter effects seem to reflect the impact of the morphine molecule on another part of the brain, the *locus coeruleus* (Gold, 1993; Jaffe, 1992), a region of the brain that is thought to play a role in the perception of anxiety. The locus coeruleus is also involved in the perception of pain (Miller & Gold, 1993). It appears that this is the area of the brain where the narcotic analgesics are able to reduce the individual's anxiety level and promote sleep by mimicking the actions of a naturally occurring opioid peptide normally found there.

As we discussed earlier, narcotic analgesics also suppress the cough reflex. Physicians usually prescribe codeine, a close chemical relative to morphine, for this purpose. Research has shown that codeine suppresses the action of the medulla, a portion of the brain responsible for the maintenance of the body's internal state (Jaffe, 1992; Jaffe & Martin, 1990).

Effects of Narcotic Analgesics at Normal Dosage Levels

For the person who is using narcotics for medical reasons at normal dosage levels, these drugs will change the individual's perception of pain (Thomason & Dilts, 1991). To understand how this is achieved, one must understand that pain is a multi-faceted phenomenon. According to Melzack (1990), there are actually two forms of pain. The first form of pain, what Melzack terms *phasic* pain, is a sharp expression of discomfort experienced at the instant of injury. This is followed by a steady, less intense, but more enduring form of pain called *tonic* pain.

Not surprisingly, given the complexity of the central nervous system, there appear to be different neurological pathways for each form of pain. The neuropathways for phasic pain are naturally dampened quickly (Melzack, 1990), warning the organism that injury has occurred without overwhelming it with needless pain messages. Tonic pain, on the other hand, seems to serve the function of warning the organism to rest until recovery can take place. Although morphine is of little value in the control of phasic pain, it seems to be well suited for controlling the enduring tonic form of pain (Fulton & Johnson, 1993; Melzack, 1990).

When therapeutic doses of morphine are given to a patient in pain, he or she usually reports that the pain is less intense, less discomforting, or entirely gone (Jaffe, 1992; Jaffe & Martin, 1990). However, many factors affect the degree of analgesia achieved through the use of morphine. Fishman and Carr (1992) identified several variables, including (1) the route by which the medication is administered, (2) the interval between doses, (3) the dosage level being used, and (4) the half-life of the specific medication being used.

People's experience of pain is also influenced by their anxiety level, their expectations for the narcotic, the length of time they have been receiving narcotic analgesics, and their general state of tension. The more tense, frightened, and anxious a person is, the more likely he or she is to experience pain in response to a given stimuli. The opiates raise the individual's pain threshold by moderating some of the fear, anxiety, and tension that normally accompany pain states (Gold, 1993; Jaffe & Martin, 1990). Because patients on opiates do not attach as much importance to the pain, they experience less distress than before.

Some patients who receive narcotic analgesics for the control of pain also report a sense of euphoria (Bushnell & Justins, 1993; Jaffe, 1992; Jaffe & Martin, 1990). As we discussed earlier, opiates seem to mimic the action of naturally occurring neurotransmitters in several different regions in the brain. Two regions of the limbic system of the brain, the *nucleus accumbens* and the *ventral tegmentum*, seem to be associated with the pleasurable response that many patients report (Restak, 1994). Researchers believe that, by flooding these regions of the brain with a narcotic analgesic, the brain reacts as if massive amounts of endorphins were released. If the patient is not in pain, he or she will often experience a sense of euphoria and, in some cases, a "rush" or "flash" similar to sexual orgasm (Hawkes, 1992). This unintended but pleasant side effect contributes to the abuse potential of narcotic analgesics.

Complications from Narcotic Analgesics at Normal Dosage Levels

Even at therapeutic dosage levels, narcotic analgesics cause some degree of constriction of the pupils. Some patients experience constriction of the pupils even in total darkness (Shannon, Wilson, & Stang, 1992). This abnormal constriction, or "pinpoint" pupils, is one of the diagnostic signs a physician looks for when the patient is suspected of abusing narcotic analgesics.

Another side effect that occurs at therapeutic

dosage levels is some amount of respiratory depression. Although the degree of respiratory depression is not as significant when narcotics are given to a patient in pain (Bushnell & Justins, 1993), respiration may be affected for 4 to 5 hours, even following a therapeutic dose. For this reason, many experts advise that narcotic analgesics be used with caution in individuals who suffer from respiratory problems such as asthma, emphysema, chronic bronchitis, and pulmonary heart disease.

Supernaw (1991), however, challenged this belief, concluding that the "fear of respiratory depression appears to be misplaced" (p. H-11). Certainly, when used for extended periods of time, the patient can become tolerant to the respiratory depressive effects of narcotic analgesics (Fishman & Carr, 1992). Physicians are still not sure how much respiratory depression may be caused by narcotic analgesics, or whether this is a problem for patients with respiratory disorders. Thus, until a definitive answer is found to the question of whether narcotic analgesics cause respiratory depression, health care workers should anticipate that the narcotics will cause the respiratory center of the brain to become less sensitive to rising blood levels of carbon dioxide, and thus some degree of respiratory depression will occur (Bushnell & Justins, 1993; Thomason & Dilts, 1991).

When used at therapeutic dosage levels, narcotic analgesics can cause some degree of nausea and vomiting (Fishman & Carr, 1992). At normal dosage levels, approximately 40% of ambulatory patients will experience some degree of nausea and approximately 15% will vomit (Jaffe & Martin, 1990). Surprisingly, it is ambulatory patients who seem to be most likely to experience nausea or vomiting after receiving a narcotic analgesic. Thus, patients should not walk around immediately after receiving a narcotic analgesic.

These side effects are dose-related; as the dosage level increases, these side effects are seen in a greater percentage of the population. Some individuals are quite sensitive to the opiates and

will experience adverse reactions to narcotics at even low dosage levels. Melzack (1990) advanced the theory that the individual's response to the narcotics may be genetically mediated, and went on to hypothesize that a genetic mechanism may also account for the phenomenon of narcotics addiction. In other words, Melzack suggests that some people are more likely to become addicted because their genetic heritage predisposes them to narcotics addiction. This theory will be discussed in more detail in Chapters 17 and 18.

At therapeutic dosage levels, morphine and similar drugs have been found to decrease the secretion of hydrochloric acid in the stomach. Peristalsis, the muscle contractions that push food along through the intestines is also restricted (Shannon, Wilson, & Stang, 1992), possibly to the point of spasm in the muscles involved (Jaffe & Martin, 1990). (This is the side effect that made morphine so useful in the treatment of dysentery.) This restriction causes some degree of constipation for individuals using narcotic analgesics.

Another troublesome side effect of the narcotic analgesics is a stimulation of the smooth muscle tissue surrounding the bladder. This effect, in combination with the narcotic analgesics' tendency to reduce the voiding reflex, may result in urinary retention (Tyler, 1994; Jaffe, 1992).

Some patients who receive narcotic analgesics complain of excessive sedation, and morphine sometimes causes nightmares. Furthermore, tolerance to the analgesic action of narcotic analgesics develops quickly, possibly in as little as 1 to 2 weeks of regular use (Tyler, 1994). After that point, it is necessary to increase the daily dose to achieve the same degree of analgesia that was once accomplished at a lower dose.

Finally, although narcotic analgesics are usually used to control acute episodes of pain, they also have a role in the control of chronic, intense levels of pain such as those associated with some forms of terminal cancer. However, the dosage levels utilized with cancer patients are often quite high. When they use narcotic analgesics for extended periods of time, patients will become tolerant to the analgesia provided by the drug (McCaffery & Ferrell, 1994; Fulton & Johnson, 1993). This tolerance, according to McCaffery and Ferrell (1994), is a normal phenomenon and should not automatically be interpreted as a sign that the patient is addicted to painkillers. Sometimes switching to another form of narcotic analgesic effectively combats tolerance to the analgesic effect. Because the chemical structures of different drugs vary, patients often do not develop the same degree of tolerance to different narcotic analgesics.

Another approach is to increase the dose of the original drug until the patient once again is able to tolerate the pain. In some cases, the daily dosage level could be raised to levels that would literally kill a nontolerant patient. For example, a single intravenous dose of 60 mg of morphine is potentially fatal to the opiate-naive person (Kaplan, Sadock, & Grebb, 1994). In contrast, Fulton and Johnson (1993) offer an example of a cancer patient whose daily morphine levels gradually increased from 60 mg a day of morphine to 3,200 mg a day before the patient died of cancer.

Administration of the Narcotic Analgesics

The narcotic analgesics are well absorbed from the gastrointestinal tract, but when they are administered orally, uneven blood levels of the medication are obtained (Shannon, Wilson, & Stang, 1992). This is a result of the "first-pass metabolism" effect. For example, the liver metabolizes at least 80% of the morphine absorbed through the gastrointestinal tract *before* it reaches the brain (Tyler, 1994). The first-pass metabolism effect makes it difficult to determine how much of an oral dose of a narcotic analgesic will actually reach the brain. For this reason, orally administered narcotic analgesics are used only for mild to moderate levels of pain.

The intravenous administration of narcotics actually allows for the greatest degree of control over the amount of drug that actually reaches the brain. For this reason, intravenous injection is the primary method of administration for narcotic analgesics (Jaffe & Martin, 1990). There are exceptions to this rule. For example, a new transdermal patch has been developed for the narcotic fentanyl. (This will be discussed in more detail in the section on fentanyl.)

Methods of Narcotics Abuse

Although the narcotic analgesics are quite useful in the control or treatment of a range of conditions, they are also popular drugs of abuse. When narcotics are abused, they are usually either injected under the skin (a subcutaneous injection, or "skin popping"), injected directly into a vein ("mainlining"), smoked, or inhaled intranasally. Narcotics are well absorbed through the lungs (as in when heroin or opium are smoked) and through the nasal mucosa (when heroin powder is inhaled).

Historically, the practice of smoking opium has not been common in the United States since the turn of the 19th century. Supplies of opium are quite limited in the United States, and opium smoking wastes a great deal of the chemical. However, in parts of the world where supplies of opium are more plentiful, the practice of smoking opium remains quite popular. Both "snorting" heroin powder and smoking heroin have become common methods of administering the drug in the United States. This change in heroin use patterns is apparently an attempt by heroin abusers and addicts to avoid exposing themselves to contaminated intravenous needles (Smolowe, 1993).

When heroin is smoked, the heroin powder is heated in a piece of aluminum foil, using a cigarette lighter or match as a heat source. The fumes are inhaled, allowing users to get "high" without exposing themselves to contaminated needles (*Alcoholism & Drug Abuse Week*, 1991c;

Pinkney, 1990; Scaros, Westra, & Barone, 1990). This practice is known as "chasing the dragon" (Strang, Griffiths, Powis, & Gossop, 1992) and has been found in London and some isolated areas of the United States.

The practice of snorting heroin is quite similar to the way that cocaine powder is inhaled. A razor blade or knife is used to "dice" the powder until it is a fine, talcumlike consistency. The powder then is arranged in a small pile or a line and inhaled through a straw.

Narcotics users obtain their daily supply of the drug from many sources. Unless the addict has access to "pharmaceuticals," the usual practice is to buy "street" narcotics. The street narcotic is a drug that usually has been smuggled into the country and then distributed for sale on the local level. The narcotics are usually sold in powder form in small packets, which are then sold individually. The powder is mixed with water, heated in a small container (usually a spoon) over a flame, and the mixture is then injected.

"Pharmaceuticals" are medications intended for legal use that have been diverted to the streets. Some health care professionals with access to pharmaceutical supplies divert medications to themselves. Other addicts may purchase pharmaceuticals through the illicit drug market. The pharmaceutical tablet is crushed or capsule taken apart and the powder is mixed with water. Again, the mixture is heated in a small container (such as a spoon or bottlecap) over a flame to mix the powder with the water. The resulting mixture is then injected.

The narcotic addict's method of injection differs from the manner in which a physician or nurse injects medication into a vein. Lingeman (1974) describes the process, called "booting," as one in which the narcotic is injected into the vein

> a little at a time, letting it back up into the eye dropper, injecting a little more, letting the blood-heroin mixture back up, and so on. The addict believes that this technique prolongs the initial pleasurable sensation of the heroin as it first takes effect—a feeling of warmth in the abdo-

men, euphoria, and sometimes a sensation similar to an orgasm. (p. 32)

In the process, however, the hypodermic needle and the syringe (or the eye dropper attached to a hypodermic needle, a common substitute for a hypodermic needle) become contaminated with the individual's blood. When other addicts use the same needle, as is commonly done both by cocaine and opiate addicts, contaminated blood from one individual is passed to the next, and the next, and the next. . . . For this reason, many heroin addicts now choose to either smoke heroin and inhale the fumes or snort heroin powder, rather than run the risk of exposing themselves to AIDS through a contaminated needle.

Sometimes, addicts who inject narcotics that were originally intended for oral ingestation also inject accompanying starch or other "fillers" directly into the bloodstream (Wetli, 1987). These "fillers," which are not meant to reach the blood, are mixed with oral medications to give them body and form. The chemical properties of these fillers are such that they usually are destroyed by stomach acid when the medication is taken orally or harmlessly pass through the body and are excreted. But when injected with the narcotic, these fillers cannot be inactivated by the body's defenses. Street narcotics sold for intravenous injection may be adulterated with a variety of substances (for more information on this practice, see Chapter 33). Repeated exposure to pharmaceutical fillers or adulterants from street drugs can cause extensive scarring at the point of injection. These scars form the famous "tracks" caused by repeated injections of narcotics.

Even a single dose of opiates reduces anxiety and provides a feeling of increased self-esteem. When abused, many opiates produce a "rush" or a "flash." This sudden, brief, pleasurable sensation, described as similar to the sexual orgasm, lasts about 30 to 60 seconds (Lingeman, 1974; Jaffe, 1986, 1989; Mirin, Weiss, & Greenfield, 1991; Hawkes, 1992). The individual then experiences a feeling of drowsiness and euphoria that lasts for several hours (Scaros, Westra, & Barone, 1990).

Opiate users report that, as their tolerance develops, they do not experience the "rush" or "flash" from the drug with the same intensity as they did when they first started to use narcotics. Apparently, repeated use of narcotics causes the brain to reduce the amount of endorphins it produces (Klein & Miller, 1986). In other words, over time, the brain substitutes the chemical opiates for natural endorphins, and as tolerance develops, the effect of the narcotics becomes less intense.

When the supply of opiates is eliminated from the body, the brain no longer has the necessary amounts of either natural endorphins or chemical opiates to utilize in the regulation of the emotions and pain. In time, the brain will again produce endorphins on its own. However, until it does, the individual will experience withdrawal symptoms. (Withdrawal from the opiates will be discussed later in the chapter.)

Over time, the individual becomes tolerant to some of the effects of the opiates, but tolerance does not develop equally to each of the effects (Jaffe, 1989). The individual can develop "remarkable tolerance" (Jaffe, 1989, p. 649) to both the analgesic and respiratory depressant effects of opiates but less to the constipation that can result from opiate use. Thus, chronic use of narcotics often results in significant problems with constipation.

Narcotics abusers also quickly become tolerant to the drugs' ability to bring about euphoria. Initially, the narcotics user increases the dose to try to reachieve the initial "rush." But the tolerance to the drug's euphoric effects is not "an infinite process" (Parry, 1992, p. 350). There seems to be a "threshold effect" (p. 350) for both narcotics abusers and long-term heroin addicts, which allows the individual to achieve a "stable genial state" (p. 350) without becoming "high" on the narcotic. Thus, long-term opioid addicts learn to regulate their drug use. They use dosage levels large enough to prevent withdrawal and provide themselves some degree of pleasure from the drug, but they will avoid levels so large that they become "high" on the drug.

Narcotics Abuse and Addiction

As stated earlier, the narcotic family of drugs possesses a significant potential for addiction. Indeed, the potential for addiction is so serious that this is one of the major factors limiting the medical uses of narcotic analgesics (Jaffe & Martin, 1990). Unfortunately, many health care workers hesitate to utilize narcotic analgesics in the most effective manner because they fear the patient will become addicted (Melzack, 1990). However, patients who receive narcotics for the control of pain are unlikely to become addicted unless they have a prior history of drug dependency. Statistically, fewer than 1% of those patients who receive narcotic analgesics for the control of pain, even if they do so for extended periods of time, become addicted to these medications (McCaffery & Ferrell, 1994).

Individuals who use a narcotic for its "psychological effects" are the most likely to become addicted (Melzack, 1990, p. 27). But only a fraction of those who *briefly* experiment with opiates for recreational purposes will become addicted (Jaffe, 1989).[3] At most, "opioid dependence develops in about half of the individuals who engage in opioid abuse" (Jenike, 1991, p. 4). But Jenike also points out that addiction to narcotics can develop in "less than two weeks" (p. 4) if the drugs are used on a daily basis in regularly increasing doses. Thus, although opioids do not seem to be quite as addictive as the popular press portrays them, they *do* have a significant addictive potential.

In the traditional psychoanalytic view of ad-

---

[3]However, because it is not possible to predict in advance who will become addicted, the recreational use of narcotic analgesics is *not* recommended.

diction, there is a dynamic interaction between a person's psychological distress and that person's vulnerability to develop an addiction. The psychoanalytic perspective views opiate addicts as being drawn to the drug because of its ability to help them control powerful feelings of rage and anger.

Although to date, clinical research data do not fully support the psychological vulnerability hypothesis, research does suggest perhaps as many as 50% of those who abuse narcotics have suffered from periods of depression (Melzack, 1990). Furthermore, individuals who actively use narcotics on a daily basis are significantly more depressed than those who occasionally abuse opioids, and both groups are more depressed than those who do not use narcotics at all (Maddux, Desmond, & Costello, 1987). However, the dysphoria so common in chronic opioid users is probably a "pharmacological consequence" (Handelsman, Aronson, Ness, Cochrane, & Kanof, 1992, p. 284) of the chronic use of narcotics, not a result of the abuse of opiates. Further support for this theory is provided by Kanof, Aronson, and Ness (1992), who found that addicts with long-term involvement in a methadone maintenance program who were gradually withdrawn from methadone experienced episodes of depression that could last for several weeks after detoxification. They attributed this finding to the individual's prior use of narcotics, rather than to either the process of withdrawal or a preexisting depressive state.

One consequence of the drug-related depression of the recovering addict is that feelings of dysphoria may serve to trigger further narcotics use. Unless the individual is aware that dysphoric feelings are a consequence of prolonged heroin use, he or she may confuse the withdrawal-related dysphoria with "unhappy feelings that might have prompted experimentation with heroin in the first place" (Handelsman et al., 1992, p. 285).

The final answer to the question of whether narcotics addicts use opioids because they are attempting to self-medicate emotional pain, or whether narcotics addicts experience emotional pain as a pharmacological consequence of prolonged chemical use, has yet to be answered to the satisfaction of all involved.

Withdrawal from Narcotics

Following an extended period of use, the exact length of which is unknown, the opiates will bring about a classic pattern of withdrawal symptoms when discontinued. The typical heroin addict becomes fully addicted 2 years after first abusing the drug (Hoegerman & Schnoll, 1991). However, there are many variations on this pattern and ultimately as many different roads to addiction as there are narcotics addicts.

The symptoms of withdrawal from narcotics vary in intensity, depending on (1) the dose of the opiate that was abused, (2) the length of time the person has used the drug, and (3) the speed with which withdrawal is attempted (Jaffe, 1989). In theory, an opiate addict who has been using the equivalent of 50 mg of morphine a day for 3 months will have an easier detoxification than would someone who has been using the equivalent of 50 mg of morphine a day for 3 years. Also, an opiate addict who is gradually withdrawn from opiates at the rate of the equivalent of 10 mg of morphine a day will have an easier detoxification than would an addict who suddenly stops using the drug ("cold turkey").

The popular belief is that withdrawal from narcotics is extremely uncomfortable, but Jay, Elliott, and Varni (1986) state that this may not always be true. The individual's perception of pain and discomfort is actually the result of a complex interaction between factors such as knowledge, attention, motivation, and suggestibility. Thus the individual's perception of and response to the withdrawal process is influenced to a large degree by his or her cognitive "set."

The discomfort experienced during withdrawal is, to some degree, a learned phenomenon. As Peele (1985) notes:

> In all cases, what is identified as pathological withdrawal is actually a complex self-labeling

process that requires users to detect adjustments taking place in their bodies, to note this process as problematic, and to express their discomfort and translate it into a desire for more drugs. (p. 19)

This phenomenon has also been observed in real-life settings, where narcotics addicts are forced to go through the withdrawal process "cold turkey." For example, in a therapeutic community that actively discourages reports of withdrawal discomfort, narcotics addicts do not go through the dramatic withdrawal displays so often noted in methadone detoxification programs (Peele, 1985). Furthermore, incarcerated narcotics addicts who are denied further access to the drug are often able to go through withdrawal without the dramatic symptoms common in detoxification programs.

Thus, the withdrawal process following addiction to narcotics is not simply a physical phenomenon. Nor are the withdrawal symptoms automatic; rather, they are influenced by such factors as the individual's expectations, level of anxiety, attention to (or away from) the withdrawal symptoms, and motivation for detoxification and withdrawal from narcotics.

A rarely studied aspect of narcotics abuse is the tendency for addicts to attempt withdrawal on their own. Gossop, Battersby, and Strang (1991) examined a group of 47 narcotics addicts in England and found a total of 212 "informal" detoxification episodes. The most common method for self-detoxification was simply going "cold turkey," although a significant number of these attempts used either benzodiazepines or other narcotics to control the withdrawal symptoms. The authors conclude that very little is known about the phenomenon of self-detoxification and suggest that written guidelines for self-withdrawal may be of value.

Narcotics Use During Pregnancy

The narcotics, like a large number of other drugs, cross the placenta in the woman who is pregnant. Thus, when a woman who is pregnant uses narcotics, both the mother and the fetus are exposed to opiates. These infants are, in a very real sense, hidden victims of addiction, which will be discussed in more detail in Chapter 20.

The Scope of the Problem of Narcotics Abuse and Addiction

In the late 1960s it was hypothesized that "the majority [of those who abuse opiates] go on to mainlining" (Lingeman, 1974, p. 106). As we've mentioned before, it is currently thought that only a fraction of those who *briefly* experiment with opiates will actually become addicted (Jaffe, 1989, 1990). For example, between 1 and 3% of the 18- to 25-year-olds in the United States have tried heroin at least once (Hoegerman & Schnoll, 1991), and certainly not all these people are addicted to heroin. The actual percentage of heroin abusers who go on to become addicted is not known.

Various authors estimate that, in addition to those who are addicted to narcotics, between 1 million (Foley, 1993) and 2 million people in the United States (American Academy of Family Physicians, 1989) abuse heroin occasionally. Dygert and Minelli give an even higher estimate of 3.5 million intravenous heroin abusers who are not addicted to the drug. Gold (1993) estimates that just under 3 million people in the United States have used heroin at some point in their lives but does not give an estimate of the number of current users. The Council on Addiction Psychiatry of the American Psychiatric Association estimates that there are "over 1 million chronic, hard-core intravenous heroin abusers" (1994, p. 792) in the United States, without attempting to determine what percentage of this number were addicted to the drug.

One aspect of narcotics abuse that has not been studied in detail is the number of people who apparently use narcotics only occasionally, without becoming addicted (Shiffman, Fischer, Zettler-Segal, & Benowitz, 1990). These individuals, called "chippers," may constitute 40% to 50% of the number of heroin users (Sabbag, 1994). They seem to use narcotics more in response to social stimuli than for internal or pharmacological reasons. In other words, these "chippers" use narcotics in a certain social "set," and they feel no urge to use chemicals when they are in other social settings.

Eisenhandler and Drucker (1993) identified another subpopulation of narcotics addicts about whom virtually nothing is known. These are those addicts who hold stable jobs with health insurance benefits and who receive health care through private health providers. The authors examined the records of 6.5 million hospital admissions over a 10-year period starting in 1982 and identified 31,810 cases of opiate dependency in which patients hospitalized for treatment had private health care insurance. The authors also estimate that between 1 and 2% of those insured by private health care insurance are actually intravenous drug users. They suggest that there may be a significant number of narcotics addicts who are employed, have private health care coverage, and have never been identified as narcotics addicts by public service agencies.

Although there is little real information about the problem of narcotics abuse in the United States, heroin is thought to be the most common narcotic of abuse, constituting perhaps as much as 90% of the problem of narcotics addiction (Dygert & Minelli, 1993). Estimates of the number of people addicted to heroin range from between 400,000 to 600,000 (Kaplan, Sadock, & Grebb, 1994; Brust, 1992; The American Academy of Family Physicians, 1989) and 1 million (*Fighting Drug Abuse*, 1992) people. Researchers suspect that there is a large but unknown number of people who abuse heroin but are not actually addicted. There is also a subpopulation of narcotics abusers, about whom little is known, who limit themselves to pharmaceuticals.

Heroin addicts seem to be concentrated on the coasts. It is estimated that between 200,000 (Eisenhandler & Drucker, 1993; Ross, 1991) and 300,000 (Kaplan, Sadock, & Grebb, 1994) heroin addicts—which is to say fully half of all heroin addicts in the United States—live in New York City (Sabbag, 1994). Another 275,000 are believed to reside in California (Pinkney, 1990).

In spite of the much publicized "war on drugs" of the past generation, the number of active narcotics addicts has remained relatively constant over the past decade (*Alcoholism & Drug Abuse Week*, 1991c; Horgan, 1989). There are even reports that the number of active narcotics addicts in this country has increased in recent years (Smolowe, 1993; *Fighting Drug Abuse*, 1992).

The popular image of the heroin addict is that of a male, usually in his early twenties. Actually, males *do* make up the majority of the heroin addicts in the United States, by a ratio of 3:1 (Kaplan & Sadock, 1990). But this ratio also suggests that, of the estimated 600,000 heroin addicts, perhaps 350,000 are males and 150,000 are female. If the higher estimate of 1 million active narcotics addicts is used, then some 250,000 women in the United States are addicted to narcotics.

Much of the heroin found in the United States originates in Afghanistan, which is surprising, in light of the recent political history of that country. The United States provided weapons, medical supplies, and other forms of aid during the Soviet Union's invasion of Afghanistan in the 1970s. Now, farmers in Afghanistan are growing large crops of opium poppies, and hugh supplies of heroin are reaching the United States. These signs suggest that a new wave of heroin addiction may be starting in this country, and possibly in Europe as well.

Symptoms of Opiate Withdrawal

Acute Withdrawal

In general, opiate withdrawal symptoms begin 8 to 12 hours after the last dose of the drug (Gold, 1993; Jaffe, 1989), depending on the speed with which the individual's body is able to metabolize the specific chemical being used. In some cases, withdrawal symptoms will appear sooner than 8 to 12 hours after the last dose. To avoid these withdrawal symptoms, the addict must either inject the drug again or substitute the use of another drug.

The withdrawal symptoms include a "craving" for more narcotics, tearing of the eyes, running nose, repeated yawning, sweating, restless sleep, dilated pupils, anorexia, irritability, insomnia, weakness, abdominal pain, nausea, vomiting, gastrointestinal upset, chills, diarrhea, muscle spasms and muscle aches, irritability, and possible ejaculation in male addicts (Gold, 1993; Hoegerman & Schnoll, 1991; Scaros, Westra, & Barone, 1990). Constipation is a potential complication of narcotics withdrawal and in rare cases can result in fecal impaction and intestinal obstruction (Jaffe, 1989, 1990).

It has been suggested that these withdrawal symptoms can make the person so uncomfortable as to reinforce continued drug use (Bauman, 1988). This is true even if drug tolerance precludes the initial "rush" (Jaffe, 1986, 1989). Research indicates that perhaps 22% to 35% of opioid addicts have a pathologic fear of detoxification of phobic proportions (Milby et al., 1994).

Opiate addicts in a medical setting often emphasize the distress that they experience during withdrawal, possibly as a ploy to obtain additional medications. Jenike (1991) offers several examples of the manipulativeness demonstrated by addicts in maintaining their drug habits. However, although withdrawal from narcotics may be uncomfortable, it is not fatal, except possibly for infants born addicted to narcotics (Group for the Advancement of Psychiatry, 1990). Narcotic withdrawal is thus "seldom a medical emergency" (Kaplan & Sadock, 1990, p. 40). Symptoms of the opiate withdrawal syndrome will eventually abate in the healthy individual, even in the absence of treatment.

Extended Withdrawal

There is evidence of a second phase of withdrawal from narcotics that lasts beyond the phase of acute withdrawal. During this extended phase of withdrawal, which can last for several months, the individual may experience feelings of fatigue, heart palpitations, and a general feeling of restlessness (Satel, Kosten, Schuckit, & Fischman, 1993).

Satel et al. also found evidence that a phase of "protracted abstinence" (p. 699) may extend for up to 30 weeks after acute withdrawal, during which time the addict's physical functioning slowly returns to normal. Satel et al. cite research studies that have found significant changes in respiration rate, size of the pupils of the eyes, blood pressure changes, and body temperature changes in recovering narcotics addicts more than 17 weeks after the last dose of narcotics. Thus, it appears that the withdrawal process for narcotics addicts takes far longer than the 1 to 2 weeks originally thought.

Complications from Narcotics Abuse and Addiction

Surprisingly, in light of the reputation that narcotics have for destroying lives, there is relatively little evidence to suggest that permanent organ damage occurs from the chronic administration of pharmaceutical opiates (Jaffe, 1992). Indeed, patients in extreme pain, as with some forms of cancer, receive massive doses of narcotic analgesics for extended periods of time without showing evidence of opiate-induced damage to any of the organ systems.

Earlier this century, before the implementation of strict government guidelines for the accountability of each dose of narcotic analgesic purchased by a physician or health care facility, it was not uncommon for medical professionals to be addicted to morphine for years or even decades. The professional involved took care to utilize proper "sterile" techniques and, with the exception of the addiction, appeared to be in good health. For example, the famed surgeon William Halsted was addicted to morphine for 50 years without apparent problems (Smith, 1994).

However, these health care professionals were injecting pharmaceutical-quality narcotic analgesics, not street drugs purchased from illicit sources. The abuse of street narcotics carries with it serious health risks. Heroin users have been known to suffer from cerebral vascular accidents (CVAs, or "strokes"), infectious endocarditis, liver failure, disorders of the body's blood-clot formation mechanisms, malignant hypertension, heroin-related nephropathy (abnormal kidney function), and uremia (a toxic kidney condition) (Brust, 1992). However, it is not clear whether these effects are the direct result of heroin abuse or are caused by added "fillers" (for more information on drug fillers, see Chapter 33).

There are two possible exceptions to the observed lack of toxic effects from the chronic use of narcotics. First, some researchers believe that "prolonged exposure to opioids induces, in some individuals, long-lasting adaptive changes that require continued administration of an opioid to maintain normal mood states and normal responses to stress" (Jaffe, 1992, p. 193). As we will discuss later in this book, some believe that even a single dose of narcotics will bring about physical changes within the brain (Dole, 1988, 1989; Dole & Nyswander, 1965). After these physical changes supposedly take place, it is thought that the individual will require a constant supply of opioids to function on a normal level; this is the theory behind methadone maintenance programs. However, this theory has been challenged (Peele, Brodsky, & Arnold, 1991; Peele, 1989) and it is not universally accepted.

Second, when abused at high dosage levels, narcotics have caused seizures (Foley, 1993). This rare complication of narcotics use is apparently caused by the high dosage level of the opioid, and Foley reports that patients usually respond to the effects of a narcotics blocker such as Narcan (naloxone). However, with seizures caused by the drug meperidine, naloxone may actually reduce the patient's seizure threshold, making it more likely that he or she will continue to experience meperidine-induced seizures (Foley, 1993). Thus, the physician must identify the specific narcotic(s) being abused to initiate the proper intervention for opioid-induced seizures.

In spite of these effects, however, there is little evidence to suggest that the narcotics are, by themselves, able to bring about the same level of toxic effects associated with the chronic use of alcohol.

Narcotics Overdose

The abuse of narcotics may result in serious illness and possibly death. Indeed, in 1990, at least 33,700 heroin-related emergency room admissions were reported to the Drug Abuse Warning Network (*Alcoholism & Drug Abuse Week*, 1991a). This number does not include those who died after injecting narcotics but never lived long enough to reach the hospital emergency room.

A common cause of death from narcotics is opiate overdose. The exact mechanism of death in a narcotics overdose appears to be respiratory arrest (Thomason & Dilts, 1991). However, this is true only for cases of overdose with pharmaceutical opiates. There is some question whether fatal overdoses from street narcotics are caused by the narcotics themselves or by the multitude of chemicals added to dilute them (Khuri, 1989).

For example, Scaros, Westra, and Barone (1990) report that a typical sample of street heroin also contains between 68 and 314 mg of quinine, a common adulterant added to heroin. If the injection of heroin is drawn out for a 10-second period by "booting" the drug, the addict will be injecting up to *182* times the maximum recommended rate of injection of quinine. This rate of quinine injection is in itself capable of causing a fatal reaction in many individuals. Thus, some question exists as to whether deaths by "narcotics overdoses" are indeed caused by the narcotics or by other substances that are mixed with narcotics sold on the streets.

Street Myths and Narcotics Overdose

There are several street myths about the treatment of opiate overdose. First, there is the myth that cocaine (or another CNS stimulant) will help control an opiate overdose. Another myth is that the symptoms of an overdose can be controlled by putting ice packs under the arms and on the groin of the overdose victim. Yet another myth is that the person who had the overdose should be kept awake and kept walking around until the drug wears off.

Unfortunately, the treatment of an opiate overdose is a complicated matter that does not lend itself to such easy solutions. Even in the best-equipped hospital, a narcotics overdose may result in death. The current treatment of choice for a narcotics overdose is Narcan (naloxone hydrochloride) (Khuri, 1989). Naloxone hydrochloride is thought to bind at the narcotic receptor sites within the brain, preventing the narcotic molecules from reaching the receptors and causing respiratory depression. But even with the use of naloxone, oxygen and possibly mechanical ventilation may also be necessary (Sheridan, Patterson, & Gustafson, 1982). The effects of naloxone are also short-lived, as the drug has a half-life of only 60 to 90 minutes (Khuri, 1989). Thus, the patient may need to receive several doses to become fully recovered from the narcotics overdose. *Any known or suspected opiate overdose is a life-threatening emergency that always requires immediate medical support and treatment.*

Fentanyl and Related "Designer" Drugs

In 1968, a new synthetic narcotic known as Sublimaze (fentanyl) was introduced. Like other opiates, fentanyl is utilized in the medical setting for the control of pain. Because of its short duration of action, this drug is especially useful as an analgesic during and immediately after surgery (Shannon, Wilson, & Stang, 1992).

Fentanyl is highly lipid soluble and so has a rapid onset of action when administered by intravenous injection. This characteristic makes fentanyl especially attractive as a surgical anesthetic. Fentanyl is also absorbed through the lungs and through the skin, and so it can be smoked, applied topically, or injected into muscle tissue.

A transdermal fentanyl patch was developed on the theory that the slow absorption of small amounts of fentanyl through the skin would offer relief from pain without the need for repeated injections of the medication. Unfortunately, the medication is so slowly absorbed through the skin that therapeutic blood levels of fentanyl are not achieved until up to 12 hours after the individual first starts to use the "patch" (Tyler, 1994).

However, fentanyl-laced candy was recently introduced for use as a premedication for children about to undergo surgery (*Forensic Drug Abuse Advisor*, 1994b). Just as opium was once used in Rome to calm infants who were crying (Ray & Ksir, 1993), after thousands of years of medical progress, we have returned to using opiates to calm the fears of children.

Fentanyl is known to be extremely potent, but there is some controversy over exactly how potent fentanyl actually is. For example, the *Forensic Drug Abuse Advisor* (1994b) suggests that fentanyl is 50 times as powerful as morphine. However, Stix (1994) claims that fentanyl is 100 times as powerful as morphine, and Ashton (1992) believes it is 1,000 times as potent as morphine. Kirsch (1986) went even further, estimating that fentanyl is "approximately 3,000 times stronger than morphine, [and] 1,000 times stronger than heroin" (p. 18). Kirsch notes that the active dose in humans is one microgram, offering as a basis of comparison the observation that the average postage stamp weighs 60,000 micrograms.

Although there is some disagreement as to its exact potency, there is little dispute over the fact that fentanyl is quite powerful. Even more frightening is its significant abuse potential. Fentanyl need not be injected; it can also be snorted or smoked. When inhaled intranasally, the drug is deposited on the blood-rich tissues of the sinuses where it is absorbed into the general circulation. When fentanyl is smoked, the molecules easily cross into the general circulation through the lungs. Indeed, so rapidly is fentanyl absorbed through the lungs that it is possible for the user to overdose on the medication after just one inhalation (*Forensic Drug Abuse Advisor*, 1994b).

Law enforcement officials have struggled with the problem of illicit fentanyl users almost from the moment the drug was introduced. The drug is so powerful that even small amounts have a value to illicit drug users. For example, some addicts scrape the residual medication from transdermal fentanyl patches and then smoke the small amounts obtained. But fentanyl is not the most powerful narcotic analgesic being used by illicit drug abusers. By manipulating the chemical structure of fentanyl, it is possible to produce a drug "analog" that is 2,000 to 6,000 times as potent as morphine (Gallagher, 1986). (The subject of "designer" drugs and drug analogs will be discussed in more detail in Chapter 33.)

A special test procedure must be utilized to detect fentanyl in the blood or urine (Evanko, 1991). Because fentanyl is so potent that extremely small doses are effective, routine drug toxicology screens easily overlook the presence of fentanyl in the blood or urine of a suspected drug user (*Forensic Drug Abuse Advisor*, 1994b). Thus, even a "clean" urine or blood drug screen may not rule out fentanyl use.

Adverse Effects of Fentanyl

When used in a medical setting for the control of pain, some side effects of fentanyl include blurred vision, a sense of euphoria, nausea, vomiting, dizziness, delirium, lowered blood pressure, constipation, possible respiratory depression, respiratory arrest, and cardiac arrest (Shannon, Wilson, & Stang, 1992). At high dosage levels, muscle rigidity is possible (Foley, 1993). Blood pressure may drop by as much as 20% and heart rate may drop by as much as 25% (Beebe & Walley, 1991).

In addition to experiencing any of these side effects, fentanyl abusers also run the risk of other complications not normally seen when the drug is used in a medical setting. Because of its potency, fentanyl abuse carries with it a significant risk of fatal overdose, especially for individuals who expect the drug to be only about as potent as street heroin. Some addicts have been known to die so rapidly after using fentanyl that they were found with the needle still in their arms (Evanko, 1991). Some researchers attribute the rapid death to the narcotic itself, whereas others postulate that death is brought on by the various chemicals added to the drug to "cut" or dilute it on the street.

The Subjective Effects of Fentanyl

Although it is entirely synthetic, fentanyl is still a member of the opiate family of analgesics. As such, fentanyl will produce analgesia, for which it is utilized in medical settings. When abused, it will also produce a sense of drowsiness and euphoria. Addicts also report a short-lived rush that is apparently of a shorter duration than the rush from heroin abuse (Kirsch, 1986).

The biological half-life of fentanyl is rather short; according to Laurence and Bennett (1992), the half-life period of a single intravenous dose of fentanyl is 3 hours. Although the duration of fentanyl's analgesic effect lasts only between 30 minutes and 2 hours, the effects on the individual's respiration may last longer (Shannon, Wilson, & Stang, 1992). Fentanyl does offer one medical advantage over more traditional narcotic analgesics: Fentanyl produces a more rapid analgesic response than does morphine, often causing analgesia in just minutes.

It is difficult to understand the addictive potential of fentanyl. Dr. William Spiegelman (quoted in Gallagher, 1986) observed that "it can take years to become addicted to alcohol, months for cocaine, and one shot for fentanyl" (p. 26). To further complicate matters, "street chemists" are manipulating the chemical structure of fentanyl, adding a few atoms to the basic fentanyl chain here and snipping a few atoms there to produce what are known as "drug analogs." Unfortunately, in the past decade, fentanyl and its analogs have become a significant part of the drug abuse problem in the United States, and there is no end in sight to this problem.

The Treatment of Narcotics Addiction

Popular belief is that once an opiate addict, always an addict. Indeed, there does seem to be some basis for this pessimism. Research suggests that some 90% of those addicts who achieve abstinence return to chemical use within 6 months (Schuckit, 1989). Hser, Anglin, and Powers (1993) interviewed 581 individuals originally identified as narcotics addicts by the criminal justice system in the period from 1962 until 1964; 24 years later, only 22% of the original sample of 581 narcotics addicts were opiate-free, 7% were involved in a methadone maintenance program, and 10% engaged in only occasional narcotics use. Almost 28% of the original sample had died, with the main causes of death being homicide, suicide, and accident, in that order. Thus, a greater percentage of addicts had died than had achieved abstinence by 1986.

This is indeed a rather pessimistic view of the course of narcotics addiction. However, other studies have found that more than a third of all opiate addicts will ultimately be able to achieve and retain sobriety. For those addicts who survive their addiction, abstinence from opiate use is finally achieved between 6 years (T. Smith, 1994) and 9 years (Jenike, 1991; Jaffe, 1989) after the addiction first develops.

Summary

Physicians have been using narcotics to treat pain and disease for thousands of years. Indeed, after alcohol, the narcotics can be considered our oldest drug. Various members of the narcotic family of drugs have been found to be effective in the control of severe pain, severe cough, and severe diarrhea. The only factor that limits their application in less severe conditions is their addiction potential.

Although narcotics addiction has been a problem for some time, synthetic narcotics have made new forms of narcotic analgesics available to drug users. Fentanyl and its chemical cousins are products of the pharmacological revolution that began in the late 1800s, and they promise to remain a part of the drug abuse problem for generations to come.

CHAPTER TWELVE

Over-the-Counter Analgesics

Medications used to control pain can be classified into three groups. First, there are the *local anesthetics*, which interfere with the transmission of pain messages from the site of the injury to the brain. Cocaine was once the local anesthetic of choice, and even now it is still used under special medical circumstances.

The second group are the *global analgesics*. These drugs work within the brain to nonselectively alter the individual's perception of pain. The narcotic family of drugs are the most frequently utilized global analgesics.

Finally, there are the *nonnarcotic analgesics*, which are thought to interfere with the chemical sequence that results in pain at the site of an injury. This class of medications includes aspirin[1] ibuprofen, naproxen,[2] and acetaminophen, chemicals that are normally considered over-the-counter (OTC) medications.[3] Cocaine and the narcotic analgesics have been reviewed in earlier chapters. In this chapter, we will discuss the most popular OTC analgesics.

----

[1]Aspirin is one of a family of related compounds, many of which have some analgesic, antiinflammatory, antipyretic (antifever) action. However, because none of these aspirinlike chemical compounds is as powerful as aspirin, they will not be discussed in this text.

[2]Naproxen was available only by prescription until 1994, when it was approved for use as an over-the-counter medication, in modified dosage levels.

[3]An over-the-counter medication is one that can be legally purchased without a prescription.

A Short History of Pain Management

Until the introduction of aspirin in the late 1800s, physicians were forced to use narcotic-based analgesics to control even mild to moderate levels of pain. However, the opiates are addictive and have a depressant effect on the central nervous system—factors that limit their usefulness in controlling pain. Physicians now hesitate to utilize narcotic-based analgesics except in the case of severe pain (Giacona, Dahl, & Hare, 1987).

Aspirin, or *acetylsalicylic acid*, was first developed in 1827 from silicin, which is found in the bark of certain willow trees; however, it was not commercially marketed until 1898 (Gay, 1990; Mann & Plummer, 1991). The term *Aspirin* (with a capital *A*) was introduced by the Bayer pharmaceuticals company as the brand name for acetylsalicylic acid around the turn of the century. Over time, however, the term *aspirin* (with a small *a*) has come to mean *any* preparation of acetylsalicylic acid. The manner in which this happened lies beyond the scope of this chapter, but it is reviewed in excellent detail by Mann and Plummer (1991).

Shortly after it was isolated, researchers quickly discovered that aspirin is effective in controlling mild to moderate levels of pain without the risk of addiction associated with the narcotic family of analgesics. Aspirin was also found to have other applications that the narcotic family of analgesics do not, such as the control of inflammation and the ability to reduce fever. Because of its multiple uses, aspirin has become the most frequently used drug in the world (Mann & Plummer, 1991). In 1993, the estimated worldwide consumption was 38,000 *tons* (or 76 million pounds) (Castleman, 1994). In the United States alone, 80 *million* aspirin tablets are consumed each day (Stolberg, 1994; Graedon & Ferguson, 1993).

Since the 1950s, three other OTC analgesics have also been introduced: acetaminophen, ibuprofen, and naproxen. These aspirinlike analgesics collectively represent the lion's share of the $2.7 billion spent in 1990 on OTC analgesics in the United States. However, aspirin remains popular and accounts for 28% of the OTC analgesic sales in the United States (*U.S. News & World Report*, 1994).

Acetaminophen was introduced as an OTC analgesic in the United States in the 1950s. The term "acetaminophen" is actually a form of chemical shorthand for *N-acetyl-para-aminophenol*. The drug was actually first isolated in 1878, and its ability to reduce fever was identified shortly after its discovery. But at the time it was thought that acetaminophen would share the dangerous side effects found in a close chemical cousin, para-aminophenol. So it was set aside, and chemists did not pay much attention to this chemical until the early 1950s (Mann & Plummer, 1991). By that time, sufficient evidence had accumulated to show that acetaminophen was quite a bit safer than para-aminophenol and did not have the same potential for harm found in aspirin. A massive advertising campaign played on the fact that aspirin could irritate the stomach, whereas acetaminophen does not. By the early 1970s, acetaminophen had carved a small but respectable niche for itself in the OTC analgesic market.

Ibuprofen was introduced in the United States as a prescription-only drug in 1974, although it was available in Europe as a prescription drug before then. In 1984, the Food and Drug Administration approved the sale of ibuprofen without prescription in modified dosage forms. Since its introduction as an OTC medication, ibuprofen has captured more than 20% of the nonprescription painkiller market (Squires, 1990).

The U.S. Food and Drug Administration granted permission for *naproxen* to be classified as an over-the-counter medication in 1994. Previously, naproxen had been available only as a prescribed medication. In its OTC form, naproxen will probably be recommended for treating the common cold, headache, minor dental pain, menstrual cramps, and for reducing fever (Gannon, 1994). Naproxen has not been available as an OTC medication long enough to determine how appealing it will be to consumers. However, there is a very good chance that it will become a popular OTC medication and will capture some of the market now held by aspirin and ibuprofen (Gannon, 1994).

Although these medications are indeed quite useful, each has the potential for adverse and possibly fatal side effects, even at normal dosage levels (Aronoff, Wagner, & Spangler, 1986). Aspirin itself was introduced before the modern rules and regulations that govern medication distribution in this country were developed. In fact, aspirin is such a potent drug that, had it been discovered today rather than a century ago, it would be available by prescription only (Graedon & Ferguson, 1993).

Aspirin, acetaminophen, and ibuprofen have all been known to be abused. Even naproxen has a history of occasionally being abused by patients who were taking it under a physician's supervision. And each chemical has been found to have potentially harmful side effects under certain conditions. Thus chemical dependency professionals should have a working knowledge of the OTC analgesics.

Medical Uses of the OTC Analgesics

Although aspirin has been in use for more than a century, scientists are still discovering new uses for aspirin. Aspirin is used to control mild to moderate levels of pain (Supernaw, 1991;

Giacona, Dahl, & Hare, 1987) and has also been found effective in treating common headaches, neuralgia, the pain associated with oral surgery, toothache, and various forms of musculoskeletal pain (Giacona, Dahl, & Hare, 1987). Patients who suffer from migraine headaches and take just one aspirin tablet every other day have been found to have 20% fewer migraines (Graedon & Ferguson, 1993; Gilman, 1992; Graedon & Graedon, 1991). Aspirin may also be of value in controlling a form of hypertension that occasionally complicates pregnancy (Patrono, 1994; Graedon & Ferguson, 1993; Graedon & Graedon, 1991). Furthermore, aspirin is helpful in relieving the symptoms of dysmenorrhea (painful menstruation) and in reducing inflammation and fever.

Aspirin's fever-reduction capability is effected, in part, by causing peripheral vasodilation and sweating, which helps lower the body temperature (Shannon, Wilson, & Stang, 1992). Aspirin is also thought to interfere with prostaglandin production in the hypothalamus, a region of the brain that helps control temperature (Laurence & Bennett, 1992). This effect, in turn, helps limit fever but does not lower the body temperature below normal.

Surprisingly, physicians have only recently discovered that aspirin may be an important adjunct to the treatment of either initial or subsequent heart attacks (American Society of Hospital Pharmacists, 1994; Shannon, Wilson, & Stang, 1992; *The Medical Letter*, 1989; *Internal Medicine Alert*, 1989). Indeed, there is even evidence that low doses of aspirin may be of value in the treatment of an evolving myocardial infarction in which a blood vessel is blocked by a blood clot (Stolberg, 1994; Hennekens, Jonas, & Buring, 1994; Patrono, 1994).

Aspirin's value in the fight against cardiovascular disease was discovered in a 1980s research project involving 22,000 male physicians (*Psychiatry Drug Alerts*, 1989). After a 5-year period, physicians who took just one 325 mg aspirin tablet every other day suffered 44% fewer heart attacks compared to the physicians who took a placebo. This beneficial effect was noted only for

individuals over the age of 50 and was strongest for those individuals with low blood cholesterol levels.

Physicians have also discovered that aspirin is of value in the treatment of a rare neurological disorder known as *transient ischemic attacks* (TIAs), in which the patient loses his or her memory for a short period of time. In addition, aspirin is useful in the control of inflammation caused by rheumatoid arthritis, osteoarthritis, and other forms of arthritis (Graedon & Graedon, 1991; McGuire, 1990; Giacona, Dahl, & Hare, 1987).

In addition to all of its known uses, some research evidence suggests that aspirin may be of value in the prevention of both gallstones and cataracts (Graedon & Ferguson, 1993). Indeed, some researchers even believe that aspirin may be helpful in treating HIV infection (Stolberg, 1994). Preliminary laboratory research suggests that, in some unknown manner, aspirin may prevent the AIDS virus from replicating. Researchers are now exploring this effect to see whether it can be applied to treat those infected with HIV.

Aspirin, ibuprofen, and naproxen all have a chemical structure different from the steroids, another class of antiinflammatory drugs. For this reason, they are often called *Nonsteroidal antiinflammatory drugs* (or NSAIDs). Because acetaminophen has no significant antiinflammatory effect, it is not usually classified as a NSAID (Supernaw, 1991; Morgenroth, 1989), but it is not without its uses. Acetaminophen has been found to be as effective in the control of fever as aspirin (American Society of Hospital Pharmacists, 1994). Furthermore, as an OTC analgesic, acetaminophen is as potent as aspirin and can be used for virtually every painful condition that aspirin is used for.

Ibuprofen was the result of an intensive search by pharmaceutical companies to find a drug with the analgesic, antipyretic (fever reducing), and antiinflammatory actions of aspirin that was safer to use. As we will discuss later in this chapter, aspirin is a potentially dangerous chemical that can even have fatal side effects. Ibuprofen is thought to be about 30 times as effective as aspirin in both combating inflammation and in controlling pain and about 20 times as effective as aspirin in controlling fever (Mann, 1994).

Naproxen is another chemical compound that emerged from the search for compounds that offered the advantages of aspirin without its dangerous side effects. Long available only by prescription, naproxen has been found to be able to control mild to moderate levels of pain. Naproxen also has an antiinflammatory effect that makes it useful in treating such conditions as rheumatoid arthritis, dysmenorrhea, gout, tendinitis, and bursitis. As an OTC analgesic, naproxen is recommended for the treatment of headaches, the aches of the common cold, backache and muscle aches, arthritis, and the discomfort of menstrual cramps in addition to the control of fever (Gannon, 1994).

One exciting application of ibuprofen's antiinflammatory action is in the control of the tissue inflammation caused by cystic fibrosis, a disease that strikes children. Konstan, Hoppel, Chai, and Davis (1991) found that, like the anabolic steroids, dosage levels of 300 to 600 mg of ibuprofen were effective in controlling the inflammation of the lung tissues that is so often part of this disorder. However, when dosage levels were adjusted to match the child's body size, the authors found that ibuprofen was able to achieve acceptable levels of inflammation control without the harsh side effects often seen with anabolic steroid use.

Aspirin, acetaminophen, and ibuprofen have all been found to be effective in helping to control the pain associated with some forms of cancer (Fishman & Carr, 1992). Researchers have further concluded that aspirin and ibuprofen, when used in combination with narcotic analgesics, may actually lower the patient's need for narcotic painkillers after surgery, at least in some cases (Murphy, 1993).

Although not technically a recognized medical application of aspirin, the regular use of aspirin may inhibit the growth of tumors in the colon. Giovannucci, Rimm, Stampfer, Colditz,

Ascherio, and Willett (1994) reported on an ongoing project involving 47,900 male health care professionals who responded by mail to questionnaires in 1986, 1988, and again in 1990. The questionnaires included inquiries about aspirin use and the respondent's health status. The responses revealed that regular aspirin users (more than twice a week) had a significantly lower risk for colorectal cancer than did occasional aspirin users, after factoring out the impact of such variables as diet and parental history of cancer.

The exact mechanism by which aspirin may inhibit the growth of colorectal cancer is still not clear at this time. Thun, Namboodiri, and Heath (1991) suggest that aspirin's ability to inhibit prostaglandin synthesis (a process that will be discussed in the next section) may interfere with tumor cell growth through some unknown process. Another theory is that aspirin may stimulate the body's immune response in some unknown manner, allowing the body to fight the invading cancer more effectively.

Yet another possibility advanced by Thun, Namboodiri, and Heath (1991) is that, because aspirin increases the possibility of gastrointestinal bleeding, it may increase the tumor's tendency to bleed, which makes the tumor easier to detect. Thus it may be possible to discover a tumor at an earlier stage than would normally be the case. However, Giovannucci et al. (1994) found that the total number of colorectal cancers detected among aspirin users was significantly lower in their research sample, even after the variable of tumor bleeding was controlled for. They called for further research to determine the exact mechanism by which aspirin may inhibit the growth of tumors in the colon.

Unfortunately, given its popularity as an analgesic, acetaminophen does not seem to have any impact on tumor growth or the detection of colon tumors. Physicians are still learning about naproxen as well. There is strong evidence to suggest that, in addition to its antiinflammatory effects, naproxen may have other uses. For example, when used in combination with the antibiotic ampicillin, naproxen seems to reduce the distress felt by children with respiratory infections. As medical researchers continue to seek new uses for the OTC analgesics, these "old" drugs will prove of value in the treatment of disease well into the next century.

The Pharmacology of the OTC Analgesics

Aspirin

Aspirin is usually administered by mouth and is ultimately metabolized in the liver, although preliminary biotransformation takes place in the gastrointestinal tract. When taken on an empty stomach, aspirin begins to reach the blood-stream in as little as 1 minute (Rose, 1988). However, its primary site of absorption is the small intestine. After a single dose, peak blood levels of aspirin are achieved in between 15 minutes (Shannon, Wilson, & Stang, 1992) and 1 to 2 hours (McGuire, 1990).

Aspirin is biotransformed mainly in the liver. Although aspirin has a half-life of 15 to 20 minutes, one metabolite of aspirin—salicylate— has a half-life of 2 hours (or more if the person is using aspirin in high doses) (Shannon, Wilson, & Stang, 1992). Excretion of aspirin and its metabolites takes place through the kidneys, and only about 1% of the drug is eliminated unchanged in the urine.

Unlike the narcotic analgesics, which seem to work mainly within the brain, aspirin seems to have a different mechanism of action. First, rather than working within the brain itself (Gazzaniga, 1988), aspirin appears to work both at the site of the injury and within the spinal cord (Fishman & Carr, 1992). Although researchers have found evidence that aspirin reduces pain perception by acting on the spinal cord, the exact mechanism by which this is accomplished is still not clear (Graedon & Ferguson, 1993; Fishman & Carr, 1992). To understand how aspirin works, it is necessary to examine how the human body functions.

When damaged, each cell in the human body releases several chemicals to warn neighboring cells of the damage and to activate the body's repair mechanisms. Some of these chemicals include histamine, bradykinin, and a group of chemicals known as the prostaglandins. The inflammation and pain that results when these chemicals are released serves both to warn the individual of the injury and to activate the body's repair mechanisms.

Aspirin's analgesic effect at the site of the injury may be attributed to its power to inhibit the production of prostaglandins (American Society of Hospital Pharmacists, 1994; Bushnell & Justins, 1993). Aspirin inhibits the production of *cyclooxygenase*, an enzyme involved in prostaglandin production. By blocking the action of cyclooxygenase, aspirin is able to block prostaglandin production, lowering the level of pain and reducing inflammation.

Aspirin's ability to inhibit the formation of blood clots appears to be caused by indirectly inhibiting synthesis of the protein *thromboxane A_2* (Patrono, 1994). This protein is found in blood platelets and is essential to the formation of blood clots. Blood platelets have a normal lifetime of between 8 and 10 days, and the body is constantly manufacturing new platelets to replace those that have died. Because blood platelets cannot manufacture the protein thromboxane A_2, aspirin reduces the ability of all existing blood platelets to form clots. This is thought to be the mechanism through which aspirin is so useful in the treatment of heart attacks, strokes, and other conditions (Patrono, 1994). Eventually, these aspirin-inhibited blood platelets will be replaced with new ones as part of the normal process of platelet replacement. Thus, doses of aspirin must be taken every day or every other day to provide optimal inhibition of blood clot formation.

Acetaminophen

Acetaminophen is usually administered orally, although it may also be administered as a rectal suppository. Oral preparations include tablet, capsule, or liquid forms, and virtually 100% of the medication is absorbed through the gastro-intestinal tract (Shannon, Wilson, & Stang, 1992). Its peak effects occur 30 minutes to 2 hours after a single dose. Acetaminophen is metabolized in the liver, and virtually 100% of the drug is eliminated in the urine, although it may also be found in breast milk of nursing mothers.

Acetaminophen is thought to be as powerful as aspirin in its analgesic and fever-reducing potential (Supernaw, 1991). Indeed, as an anal-gesic or antifever medication, acetaminophen can be substituted for aspirin on a milligram-for-milligram basis. But the exact manner by which acetaminophen reduces pain or fever remains unknown (Shannon, Wilson, & Stang, 1992; Morgenroth, 1989). Unlike aspirin, acet-aminophen does not interfere with the normal blood clotting (Shannon, Wilson, & Stang, 1992). Nor does acetaminophen possess a significant antiinflammatory potential. Although acet-aminophen is able to control mild to moderate levels of pain, it does not seem to inhibit the formation of prostaglandins. Finally, individu-als who are allergic to aspirin do not usually suffer from adverse reactions when they take acetaminophen. These features often make acet-aminophen an ideal substitute for individuals who are unable to take aspirin.

Ibuprofen

Ibuprofen is usually administered orally, and about 80% of a single dose is absorbed from the gastrointestinal tract. Ibuprofen is metabolized in the liver, and its half-life is between 2 and 4 hours (Shannon, Wilson, & Stang, 1992). About 99% of the ibuprofen molecules become protein-bound following absorption into the general circulation (Olson, 1992). Ibuprofen and its me-tabolites are mainly eliminated by the kidneys, although a small amount of ibuprofen is elimi-nated through the bile.

Like aspirin, ibuprofen has been found to be effective in the control of mild to moderate levels of pain and in the control of fever (Shan-non, Wilson, & Stang, 1992). And, like aspirin, ibuprofen's analgesic action is thought to result from its ability to interfere with the production of the prostaglandins (Squires, 1990). This does not mean that ibuprofen can automatically be substituted for aspirin to control inflammation. Indeed, there is disagreement as to ibuprofen's effectiveness as an antiinflammatory agent.

Morgenroth (1989) suggests that ibuprofen is somewhat less effective than aspirin in treating inflammation, but Graedon (1980) disagrees. Graedon points out that ibuprofen is equally as effective as aspirin, but only at dosage levels of between 1,600 and 2,400 mg a day. And, as noted earlier in this chapter, Mann (1994) be-lieves that ibuprofen is 30 times as effective as aspirin in fighting inflammation.

No matter how powerful ibuprofen may be in fighting inflammation, ibuprofen's antiin-flammatory effects may not occur until after 2 to 4 weeks of continuous drug use, and then only at close to the maximum recommended dosage levels for this analgesic (Fischer, 1989). Although this suggests that one would do better to utilize aspirin for the control of inflammation, one must remember that aspirin is quite irritat-ing to the stomach. Ibuprofen, on the other hand, is about one-fifth to one-half as irritating to the stomach as aspirin (Giacona, Dahl, & Hare, 1987). Thus, ibuprofen is often utilized in cases where the individual is unable to toler-ate the gastrointestinal irritation caused by as-pirin.

Still, it has been estimated that between 4 and 14% of those who use ibuprofen will also expe-rience some degree of gastrointestinal irritation (Graedon, 1980). And just as aspirin can cause gastrointestinal bleeding when used for pro-longed periods of time, researchers estimate that approximately 3 out of every 1,000 people will also experience some degree of ibuprofen-induced gastrointestinal bleeding (Carlson et al., 1987). Taha, Dahill, Sturrock, Lee, and Russell (1994) found that 27% of their sample who had used ibuprofen for an extended period of time had evidence of ulcer formation in the gastrointestinal tract. However, the number of ibuprofen-using subjects in their sample was quite small, and it is not clear how representative these findings are of the ability of ibuprofen to contribute to gastrointestinal ulcer formation.

Naproxen

The latest arrival in the OTC analgesic market, naproxen, has a mechanism of action that is very similar to that of aspirin (American Society of Hospital Pharmacists, 1994) by interfering with the production of prostaglandins. However, naproxen may be more effective than aspirin as an antiinflammatory agent (American Society of Hospital Pharmacists, 1994; Graedon & Graedon, 1991). Although this characteristic would make it of value for the treatment of inflammatory conditions, it is not yet clear whether naproxen will be marketed as an antiinflammatory agent in the OTC market.

Like aspirin, naproxen has an antipyretic effect. Researchers are not sure of the exact mechanism through which naproxen reduces fever, but it is believed that naproxen may suppress the synthesis of prostaglandins in the hypothalamus (American Society of Hospital Pharmacists, 1994), a region of the brain that helps to regulate body temperature.

The half-life of naproxen in the healthy adult is approximately 10 to 20 hours. An estimated 30% of a given dose of naproxen is metabolized by the liver into the inactive metabolite *6-desmethylnaproxen*; only 10% is excreted unchanged, and 5% is excreted in the feces (American Society of Hospital Pharmacists, 1994). The majority of a standard dose of naproxen is excreted in the urine as either metabolized or unmetabolized drug.

As stated earlier, naproxen binds to proteins in the blood plasma, which can absorb only so much of the medication before reaching a saturation point. Research suggests that the concentration of naproxen reaches a plateau if the patient takes 500 mg twice daily for 2 to 3 days (American Society of Hospital Pharmacists,

1994).[4] Thus, the typical dosage level does not exceed 500 mg every 12 hours.

All the OTC analgesics can control mild to moderate levels of pain. These effects are both an advantage and a danger for the patient. The control of pain or fever provides only symptomatic relief. Even when pain or fever has been controlled, its cause must still be identified and treated to ensure adequate medical care (Fishman & Carr, 1992).

Effects of OTC Analgesics at Normal Dosage Levels

Aspirin

There is conflicting evidence as to whether aspirin's analgesic effects are dose-related (Giacona, Dahl, & Hare, 1987), and there is mixed evidence suggesting little or no additional analgesic benefits from increasing adult dosage levels above 600 mg every 4 hours. At this dosage level, both aspirin and acetaminophen have a significant analgesic potential. McGuire (1990) reports that 650 mg of aspirin or acetaminophen, a standard dose of two regular strength tablets of either medication, provides an analgesic effect equal to 50 mg of the narcotic painkiller meperidine (Demerol). Kaplan and Sadock (1990) suggest that 650 mg of aspirin has the same analgesic potential as 32 mg of codeine, 65 mg of Darvon (propoxyphene), or a 50 mg oral dose of Talwin (pentazocine).

In a study by Kacso and Terezhalmy (1994), a single dose of 1,300 mg of aspirin seemed to provide a greater degree of relief from pain than did a single dose of 600 mg. However, dosage levels above 1,300 mg in a single dose did not provide any greater degree of analgesia, and actually put the user at risk for a toxic reaction.

---

[4]Patients should not take 500 mg of naproxen twice a day, however, except under a physician's supervision.

In contrast, Aronoff, Wagner, and Spangler (1986) postulate that there is a "ceiling effect" (p. 769) for aspirin, beyond which higher dosage levels will not provide greater pain relief. They put this ceiling at "approximately 1,000 mg every 4 hr" (p. 769). A dosage level of aspirin higher than this "only increases the threat of a toxic reaction" (McGuire, 1990, p. 30).

The American Society of Hospital Pharmacists (1994) recommends a normal adult oral dosage level of 325 to 650 mg of aspirin every 4 hours as needed for the control of pain. This recommendation includes a warning that aspirin should not be continuously used for longer than 10 days by an adult or longer than 5 days by a child under the age of 12, except under a doctor's orders.[5]

When taken by mouth, aspirin is rapidly and completely absorbed from the gastrointestinal tract and distributed by the blood to virtually every body tissue and fluid. The actual speed at which aspirin is absorbed depends on the acidity of the stomach contents (Sheridan, Patterson, & Gustafson, 1982). When taken on an empty stomach, the rate at which aspirin is absorbed depends on how quickly the tablet crumbles after reaching the stomach (Rose, 1988). After the tablet crumbles, the individual aspirin molecules pass through the stomach lining into the general circulatory system.

When taken with food or immediately after eating, aspirin may take 5 to 10 times longer to reach the bloodstream and have a therapeutic effect on the individual (Pappas, 1990). Ultimately, however, *all* the aspirin is absorbed from the gastrointestinal tract. Therefore, Rodman (1993) suggests that aspirin be taken with food to limit aspirin-induced irritation to the stomach lining. However, in some cases, it is desirable to achieve as high a blood level of aspirin as soon as possible. Patients should

consult a pharmacist or physician before attempting to use this technique to limit stomach irritation.

Aspirin is sold both alone and in combination with agents designed to reduce irritation to the stomach. In theory, timed-released and enteric coated tablets have the potential for reducing the irritation to the gastrointestinal tract. However, both forms of aspirin have been known to bring about erratic absorption rates, making it harder to achieve the desired effect (Shannon, Wilson, & Stang, 1992).

Some patients take aspirin with antacids to reduce irritation to the stomach. When antacids are mixed with aspirin, however, the blood level of aspirin is 30% to 70% lower than when aspirin is used without antacids (Rodman, 1993; Graedon, 1980). This is a matter of some concern for individuals who are taking the drug for the control of inflammation or pain, because lower blood levels of aspirin mean that less of the drug is available to help control the pain.

Acetaminophen

The usual adult dose of acetaminophen is also 325 to 650 mg every 4 hours, as needed for the control of pain (American Society of Hospital Pharmacists, 1994). In many ways, dosage recommendations for aspirin and acetaminophen are very similar. For example, Aronoff, Wagner, and Spangler (1986) observe that acetaminophen's antipyretic and analgesic effects are equal to those of aspirin, and the ceiling level is the same for these two drugs.

Peak blood concentrations are achieved 30 minutes to 2 hours after an oral dose of acetaminophen (Shannon, Wilson, & Stang, 1992). The half-life of an oral dose of acetaminophen is normally from 1 to 4 hours. However, because this chemical is metabolized in the liver, people with significant liver damage may experience a longer acetaminophen half-life than what is normally the case and should use acetaminophen only under a physician's supervision. Sands, Knapp, and Ciraulo (1993) go even further, recommending that patients with alcohol-

---

[5] When used in the treatment of arthritis, aspirin may be used at higher than normal dosage levels for extended periods of time. These dosage levels are used under a doctor's supervision, and the dangers associated with these high dosage levels are weighed against the benefits that the medication offers.

related liver damage totally avoid the use of acetaminophen because enzymes produced by the alcohol-damaged liver transform acetaminophen into a toxin, even when the drug is used at recommended dosage levels.

Ibuprofen

Ibuprofen occupies a unique position in that it is available both over the counter and as a prescription medication. When used as a nonprescription analgesic, the recommended dose of ibuprofen is 200 to 400 mg every 4 hours (Dionne & Gordon, 1994). As a prescription medication, doses of 400 to 800 mg are often prescribed, depending on the specific condition being treated.

Shannon, Wilson, and Stang (1992) recommend that 300 to 600 mg of ibuprofen be used 3 to 4 times a day for the control of rheumatoid arthritis and 200 to 400 mg every 4 to 6 hours for the control of mild to moderate pain. However, there is some disagreement about ibuprofen's analgesic potential. Dionne and Gordon (1994) note that the greatest degree of relief from pain is achieved with doses of 400 to 600 mg, and that ibuprofen above this level is unlikely to result in greater levels of analgesia. In contrast, however, Rosenblum (1992) states that 800 mg of ibuprofen provides greater control of postoperative pain than therapeutic doses of the narcotic fentanyl in a small sample of women recovering from laparoscopic surgery.

It is important to keep in mind the fact that the *OTC* dosage levels of ibuprofen are limited to 200 to 400 mg every 4 hours; a physician may prescribe a higher dosage level. However, even when it is used as a prescription medication, the total daily dosage level should not exceed 3,200 mg per day, in divided doses (Dionne & Gordon, 1994).

When used orally, ibuprofen is rapidly absorbed and distributed throughout the body. After a single dose, peak blood plasma levels are achieved 1 to 2 hours after ingesting the drug (American Society of Hospital Pharmacists, 1994). Within 4 hours of ingesting a normal

dose, blood plasma levels will fall to about half the peak plasma level (Shannon, Wilson, & Stang, 1992).

Naproxen

Although naproxen was available by prescription in the United States for a number of years, it was finally approved for over-the-counter use in 1994. One brand name of OTC naproxen is "Aleve," sold in tablets of 200 mg of naproxen and 20 mg of sodium (Gannon, 1994). According to a package insert, users are advised to take up to 3 tablets, twice a day.

Complications from OTC Analgesic Use

The OTC analgesics are hardly "safe" medications. In general, these drugs can "be harmful, even deadly, if used too often, in combination with one another, or by the wrong people at the wrong time" (Morgenroth, 1989, p. 36). Although they are available without a prescription, the OTC analgesics pose a significant potential for harm, a fact that many people tend to forget.

Aspirin

Aspirin is the most commonly used drug in the United States, where between 20 billion (Rapoport, 1993) and 40 billion (Talley, 1993) tablets of aspirin are consumed a year. Steele and Morton (1986) estimate that between 30 to 74 *million pounds* of aspirin are consumed each year. Worldwide, 100 million pounds of aspirin are consumed each year (Mann & Plummer, 1991).

Because aspirin is a popular over-the-counter medication, many people underestimate both its usefulness and its potential for causing serious side effects (Jaffe & Martin, 1990). Consider that after just a single dose, virtually every user will experience some degree of gastrointestinal bleeding (Talley, 1993; Pappas, 1990). This aspirin-induced gastrointestinal bleeding is usually minor after a single dose. But up to 15% of those individuals who occasionally take aspirin at recommended dosage levels will experience a significant adverse side effect (Rapoport, 1993). When it is used on a chronic basis, a significant percentage of individuals will experience adverse aspirin-related side effects. Forty percent of the patients who use aspirin at recommended doses on a chronic basis will experience an erosion in their stomach lining, and between 17% (Kitridou, 1993) and 30% (Taha, Dahill, Sturrock, Lee, & Russell, 1994) will actually develop stomach ulcers.

Thus, it should not be surprising to learn that, when used on a regular basis, aspirin may contribute to the formation of a "bleeding" ulcer.[6] Indeed, in more than 20% of cases of "bleeding" ulcers, doctors conclude that the patient's use of aspirin was a major contributing factor (Talley, 1993). Wilcox, Shalek, and Cotsonis (1994) give an even higher estimate, noting that 41% of the patients admitted to the hospital for a gastrointestinal (GI) hemorrhage had consumed aspirin in the week prior to admission. The regular use of aspirin can also contribute to the formation of potentially life-threatening ulcers in the small intestine (Allison, Howatson, Torrance, Lee, & Russell, 1992). Therefore, aspirin should not be used by anyone with a history of ulcers, bleeding disorders, or other gastrointestinal disorders (American Society of Hospital Pharmacists, 1994). It is further suggested that people not take aspirin with acidic foods such as coffee, fruit juices, or alcohol, which may further irritate the gastrointestinal system (Pappas, 1990).

Not every patient who uses aspirin for a protracted period of time will experience a major gastrointestinal hemorrhage or ulcers. But a significant number who do use aspirin for extended periods will develop bleeding severe

enough to require hospitalization. Furthermore, many of the ulcers that form as a result of aspirin use fail to produce major warning symptoms (Taha et al., 1994). Thus, the potential benefit for the use of aspirin must be weighed against the potential harm the drug can cause.

Aspirin's ability to cause gastric irritation is thought to be a side effect of aspirin's nonselective ability to interfere with production of prostaglandins (Mortensen & Rennebohm, 1989). Because aspirin is a nonselective antiprostaglandin, it can disrupt the production of the prostaglandins necessary for the proper function of the gastric lining. Thus, while blocking the production of prostaglandins at the site of an injury, aspirin can cause irritation and bleeding in the stomach and gastrointestinal tract. This is why such a large percentage of chronic aspirin users experience gastrointestinal problems.

When used at recommended dosage levels for extended periods of time, aspirin has also been known to cause breathing problems in up to 33% of patients (Kitridou, 1993), probably as a result of allergic reactions to aspirin. Approximately 2% of the general population is allergic to aspirin. However, of those individuals with a history of allergic disorders, approximately 20% are allergic to aspirin. Patients who are sensitive to aspirin are likely also to be sensitive to ibuprofen, as cross-sensitivity between these two drugs is common (Shannon, Wilson, & Stang, 1992; Fischer, 1989).

Symptoms of an allergic reaction to aspirin might include rash, breathing problems, and asthmalike reactions that may be fatal (Zuger, 1994). Patients with symptoms of the "aspirin triad"—a history of nasal polyps, asthma, and sensitivity to aspirin—should not use either aspirin or ibuprofen (Shannon, Wilson, & Stang, 1992). Anyone with a history of chronic rhinitis should not use aspirin except under a physician's supervision (Shannon, Wilson, & Stang, 1992). These conditions are warning signals for individuals "at risk" for an allergic reaction to aspirin or similar agents.

Aspirin can cause a number of other side effects, including anorexia, nausea, and vomit-

---

[6] This is the formation of a stomach ulcer over a blood vessel in the stomach wall. As the surrounding tissue is destroyed by the stomach acid, the blood vessel is gradually exposed and ultimately ruptures. This is a serious medical emergency, which may result in the patient's death.

ing (Sheridan, Patterson, & Gustafson, 1982). Because aspirin can cause gastrointestinal bleeding, individuals who use aspirin on a regular basis may actually develop anemia as a result of the constant internal blood loss.

Because of their effects on blood clotting, neither aspirin, naproxen, nor ibuprofen should be used by individuals with a bleeding disorder such as hemophilia (American Society of Hospital Pharmacists, 1994; Shannon, Wilson, & Stang, 1992). Even in a normal patient, a single dose of aspirin can prolong bleeding time for between 3 to 7 days after the last use of the drug (Shannon, Wilson, & Stang, 1992). People undergoing anticoagulant therapy involving such drugs as heparin or warfarin should not use aspirin except when directed by a physician (Rodman, 1993). The combined effects of aspirin and the anticoagulant may result in significant, unintended blood loss.

Patients being treated for hyperuricemia (a buildup of uric acid in the blood often found in gout as well as other conditions) should not use aspirin. When used at normal dosage levels, aspirin reduces the body's ability to excrete uric acid, contributing to the problem of uric acid buildup. If the individual is taking the prescription medication probenecid, one of the drugs used to treat hyperuricemia, he or she should not take aspirin. At therapeutic doses, aspirin inhibits the action of probenecid, allowing uric acid levels to build up in the blood. Acetaminophen has been advanced as a suitable substitute for patients who suffer from gout and need a mild analgesic (Shannon, Wilson, & Stang, 1992).

Aspirin also should not be used in patients who are receiving medications to control their blood pressure, except under a physician's supervision. It has been found that aspirin may interfere with the effectiveness of some antihypertensive medications (Fischer, 1989). Although the exact mechanism by which this happens is unclear, it may reflect the impact of aspirin use on prostaglandin production within the kidneys.

Patients taking other NSAIDs such as ibuprofen or naproxen should not take aspirin, except under a physician's supervision. The combined effects of these medications can cause significant gastrointestinal tract irritation (Rodman, 1993).

Aspirin, naproxen, and ibuprofen can all bring about a loss of hearing and a persistent "ringing" in the ears known as "tinnitus." The patient's hearing usually returns to normal when the offending medication is discontinued. A very rare side effect of aspirin use is *hepatotoxicity*, in which the aspirin may prevent the liver from filtering the blood effectively (Gay, 1990). This allows the buildup of certain toxins in the blood, which may appear suddenly. The available literature suggests that hepatotoxicity caused by the use of aspirin or ibuprofen is extremely rare but has been documented (Gay, 1990). Another rare complication from aspirin use is a drug-induced depression (Mortensen & Rennebohm, 1989).

For reasons that are not entirely clear, the elderly are especially susceptible to toxicity from aspirin and similar agents, perhaps because their bodies are unable to metabolize and excrete this family of drugs as effectively as younger adults. Bleidt and Moss (1989) attribute this to the reduced blood flow to the liver and kidneys. Another complication of aspirin use in the elderly is the development of drug-induced anxiety states (Sussman, 1988).

Aspirin or related compounds should not be given to children who are suffering from a viral infection, unless under a physician's supervision. Research strongly suggests that aspirin increases the possibility of the child developing *Reye's syndrome* (Morgenroth, 1989; Sagar, 1991). Reye's syndrome is a serious, potentially fatal condition that affects children between the ages of 2 and 12, for the most part (Sagar, 1991), and usually follows a viral infection such as influenza or chicken pox. Symptoms include swelling of the brain, seizures, disturbance of consciousness, and a fatty degeneration of the liver (*Dorland's Illustrated Medical Dictionary*, 1988) as well as coma and possible death (Sagar, 1991).

Individuals who plan to consume alcohol should avoid using aspirin immediately prior to or while actively drinking. According to Roine et al. (1990) the use of aspirin prior to the ingestion of alcohol decreases the activity of gastric alcohol dehydrogenase, an enzyme produced by the stomach that starts to metabolize alcohol even before it reaches the bloodstream. This action results in a higher than normal blood alcohol level, even in the rare social drinker.

Surprisingly, aspirin has also been implicated in the failure of the intrauterine devices (IUDs) to prevent pregnancy. The antiinflammatory action of aspirin is thought to be the agent that interferes with the effectiveness of intrauterine devices.

Aspirin has also been implicated in fertility problems for couples who wish to have children. The use of aspirin even at therapeutic dosage levels may reduce sperm motility (ability to move) by up to 50%. Although this is not to suggest that aspirin might serve as a method of birth control, the reduction in sperm motility could interfere with the couple's ability to conceive.

Ibuprofen

Ibuprofen has been implicated as the cause of blurred vision in some patients (Nicastro, 1989). Graedon (1980) suggests that people using ibuprofen who experience some change in their vision should discontinue the medication and consult with their physician immediately. In addition to the 3% to 9% of the patients on ibuprofen who experience skin rashes or hives, ibuprofen has been implicated in the formation of cataracts (Graedon, 1980) and as the cause of migraine headaches in both men and women (Nicastro, 1989).

The Upjohn Company (the manufacturers of Motrin) warns that ibuprofen has been found to cause a number of side effects, including heartburn, nausea, diarrhea, vomiting, nervousness, hearing loss, changes in vision, and elevated blood pressure (Medical Economics Company,

1995). It has also been known to cause congestive heart failure in people with preexisting heart problems.

Recent research also shows that ibuprofen can cause or contribute to kidney failure in people with high blood pressure, kidney disease, or other health problems (Squires, 1990). This may be a side effect of ibuprofen's ability to block the production of prostaglandin. By blocking the body's production of prostaglandin, ibuprofen also reduces the blood flow throughout the body, especially to the kidneys. If the individual is already suffering from a reduction in blood flow to the kidneys for any reason, including "normal aging, liver or cardiovascular disease or simply dehydration from vomiting, diarrhea and fever accompanying the flu" (Squires, 1990, p. 4E), ibuprofen may cause or contribute to acute kidney failure.

Patients who are suffering from *systemic lupus erythematosus* (often simply called "lupus" or SLE) should not use ibuprofen, except under a physician's supervision. Occasionally, ibuprofen has caused a condition known as *aseptic meningitis* within hours of the time that a patient with SLE had ingested the ibuprofen. Aseptic meningitis is also a complication in extremely rare cases in which a patient who does *not* have SLE ingests ibuprofen (Zuger, 1994). However, there have been fewer than 40 reported cases of this side effect in patients who do not have SLE or some other autoimmune disorder.

If a person is also taking lithium, ibuprofen may increase the blood levels of lithium by 25% to 60% (Rodman, 1993; Jenike, 1991). This effect is most pronounced in older individuals and may contribute to lithium toxicity. Close monitoring of blood lithium levels is critical for patients who use both lithium and ibuprofen concurrently, even if the OTC ibuprofen is taken at recommended dosage levels.

Ibuprofen also reduces the rate at which the prescription medication methotrexate is excreted from the body (Rodman, 1993). Reduced excretion rates may result in the buildup of toxic levels of methotrexate. If an OTC analgesic should be required, Rodman (1993) recommends the use of acetaminophen.

Ibuprofen should not be used in conjunction with other NSAIDs, including aspirin, except under a physician's supervision (Rodman, 1993). The combined effects of NSAIDs may result in excessive irritation to the gastrointestinal tract and possibly severe bleeding.

Acetaminophen

Acetaminophen is metabolized by the liver. As outlined in Chapter Five, the liver may be damaged by the chronic use of alcohol. It has been observed (Morgenroth, 1989) that chronic alcohol use may lower the dosage level at which acetaminophen becomes toxic. According to Mitchell (1988), there are a few cases in which chronic alcoholics have suffered from toxic effects of acetaminophen at dosage levels only slightly higher than the normal recommended dose. Thus, active or recovering alcoholics are advised not to use acetaminophen for any reason, except under a doctor's supervision (Shannon, Wilson, & Stang, 1992).

Naproxen

Much of the information available on naproxen and its effects is based on experiences with prescription forms of this chemical. In some users, naproxen has been found to be a factor in potentially fatal allergic reactions. Patients with the "aspirin triad" (discussed earlier) should not use naproxen, and naproxen may also contribute to the formation of peptic ulcers and gastrointestinal bleeding. Animal research suggests the possibility of damage to the eyes as a result of naproxen use, although it is not clear at this time whether this applies to humans as well.

Naproxen has occasionally contributed to drowsiness, dizziness, feelings of depression, and vertigo, and patients have been known to experience diarrhea, heartburn, constipation, and vomiting. Indeed, between 3 and 9% of the patients who used prescription-strength naproxen experienced such side effects as constipation, heartburn, abdominal pain, and nausea. Taha et al. (1994) found that 44% of their sample who had used naproxen for extended periods of time showed evidence of gastrointestinal ulcers. Although it is not clear how representative these findings are of naproxen's ability to contribute to the formation of ulcers, naproxen should not be used by patients with a history of peptic ulcer disease (Dionne & Gordon, 1994).

There have been rare reports of patients who developed side effects such as skin rash, diarrhea, headache, insomnia, sleep problems, problems with their hearing, and/or tinnitus after using naproxen. There have also been reports of potentially fatal liver dysfunctions that seem to have been caused by naproxen. Thus, although this medication has been approved for OTC use, it is hardly without its dangers.

OTC Analgesic Overdose

Aspirin

Although scientists have made great strides in understanding and thus countering the effects of an aspirin overdose, this medication remains potentially dangerous in an overdose situation. The average dosage level necessary to produce a toxic reaction is about 10 grams of aspirin for an adult and about 150 mg of aspirin for every kilogram of body weight for children. A dose of 500 mg per kilogram of body weight is potentially fatal.

In the past 40 years, scientists have learned a great deal about how an aspirin overdose affects the body (Yip, Dart, & Gabow, 1994). Although medical researchers have developed methods to treat an aspirin overdose, it has been estimated that in 1990 aspirin caused approximately as many deaths in the United States as did heroin overdoses (Playboy, 1991).

Symptoms of an aspirin toxicity are usually

found in patients who take large doses of aspirin, but even small doses may result in toxicity for the individual who is aspirin-sensitive. Symptoms of aspirin toxicity include headache, dizziness, tinnitus, mental confusion, increased sweating, thirst, dimmed vision, and hearing impairment (Shannon, Wilson, & Stang, 1992). Other symptoms of aspirin toxicity include restlessness, excitement, apprehension, tremor, delirium, hallucinations, convulsions, stupor, coma, and—at higher dosage levels—possible death.

Acetaminophen

Acetaminophen overdoses account for over 100,000 telephone calls to regional poison control centers each year in the United States (Anker & Smilkstein, 1994). Acetaminophen is the drug most commonly ingested in an overdose attempt (Anker & Smilkstein, 1994; Lipscomb, 1989); unfortunately, it is also potentially deadly.

Adolescents often ingest acetaminophen when they make suicide gestures (Morgenroth, 1989). Although suicide is rarely intended, the relatively low dose necessary to produce a toxic reaction to acetaminophen makes it a poor choice for such a gesture. Because the effects of a toxic dose of acetaminophen are not always immediately apparent, medical assistance may not be sought until several days after the initial overdose, well after the time for effective countermeasures has passed.

Acetaminophen is effective and relatively safe when used at recommended dosage levels, but when taken to excess, it is quite toxic to the liver. Large doses of acetaminophen destroy the enzyme *glutathione*, a chemical produced by the liver to protect itself from various toxins (Anker & Smilkstein, 1994). A dose of just 7.5 to 15 grams of acetaminophen (15 to 30 extra-strength tablets) is enough to cause a toxic reaction in a healthy adult (Morgenroth, 1989). For children, the toxic level is approximately 140 mg per kilogram of body weight. The danger is not limited to individuals who take a single large dose of acetaminophen; individuals who use acetaminophen at high dosage levels for extended periods of time (5,000 mg a day for 2 to 3 weeks) are also likely to develop liver damage (Supernaw, 1991).

Unfortunately, although an antidote to acetaminophen is available, it must be administered *within 12 hours* of the overdose to be fully effective. When administered within several hours of the initial overdose, the antidote—*N-acetylcysteine*—is quite effective in the treatment of acetaminophen poisoning (Mitchell, 1988). If, as all too often happens, the individual waits until the symptoms of acetaminophen toxicity develop before seeking help—a process that may take 2 to 3 days—it may be too late to prevent permanent liver damage or even death.

Ibuprofen

Ibuprofen's popularity as an OTC analgesic has resulted in an increasing number of overdoses of this drug (Lipscomb, 1989). Symptoms of overdose include seizures, acute renal failure, abdominal pain, nausea, vomiting, drowsiness, and metabolic acidosis (Lipscomb, 1989). There is no specific antidote for ibuprofen toxicity, and medical care is often aimed at supportive treatment only.

Summary

Over-the-counter analgesics are often discounted by many as not being "real" medications. But aspirin is still the most popular "drug" in the United States. Each year, more than 20,000 tons of aspirin are manufactured and consumed in this country alone, and aspirin accounts for only about 28% of the OTC analgesic sales.

Aspirin, acetaminophen, ibuprofen, and naproxen are all effective in the control of mild to moderate levels of pain, without the side effects found with narcotic analgesics. Some

OTC analgesics are also useful in controlling the inflammation of autoimmune disorders and postsurgical pain, and the pain associated with cancer. Aspirin may even contribute to the early detection of some forms of cancer. Medical researchers are still discovering new applications for these potent medications.

Even though they are available without a prescription, the OTC analgesics do carry signif-icant potential for harm. Acetaminophen has been implicated in toxic reactions in chronic alcoholics at near-normal dosage levels. It also has been implicated as the cause of death in acetaminophen overdoses. Aspirin and ibu-profen have been implicated in fatal allergic reactions, especially in those who suffer from asthma.

CHAPTER THIRTEEN

The Hallucinogens

It has been estimated that about 6,000 different species of plants can be used for their psycho-active properties (Brophy, 1993). Several species of mushrooms can produce hallucinations (Rold, 1993), and many of these plants and mushrooms have been used for centuries in religious ceremonies, healing rituals, for pre-dicting the future (Kaplan & Sadock, 1990; Berger & Dunn, 1982), and to prepare warriors for battle (Rold, 1993). Even today, certain religious groups use mushrooms with hallucinogenic properties as part of their worship, although this practice is illegal in the United States (Rold, 1993).

Over the years, researchers have identified approximately 100 different hallucinogenic compounds that can be found in various plants or mushrooms. Many of these compounds have been extensively studied by scientists. Indeed, it was through a medical experiment that the effects of *lysergic acid diethylamide-25* (LSD-25, or simply LSD) were discovered. LSD is a substance obtained from the rye ergot fungus *Claviceps purpurea* (Lingeman, 1974). In 1943, a scientist accidentally ingested a small amount of LSD-25 while conducting an experiment and experienced its hallucinogenic effects.

After World War II, there was a great deal of scientific interest in the various hallucinogenics, especially given the similarities between the subjective effects of these chemicals and various forms of mental illness. Because these sub-stances were so potent, certain agencies of the U.S. government experimented with various chemical agents, including LSD, as possible chemical warfare weapons (Budiansky, Goode, & Gest, 1994). At one point scientists questioned whether LSD might be useful in the treatment of alcoholism (Henderson, 1994a).

The hallucinogens were hardly a well-kept secret, and in the 1960s, they moved from the laboratory into the streets, where they quickly became popular drugs of abuse (Brown & Braden, 1987). The popularity and widespread abuse of LSD in the 1960s prompted its classifi-cation as a controlled substance in 1970 (Jaffe, 1990). But this classification did not solve the problem of its abuse. Over the years, LSD has waxed and waned in popularity, and now ap-pears to be increasing once more (Henderson, 1994a; *Mayo Clinic Health Letter*, 1989).

The hallucinogen phencyclidine (PCP) de-serves special mention. Because of its toxicity, PCP fell into disfavor in the early 1970s (Jaffe, 1989). But, in the 1980s, a form of PCP that could be smoked was introduced, and it again became a popular drug of abuse. Currently, PCP seems to have fallen out of favor again, although it is still being used.

Another drug, *N, alpha-dimethyl-1,3 benzodi-oxole-t-ethanamine* (MDMA), became quite pop-ular as a chemical of abuse in the late 1970s and early 1980s. This drug is frequently sold on the streets under the name of "Ecstasy." Both PCP and MDMA will be discussed in later sections of this chapter.

The Scope of the Problem of Hallucinogen Abuse

It is difficult to estimate the number of casual hallucinogenic users in this country. Evidence suggests that LSD is gaining in popularity with adolescents (Kaminer, 1994; Gold, Schuchard, & Gleaton, 1994). Indeed, Gold et al. report that 5.3% of the high school seniors questioned admitted to having used LSD at least once. Johnston, O'Malley, and Bachman (1994) found that 10.3% of the seniors of the class of 1993 admitted to having used LSD at least once, a significant increase over the previous year.

These figures suggest that high school seniors are more likely to accept experimental LSD use than were students from past years; these figures also suggest a trend toward increasing acceptance of LSD use by adolescents. In the past, the majority of those who used hallucinogens experimented with the drug and then either totally avoided further hallucinogen use or went on to use hallucinogens on only an episodic basis (Jaffe, 1989). However, LSD has recently been "repackaged" and "reformulated," so that current preparations contain lower dosages than were typical in past years (Gold, Schuchard, & Gleaton, 1994). Thus, much of what was discovered about the effects of LSD in the 1960s and 1970s may not apply to the current user, since he or she may ingest a far smaller dose of LSD than was typical 20 years ago.

The Pharmacology of the Hallucinogens

The commonly abused hallucinogenics can be divided into two major groups on the basis of their chemical structure (Jaffe, 1989). First, there are the hallucinogens that bear a structural resemblance to the neurotransmitter serotonin. Hallucinogens in this group include LSD, psilo-

cybin, and the chemical dimethyltryptamine (DMT).

A second group of hallucinogenics is chemically related to the neurotransmitters dopamine and norepinephrine. The chemical structure of these agents also resembles that of the amphetamine family of drugs (Jaffe, 1989). These hallucinogens include, among others, mescaline, MDMA, and DOM (which is also known as STP).

Despite the chemical differences between hallucinogens, their effects are remarkably similar. A possible exception to this rule is DMT. The effects of DMT last only about 20 minutes, which is why it is often called a "businessman's high"; it easily fits into a typical half-hour lunch break. Aside from this exception, DMT is very similar to the other hallucinogens discussed in this chapter.

Although it is common for a person under the influence of one of the hallucinogens to believe that he or she has a new insight into reality, these drugs do not generate new thoughts so much as alter one's perception of existing sensory stimuli (Snyder, 1986). And, in spite of their chemical differences, these drugs all produce hallucinations or hallucinatorylike experiences that are usually recognized by the user as being drug-induced (Lingeman, 1974). Thus, the terms "hallucinogen" or "hallucinogenic" are usually applied to this class of drugs.

LSD has long been considered the standard hallucinogenic, and the effects of other hallucinogens are often compared to those of LSD. To avoid duplication of material, the major focus of this chapter will be on the hallucinogens LSD, MDMA, and PCP; other hallucinogens will be discussed only briefly.

The Pharmacology of LSD

In terms of relative potency, LSD is perhaps the most potent chemical known to man. Research has shown that LSD is effective at doses as low as 50 micrograms (Mirin, Weiss, & Greenfield, 1991). The usual street dose of LSD is about 0.05 mg (Restak, 1994). Although it is possible to administer LSD by intravenous injection, this is quite rare (Henderson, 1994a). The usual method of administration is orally. It is not possible to absorb LSD through the skin (Henderson, 1994a).

The LSD molecule is water-soluble. When taken by mouth, LSD is rapidly absorbed from the gastrointestinal tract and quickly distributed to all body tissues including the brain (Mirin, Weiss, & Greenfield, 1991). Because it is distributed throughout the body, only about 0.01% of the drug actually reaches the brain (Lingeman, 1974). Thus, if the user were to ingest a 50-microgram dose of LSD, only five-tenths of a microgram would actually reach the brain.

The chemical structure of the LSD molecule is very similar to that of the neurotransmitter serotonin, and in the brain, the LSD molecules seem to use some of the same receptor sites normally utilized by serotonin. This probably accounts for the ability of LSD to cause perceptual and mood distortions, as serotonin is a neurotransmitter involved in the process of perception and mood modification (Henderson, 1994a).

One theory is that LSD inhibits the activity of serotonin in the region of the brain known as the *dorsal midbrain raphe* (Mirin, Weiss, & Greenfield, 1991). Jaffe (1989) challenged this theory and suggested that LSD exerts an effect at various sites in the central nervous system, ranging from the cortex of the brain to the spinal cord and including (but not limited to) the midbrain sites identified by Mirin, Weiss, and Greenfield (1991). Another theory is that LSD's psychoactive effects are caused by the drug's actions in the region of the brain known as the *temporal lobe* (Restak, 1994). Restak supports this theory with the observation that individuals who suffer from temporal lobe epilepsy often report experiences similar to those of LSD users. However, after more than 50 years of research, the exact mechanism of action for LSD is still unknown (Henderson, 1994a; Jaffe, 1989).

The user begins to feel the effects of a dose of LSD in 30 minutes to 1 hour (Henderson, 1994a). In addition to a sense of euphoria, some of the physical effects of LSD include tachycardia, increased blood pressure, increased body temperature, pupillary dilation, nausea, and muscle weakness (Jaffe, 1989). Other side effects of LSD include an exaggeration of normal reflexes (a condition known as hyperreflexia), dizziness, and some degree of muscle tremor (Jaffe, 1989). Lingeman (1974) characterized these changes as "relatively minor" (p. 133), although they may cause some degree of anxiety for the inexperienced user.

Tolerance to the effects of LSD develop quickly, often within 2 to 4 days of continual use (Henderson, 1994a; Mirin, Weiss, & Greenfield, 1991; Brown & Braden, 1987). If the user becomes tolerant to the effects of LSD, increasing the dosage level will have little if any effect (Henderson, 1994a). However, tolerance to LSD's effects abates after just 2 to 4 days of abstinence (Henderson, 1994a; Jaffe, 1989; Lingeman, 1974). Cross-tolerance between the different hallucinogens is also quite common (Jaffe, 1989; Lingeman, 1974). Therefore, most users of hallucinogens limit their use of these chemicals to just a few days at a time, interspaced with periods of abstinence to allow their bodies to lose the tolerance acquired during the last period of hallucinogenic use.

In terms of direct physical mortality, LSD is perhaps the safest drug known to modern medicine (Brown & Braden, 1987; Weil, 1986); however, Lingeman (1974) reports that an elephant who received a massive dose of LSD (297,000 micrograms, or 5,940 doses at 50 micrograms each) died.[1] Although this suggests that LSD may prove toxic to the user, the lethal dose of LSD for humans is simply not known.[2] Indeed, Henderson (1994a) states that "the risk of death from an overdose of LSD is virtually nonexistent" (p. 43). But, indirectly, LSD has been implicated as the cause of death in some users, usually as a result of accidents.

---

[1] Lingeman (1974) did not mention how the elephant happened to ingest the LSD in the first place.

[2] It should be noted that this margin of safety does not extend to the other hallucinogens; it is possible both to overdose and to die from some of the other popular hallucinogens.

The half-life of LSD is not known, but estimates range from 2 to 3 hours (Shepherd & Jagoda, 1990; Jaffe, 1989, 1990) to 5 hours (Henderson, 1994a). Approximately half of the original dose of LSD is metabolized by the liver, and only about 1% is excreted unchanged. The rest is biotransformed by the liver and excreted in the bile (Henderson, 1994a). Surprisingly, given its short half-life, the effects of LSD in humans seem to last about 8 to 12 hours (Kaplan & Sadock, 1990), a phenomenon that is not understood at this time.

Although it has been in use for more than 50 years, researchers are continually discovering more about LSD. It is now known that only a small portion of a given dose of LSD actually enters the brain. But, as we will discuss in the next section, the drug has a profound impact on consciousness.

Subjective Effects of the Hallucinogens

The effects of the hallucinogens vary, depending on a range of factors such as the individual's personality makeup, the user's expectations for the drug, and the environment in which the drugs are used (Kaplan & Sadock, 1990).

Users often refer to the effects of LSD as a "trip," and each LSD trip moves through several distinct phases (Brophy, 1993). First, within a few minutes of taking LSD, there is a release of inner tension. This stage, which lasts 1 to 2 hours (Brophy, 1993) is characterized by either laughter or crying, as well as a feeling of euphoria (Jaffe, 1989). The second stage usually begins from 30 to 90 minutes (Brown & Braden, 1987) to 2 to 3 hours (Brophy, 1993) after the drug is ingested. During this portion of the LSD trip, the individual experiences the perceptual distortions, such as visual illusions and hallucinations, that are the hallmark of the hallucinogenic experience.

Mirin, Weiss, and Greenfield (1991) describe this phase as marked by "wavelike perceptual changes" (p. 290) and often synesthesia. *Synes-*

thesia refers to the "slipping over" of information from one sensory system to another. For example, a person experiencing synesthesia may report "tasting" colors or "seeing" music.

The third phase of the hallucinogenic experience begins 3 to 4 hours after the drug is ingested (Brophy, 1993), during which time the person experiences a distortion of the sense of time. The person may also experience marked mood swings and a feeling of ego disintegration. Feelings of panic are often experienced during this phase, as are occasional feelings of depression (Lingeman, 1974). (These LSD-related anxiety reactions will be discussed in the next section.) Individuals in this stage often believe that they possess quasimagical powers or are magically in control of events around them (Jaffe, 1989). This loss of contact with reality has resulted in fatalities; for example, individuals have jumped from windows, believing they could fly. It is for this reason that LSD has been indirectly implicated as the cause of death in a number of cases.

The effects of LSD start to wane 4 to 6 hours after ingestion. As the individual begins to recover, he or she experiences "waves of normalcy" (Mirin, Weiss, & Greenfield, 1991, p. 290) that gradually blend into the normal state of awareness. Within 12 hours, the acute effects of LSD clear, although the individual may experience a "sense of psychic numbness, [that] may last for days" (Mirin, Weiss, & Greenfield, 1991, p. 290).

The "Bad Trip"

As noted earlier, it is not uncommon for the individual who has ingested LSD to experience significant levels of anxiety, which may reach the levels of panic reactions; this is known as a "bad trip." The likelihood of a bad trip is determined by three factors: (1) the individual's expectations for the drug (which is known as the "set"), (2) the setting in which the drug is used, and (3) the user's psychological health (Mirin, Weiss, & Greenfield, 1991).

According to Mirin, Weiss, and Greenfield

(1991), a bad trip is most likely to occur with inexperienced LSD users. If the person does develop a panic reaction to the LSD experience, she or he will often respond to calm, gentle reminders from others that these feelings are caused by the drug and that they will pass. This is known as "talking down" the LSD user.

In extreme cases, an individual may require pharmacological support to deal with the LSD-induced panic attack. But there is some disagreement as to which antianxiety medications offer the greatest potential for relief during an LSD-related panic reaction. Kaplan and Sadock (1990) recommend administering diazepam or, in extreme cases, haloperidol. However, Jenike (1991) warns *against* using benzodiazepines (such as diazepam) because the benzodiazepines tend to distort the individual's sensory perception. Normally, this distortion is so slight as to be unnoticed by the typical patient, but when combined with the effects of LSD, the benzodiazepine-induced sensory distortion may cause even more anxiety than before (Jenike, 1991). Instead, Jenike suggests that low doses of the antipsychotic medication haloperidol may be used by medical personnel to abort the LSD-related panic attack.

Many hallucinogens are adulterated with belladonna or other anticholinergics (Henderson, 1994a; Kaplan & Sadock, 1990). When mixed with phenothiazines, these substances may bring about coma and death through cardio-respiratory failure. Thus, it is imperative that the physician treating a bad trip know what drugs have been used (and if possible be provided with a sample) to determine what medication to use in treatment.

The LSD-induced bad trip normally lasts only a few hours and typically resolves itself as the drug's effects wear off (Henderson, 1994b). However, LSD may have long-lasting effects on some users. Some researchers believe that in rare cases LSD is capable of activating a latent psychosis (Henderson, 1994b), but it's not clear whether this reflects the activation of a preexisting psychiatric disorder or whether it represents a drug-induced psychotic break. One reason it is so difficult to identify LSD's relationship to the development of psychiatric disorders is that the "LSD experience is so exceptional that there is a tendency for observers to attribute *any* later psychiatric illness to the use of LSD" (Henderson, 1994b, p. 65, italics added).

The LSD "Flashback"

The "flashback" is another long-term consequence of LSD use that is not well understood. Approximately 25% of those who use hallucinogenic drugs will experience some form of flashback (Kaplan & Sadock, 1990). In brief, the flashback is a "spontaneous recurrence" (Mirin, Weiss, & Greenfield, 1991, p. 292) of the drug experience that may take place days, weeks, or in some cases even months after the last time LSD was used. Flashback experiences may be brought on by stress, fatigue, marijuana use, sudden bright light (as when emerging from a dark room), illness, and occasionally by intentional effort. Flashbacks usually last a few seconds to a few minutes, although they occasionally last a day or two or even longer (Kaplan & Sadock, 1990).

Flashback experiences are often frightening, prompting some people to become depressed, develop a panic disorder, or, occasionally, become suicidal (Kaplan & Sadock, 1990). However, some LSD users enjoy the visual hallucinations—"flashes" of color, halos around different objects, the perception that things are growing smaller or larger—and feelings of depersonalization common in flashbacks (Mirin, Weiss, & Greenfield, 1991).

In about 50% of the cases, the flashbacks gradually cease over a period of months. However, some individuals experience flashback episodes for as long as 5 years following the last use of a hallucinogen. Usually, the only treatment needed for a patient having an LSD flashback is reassurance that it will end, but occasionally benzodiazepines may be needed to help control anxiety.

There still is a lot that remains to be discovered about this elusive chemical. Unfortunately, even before scientists were able to learn all that there is to know about LSD, another popular hallucinogen appeared. This new hallucinogen is called PCP.

Phencyclidine (PCP)

The drug *phencyclidine* (PCP) was first introduced in 1957 as an experimental intravenously administered surgical anesthetic (Milhorn, 1991). By the mid-1960s, researchers had discovered that 10 to 20% of the patients who had received PCP experienced a drug-induced delirium, and the decision was made to discontinue using the drug with humans (Milhorn, 1991; Brown & Braden, 1987). However, phencyclidine continued to be used in veterinary medicine in the United States until the mid-1970s.

In 1978, all legal production of PCP in the United States was discontinued, and the drug was declared a controlled substance under the Comprehensive Drug Abuse Prevention and Control Act of 1970 (Slaby, Lieb, & Tancredi, 1981). However, it continues to be used as a veterinary anesthetic and is legally manufactured by pharmaceutical companies in other parts of the world (Kaplan, Sadock, & Grebb, 1994).

Although clinical interest in PCP as an anesthetic for human use ended in the mid-1960s, PCP became a popular drug of abuse and for two important reasons. First, PCP is easily manufactured in illicit laboratories (Slaby, Lieb, & Tancredi, 1981). Because it is so easy to produce, PCP is either mixed into other street drugs or sold under the guise of other chemicals that are more difficult to manufacture (Brophy, 1993). It is quite common for a person who thought that they had purchased LSD, for example, to have unknowingly purchased PCP. The drug is also often mixed with marijuana to make it seem more potent.

Second, users discovered that by smoking PCP it was possible to more easily control some of PCP's harsh effects. If the symptoms become too harsh and aversive, the user can simply stop smoking the PCP-laced cigarette for a while. This ability to titrate the effects cannot be achieved through the other methods of PCP abuse, which include intranasal inhalation, oral administration, and intramuscular or intravenous injection (Brown & Braden, 1987; Slaby, Lieb, & Tancredi, 1981).

Pharmacology of PCP

Chemically, phencyclidine is a weak base that is both water soluble and lipid soluble. As a weak base, it is absorbed mainly through the small intestine rather than through the stomach (Zukin & Zukin, 1992). This slows the absorption of the drug into the body, because the drug molecules must pass through the stomach to reach the small intestine. Still, the effects of an oral dose of PCP generally appear in just 20 to 30 minutes.

When smoked, PCP is rapidly absorbed through the lungs, and the user begins to experience symptoms of PCP intoxication within about 2 to 3 minutes (Milhorn, 1991; Shepherd & Jagoda, 1990). However, only about 30% to 50% of the PCP in the cigarette is actually absorbed; much of the rest is converted into the chemical *phenylcyclohexene* by the heat of the cigarette (Shepherd & Jagoda, 1990).

PCP's lipid solubility is quite high, and so PCP tends to accumulate in fatty tissues and in the tissues of the brain. Indeed, because PCP molecules tend to concentrate in the brain, the level of PCP in the brain may reach 31 to 113 times as high as blood plasma levels (Shepherd & Jagoda, 1990). Once in the brain, PCP acts at a number of different receptor sites, including blocking those utilized by the neurotransmitter *N-methyl-D-aspartic acid* (NMDA) (Zukin & Zukin, 1992). This seems to be the receptor site most strongly affected at low doses. PCP also binds to one of the numerous opioid receptor sites (the sigma receptor site) (Daghestani & Schnoll, 1994).

Because PCP also concentrates in the body's adipose (fat) tissues, it can remain for days or weeks following the last dose of the drug. This is one reason PCP's effects last for such a long time. Furthermore, if a user loses weight, it is possible for unmetabolized PCP still in the adipose tissue to be released back into the general circulation, causing flashback experiences (Zukin & Zukin, 1992).

Once in the human body, PCP has some rather unusual effects. Depending on the dosage level and the route of administration, PCP can function as an anesthetic, a stimulant, a depressant, or a hallucinogenic (Weiss & Mirin, 1988; Brown & Braden, 1987). As Jaffe (1990) observed, "few drugs seem to induce so wide a range of subjective effects" as PCP (p. 557).

Some of the desired effects of PCP intoxication include a sense of euphoria; decreased inhibitions; a feeling of immense power; a reduction in the level of pain; and altered perception of time, space, and body image (Milhorn, 1991). However, "most regular users report unwanted effects" (Mirin, Weiss, & Greenfield, 1991, p. 295) caused by PCP. Some of the more common negative effects include feelings of anxiety, restlessness, and disorientation. In some cases, the user retains no memory of the period of intoxication, a reflection of the anesthetic action of the drug (Ashton, 1992). Other negative effects of PCP include disorientation, mental confusion, assaultiveness, anxiety, irritability, and paranoia (Weiss & Mirin, 1988). PCP may also contribute to suicidal thinking on the part of the user (Jenike, 1991; Weiss & Mirin, 1988). Berger and Dunn (1982), in drawing on the wave of PCP abuse that took place in the 1970s, report that drug-induced depression is common and that the drug would bring the user either to "the heights, or the depths" (p. 100) of emotional experience. Indeed, so many people have experienced so many different undesired effects from PCP that researchers are at a loss to explain why the drug is so popular (Newell & Cosgrove, 1988).

Only a limited degree of tolerance is thought to develop to the effects of PCP (Jenike, 1991), and there is no evidence of physical dependence on PCP (Newell & Cosgrove, 1988). PCP is biotransformed by the liver into a number of inactive metabolites, which are then excreted mainly by the kidneys (Zukin & Zukin, 1992). Only about 10% of the drug is excreted unchanged (Shepherd & Jagoda, 1990). Unfortunately, one characteristic of PCP is that it takes the body an extended period of time to biotransform and excrete the drug. The half-life of PCP following an overdose may be as long as from 20 hours (Kaplan, Sadock, & Grebb, 1994) to 72 hours (Jaffe, 1990) up to a period of weeks (Grinspoon & Bakalar, 1990).

Some physicians believe that it is possible to reduce the half-life of PCP in the body by acidifying the urine. This is done by having the patient ingest large amounts of ascorbic acid or cranberry juice (Kaplan & Sadock, 1991; Grinspoon & Bakalar, 1990). However, one potentially dangerous complication of this technique is the possible development of a condition known as *myoglobinuria*, which may cause the kidneys to fail (Brust, 1993). Because of this potential complication, many physicians do not recommend the acidification of the patient's urine.

Symptoms of Mild Levels of PCP Intoxication

In small doses, usually less than 5 mg, PCP produces a state resembling alcohol intoxication (Mirin, Weiss, & Greenfield, 1991) or CNS depressant intoxication (Weiss & Mirin, 1988). The individual experiences muscle incoordination, staggering gait, slurred speech, and numbness of the extremities (Jaffe, 1989). Other effects of mild doses of PCP include agitation, some feelings of anxiety, flushing of the skin, visual hallucinations, irritability, possible sudden outbursts of rage, and feelings of euphoria or depression (Milhorn, 1991; Beebe & Walley, 1991).

The acute effects of a small dose of PCP last between 4 to 6 hours. The post-PCP recovery period can last 24 to 48 hours (Milhorn, 1991; Beebe & Walley, 1991), during which time the user "comes down," or gradually returns to normal.

Symptoms of Moderate Levels of PCP Intoxication

As the dosage level increases to between 5 and 10 mg, many users experience a range of symptoms, including a disturbance of body image, in which different parts of the body no longer seem "real" (Brophy, 1993). The user may also experience slurred speech, nystagmus (twitching of the eyes), dizziness, ataxia, tachycardia, and an increase in muscle tone (Brophy, 1993; Weiss & Mirin, 1988). Other symptoms of moderate levels of PCP intoxication include paranoia, severe anxiety, belligerence, and assaultiveness (Grinspoon & Bakalar, 1990) as well as unusual feats of strength (Brophy, 1993; Jaffe, 1989). Some people have experienced drug-induced fever, an excess of salivation, drug-induced psychosis, and violence.

Symptoms of Severe Levels of PCP Intoxication

As the dosage level reaches 10 to 25 mg or higher, the individual's life is in extreme danger. At this dosage level, PCP can cause coma, seizures, hypertension, and severe psychotic reactions similar to schizophrenia (Kaplan & Sadock, 1990; Grinspoon & Bakalar, 1990; Weiss & Mirin, 1988). A PCP-induced coma can last up to 10 days (Mirin, Weiss, & Greenfield, 1991).

In addition to the possibility of a coma, the individual may develop cardiac arrhythmias, encopresis (involuntary defecation), visual and tactile hallucinations, and a drug-induced paranoid state. Death from respiratory arrest, convulsions, and hypertension have all been reported in cases of PCP overdose (Brophy, 1993). Because of the assaultiveness frequently induced by PCP, many users become either the victims or perpetrators of homicide (Ashton, 1992).

Complications from PCP Abuse

As we noted earlier, PCP has been implicated as causing a drug-induced psychosis which may last for days, weeks (Jenike, 1991; Jaffe, 1989; Weiss & Mirin, 1988), or even months following the last use of the drug (Ashton, 1992). This drug-induced psychosis seems to be most likely for users who either have suffered a previous schizophrenic episode (Mirin, Weiss, & Greenfield, 1991) or are vulnerable to such an episode (Jaffe, 1989).

Unfortunately, there is no way to predict in advance who may develop a PCP-induced psychosis. But Grinspoon and Bakalar (1990) report that 6 out of 10 patients who had developed a PCP psychosis went on to develop chronic schizophrenia. This may suggest a predisposition for schizophrenia in at least some people who experience a PCP psychosis. Ashton (1992), on the other hand, suggests that the apparent PCP-induced psychosis may result from organic brain damage caused by chronic PCP use. At this time, there is no clear understanding of the mechanism through which PCP induces a psychotic reaction.

The PCP psychosis usually progresses through three different stages, each of which lasts approximately 5 days (Mirin, Weiss, & Greenfield, 1991; Weiss & Mirin, 1988). The first stage of the PCP psychosis is usually the most severe and is characterized by paranoid delusions, anorexia, insomnia, and unpredictable assaultiveness. During this phase, the individual is extremely sensitive to external stimuli (Mirin, Weiss, & Greenfield, 1991; Jaffe, 1989), and the "talking down" techniques that may work with a bad LSD trip do not usually calm a person experiencing a PCP psychosis (Brust, 1992; Jaffe, 1990).

The middle phase of the PCP psychosis is marked by continued paranoia and restlessness, but the individual is usually calmer and in intermittent control of his or her behavior (Mirin, Weiss, & Greenfield, 1991; Weiss & Mirin, 1988). This phase also usually lasts 5 days, and will gradually blend into the final phase of the PCP psychosis recovery process. The final phase is marked by a gradual recovery over 7 to 14 days, although in some patients the PCP psychosis may last for months (Mirin,

Weiss, & Greenfield, 1991; Weiss & Mirin, 1988; Slaby, Lieb, & Tancredi, 1981). Social withdrawal and severe depression are also common consequences of chronic PCP use (Jaffe, 1990).

There appear to be some minor withdrawal symptoms following prolonged periods of hallucinogen use. Chronic PCP users have reported memory problems that seem to clear when they stop using the drug (Jaffe, 1990; Newell & Cosgrove, 1988). Recent evidence suggests that chronic PCP users demonstrate the same pattern of neuropsychological deficits found in other forms of chronic drug use, indicating that PCP may cause chronic brain damage (Newell & Cosgrove, 1988; Grinspoon & Bakalar, 1990).

Research has also revealed that, at high dosage levels, PCP can cause hypertensive episodes (Lange, White, & Robinson, 1992). These periods of unusually high blood pressure may then cause the individual to experience a cerebral vascular accident (CVA, or "stroke") (Daghestani & Schnoll, 1994; Brust, 1992). Although research into this area is lacking, the possibility does exist that this is the mechanism through which PCP is able to bring about brain damage on the part of the user.

Ecstasy: Latest in a Long Line of "Better" Hallucinogens?

In the past two decades, substance abuse professionals have been dealing with a "new" hallucinogenic, the chemical formula for which is *N, alpha-dimethyl-1,3 benzodioxole-t-ethanamine.* On the streets, this drug is called "Ecstasy," "XTC," "M&M" or "Adam" (Beebe & Walley, 1991), "rave," or simply the letter *E* (Henry, Jeffreys, & Dawling, 1992). Clinicians and chemists refer to the drug by the initials "MDMA."

Although classified by some as a new "designer" drug, MDMA is hardly new; it was first synthesized by scientists in 1914. But a medical use for MDMA was never identified, and the chemical remained little more than a curiosity until the 1970s (Sternbach & Varon, 1992; Mirin, Weiss, & Greenfield, 1991; Climko, Roehrich,

Sweeney, & Al-Razi, 1987). The one place it did get attention was in the U.S. Army, which briefly considered MDMA as a possible chemical warfare agent in the 1950s before moving on to other compounds (Abbott & Concar, 1992). Because no one seemed interested in MDMA, it was not classified as a controlled substance in the early 1970s, when the drug classification system currently in use was set up. Although the British government banned MDMA in 1977 (Abbott & Concar, 1992), the U.S. Drug Enforcement Administration did not classify MDMA as a controlled substance until July 1, 1985 (Climko et al., 1987).

Chemically, MDMA resembles the amphetamines and is related to another hallucinogen, MDA (Kirsch, 1986; Creighton, Black, & Hyde, 1991). MDMA briefly surfaced as a drug of abuse during the 1960s, but because LSD was more potent and did not cause the nausea or vomiting often experienced by MDMA users, LSD became more popular. MDMA was all but forgotten for almost 20 years.

Then, during the mid-1970s, illicit drug manufacturers in the United States "decided to resurrect, christen, package, market, distribute, and advertise" (Kirsch, 1986, p. 76) MDMA. Because MDMA was not yet classified as a controlled substance, it could be manufactured without fear of the harsh penalties associated with the manufacture of LSD or the amphetamines. For a time, the name "Empathy" was considered, however "Ecstasy" was finally selected. In effect, the techniques of big business entered the drug world; unknown drug manufacturers first created a demand for a "product" and then conveniently met the demand they had created. According to Kirsch (1986), the original samples of Ecstasy included a "package insert" that "included unverified scientific research and an abundance of 1960s mumbo-jumbo" (p. 81). However, these same package inserts warned the user not to mix Ecstasy with other chemicals (including alcohol), to use the drug only occasionally, and to take care to ensure a proper "set."

MDMA soon became a popular drug of

abuse, which led to its classification as a controlled substance: "trafficking in MDMA [was made] punishable by fifteen years in prison and a $125,000 fine" (Kirsch, 1986, p. 84). Several "labs" known to be involved in the production of MDMA were immediately shut down by the DEA. Unfortunately, by this time, the demand for MDMA was being met by street "chemists" who were more than happy to supply the drug . . . for a price.

Scope of the Problem of MDMA Abuse

In the past decade, MDMA has remained a popular drug of abuse for a number of people. Indeed, within the "rave" subculture in both the United States and the United Kingdom, MDMA use is considered socially acceptable. The "rave" subculture centers around parties that are frighteningly similar to the LSD parties of the 1960s and early 1970s, where MDMA is supplied to all participants (Randall, 1992). The drug is sometimes referred to as a "dance-making drug," because users are able to dance for extended periods of time (*Medical Update*, 1994).

One measure of MDMA's popularity is its rate of production. In 1976 one drug "lab" was known to have manufactured and distributed an estimated 10,000 doses of MDMA per month (Kirsch, 1986); by 1984, the same lab was manufacturing and distributing approximately 30,000 doses of the drug per month. In 1985, when the manufacture of MDMA was finally declared illegal, the same lab was thought to be turning out some 500,000 doses per month.

Underground laboratories now produce the drug. In the United States, the demand for MDMA has been fueled by news stories about Ecstasy's supposed value in psychotherapy (*Health News*, 1990). Although no one knows how many people are using MDMA here in this country, one study found that "a significant number of students" at Stanford University admitted to having used MDMA at least once (Peroutka, 1989, p. 191). In England, MDMA is used by an estimated 500,000 people each week (Abbott & Concar, 1992).

MDMA users tend to have drug-use patterns that differ from those used with other chemicals of abuse. During the mid-1980s, the *median* number of MDMA doses ingested by students who had used this drug was 4.0; the *average* number of doses was 5.4 per student (Peroutka, 1989). The dosage levels reported were between 60 and 250 mg. Furthermore, Peroutka discovered that recreational users of MDMA tend to use the drug only once every 2 to 3 weeks, if not less frequently. This rather unusual pattern reflects the fact that MDMA users quickly become tolerant to the drug's effects. As the individual becomes tolerant to MDMA, he or she is more likely to experience the negative side effects associated with its use. Surprisingly, taking a double dose of the drug increases not the desired effects but rather the unpleasant side effects of MDMA (Peroutka, 1989). Doubling the dose also increases the chances of suffering MDMA-induced brain damage (McGuire & Fahy, 1991). However, the high cost of the chemical ($20 to $25 per dose) has caused some users to turn to amphetamines as an alternative to MDMA (*Medical Update*, 1994).

The Subjective Effects of MDMA

To date, there has been little objective research into the behavioral effects of MDMA in humans. Abbott and Concar (1992) suggest that the lowest effective dose is between 75 and 100 mg for individuals who are not tolerant to MDMA. At this dosage level, the individual experiences a sense of euphoria, improved self-esteem (Beebe & Walley, 1991), and possibly some mild visual hallucinations (Evanko, 1991).

Some psychiatrists once advocated the use of MDMA as an aid to psychotherapy (Price, Ricaurte, Krystal, & Heninger, 1989, 1990). According to Climko et al. (1987), one "uncontrolled study" (p. 365) found that MDMA brought about a positive change in mood. But they further point out that MDMA has also been reported to cause "tachycardia, an occasional "wired" feeling, jaw clenching, nystagmus, a nervous desire to be in motion, transient anorexia, panic attacks, nausea and vomiting, ataxia, urinary urgency . . . insomnia, tremors, inhibition of ejaculation, and rarely, transient hallucinations" (p. 365).

Some of the effects of a "typical" dose of MDMA include an increase in heart rate, muscle tremor, tightness in jaw muscles, bruxism (grinding of teeth), nausea, insomnia, headache, and sweating. People who are sensitive to the effects of MDMA may experience numbness and tingling in the extremities, vomiting, increased sensitivity to cold, visual hallucinations, ataxia, crying, blurred vision, nystagmus, and the feeling that the floor is shaking.

Complications from MDMA Use

There have been a number of fatal reactions to MDMA, usually as a result of cardiac arrhythmias (Beebe & Walley, 1991). There have also been reports of intracranial hemorrhaging (Sternbach & Varon, 1992), and one case report of a young woman who developed a condition known as *cerebral venous sinus thrombosis* (a blood clot in the brain) after ingesting MDMA at a "rave" party (Rothwell & Grant, 1993). The authors speculate that dehydration may have been a factor in this case, and warn of the need to maintain adequate fluid intake after MDMA use.

Some MDMA users have experienced extreme temperature elevations, which are potentially fatal. These temperature elevations are most common in those who engage in heavy exercise—such as prolonged, vigorous dancing—after taking the drug (Ames, Wirshing, & Friedman, 1993; Randall, 1992; Beebe & Walley, 1991). There are also isolated reports of liver toxicity, although it is not clear whether the toxic reactions were the result of MDMA itself or from one or more contaminants in the drug (Henry, Jeffreys, & Dawling, 1992). Creighton, Black, and Hyde (1991) also question whether reported MDMA flashbacks, similar to those seen with LSD use, are caused by the MDMA or by contaminants. The authors call for further research into the effects of MDMA on the user.

Another interesting drug effect seen at normal dosage levels is that the user will occasionally "relive" past memories. These memories had often been suppressed because of the pain associated with the experiences (Hayner & McKinney, 1986). Thus, individuals may find themselves reliving experiences they wanted to forget. This phenomenon, which many psychotherapists thought might prove of benefit to the patient in the confines of the therapeutic relationship, may be so frightening as to be "detrimental to the individual's mental health" (p. 343).

Long-time MDMA use has also been connected to episodes of violence and to suicide (*Medical Update*, 1994). Furthermore, it is possible to overdose on MDMA. Some of the symptoms of an MDMA overdose are tachycardia, hypertension, hypotension, heart palpitations, hyperthermia, renal failure, and visual hallucinations (Hayner & McKinney, 1986). MDMA use may be fatal, and research suggests that this drug "can potentially kill at doses that were previously tolerated in susceptible individuals" (Hayner & McKinney, 1986, p. 342). Some potential treatments for toxic reactions to MDMA may be the use of methysergide maleate, or Beta-blockers (Ames, Wirshing, & Friedman, 1993). However, the exact mechanism through which MDMA might cause death is still not certain.

The drug can also bring about residual effects, including anxiety attacks, persistent insomnia, rage reactions and a drug-induced psychosis (McGuire & Fahy, 1991; Hayner & McKinney, 1986). This MDMA-induced psychosis is thought to be most common in chronic MDMA users, and it clinically resembles the psychiatric condition paranoid schizophrenia (Sternbach & Varon, 1992). MDMA apparently induces psychotic reactions much the way MDMA's chemical cousins, the amphetamines, do. Like the amphetamines, MDMA probably activates a psychotic reaction in a person who is predisposed to psychosis because of biochemical vulnerability (McGuire & Fahy, 1991).

It is not clear how MDMA works in the brain (Climko et al., 1987). Animal research indicates that MDMA influences the action of serotonin, a neurotransmitter found in many different regions of the brain. There is also evidence that MDMA alters the function of those neurons that use dopamine, although exactly how this occurs is not known (Ames, Wirshing, & Friedman, 1993). However, animal research strongly suggests that MDMA is a neurotoxic chemical—a chemical that destroys nerve cells, or neurons. Exactly how MDMA functions as a neurotoxin is unclear, but it appears to be specifically toxic to neurons that use serotonin as a neurotransmitter (Sternbach & Varon, 1992). MDMA is quite toxic as compared to traditional hallucinogens such as LSD. Whereas a rat can receive 10,000 times the normal human dose of LSD and not demonstrate any signs of neurotoxicity, rats, guinea pigs, and monkeys that receive only 2 or 3 times the normal dose of MDMA develop symptoms of neurotoxicity (Roberts, 1986; McGuire & Fahy, 1991).

The implications of this research are rather frightening when one stops to consider that, of those college students who admitted to using MDMA, the average dose was 60 to 250 mg, a dosage level found to cause neurotoxicity in animals (Peroutka, 1989). Clinical evidence now suggests that this drug is neurotoxic in humans as well, although there is no information on whether this brain damage is permanent (Mann, 1994; Grob, Bravo, & Walsh, 1990; *Health News*, 1990). Peroutka (1989) argues that, although there is no evidence to suggest that MDMA is addictive, there is evidence of "a long-term, and potentially irreversible, effect of MDMA on the human brain" (p. 191).

Price et al. (1989, 1990) found that MDMA users responded differently than normal subjects on a test designed to measure serotonin levels in the body. Admittedly, the measured differences between MDMA users and normal control subjects were not statistically significant, but the authors concluded that the results were indeed suggestive of neurotoxicity caused by MDMA.

Thus, current research evidence suggests that MDMA is toxic to certain brain cells in animal brains. By extension, one would expect that MDMA is also toxic to portions of the human brain, especially those that utilize serotonin as a neurotransmitter. The latest drug to emerge from the nation's illicit laboratories may very well cause organic brain damage, a sharp contrast to its reputation on the streets as a warm, relaxing, loving drug.

Summary

Weil (1986) suggests that people initially use chemicals to alter their normal state of consciousness. Hallucinogen use in the United States has followed a series of waves, as first one drug and then another became the current drug of choice. In the 1960s, LSD was the major hallucinogen, and in the 1970s and early 1980s it was PCP. Currently, MDMA seems to be gaining in popularity, although research suggests that MDMA may cause permanent brain damage, especially to those portions of the brain that utilize serotonin as a primary neurotransmitter.

Other hallucinogens will probably emerge over the years, as people look for a more effective way to alter their state of consciousness. In time, drugs will also fade, as they are replaced by still newer hallucinogenics. Just as cocaine faded from the drug scene in the 1930s and was replaced for a time by the amphetamines, so one might expect wave after wave of hallucinogen abuse, as new drugs become available. Thus, chemical dependency counselors will probably have to maintain a working knowledge of an ever growing range of hallucinogens in the years to come.

CHAPTER FOURTEEN

Inhalants and Aerosols

The inhalants are unlike the other chemicals of abuse. They are a diverse group of toxic substances, which include various cleaning agents, herbicides, pesticides, gasoline, kerosene, various forms of glue, lacquer thinner, and felt-tipped pens, to name a few. These agents are not intended to function as recreational substances, but many of the chemicals in these compounds will, when inhaled, alter the manner in which the brain functions. Because these chemicals are inhaled, they are often called *inhalants* although Esmail, Meyer, Pottier, and Wright (1993) make a case for calling this class of chemicals "volatile substances." For the purpose of this text, we will use the term *inhalants*.

At low doses, the inhalants produce a sense of euphoria. In part because of this characteristic, and in part because they are so easily accessible to children and adolescents, inhalant abuse has become the most rapidly growing form of chemical abuse in the United States (Heath, 1994).

The History of Inhalant Abuse

In the past century, historical accounts of inhalant abuse involved the practice of anesthetic abuse. Indeed, the earliest documented use of the anesthetic gases appears to have been for recreation, and historical records from the 1800s document the use of such agents as nitrous oxide for "parties." The use of gasoline fumes to get "high" is thought to have started before World War II (Morton, 1987), and record of this practice was made in the early 1950s (Blum, 1984). Currently, inhalant abuse is thought to be a worldwide problem (Brust, 1992).

By the mid-1950s and early 1960s, the popular press brought attention to the practice of "glue sniffing" (Anderson, 1989a; Morton, 1987; Westermeyer, 1987), whereby a "high" was obtained by inhaling model-airplane glue. The active agent of model glue in the 1950s was often toluene. Nobody knows how the practice of glue sniffing first started, but there is evidence that this practice began in California, when teenagers accidentally discovered the intoxicating powers of toluene-containing model glue (Berger & Dunn, 1982).

The first known reference to this practice was in 1959, in the magazine section of a Denver newspaper (Brecher, 1972). Local newspapers soon began to carry stories on the dangers of inhalant abuse, in the process giving explicit details on how to use airplane glue to become intoxicated and what effects to expect. Within a short period of time, a "nationwide drug menace" had emerged (Brecher, 1972, p. 321). However, Brecher suggests that this inhalant abuse "problem" was essentially manufactured through distorted media reports. He points out that one newspaper tracked down several stories of deaths due to glue sniffing and found only nine deaths that could be attributed to glue sniffing. Of this number, three deaths were not positively attributed to inhalant use, and six deaths were clearly due to asphyxiation—each victim had used an airtight plastic bag and had suffocated. Furthermore, Brecher (1972) notes that "among tens of thousands of glue-sniffers prior to 1964, no death due unequivocally to glue vapor had as yet been reported. The lifesaving advice children needed was not to sniff glue with their heads in plastic bags" (p. 331).

Brecher does raise the question of how serious the glue-sniffing problem was before the news media began to publish reports about it. Indeed, one is left with the impression that this "problem" was manufactured by the media, at least to some degree. However, subsequent research has found that the use of inhalants may introduce toxic chemicals into the body that can cause damage to many different parts of the body (Brunswick, 1989; Jaffe, 1989). Thus, inhalant abuse is a legitimate health issue today.

The Pharmacology of the Inhalants

Many chemical agents reach the brain more rapidly and efficiently when they are inhaled than when ingested by mouth or injected. When a chemical is inhaled, it is able to enter the bloodstream without its chemical structure being altered in any way by the liver. Once in the blood, the lipid solubility of many inhalants allows them to reach the brain in an extremely short period of time, usually within seconds (Heath, 1994; Watson, 1984; Blum, 1984).

Cone (1993) groups all the inhalants into two broad classifications: anesthetic gases and volatile hydrocarbons. Anderson (1989a), however, suggests four classes of inhalants: (1) volatile organic solvents, such as those found in paint and fuel; (2) aerosols, such as hair sprays, spray paints, and deodorants; (3) volatile nitrites, such as amyl nitrite (or its close chemical cousin, butyl nitrite); and (4) general anesthetic agents, such as nitrous oxide.

Of the different classes of inhalants commonly abused, children and adolescents most often abuse the first two classes of chemicals. Children and adolescents have limited access to the third category[1] and extremely limited access to general anesthetics, the final class of inhalants.

The chemistry of inhalants is quite complex. For a number of reasons, it is difficult to talk about the "pharmacology" of inhalants. Many different agents can be used as an inhalant, each of which has a unique chemical structure. Multiple chemical agents are often combined to meet the needs of industry. The exact combination of chemicals included in any mixture depends on its intended purpose and the conditions under which it is to be used. And because many of the chemicals used as inhalants are designed for industrial or household use, not for human consumption, there is little research into the specific effects of many inhalants on the human body.

All the chemicals in a compound are introduced into the body when the individual breathes fumes from any inhalant. There are so many different chemicals in the mixture that it is difficult to identify the agent or agents that cause euphoria or physical damage (Anderson, 1989a; Morton, 1987; Jaffe, 1989). But, as a general rule, the inhalants are *all* toxic to the human body to one degree or another (Fornazzari, 1988; Morton, 1987; Blum, 1984). One must wonder what potential for harm exists to an individual who willingly inhales concentrations of toxic chemicals that are often *100 times higher* than the permitted level of exposure for industrial workers (Blum, 1984; Morton, 1987; Fornazzari, 1988).

The Scope of the Problem

The sporadic use of inhalants is usually a "fad" among teenagers that lasts for a year or two (Schuckit, 1989). Newcomb and Bentler (1989) note that these agents are usually the first consciousness-altering agents utilized by children. The inhalants tend to be most popular among boys in their early teens, especially in poor or

[1]Butyl nitrite is sold without a prescription, in some states, where children and adolescents will potentially have access to the volatile nitrites.

rural areas where more expensive drugs of abuse are not easily available (Jaffe, 1989). However, there has been at least one report of children as young as 5 years old abusing inhalants (Beauvais & Oetting, 1988), and Johnston, O'Malley, and Bachman (1993) found that 4% of the students in the fourth grade had already abused inhalants at least once.

There is some disagreement as to the upper age limits at which inhalant abuse is found. McHugh (1987) suggests that after a year or two, and certainly by adolescence, most youths have abandoned the use of inhalants. However, Johnston, O'Malley, and Bachman (1993) found that a significant minority of students admitted to *starting* to abuse inhalants in the eighth through eleventh grades, indicating that inhalant abuse may continue well past the onset of adolescence.

Morton (1987) found that, of those adolescents who did abuse inhalants, between 30 and 40% did so only on a few occasions. Another 40% to 50% abused inhalants over a period of a few weeks to a few months before stopping, and only about 10% became "habitual abusers" (p. 454). Some individuals have continued the practice of using inhalants for 15 years or more (Schuckit, 1989; Westermeyer, 1987).

The actual percentage of people who are using solvents remains unknown (Miller & Gold, 1991b), although the practice seems to involve boys more often than girls (Morton, 1987)—usually between the ages of 10 and 15 (Miller & Gold, 1991b). One study found that 20% of the adolescent girls and 33% of the adolescent boys questioned admitted to using solvents at least once (Schuckit, 1989). In England, between 3 and 10% of the adolescents asked admitted to using inhalants at least once, and about 1% are thought to be current users (Esmail, Meyer, Pottier, & Wright, 1993).

Unfortunately, for a minority of those who abuse them, the inhalants appear to function as a "gateway" chemical, opening the way to further drug use in later years (Anderson, 1989a). Research also suggests that approximately one-third of the children who abuse inhalants go on to abuse one or more other drugs within 4 years

(Brunswick, 1989). Inhalant abuse may thus be the first warning sign of a potential for later substance abuse.

Cohen (1977) identified several different reasons the inhalants are popular chemicals of abuse. First, they have a rapid onset of action, usually on the order of a few seconds. Second, inhalant users report pleasurable effects, including a sense of euphoria, when they use these chemicals. Third, and perhaps most important, the inhalants are relatively inexpensive and easily obtained by teenagers. Indeed, they are so easily available that they have been called a "household drug" (Wisneiwski, 1994).

Virtually all the commonly used inhalants can be freely purchased by anyone. An additional advantage for the user is that inhalants are usually available in small, easily hidden packages. Brunswick (1989) identified some of the more popular inhalants as

> accessible and cheap. They are found at the corner drug store, in the garage, or under the kitchen sink. They take the form of magic markers, glue and fingernail polish. They produce a short but intense high that some have likened to the rush from rock cocaine, or "crack." (p. 6A)

Unfortunately, many inhalants are capable of causing the user harm, if not actually causing death. The inhalant abuser thus runs a serious risk whenever he or she begins to "huff."[2]

How Inhalants Are Used

McHugh (1987) describes inhalant abuse as "a group activity" (p. 334). There are a number of ways that inhalants can be abused, depending on the specific chemical involved. Glue and adhesives are commonly poured into a plastic bag or milk carton, which is placed tightly over the mouth and nose, and the fumes inhaled (Esmail et al., 1993). Liquids such as cleaning fluids are often inhaled from a cloth or plastic container (such as an empty plastic bottle). Fumes from

---

[2]"Huff" is a street term for inhaling the fumes of an inhalant.

aerosol cans may be directly inhaled sprayed into the mouth.

There are a multitude of other ways in which users inhale fumes from various household chemicals, far too many to list in this text. However, a common feature of each method of abuse is that the user inhales concentrated fumes from a chemical not normally meant to be admitted into the body.

Subjective Effects of the Inhalants

The initial effects of the fumes include a feeling of hazy euphoria, somewhat like the feeling of intoxication caused by alcohol (Blum, 1984). This feeling of euphoria usually lasts only 30 minutes. Other symptoms emerge after a period of time and include slurred speech, excitement, double vision, ringing in the ears, and hallucinations (Kaminski, 1992; Blum, 1984; Morton, 1987). Occasionally, the individual feels omnipotent, and episodes of violence have been reported (Morton, 1987). In most cases, the effects of a single exposure to an inhalant may last up to 45 minutes (Mirin, Weiss, & Greenfield, 1991).

As noted, one of the initial experiences of inhalant abuse is a feeling of euphoria, although nausea and vomiting may also occur (McHugh, 1987). After the initial euphoria, depression of the central nervous system develops. The individual may become confused or disoriented, develop a headache, and experience a loss of inhibitions (Kaminski, 1992; McHugh, 1987). If the individual continues to inhale the fumes beyond this stage, stupor, seizures and cardiorespiratory arrest may occur (McHugh, 1987).

Although the inhalants are noted for their ability to cause rapid mental changes, the mental changes that follow inhalation of glue, solvents, or aerosol gases disappear "fairly quickly, and, with the exception of headache, serious hangovers are usually not seen" (Schuckit, 1989, pp. 184–185). What little hangover effect may occur usually clears "in minutes to a few hours" (Westermeyer, 1987, p. 903). However, in some cases, the user experiences a residual sense of drowsiness or stupor, which lasts for several hours after the last use of inhalants (Kaplan, Sadock, & Grebb, 1994; Miller & Gold, 1991b). There have also been reports of postinhalant headaches lasting for several days after the last use of the inhalant (Heath, 1994).

Complications from Inhalant Abuse

Although Lingeman (1974) believes that there are no withdrawal symptoms associated with these substances, Blum (1984) documents a surprising "delirium tremens-like" (p. 223) withdrawal syndrome following inhalant abuse. Miller and Gold (1991b) state that the nature of the withdrawal syndrome depends on the specific chemicals abused, the duration of inhalant abuse, and the dosage levels utilized. They suggest that some of the symptoms of inhalant withdrawal could include tremors, irritability, anxiety, insomnia, muscle cramps, and possibly seizures.

According to Schuckit (1989), damage to various organ systems as a result of inhalant abuse is rare but not unknown. Physical complications from inhalant abuse include possible cardiac arrhythmias (irregularities in the heart beat that may be fatal if not corrected), possible damage to the liver, kidney failure, transient changes in lung function, reduction in blood cell production possibly to the point of aplastic anemia, possible permanent organic brain damage, and respiratory depression (Anderson, 1989a; Brunswick, 1989; Morton, 1987). In addition, inhalants have been known to cause damage to the central nervous system, including cerebellar ataxia (loss of coordination) and deafness (Maas, Ashe, Spiegel, Zee, & Leigh, 1991; Fornazzari, 1988). The possibility exists that various inhalants can cause coma, convulsions, brain damage, or even death when abused (McHugh, 1987; Mirin, Weiss, & Greenfield, 1991). Esmail et al. (1993) report that abuse of volatile agents is "one of the leading causes of death in those under 18" (p. 359). Nationally, it is estimated that inhalants are responsible for between 100 and 1,000 deaths each year (Wisneiwski, 1994).

Parras, Patier, and Ezpeleta (1988) found that gasoline "sniffing" by children has sometimes resulted in lead poisoning, a serious condition that may have long-term consequences for the child's physical and emotional growth. Inhalant abuse may also cause liver damage and damage to the bone marrow, as well as sinusitis (irritation of the sinus membranes), erosion of the nasal mucosal tissues, and laryngitis, among other things (Westermeyer, 1987). These complications of inhalant abuse "usually resolve after some weeks of abstinence" (Westermeyer, 1987, p. 903), but permanent organ damage, although rare, is possible (Schuckit, 1989).

Neurological Complications

There is increasing evidence that inhalant abuse may cause permanent damage to the central nervous system. In a study of 37 chronic inhalant users, Sharp and Brehm (1977) found that 40% scored in the brain-damaged range on a test designed to detect neurological dysfunction. The authors were hesitant to attribute their findings to chronic inhalant use, suggesting instead that the results may reflect preexisting brain damage. In any case, Westermeyer (1987) recommends that patients known to abuse inhalants should be routinely assessed for damage to the central nervous system, peripheral nervous system, kidneys, liver, lungs, heart, and bone marrow.

Mirin, Weiss, and Greenfield (1991) note that some chronic users of inhalants have exhibited a condition similar to the delirium tremens (DTs) of alcoholism. The chronic exposure to toluene (the solvent that is found in various forms of glue) may result in intellectual impairment, ataxia secondary to damage to the cerebellum, deafness, and a loss of the sense of smell (Maas et al., 1991; Rosenberg, 1989). In fact, chronic exposure to toluene may result in such extensive injury to the brain that it is visible on magnetic resonance imaging (MRI) procedures physicians use to examine the physical structure of the brain.

The Abuse of Anesthetic Gases

Nitrous oxide and *ether*, the first two gases to be used as surgical anesthetics, were initially introduced as recreational drugs (Berger & Dunn, 1982). Indeed, these gases were routinely utilized as intoxicants for quite some time before they were utilized in medicine. Horace Wells, who introduced nitrous oxide to medicine, noted the pain-killing properties of this gas when he observed a person under its influence trip and gash his leg, without any apparent pain (Brecher, 1972).

As medical historians know, the first planned demonstration of nitrous oxide as an anesthetic was something less than a success. The patient returned to consciousness in the middle of the operation and started to scream in pain. However, in spite of this rather frightening beginning, physicians learned to properly use nitrous oxide and it is now an important anesthetic agent (Brecher, 1972).

As Julien (1992) points out, the pharmacological effects of the general anesthetics are the same as those of the barbiturates. There is a dose-related range of effects from an initial period of sedation and relief from anxiety on through sleep and analgesia. At extremely high dosage levels, the anesthetic gases can cause death. One of the most commonly abused anesthetic gases is nitrous oxide.

Nitrous Oxide

Nitrous oxide presents a special danger, and special precautions must be taken to maintain a proper oxygen supply to the individual's brain. It is for this reason that nitrous oxide is rarely used as an anesthetic unless it is combined with other agents (Lingeman, 1974). Julien (1992) warns that ordinary room air will not provide sufficient oxygen to the brain when nitrous oxide is used. Unless the person uses a special mixture of oxygen and nitrous oxide, the person runs the risk of *hypoxia*, a decreased oxygen level in the blood that can cause permanent brain damage if not corrected immediately. In surgery, the anesthesiologist takes special precautions to ensure that the patient always has an adequate oxygen supply. However, a person using nitrous oxide for recreational purposes lacks the support resources available to the surgical team, thus risking serious injury or even death. It is possible to develop hypoxia from any of the inhalants, not just from nitrous oxide (McHugh, 1987).

Recreational users report that nitrous oxide brings about a feeling of euphoria, giddiness, hallucinations, and a loss of inhibitions (Lingeman, 1974), and nitrous oxide is a popular drug of abuse in some circles (Schwartz, 1989). Dental students, medical school students, dentists, and anesthesiologists, all of whom have access to this gas through their professions, occasionally abuse it, along with ether, chloroform, trichlorothylene, and halothane. Also, because nitrous oxide is also used as a propellant in certain whipping cream cans, children and adolescents occasionally abuse this chemical by finding ways to release the gas from the container.

The volatile anesthetics are not metabolized by the body to any significant degree; rather, enter and leave the body essentially unchanged (Glowa, 1986). Once the source of the gas is removed, the concentration of the gas in the brain begins to drop and normal circulation brings the brain to a normal state of consciousness within moments. While the person is under the influence of the anesthetic gas, however, the ability of the brain cells to react to painful stimuli seems to be reduced.

The use of nitrous oxide, chloroform, and ether is confined, for the most part, to dental or general surgery. Rarely, however, one encounters a person who has used or is currently using these agents. There is little information available about the dangers of this practice, nor is there much information concerning the side effects of prolonged use.

The Abuse of Nitrites

Two different forms of nitrites commonly abused are *amyl nitrite* and its close chemical cousin *butyl nitrite*. When inhaled, amyl nitrite functions as a coronary vasodilator; that is, it causes the coronary arteries to dilate, allowing more blood to flow to the heart. For this reason, amyl nitrite was once commonly used in the control of angina pectoris. The drug was administered in small glass containers embedded in cloth layers. The user would "snap" or "pop" open the container with his or her fingers, and inhale the fumes to control the chest pain.[3]

With the introduction of nitroglycerine preparations, which are equally as effective as amyl nitrite and lack many of its disadvantages, few people now use amyl nitrite for medical purposes (Schwartz, 1989). It does continue to have a limited role in diagnostic medicine and the emergency treatment of cyanide poisoning. But for the most part, the medical uses of amyl nitrite have been superseded (Schwartz, 1989).

Although amyl nitrite is available only by prescription, butyl nitrite is often sold legally by mail-order houses or in specialty stores, depending on specific state regulations. In many areas, butyl nitrite is sold as a "room deodorizer," packaged in small bottles and sold for less than $10. Both drugs are thought to provide a prolonged, more intense orgasm when inhaled just before orgasm is reached. Aftereffects include an intense, sudden, headache, increased pressure of the fluid in the eyes (a danger for those with glaucoma), possible weakness, nausea, and possible cerebral hemorrhage (Schwartz, 1989).

When abused, both amyl nitrite and butyl nitrite will cause a brief (90-second) rush that includes dizziness, giddiness, and the rapid dilation of blood vessels in the head (Schwartz, 1989). This, in turn, causes an increase in intracranial pressure (*AIDS Alert*, 1989) that may contribute to the rupture of unsuspected aneurysms, causing a cerebral hemorrhage (stroke).

The use of nitrites is common among male homosexuals and may contribute to the spread of the virus that causes AIDS (Schwartz, 1989;

---

[3]It was from the distinctive sound of the glass breaking that both amyl nitrite and butyl nitrite have come to be known as "poppers" or "snappers."

AIDS Alert, 1989). It has been suggested that, by causing the dilation of blood vessels in the anus, the use of either amyl or butyl nitrite may actually aid the transmission of the HIV virus from the active to the passive partner during anal intercourse (*AIDS Alert*, 1989).

Summary

The inhalants are often the first chemicals a person abuses for recreational purposes. For the most part, inhalant abuse seems to be a teenage phase, engaged in on an episodic basis for only a year or two. A minority of users, however, will continue to inhale the fumes of gasoline, solvents, and certain forms of glue for many years.

The effects of the inhalants appear to be short-lived. There is evidence, however, that prolonged use of certain agents can result in permanent damage to the kidneys, brain, and liver. Death, either through hypoxia or prolonged exposure to inhalants, is possible. Very little is know about the effects of prolonged use of this class of chemicals.

CHAPTER FIFTEEN

Anabolic Steroid Abuse

Unlike alcohol, marijuana, or virtually any other drug of abuse, the anabolic steroids (or simply, steroids) are not primarily abused for their ability to bring about a sense of euphoria. Rather, the anabolic steroids are abused because of persistent rumors that these chemicals enhance athletic performance. Indeed, so common has the use of steroids become in certain athletic training programs that some athletes consider these drugs a "nutritional supplement" (Breo, 1990, p. 1697), not potent chemical agents.

Very little is actually known about the problem of anabolic steroid abuse (Bower, 1991). This is unfortunate, because a large number of teenagers and young adults are abusing one or more steroids in spite of their considerable potential to cause harm. Because of the growing recognition of the problem of anabolic steroid abuse, mental health and chemical dependency professionals should have a working knowledge of the effects of this class of medications.

An Introduction to the Anabolic Steroids

The term *anabolic* refers to the action of this family of drugs to increase the speed of body tissue growth; the term *steroids* refers to their chemical structure (Redman, 1990). These drugs are chemically similar to testosterone, the male sex hormone, and so have a masculinizing (androgenic)

effect on the user (Hough & Kovan, 1990; Landry & Primos, 1990). At times, this class of chemicals is referred to as the *anabolic-androgenic steroid* family of drugs.

It has been suggested that these drugs may, when abused, bring about a feeling of euphoria (Lipkin, 1989; Johnson, 1990; Kashkin, 1992; Schrof, 1992). However, this is not the primary reason most people abuse the anabolic steroids. Steroids are mainly abused either to stimulate the growth of muscle tissue or to slow the process of muscle tissue breakdown. Repeated, heavy physical exercise can damage muscle tissues. The anabolic steroids stimulate protein synthesis—a process that indirectly helps muscle tissue development, may increase muscle strength, and limits the amount of damage done to muscle tissues through heavy physical exercise (Gottesman, 1992; Pettine, 1991; Pope & Katz, 1990; Hough & Kovan, 1990).

Many nonathletic users believe that steroid use will enhance their physical attractiveness (Brower, 1993; Schrof, 1992; Pettine, 1991; Johnson, 1990; Bahrke, 1990; Pope, Katz, & Champoux, 1986). Indeed, between 25% (Fultz, 1991) and 40% (Whitehead, Chillag, & Elliott, 1992) of adolescent steroid abusers take the drug because they believe it will make them look better. Another group of people, which includes some law enforcement officers, abuse steroids to increase their strength and aggressiveness (Schrof, 1992; Bahrke, 1990).

Medical Uses of Anabolic Steroids

Although the anabolic steroids have been in use since the mid-1950s, there still is no clear consensus on how they work (Wadler, 1994). It is thought that the steroids force the body to increase protein synthesis and inhibit the action of *glucocorticoids,* chemicals that cause tissue breakdown. In a medical setting, the anabolic steroids are used to promote tissue growth and help damaged tissue recover from injury (Shannon, Wilson, & Stang, 1992).

According to the United States Pharmacopeial Convention (1990) physicians may also use one of the steroid family of drugs to treat certain kinds of anemia, help patients regain weight after periods of severe illness, and as an adjunct to the treatment of certain forms of breast cancer. In some cases, the steroids may also promote the growth of bone tissue following bone injuries. The Council on Scientific Affairs (1990b) of the American Medical Association suggests that the steroid family of drugs may prove useful in the treatment of osteoporosis.

In 1990, Congress outlawed the use of anabolic steroids except for medical purposes. The steroids are thus considered a "controlled substance" in much the same way that narcotics are, and they are listed under the Controlled Substances Act of 1970 as a Schedule III controlled substance. These medications are available, with a doctor's prescription, for certain medical purposes. However, the sale of any of 28 different forms of anabolic steroids for nonmedical purposes or by individuals who are not licensed to sell medications is a crime punishable by a prison term of up to 5 years (10 years if the steroids are sold to minors) (Fultz, 1991).

The Scope of the Problem of Steroid Abuse

There has been very little research into the scope of the problem of steroid abuse in the United States (Brower, 1993; Kashkin, 1992). But it does appear that between 4 and 12% of male high school students have abused anabolic steroids at some point in their lives (DuRant, Rickert, Ashworth, Newman, & Slavens, 1993; Yesalis, Kennedy, Kopstein, & Bahrke, 1993; Daigle, 1990; Whitehead, Chillag, & Elliott, 1992; Dreyfuss, 1989). In actual numbers, it is estimated that between 250,000 (DuRant et al., 1993) and 500,000 (Wadler, 1994; Schrof, 1992; Bahrke, 1990) high school students are either current or former users of anabolic steroids.

The problem of anabolic steroid abuse is not limited to high school students. Approximately 20% of college athletes are thought to have used steroids on at least one occasion (Hough & Kovan, 1990), and Brower (1993) suggests that a majority of athletes who abuse steroids began to do so in college. Overall, when one combines the number of estimated steroid users in school with those who are no longer in school, it has been estimated that 1 million people have abused anabolic steroids at some point, with about 300,000 people currently using these chemicals (Franklin, 1994). Other estimates are as high as "one million people" (Porterfield, 1991, p. 44; Schrof, 1992) currently abusing anabolic steroids, and an unknown number having abused the anabolic steroids at some point in their lives.

How Steroids Are Abused

Physicians often prescribe steroids with the mistaken belief that they will be able to monitor and control the use of these drugs (Breo, 1990). However, athletes frequently augment their prescribed medications with steroids obtained from other sources to increase their daily dosage.

Anabolic steroids are smuggled into the country from overseas, or diverted to the "black market" from legitimate sources.[1] Veterinary products are often sold on the street for use by humans. Whatever the source, steroids are frequently available through an informal distribution network that frequently exists in health clubs or gyms (Schrof, 1992; Johnson, 1990).

---

[1] As used here, the term *black market* is applied to any illicit source.

Bahrke (1990) estimates that between 50 and 80% of the steroids used by athletes comes from the black market. Many of the steroids smuggled into the United States originate in Mexico or Europe (Johnson, 1990). It has been estimated that illicit steroid sales are from $100 million (DuRant et al., 1993; Pettine, 1991; Miller, 1990) to $300 to $500 million a year in this country (Wadler, 1994; Council on Scientific Affairs, 1990b; Fultz, 1991).

Many users obtain steroids by "diverting" prescribed medications or by obtaining multiple prescriptions for steroids from different physicians. "Diverting" refers to a process by which medications prescribed for one person are used by someone else. Sometimes, the medications are stolen from drug stores or medicine cabinets. In other cases, an individual with a legitimate need for steroids will obtain a prescription for medications from several different doctors and then sell the excess medication to others.

Steroids can be injected into muscle tissue, taken orally, or taken in both intramuscular and oral doses simultaneously. This latter practice is known as "stacking" steroids (Brower, 1993). Injectable steroids are known as "injectables" and oral forms are known as "orals" (Bahrke, 1990) or "juice" (Fultz, 1991). In one study, fully 61% of steroid-abusing weight lifters engaged in the practice of "stacking" steroids (Brower, Blow, Young, & Hill, 1991).

Another way in which the steroids are abused is through "pyramiding" (Daigle, 1990, p. 78). In this practice, the abuser starts a cycle of abusing steroids by initially taking the smallest dose and then gradually increasing the daily dosage level, so that by midcycle the user is taking a massive amount of steroids. Then, the daily dosage level is gradually tapered, until by the last week in the cycle the abuser is again taking a relatively small daily dose. Episodes of pyramiding are interspaced with periods of abstinence from anabolic steroid use that may last several weeks or months (Landry & Primos, 1990) or perhaps even as long as a year (Kashkin, 1992). Unfortunately, during the periods of abstinence, much of the muscle mass gained is gradually lost, which

frightens many users into prematurely starting another cycle of steroid abuse (Schrof, 1992).

The Risks of Anabolic Steroid Abuse

Much of what is known about the anabolic steroids is based on clinical experience from patients who are taking steroids under a physician's care, using specific recommended dosage levels to achieve a specific goal (Medical Economics Company, 1989). Adverse side effects have been documented at relatively low doses in cases where these medications are used to treat medical conditions (Hough & Kovan, 1990), but the consequences of long-term steroid abuse are simply not known (Wadler, 1994; Kashkin, 1992; Schrof, 1992).

Most of what is known about the consequences of anabolic steroid abuse is based on clinical data obtained from male steroid abusers, in large part because most steroid abusers are male. DuRant et al. (1993) found that, of the ninth-grade students surveyed, over 5% of the boys but only 1.5% of the girls reported that they had used anabolic steroids. However, as a result of this male bias, virtually nothing is known about the long-term effects of anabolic steroid abuse on women (Gottesman, 1992).

The adverse effects of anabolic steroids are determined by (1) the route of administration, (2) the specific drugs taken, (3) the dose utilized, (4) the frequency of use, (5) the individual's health, and (6) the individual's age (Johnson, 1990). However, even at recommended dosage levels, steroids are capable of causing sore throat or fever, vomiting (with or without blood), dark-colored urine, bone pain, nausea, unusual weight gain or headache, and a range of other side effects (United States Pharmacopeial Convention, 1990).

Unfortunately, many adolescents and young adults who abuse steroids do so at dosage levels that are often 10 (Hough & Kovan, 1990), 40 (Johnson, 1990), 100 (Brower, Catlin, Blow, Eliopulos, & Beresford, 1991), or even 1,000 times the maximum recommended dosage level (Wadler, 1994; Council on Scientific Affairs, 1990b).

Brower, Blow, Young, and Hill (1991), for example, found that the dosage range of steroids used by their sample of weight lifters was between 2 and 26 times the recommended dosage level. Another study found that the *lowest* dose of anabolic steroids being used by a group of weight lifters was still 350% above the usual therapeutic dose (Landry & Primos, 1990).

There is very little information available on the effects of this family of drugs at these dosage levels (Kashkin, 1992; Johnson, 1990). It is known that the effects of the anabolic steroids on muscle tissue last for several weeks after the drugs are discontinued (Pope & Katz, 1991). Thus, muscle builders who abuse steroids may discontinue the drugs shortly before competition to avoid having their steroid use detected by urine toxicological screens. Other illicit steroid users choose specific forms of anabolic steroids that are hard to detect or that are thought to be undetectable by current laboratory tests. Thus, a "clean" urine sample does not rule out steroid use in modern sporting events nor does it rule out the possibility that the individual is at risk for any of a wide range of complications.

Complications from Steroid Abuse

The Reproductive System

Males who utilize steroids at the recommended dosage levels may experience enlargement of breasts, increased frequency of erections or continual erections (a condition known as *priapism*, which is itself a medical emergency), unnatural hair growth or hair loss, and a frequent urge to urinate. Steroid abuse may also bring about degeneration of the testicles, enlargement of the prostate gland, impotence, and sterility (Pope & Katz, 1994; Haupt, 1993; Kashkin, 1992; Hough & Kovan, 1990; Council on Scientific Affairs, 1990b). On rare occasions, steroid abuse has resulted in carcinoma (cancer) of the prostate (Johnson, 1990; Landry & Primos, 1990) and urinary obstruction (Council on Scientific Affairs, 1990b).

Women who use steroids at recommended dosage levels may experience an abnormal enlargement of the clitoris, irregular menstrual periods, unnatural hair growth or hair loss, a deepening of the voice, and a possible reduction in the size of the breasts (Redman, 1990; Hough & Kovan, 1990; Pope & Katz, 1988). The menstrual irregularities caused by steroid use often disappear when the steroids are discontinued (Johnson, 1990). The Council on Scientific Affairs (1990b) suggests that women who use steroids may experience beard growth. Another possible outcome for women is the development of "male pattern" baldness (Haupt, 1993).

The Liver, Kidneys, and the Digestive System

Steroid abusers may experience altered liver function, which can be detected through the blood tests such as the serum glautamic-oxaloacetic transaminase (SGOT) and the serum glautamic-pyruvic transaminase (SGPT) (Haupt, 1993; Johnson, 1990). However, Haupt (1993) suggests that oral forms of anabolic steroids may be more likely than injected forms to result in liver problems. The reason for this pattern of steroid effects is not clear at this time.

Anabolic steroid abuse has been implicated as a cause of hepatoxicity (liver failure). In addition, there is evidence that, when used for periods of time at excessive doses, steroids may contribute to the formation of both cancerous and benign liver tumors (Haupt, 1993; Medical Economics Company, 1989; Council on Scientific Affairs, 1990b).

The Cardiovascular System

There is evidence that steroid abuse may contribute to the development of heart disease (Johnson, 1990; Wolkowitz, 1990; Hough & Kovan, 1990). These steroid-induced complications may last for months after the drug is discontinued. This class of drugs tends to increase the levels of low-density lipoprotein cholesterol and blood pressure levels, while decreasing the levels of high-density lipoproteins (Fultz, 1991; Johnson,

1990; Council on Scientific Affairs, 1990b). These are well-documented risk factors for heart disease that may have lifelong consequences for the person abusing steroids.

In effect, the anabolic steroids may contribute to accelerated atherosclerosis of the heart and its surrounding blood vessels. There is a documented report of a 34-year-old weight lifter who suffered a stroke while using steroids (Council on Scientific Affairs, 1990b). Fultz (1991) notes that high doses of the anabolic steroids may cause blood platelets to clump together, which may contribute to both heart attacks and strokes. Recent laboratory research also suggests that steroids have a direct, dose-related, cardiotoxic (toxic to heart muscles) effect (Slovut, 1992), although the reason for this is not clear at this time.

The Central Nervous System

The anabolic steroid family of drugs is suspected to be capable of causing behavioral changes in the user. To explore this belief, Wolkowitz et al., (1990) administered a daily dose of 80 mg of the pharmaceutical steroid *prednisone* for 5 days to a sample of healthy volunteers. The authors found that "prednisone administration was associated with decreases in . . . levels of several biologically and behaviorally active neuropeptides or neurotransmitters" (p. 966). However, in spite of these measured changes in biochemical levels, they found "no significant prednisone-associated changes . . . in group mean behavioral ratings" (p. 967).

However, this study covered only a 5-day period. Individuals who abuse steroids often do so for periods of time far in excess of 5 days, and they may use daily dosage levels far above 80 mg of prednisone. As pointed out earlier, individuals who abuse steroids often do so at dosage levels between 40 (Johnson, 1990) and 1,000 times the maximum recommended dosage level (Medical Economics Company, 1989). It requires several weeks of constantly increasing dosage levels to achieve this level of steroid abuse.

At such grossly inflated dosage levels, ana-bolic steroids are suspected of causing psychotic symptoms in the chronic user (Pope & Katz, 1994; Kashkin, 1992; Johnson, 1990; Pope, Katz, & Champoux, 1986). At the very least, the unpleasant side effects of anabolic steroids may be an incentive for the person to use recreational drugs to relieve their discomfort or control the side effects of the steroids (Schrof, 1992). Kashkin (1992) reports that about 50% of steroid abusers abuse other substances in an effort to control the side effects of the anabolic steroids, including diuretics (to counteract steroid-induced "bloating") and antibiotics (to control steroid-induced acne).

Pope and Katz (1987) examined 31 weight lifters who had admitted to using steroids and found that 22% experienced some symptoms of psychosis, apparently as a side effect of their steroid use. In a later study, Pope and Katz (1988) examined 41 athletes who had used steroids and found that 9 subjects (22%) had experienced either a manic or a depressive reaction while using steroids, and another 5 subjects (12%) had experienced an apparent drug-induced psychotic reaction. In 1990, Pope and Katz reported that, in their opinion, steroid abuse had contributed to the violent behavior of three individuals, and in all three cases the end result was homicide or attempted homicide. Illicit steroid users often call this drug-induced reaction a "roid rage" (Redman, 1990; Fultz, 1991). Up to 90% of those who abuse steroids may experience an increase in aggressive or violent behaviors (Johnson, 1990).

Yesalis, Kennedy, Kopstein, and Bahrke (1993) present an interesting possible explanation for this increased level of violence. They suggest that previous studies that found a relationship between violent behavior and anabolic steroid use may have failed to establish a *causal* relationship between the two. Anabolic steroid users may have exaggerated self-reports of violence. Another possibility is that individuals who behaved in violent ways while under the influence of steroids may have been violent-prone to begin with. The authors concluded that there is a need for further research to further explore the relationship between anabolic steroid use and violence.

Steroids can cause depression in both men and women at either recommended or higher dosage levels. These drugs may also produce a toxic reaction if the individual is using too high a dose for his or her individual body chemistry. Symptoms of a toxic reaction to steroids include a drug-induced psychotic reaction, manic episodes, delirium, dementia, or a drug-induced depressive reaction that may reach suicidal proportions (Lederberg & Holland, 1989).

General Complications

Patients who have medical conditions, such as certain forms of breast cancer; diabetes mellitus; diseases of the blood vessels, kidney, liver, or heart; and males who suffer from prostate problems should not use steroids unless the presiding physician is aware of these conditions (United States Pharmacopeial Convention, 1990). The anabolic steroids are thought to be possible carcinogens (Johnson, 1990), and their use is not recommended for patients with either active tumors or a history of tumors, except under a physician's supervision.

Other side effects caused by steroid use include severe acne (especially across the back) and a foul odor on the breath (Redman, 1990). In one isolated case, unnatural bone degeneration was attributed to a weight lifter's long-term use of steroids (Pettine, 1991). Animal research also suggests that anabolic steroids may contribute to the degeneration of tendons, a finding that is consistent with clinical case reports of athletes using anabolic steroids whose tendons rupture under stress (Haupt, 1993).

Surprisingly, although anabolic steroids are often abused to improve athletic performance, the evidence to support this theory is mixed. One factor that complicates research into athletic performance is the individual's belief that these drugs will improve his or her abilities. The athlete's *expectation* of improved performance may have some impact.

Adolescents' Growth Patterns

Adolescents who use steroids run the risk of stunted growth, as these drugs may permanently stop bone growth (Haupt, 1993; Schrof, 1992; Johnson, 1990; Council on Scientific Affairs, 1990b). A further complication of steroid abuse by adolescents is that the tendons do not grow at the same accelerated rate as the bone tissues, resulting in increased strain on the tendons and a higher risk of injury (Johnson, 1990; Hough & Kovan, 1990).

Blood Infections

In addition to the complications of steroid abuse itself, individuals who abuse steroids through intramuscular or intravenous injection often share needles. These individuals run the risk of infection associated with contaminated needles. Indeed, there have been cases of athletes contracting AIDS from using a "dirty" needle (Kashkin, 1992; Scott & Scott, 1989).

Anabolic Steroids and Drug Interactions

The anabolic steroids interact with a wide range of medications, including several drugs of abuse. Potentially serious drug interactions have been noted with high doses of acetaminophen and steroids. The combination of these two drugs—steroids and acetaminophen—should be avoided except under a physician's supervision. Patients who take Antabuse (disulfiram) should not take steroids, nor should individuals who are taking Trexan (naltrexone), anticonvulsant medications such as Dilantin (phenytoin), Depakene (valproic acid), or any of the phenothiazines (United States Pharmacopeial Convention, 1990).

Are Anabolic Steroids Addictive?

In recent years, evidence has been uncovered suggesting that long-term anabolic steroid use at high dosage levels may lead to addiction. The tendency for abusers to alternate periods of high doses of steroids with steroid abstinence follows a pattern similar to other forms of drug abuse (Kashkin, 1992). Furthermore, the steroids have been known to bring about a sense of euphoria (Lipkin, 1989; Fultz, 1991), which may explain why steroid use is so attractive to some.

There also is evidence to suggest that the user may become either physically or psychologically dependent on the anabolic steroids (Johnson, 1990). In one study, Bower (1991), found that up to 57% of weight lifters who use steroids ultimately become addicted. Dreyfuss (1989) concluded that 25% of current steroids users are either physically or psychologically dependent on these drugs.

The withdrawal syndrome that accompanies anabolic steroid addiction is reported to be very similar to cocaine withdrawal. Symptoms of withdrawal from steroids include depressive reactions, possibly to the point of suicide attempts (Haupt, 1993; Kashkin, 1992; Hough & Kovan, 1990; Kashkin & Kleber, 1989). Other symptoms include sleep and appetite disturbances (which seem to be part of the poststeroid depressive syndrome; Bower, 1991), fatigue, restlessness, anorexia, insomnia, and decreased libido (Brower, Blow, Young, & Hill, 1991).

Like other drug abusers, steroid abusers require gradual detoxification from the drugs over time, as well as intensive psychiatric support to limit the impact of withdrawal and prevent a return to steroid use (Kashkin & Kleber, 1989; Hough & Kovan, 1990; Bower, 1991). Robert Dimeff, Donald Malone, and John Lombardo (cited in Bower, 1991) cite the following symptoms of steroid addiction, indicating that three or more of these symptoms would identify an individual as dependent on steroids.

- The use of higher doses than originally intended
- A loss of control over the amount of steroids used
- A preoccupation with further steroid use
- The continued use of steroids in spite of the individual's awareness of the problems caused by their use

- The development of tolerance to steroids and the need for larger doses to achieve the same effects as once brought on by lower doses
- The disruption of normal daily activities by steroid use
- The continued use of steroids to control or avoid withdrawal symptoms.

Kashkin (1992) suggests that those individuals who had gone through five or more "cycles" of steroid use were very likely to be "heavy" steroid users.

The Treatment of Anabolic Steroid Abuse

The first step in the treatment of the steroid abuser is to identify those individuals who are indeed abusing anabolic steroids, which a physician can ascertain on the basis of clinical history or blood or urine tests. Thus, a physician is often the first person to suspect that a patient is abusing steroids and is in the best position to confront the user. At this stage, the substance abuse counselor is not thought to have a significant role to play in the treatment of the anabolic steroid user.

Once the steroid abuser has been identified, close medical supervision is needed to identify and treat potential complications of steroid abuse. The attending physician may need to implement a gradual detoxification program for the steroid abuser. Most medical complications caused by steroid abuse usually clear up after the individual stops the use of steroids (Hough & Kovan, 1990); however, some of the complications (such as heart tissue damage) may be permanent. Surgical intervention may correct some side effects of steroid use (Hough & Kovan, 1990), but surgical correction is not always possible.

Following the patients' detoxification from anabolic steroids, counselors should work with patients to identify why they first began using steroids. Self-concept issues should be examined and the proper therapy initiated to help steroid users learn to accept themselves without leaning on artificial crutches such as anabolic steroids. Proper nutritional counseling may be necessary to help the athlete learn how to enhance body strength without using potentially harmful substances such as anabolic steroids. Support groups may help the individual learn to substitute social support for the chemical support of steroids.

Summary

Within the past decade, a surprising new group of drugs, the anabolic steroids, have emerged as drugs of abuse in many circles. However, steroids are not the "typical" drug of abuse. Adolescents and young adults abuse steroids because they believe these substances will increase aggressiveness, enhance athletic ability, and improve personal appearance. Little is known about the effects of these drugs at the dosage levels used by steroid abusers. The identification and treatment of steroid abusers is primarily a medical issue, but substance abuse counselors should have a working knowledge of the effects of steroid use and the complications of steroid abuse.

CHAPTER SIXTEEN

Nicotine and Tobacco Abuse

Historians believe that, long before the arrival of the first European explorers, natives of North America used tobacco in various religious ceremonies and for recreational purposes. After Europeans discovered the "New World," the art of smoking was carried back to Europe by early explorers who had adopted the habit of smoking tobacco.

In Europe, the practice of smoking tobacco was initially received with some skepticism—if not outright hostility—but eventually it became quite popular in Europe. Within a few years of its introduction, the use of tobacco spread across Europe and moved into Asia (Schuckit, 1989), but not without some harsh consequences. For example, in Germany, public smoking was once punishable by death, and in Russia, castration was the sentence for the same crime (Berger & Dunn, 1982). In Asia, the use or distribution of tobacco was a crime punishable by death, and smokers were executed as infidels in Turkey.

Tate (1989) relates the story of Rodrigo de Jerez, a member of one of Columbus' early expeditions to the New World who had adopted the habit of smoking tobacco from the American Indians. When he returned home and lit up a cigar, the townspeople thought that he had become possessed by an evil spirit. For the "good of his soul," he was imprisoned by the Inquisition for an extended period of time. History records that Rodrigo de Jerez was ultimately released from prison, but not before tobacco

smoking had become one of the most popular pastimes in Europe.

In spite of European society's strong initial response against smoking, the practice soon became at least moderately acceptable. European physicians initially thought tobacco was a medicine. More recently, smoking was viewed as a mark of sophistication. Only in the last generation or two has tobacco use been met with wide public criticism.

Tobacco today is much different from the tobacco used centuries ago. When the first European explorers arrived in the New World, tobacco was possibly "more potent and may have contained high concentrations of psychoactive substances" compared to the tobacco of today (Schuckit, 1989, p. 215). But, starting in the mid-19th century, new varieties of tobacco were planted, allowing for a greater yield than in previous years. New methods of curing the leaf of the tobacco plant were also found, speeding up the process by which the leaf was prepared for use.

The manner in which tobacco was used also changed. The advent of the industrial age brought with it machinery capable of manufacturing the cigarette, a smaller, less expensive, neater way to smoke than the hand-rolled cigar. One machine, invented by James A. Bonsack, could produce 120,000 cigarettes a day. The development of such machines greatly increased the number of tobacco products that could be produced; the increased supply reduced the price and the lower price made it possible for more people to afford tobacco products.

Changes in the tax laws made it possible to lower the price of the cigarettes, which soon became a favorite of the poor (Tate, 1989). For example, by 1890, the price of domestic cigarettes had fallen to a nickel for a pack of 20 (Tate, 1989), making them affordable to all but the poorest smoker. But this rapid acceptance of cigarettes was not universal; by 1909, no less than 10 different states had laws that prohibited cigarettes.

Before the introduction of the cigarette, the major method of tobacco use was chewing. The practice of chewing tobacco, then spitting into the ever-present cuspidor, contributed to the spread of tuberculosis and other diseases (Brecher, 1972). In response, public health officials began to campaign against the practice of chewing tobacco after the year 1910. The new cigarette, manufactured in large numbers by the latest machines, provided a more sanitary and relatively inexpensive alternative to chewing tobacco.

Smokers soon discovered that, unlike cigars or pipes, the smoke of the new cigarette was so mild that it could be fully inhaled (Burns, 1991). This allowed the nicotine to enter the lungs and bloodstream. For many, cigarette smoking became the preferred method of servicing their nicotine addiction, and the world hasn't been the same since.

The Scope of the Problem

In the United States, the use of cigarettes grew in popularity after World War I and peaked in the mid-1960s (Schuckit, 1989). Tobacco use achieved "total social acceptance" and "until quite recently, tobacco use was so common and socially acceptable . . . [that] almost everyone tried smoking" (Jaffe, 1989, p. 680). By the mid-1960s approximately 52% of adult males and 32% of adult females in the United States were cigarette smokers (Schuckit, 1989).

In 1964, the Surgeon General of the United States released a report stating that cigarette smoking was a danger to the smoker's health and outlining the various problems that may be caused by smoking. In doing so, the Surgeon General joined a battle against smoking that has been going on since the late 1800s (Tate, 1989). For a number of years since the 1964 report, the number of adult smokers in the United States gradually declined. However, evidence suggests that the number of current smokers has leveled off and may even be gradually increasing (Calabresi, Fowler, Scala, Thompson, & Willwerth, 1994).

Thus, since 1964, cigarette consumption statistics have changed. Whereas in 1963, approximately 4,300 cigarettes were smoked for every man, woman, and child in the United States, by 1983 this figure had dropped to 3,488 cigarettes per person (Brownlee, Roberts, Cooper, Goode, Hetter, & Wright, 1994). Just 7 years later, in 1990, this figure had dropped to 2,800 cigarettes per person (Fiore, 1992), and by 1993 had dropped still further to "just" 2,539 cigarettes per person (Brownlee et al., 1994).

It is thought currently that in the United States approximately 46 million people smoke cigarettes; of this number, approximately 24 million are male and 22 million are female (Brownlee et al., 1994). Unfortunately, even though the purchase of cigarettes by adolescents is illegal, 3.1 million of those who smoke are teenagers (Roberts & Watson, 1994).

In addition to the changes in smoking patterns in the United States, there is evidence that cigarette smoking is on the increase in many parts of the world. Globally, cigarette production has reached a plateau of approximately 5.4 trillion cigarettes per year (Wiley, 1993). Cigarettes are both manufactured in other countries and exported from the United States to virtually every country in the world. Thus, the problem of cigarette smoking has both national and global repercussions.

Although in 1964 it was thought that smoking was a relatively simple phenomenon, we now know that this is not the case. For example, it has been discovered that attitudes toward smoking are often established in childhood or early adolescence. This is true even if the individual does not *begin* to smoke until late adolescence or early adulthood. Furthermore, researchers have discovered that many individuals begin to smoke at an extremely early age; by the age of 12, fully 50% of the school children in Canada have already experimented with tobacco (Walker, 1993).

Thus, the first stages of nicotine addiction are established early in life. Almost 50% of cigarette smokers begin smoking on a regular basis by the age of 18 (Fiore, 1992), and 90% of tobacco smokers are addicted to nicotine before the age of 20 (Walker, 1993). In a very real sense, smoking is a lifelong problem with its deepest roots in childhood and adolescence, and the final fruits of this addictive process are often not found until later adulthood.

The Pharmacology of Tobacco Smoking

The primary method by which tobacco is used is by smoking (Schuckit, 1989), although in recent years chewing tobacco has regained some popularity. The exact pharmacology of tobacco smoking is quite complicated, as there are several variables that influence the composition of tobacco smoke. According to Jaffe (1990), some of these variables include (1) the exact composition of the tobacco being used, (2) how densely the tobacco is packed in the cigarette, (3) the length of the column of tobacco (for cigarette or cigar smokers), (4) the characteristics of the filter being used (if any), (5) the paper being used (for cigarette smokers), and (6) the temperature at which the tobacco is burned.

Tobacco smoke contains some 4,000 different compounds, of which approximately 2,550 come from the unprocessed tobacco itself, and another 1,450 come from additives, pesticides, and a range of other organic or metallic compounds that either intentionally or unintentionally find their way into cigarettes (Burns, 1991). Jaffe (1990) offers a partial list of the compounds found in tobacco smoke: "carbon monoxide, carbon dioxide, nitrogen oxides, ammonia, volatile nitrosamines, hydrogen cyanide, volatile sulfur-containing compounds, nitrites and other nitrogen-containing compounds, volatile hydrocarbons, alcohols, and aldehydes and keytones (e.g., acetaldehyde, formaldehyde and acrolein)" (p. 545). The concentrations of many of these chemicals, such as carbon monoxide, are such that "uninterrupted exposure" would result in death (Burns, 1991, p. 633). For example, Burns notes that the concentration of carbon monoxide found in cigarettes is "similar to that found in automobile exhaust" (p. 633), a known source of potentially dangerous concentrations of carbon monoxide. Cigarette smoke is also known to contain a small amount of arsenic (Banerjee, 1990).

Cigarette smoke also contains radioactive compounds such as polonium 210 (Evans, 1993; Jaffe, 1990) and lead 210 (Brownson, Novotny, & Perry, 1993). These compounds, for the most part, are found in the soil in which tobacco is grown and are incorporated into the tobacco plant. However, over a 1-year period, the cumulative radiation exposure for a 2-pack-a-day smoker is equal to the exposure of 250 to 300 chest X rays (Evans, 1993).

All these chemicals—and a multitude of others—are inhaled when a person smokes. Some of the chemicals found in tobacco smoke are documented carcinogens, or chemicals that are known to cause cancer. At least 43 known or suspected carcinogens are found in cigarette smoke (Burns, 1991) and are thus introduced directly into the body.

Nicotine

The major psychoactive effects caused by cigarette smoking are thought to be caused by nicotine. Indeed, there is evidence that tobacco companies view cigarettes as little more than a single-dose container of nicotine that will quickly administer the chemical to the user (Mondi, Hooten, & Peterzell, 1994; Benowitz & Henningfield, 1994). Mondi et al. suggest that tobacco companies are well aware of nicotine's psychoactive effects and that tobacco companies have manipulated nicotine's pharmacological properties to keep cigarette smokers from quitting.

The effects of nicotine are very similar to those of other drugs of abuse. When nicotine reaches the brain, the user experiences a "high"—a sense of release from stress or sense of euphoria (Fiore, Jorenby, Baker, & Kenford, 1992). As we will discuss in a later section of this chapter, one characteristic that nicotine shares with the other drugs of abuse is an ability to cause addiction.

In terms of immediate health consequences, nicotine itself seems to be a relatively "safe" chemical. The lethal dose of nicotine in a healthy adult is estimated to be around 60 mg (Ashton, 1992); the "typical" cigarette contains about 10 mg of nicotine (Lee & D'Alonzo, 1993). But the bioavailability of nicotine ranges from 3% to 40%, meaning that only 3% to 40% of the nicotine in the cigarette is actually absorbed by the smoker (Benowitz & Henningfield, 1994).

One reason some of the nicotine in a cigarette is not absorbed is that the level of acidity in cigarette smoke makes it difficult for the body to absorb the nicotine. However, when a person smokes a cigarette, each "puff" of tobacco smoke contains about 350 micrograms of nicotine (Mann, 1994). As the individual continues to smoke the cigarette, between 0.05 and 2.5 mg of nicotine will eventually reach the brain (Lee & D'Alonzo, 1993; Ashton, 1992). Thus, the typical smoker will receive between 1/1200 and 1/24 of the estimated lethal dose of nicotine each time he or she smokes a cigarette.

Nicotine is known to have psychoactive "properties similar to those of cocaine and amphetamine" (Rustin, 1988, p. 18). Researchers disagree as to its relative potency, however. Jaffe (1989) suggests that nicotine is a less powerful reinforcer than cocaine or the amphetamines; Weil (1986), on the other hand, claims that nicotine is a more powerful reinforcer than the amphetamines. Henningfield and Nemeth-Coslett (1988) state that intravenous nicotine is thought to be 5 to 10 times more potent than intravenous cocaine in terms of its reward potential.

Researchers agree that nicotine is a powerful reinforcer and that it reaches the brain very quickly; they disagree on its exact potency or the speed with which smoking cigarettes allows nicotine to reach the brain. Estimates of the speed which nicotine reaches the brain after the first "puff" of a cigarette range from 7 seconds (Fiore et al., 1992) to 8 seconds (Jaffe, 1990), to a high of 19 seconds (Benowitz, 1992).

Once in the body, nicotine is rapidly distributed to virtually every blood-rich tissue in the body, including the brain (Henningfield & Nemeth-Coslett, 1988). Indeed, nicotine accumulates in the brain at such high levels that the measured levels of nicotine in the brain may be twice as high as the level of nicotine found in the blood (Fiore et al., 1992). High concentrations of nicotine are also found in the lungs and spleen of cigarette smokers.

Within the brain, nicotine is thought to facilitate the release of the neurotransmitter dopamine within the region of the limbic system known as the *nucleus accumbens* (Miller & Gold, 1993). As we discussed in Chapter 1, this is a region of the brain thought to be involved in the perception of pleasure, which may explain why cigarette smokers report a sense of euphoria or pleasure when they smoke.

But another region of the brain where nicotine exerts a major effect is the *medulla*; this is the region of the brain that is responsible for such functions as swallowing, vomiting, respiration, and the control of blood pressure (Restak, 1984). This is also why many first-time smokers experience both nausea and vomiting (Jaffe, 1990). The smoker's heart rate is also modified by nerve impulses from the medulla, which accounts at least in part for nicotine's immediate effects on the cardiovascular system. These effects include an increase in heart rate, an increase in blood pressure, and an increase in the strength of heart contractions. While the heart rate is increased, the peripheral blood flow in the body is reduced, as nicotine causes the blood vessels in the outer regions of the body to constrict (Schuckit, 1989). This process contributes to nicotine's tendency to increase blood pressure levels.

In addition to its effects on the brain, nicotine

causes a decrease in the strength of stomach contractions (Schuckit, 1989). Cigarette smoke itself can cause irritation of the tissues of the lungs and pulmonary system. Cigarette smoking also deposits potentially harmful chemicals in the lungs and causes a decrease in the motion of the *cilia*, the small, hairlike projections that help clean the lungs.

The peak concentrations of nicotine are reached in the first minutes after the cigarette is smoked, and then the level of nicotine in the blood starts to drop. The biological half-life of nicotine is between 100 minutes (Rustin, 1992) and 2 hours (Fiore et al., 1992). Because only 50% of the nicotine from one cigarette is metabolized in the half-life period, a reservoir of unmetabolized nicotine is established over the course of a day, as the individual smokes cigarette after cigarette.

Only 5% to 10% of the nicotine that enters the body is excreted unchanged; the rest is metabolized by the liver. Of the nicotine that is metabolized by the liver, 90% is metabolized into *cotinine*, a metabolite of nicotine that has no known psychoactive properties. The remaining 10% is metabolized into *nicotine-n-oxide*. These chemicals are then excreted from the body in the urine.

At one point, it was thought that cigarette smokers may be able to metabolize nicotine more quickly than nonsmokers. This assumption was based on the observation that the nicotine in the smoker's blood causes the body to metabolize some medications more quickly than in the nonsmoker. It was assumed that this was one reason smokers gradually increased the frequency with which they smoked cigarettes in the first few years. However, Benowitz and Jacob (1993) tested this hypothesis and found that smokers and nonsmokers metabolize nicotine at more or less the same rate. They also concluded that their data did not support the theory that smokers would gradually smoke more frequently as they became more adept at metabolizing nicotine. Thus, the question of why beginning smokers gradually smoke more often over time remains unanswered.

Acetaldehyde

Nicotine is not the only psychoactive chemical in tobacco. Tobacco smoke also includes a small amount of acetaldehyde. Acetaldehyde is the first metabolite produced by the liver when the body breaks down alcohol. In terms of its psychoactive potential, acetaldehyde is thought to be more potent than alcohol. Also, like alcohol, acetaldehyde has a sedative effect on the user (Rustin, 1988). Thus, although nicotine is believed to have the strongest effect on the user, other compounds in tobacco smoke also have some impact on the smoker's state of mind.

Cigarette Smoking and Alzheimer's Disease

Surprisingly, in spite of all the dangers associated with cigarette smoking (which will be discussed in a later section of this chapter), there is a "negative association" (Brenner et al., 1993, p. 293) between cigarette smoking and the later development of Alzheimer's disease. The reasons are not clear, but research suggests that individuals who smoked at one point in their lives were less likely to later develop Alzheimer's disease. Brenner et al. hypothesize that low doses of nicotine may alter the sensitivity of certain neurons in the brain to acetylcholine, making them more sensitive to this neurotransmitter. This, in turn, could make it possible for the same neurons to function effectively even with reduced levels of acetylcholine.

The authors are quick to point out that their findings do not support the practice of cigarette smoking as a treatment for or preventive measure against Alzheimer's disease; the potential benefits are far outweighed by the health consequences of tobacco use. However, the authors did suggest that their findings hint at a possible treatment mechanism for Alzheimer's disease that is worthy of further investigation.

Drug Interactions

Drug interactions between nicotine and various other therapeutic agents are well documented.

Cigarette smokers, for example, require more morphine for the control of pain than do nonsmokers (Bond, 1989; Jaffe, 1990). Some suggest that smokers may experience less sedation from benzodiazepines than do nonsmokers (Bond, 1989; Jaffe, 1990). However, Creelman, Sands, Ciraulo, Greenblatt, and Shader (1989) found no evidence to support this theory, and they concluded that "smokers should not require different dosing of benzodiazepines than nonsmokers" (p. 167).

Nicotine also seems to counteract some of the sedation seen with alcohol use, and Schuckit (1989) has suggested that this may be one reason alcoholics often smoke so much. Tobacco also interacts with many anticoagulants, as well as the beta blocker propranol and caffeine, and women who use oral contraceptives and who smoke are more likely to experience strokes, myocardial infarction, and thromboembolism than are their nonsmoking counterparts (Bond, 1989).

Subjective Effects of Nicotine

The exact mechanism by which nicotine affects the central nervous system is unknown. However, nicotine is thought to bring about a dose-dependent, biphasic response at the level of the individual neurons of the brain, especially those that utilize the neurotransmitter acetylcholine (Ashton, 1992; Restak, 1991; Benowitz, 1992). Initially, nicotine stimulates these neurons, possibly contributing to the smoker's feeling of increased alertness. However, over longer periods of time, the nicotine blocks the effects of acetylcholine, reducing the rate at which those neurons "fire."

This theory seems to account for the observed effects of cigarette smoking. Smokers are known to experience stimulation of the brain (Schuckit, 1989) as well as decreased muscle tone (Jaffe, 1990). This is why many smokers find that cigarette smoking helps them to relax when they are under pressure. About 90% of cigarette smokers report a sense of pleasure when they smoke

(Ashton, 1992). As animal research suggests, this may reflect nicotine's ability to stimulate the release of the neurotransmitters norepinephrine and dopamine (Jaffe, 1990), chemicals known to be used by the brain's "pleasure system."

The first-time smoker often feels nauseous and may even vomit (Restak, 1991). However, over time, the smoker develops tolerance to these effects. The stimulation of the neurotransmitter systems outlined above eventually results in an association between smoking and the nicotine-induced pleasurable sensations. Thus, with repeated episodes of nicotine use over a period of time, the individual comes to associate smoking with pleasurable sensations, as the neurotransmitters norepinephrine and dopamine are released within the brain.

Nicotine Addiction

Although it has been known for some time that nicotine is addictive, people often underestimate its addictive potential. Cocaine, for example, has the reputation of being a profoundly addictive substance, but only 3% to 20% of those who use cocaine go on to become addicted to this chemical (Musto, 1991). In contrast, consider that Pomerleau, Collins, Shiffman, and Pomerleau (1993) estimate that between one-third and one-half of those who experiment with smoking go on to become addicted. Jaffe (1989) concludes that "a very high percentage" (p. 680) of those who smoke 100 cigarettes will go on to become daily smokers. Walker (1993) gave an even lower figure, noting that children who smoke just 4 or more cigarettes stand a 94% chance of continuing to smoke.

But not everyone who begins to smoke will go on to become addicted to nicotine (Henningfield & Nemeth-Coslett, 1988). In spite of the popular image of nicotine as an addictive substance, a small minority (perhaps 5% to 10%) of those who smoke are not addicted to nicotine (Jarvik & Schneider, 1992; Shiffman, Fischer, Zettler-Segal, & Benowitz, 1990). These individuals, who demonstrate an episodic pattern of nicotine use, are classified as cigarette "chippers."

As a group, chippers do not appear to smoke in response to social pressures or to avoid the symptoms of withdrawal (Shiffman et al., 1990). Indeed, one of the defining characteristics of tobacco "chippers" is that they do not experience withdrawal symptoms when they stop smoking. This suggests that the "chipper" is not addicted to nicotine. Unfortunately, very little beyond this is known about tobacco "chipping," and there is much to learn about this phenomenon.

However, 90% to 95% of those who smoke *are* addicted to nicotine, and they demonstrate all the typical characteristics of drug addiction: tolerance, withdrawal symptoms, and drug-seeking behaviors (Rustin, 1988, 1992). In addition, tobacco users develop highly individual drug-using rituals. These smoking rituals seem to provide the individual a sense of security and contribute to the tendency to smoke when anxious.

Nicotine addiction is a very real problem. To place the strength of nicotine addiction in perspective, Kozlowski, Wilkinson, Skinner, Kent, Franklin, and Pope (1989) asked some 1,000 individuals in treatment for a drug addiction to rate the relative difficulty of quitting smoking, as compared to giving up their drug of choice. Surprisingly, 74% rated the task of quitting cigarette use at least as difficult as giving up their drug of choice, a finding that underscores the addiction potential of tobacco.

Some researchers believe that chronic smokers tend to smoke in such a way as to regulate the nicotine level in their blood. Smokers increase or decrease their cigarette use to achieve and then maintain a person-specific blood level of nicotine (Sherman, 1994; Pomerleau et al., 1993; Benowitz, 1992; Shiffman et al., 1990). This may explain why smokers use fewer cigarettes when given cigarettes of a high nicotine content but smoke more when given low-nicotine cigarettes (Benowitz, 1992; Jaffe, 1990).

Henningfield and Nemeth-Coslett (1988) challenge this conclusion, noting that research has shown that cigarette smokers are "remark-

ably insensitive" (p. 45s) to changes in nicotine levels in the blood. They claim that the hypothesis that cigarette smokers regulate their use to maintain a constant blood plasma level of nicotine has "never been convincingly demonstrated" (p. 46s). After reviewing the rapid changes in blood plasma nicotine levels across the span of a single day, Henningfield and Nemeth-Coslett concluded that the research data does not support the constant-level hypothesis. However, the issue has not been completely resolved.

Nicotine Withdrawal

Withdrawal symptoms usually begin within 2 hours of the last use of tobacco and peak within 24 hours (Kaplan, Sadock, & Grebb, 1994). Then, they gradually decline over the next 10 days to several weeks (Hughes, 1992; Jaffe, 1989). The exact nature of the withdrawal symptoms varies from person to person. Surprisingly, in light of the horror stories often heard about the agony of giving up cigarette smoking, research has found that approximately 25% of those who quit cigarettes report no withdrawal symptoms at all (Benowitz, 1992). The exact reason for this occurrence is not clear, although it has been suggested that a higher daily intake of nicotine may be associated with stronger withdrawal symptoms (Jaffe, 1990). The reverse is also thought to be true: those who report little or no withdrawal from nicotine may have been smoking fewer cigarettes to begin with. But this is only a theory, and the exact relationship between the number of cigarettes an individual smokes and the severity of his or her withdrawal from nicotine is still unclear.

Some symptoms of nicotine withdrawal include anxiety, sleep disturbance, irritability, impatience, difficulties in concentration, restlessness, a "craving" for tobacco, hunger, gastrointestinal upset, headache, and drowsiness (Fiore et al., 1992; Hughes, 1992). Other possible symptoms of nicotine withdrawal include depression, hostility, fatigue, lightheadedness, headaches, a tingling sensation in the limbs, constipation, and increased coughing (Jarvik & Schneider, 1992).

Although it is thought that these withdrawal symptoms gradually decrease in frequency and intensity, this may not be true for everyone. In their study of nicotine withdrawal, Hughes, Gust, Skoog, Keenan, and Fenwick (1991) found that up to 25% of their sample of smokers continued to experience withdrawal symptoms from nicotine a full month after they had stopped smoking. Even 6 months after they had stopped smoking, up to 75% of those who were abstinent experienced at least an occasional craving for nicotine.

Over time, the former smoker experiences a decrease in heart rate and blood pressure and improved peripheral blood flow patterns. Jarvik and Schneider (1992) state that the heart rate will drop after about 10 days of abstinence, but Hughes (1992) contends that the heart rate begins to decline in as little as 2 days, with further decreases 7 and 14 days following the last cigarette. Thus, although the precise time frame is not clear, researchers agree that there ultimately will be an improvement in cardiac function if the individual stops smoking.

Some have suggested the possibility that the withdrawal process may exacerbate preexisting depressive disorders in some people (Breslau, Kilbey, & Andreski, 1993; Jaffe, 1990). Research has revealed that 60% of smokers who try to quit have histories of major depression. However, this does not mean that the cigarette withdrawal process caused the individual to become depressed. Rather, researchers now believe that cigarette smoking and depression are separate conditions that seem to be influenced by the same genetic factors (Glassman, 1993; Breslau, Kilbey, & Andreski, 1993). This is still only a theory, and the exact nature of the relationship between smoking and depression remains to be identified.

What *is* known is that cigarette smokers tend to use nicotine as a way to cope with negative emotional states, of which depression is a good example; other examples of negative emotional states include anxiety, boredom, or sadness (Sherman, 1994). Nicotine soon becomes an easily administered, quick method for coping with these feelings, and the smoker soon learns that he or she can control negative emotional states through the use of cigarettes.

Cigarette Cessation and Weight Gain

People who stop smoking often report a distressing increase in weight during the first few weeks of abstinence, although the exact mechanism by which this comes about remains unknown (Eisen, Lyons, Goldberg, & True, 1993). One theory is that cigarette smoking helps suppress the individual's appetite (Jaffe, 1990), so it seems logical to assume that the reverse will be true when the person stops smoking. Smokers also tend to retain less fluid than nonsmokers do, and some of the weight gain noted after a person stops smoking may reflect added fluid.

Although many ex-smokers dislike this weight gain, researchers have come to view it in a more positive light. Hughes et al. (1991) found that these individuals who gained weight were more likely to remain abstinent. Furthermore, they discovered that weight levels "returned to precessation levels at 6 months" (p. 57), suggesting that weight gain may be a time-limited side effect of abstinence.

Williamson, Madans, Anda, Kleinman, Giovino, and Byers (1991) explored the problem of weight gain in ex-smokers, using a sample of 748 male and 1,137 female smokers contrasted to 409 men and 359 women who had abstained from the use of tobacco for one year. In this sample, the average male smoker gained 2.8 kilograms (6.1 pounds)[1] and the average female smoker gained 3.8 kilograms (8.4 pounds) after stopping smoking. In a minority of ex-smokers—some 10% of the men and 13% of the women—the authors found a larger weight gain of 13 kilograms (28.6 pounds).

Williamson et al. also uncovered an interesting twist; the average smoker in their sample actually weighed less than individuals who had

[1]There are 2.2046 pounds per kilogram.

never smoked. Furthermore, by "the end of the study . . . the mean body weight of those who had quit had increased only to that of those who had never smoked" (p. 743). The implication of this study is that tobacco use interferes with weight gain, but through some unknown mechanism.

Although excessive weight is a known risk factor for cardiovascular disease, the health benefits obtained by giving up cigarette use far outweigh the potential risks associated with post-cigarette weight gain (Eisen et al., 1993). A former smoker would have to gain 50 to 100 pounds before the health risks of the extra weight would come close to the health risks inherent in cigarette smoking (Brunton, Henningfield, & Solberg, 1994). As we have seen, most former smokers gain only a modest amount of weight when they give up cigarette smoking.

Complications from Chronic Tobacco Use

Because of the various factors that influence the effects of tobacco smoke, the impact of smoking on any given individual is quite difficult to determine. The exact amount of nicotine, "tar," and carbon monoxide obtained from a specific brand of cigarette can be determined by a test machine (Hilts, 1994), but the test data has little relationship to the amount of "tar" and nicotine the average smoker will inhale. Although the machine will "smoke" a cigarette in a predictable manner, the various smoking methods utilized by different individuals causes significant variability in both the specific chemical combinations generated by each cigarette and what chemicals are absorbed into the smoker's body. For example, some smokers inhale the cigarette smoke more deeply into their lungs than other smokers do. Other smokers hold their cigarette in such a way as to block the air holes in filters (thus altering the content of the smoke). These smoker-specific behaviors make it difficult to determine exactly what chemicals, and in what concentrations, may be introduced into the body of any given individual when he or she

smokes a cigarette. Still, the Federal Trade Commission continues to rely on data provided by the tobacco industry itself to determine the content of cigarette smoke (Hilts, 1994; Cotton, 1993).

At times it seems that the tobacco industry is the only organization that continues to doubt that tobacco use causes illness. Indeed, the standard policy of the tobacco industry seems to be to attack any study that suggests that smoking causes *any* form of physical disease. However, in spite of all of the protests advanced by the tobacco industry, there is an impressive body of medical literature that associates tobacco use with an increased risk for a wide range of conditions.

Cigarette smoking did not become popular until around the turn of the century. At that time, carcinoma (cancer) of the lung was a relatively rare disorder (Bloodworth, 1987). Many physicians of a century ago went through an entire medical career without ever seeing a case of lung cancer. Even as recently as 1921—by which time cigarette smoking had become quite popular—the association between tobacco use and cancer was not recognized (Foa, 1989). Indeed, it was not until 1923 that lung cancer was included in the International Classification of Diseases (*Smithsonian*, 1989) and it was not until 1940 that the Mayo Clinic first suggested a relationship between smoking and coronary artery disease (Bartecchi, MacKenzie, & Schrier, 1994).

Thus, for a long time, tobacco use was viewed as a harmless vice. But now the association between tobacco use and a wide range of diseases is well known. It is estimated that 40% of those who are addicted to nicotine will die prematurely as a result of tobacco-induced illness (Benowitz & Henningfield, 1994). Nationally, it is estimated that between 400,000 (McGinnis & Foege, 1993) and 450,000 (American Medical Association, 1993a) cigarette smokers in the United States die each year from smoking-related illness. A smaller number of nonsmokers also die from what is known as "passive" or "environmental" smoke (to be discussed later).

It is difficult to put the problem of the risks

associated with cigarette smoking into strong enough terms. Fully 30% of *all* cancer deaths are caused by smoking (Bartecchi, MacKenzie, & Schrier, 1994; Fiore, Epps, & Manley, 1994). Specifically, the use of tobacco products is thought to be the cause of an annual 179,000 deaths from cardiovascular disease; 119,920 deaths from lung cancer; 31,402 deaths from other cancers; and 84,475 deaths from other respiratory disease (Bartecchi, MacKenzie, & Schrier, 1994).

Cigarette smoking is thought to cause more than 75% of all cases of esophageal cancer, 30% to 40% of all bladder cancers, and 30% of the cases of cancer of the pancreas (Sherman, 1991). Cigarette smoking is the single largest cause of preventable death in the United States (Bartecchi, MacKenzie, & Schrier, 1994). Fully one-fifth of all deaths in the United States and one-sixth of all deaths in the United Kingdom are caused by some form of smoking-induced cancer (*The Lancet*, 1991a). Furthermore, it has been estimated that tobacco use around the world is responsible for almost 2.5 million (Council on Scientific Affairs, 1990a) premature deaths each year. If present trends continue, it is estimated that, by the year 2030, cigarette smoking will cause 10 million premature deaths each year, or 27,300 deaths each day from cigarette-related illness worldwide (*The Lancet*, 1991a).

Cigarette smokers sometimes defend their addiction on the grounds that it is a "harmless" addiction, that it is inexpensive, or that it is legal. It is neither harmless nor inexpensive. The estimated total financial impact of smoking, in terms of lost productivity and health care costs for tobacco-related disease is in excess of $100 billion per year, and smoking causes more than 187,000 fires each year—an additional loss of $550 million in property damage (MacKenzie, Bartecchi, & Schrier, 1994b). Although cigarette smoking is legal, there is hardly a body system that is not affected by cigarette smoking. Indeed, tobacco products are the only products sold in the United States that are "unequivocally carcinogenic when used as directed" (MacKenzie, Bartecchi, & Schrier, 1994b, p. 977). What follows is just a short list of the various conditions known, or

strongly suspected, to be a result of cigarette smoking.

Complications of the Mouth, Throat, and Pulmonary System

According to Wetter, Young, Bidwell, Badr, and Palta (1994), chronic cigarette smokers are known to suffer increased rates of respiratory problems during sleep, as compared to non-smokers. The authors examined data from 811 adults who were studied at the sleep disorders program at the University of Wisconsin-Madison medical center. They found that current smokers were at greater risk for such sleep breathing disorders as snoring and sleep apnea than were nonsmokers. So strong was the relationship between smoking and sleep disorders that the authors recommend that smoking cessation be considered one of the treatment interventions for a patient with a sleeping-related breathing disorder.

Chronic smokers also have higher rates of cancer of the lung, mouth, pharynx, larynx, and esophagus than do nonsmokers. Cigarette smokers are more likely than nonsmokers to develop chronic bronchitis, pneumonia, and chronic obstructive pulmonary diseases such as emphysema. Indeed, Sherman (1991) estimates that 81% of all chronic obstructive pulmonary disease (COPD) deaths can be traced to cigarette smoking. When they do develop one or more pulmonary diseases, smokers are more likely to die from their lung disorder than are nonsmokers (Lee & D'Alonzo, 1993; Burns, 1991; Jaffe, 1990; Schuckit, 1989).

Complications of the Digestive Tract

Alcohol and cigarette smoking are both associated with an increased risk of cancer in the upper digestive and respiratory tracts (Garro, Espina, & Lieber, 1992). Research suggests that alcoholics have almost a 6-fold greater chance of developing cancer in the mouth and pharynx as compared with nondrinkers. Smokers have been found to have a 7-fold increased risk of mouth or pharynx cancer as compared with nonsmokers. However, alcoholics who *also* smoke have a 38-fold greater risk for cancer of the mouth or pharynx than do nonsmoking nondrinkers (Garro, Espina, & Lieber, 1992).

Complications of the Heart and Cardiovascular System

Smoking is a known risk factor for the development of coronary heart disease, hypertension, aortic aneurysms, and atherosclerotic peripheral vascular disease. Cigarette smoking is a known risk factor for the development of both cerebral infarction and cerebral hemorrhage (either condition may be called a "stroke") (Robbins, Manson, Lee, Satterfield, & Hennekens, 1994; Sherman, 1991). Furthermore, cigarette smokers are at increased risk for the development of adult-onset leukemia (Brownson, Novotny, & Perry, 1993). Although this is not traditionally viewed as a consequence of cigarette smoking, Brownson, Novotny, and Perry estimate that approximately 14% of all cases of adult-onset leukemia in the United States can be traced to cigarette smoking.

Cigarette smoking also causes constriction of the coronary arteries. Moliterno et al., (1994) measured the diameters of the coronary arteries of 42 cigarette smokers who were being evaluated for complaints of chest pain. They found a *7% decrease* in coronary artery diameter for those individuals without coronary artery disease who had smoked a cigarette. The coronary arteries are the primary source of blood for the muscle tissues of the heart, and anything that causes a reduction in the amount of blood that can flow through the coronary arteries, even for a short period of time, holds the potential to cause damage to the heart itself. Thus, the short-term reduction in coronary artery diameter brought on by cigarette smoking may, ultimately, contribute to cardiovascular problems for the smoker.

Complications of the Visual System

In addition to cigarette-induced cancer, smokers may experience other, nonfatal forms of illness as well. A pair of recent studies revealed that smoking was associated with a higher risk of cataract formation both in men (Christensen et al., 1992) and in women (Hankinson et al., 1992). Although the exact mechanism for cataract formation is not clear, male smokers who currently use 20 or more cigarettes a day are twice as likely to form cataracts as are nonsmokers (Christensen et al., 1992). Research also revealed that women who quit cigarette smoking, even if they had done so a decade earlier, are still at risk for cataract formation (Hankinson et al., 1992). The findings from these two studies indicate that cigarette-induced disease is far more involved than had previously been thought, and they suggest that at least some of the physical damage caused by cigarette smoking does not reverse itself after the smoker quits.

Other Complications from Cigarette Smoking

The use of tobacco products is thought to contribute to the formation of peptic ulcers (Lee & D'Alonzo, 1993; Jarvik & Schneider, 1992). Cigarette smoking is also thought to be a risk factor for the development of psoriasis, although researchers do not know why this may be true (Baughman, 1993). Researchers are also not sure why cigarette smokers suffer from higher rates of cancer of the kidneys than do nonsmokers.

Researchers have uncovered a relationship between cigarette smoking and a thyroid condition known as *Graves' disease*. Although the exact relationship is unclear, researchers suspect that cigarette smoking "might be one of these environmental stimuli capable of inducing Graves' disease in genetically predisposed individuals" (Prummel & Wiersinga, 1993, p. 479). Research into how cigarette smoking contributes to the development of Graves' disease in at least some individuals is currently in progress. However, at this time, cigarette smoking appears to be one of the risk factors for this thyroid dysfunction.

Finally, evidence suggests that smoking can cause changes in the brain that may persist for many years after the individual stops smoking (Sherman, 1994). A measurable decline in mental abilities begins about 4 hours after the last cigarette, and some former smokers report that they have never felt "right" for as long as *9 years* after their last cigarette. Although there has been no research into the long-term effects of cigarette abstinence on cognitive function (Sherman, 1994), these reports are quite suggestive.

Gender-Related Complications

At least 126,000 of those who die of smoking-related illness in the United States each year are women (University of California, Berkeley, 1990c). As the number of women smokers increases, the annual death toll among women is expected to increase to about 240,000 premature deaths in women by the mid-1990s (Peto, Lopez, Boreham, Thun, & Heath, 1992). Women who smoke are at increased risk for "invasive cervical cancer, miscarriages, early menopause, and osteoporosis, among other disorders" (University of California, Berkeley, 1990c, p. 7).

Approximately 56,000 women die each year as a result of lung cancer, as compared to 46,000 women who die each year as a result of cancer of the breast (Bartecchi, MacKenzie, & Schrier, 1994). Thus, lung cancer has surpassed cancer of the breast to become the leading cause of cancer-related deaths in women in the United States.

Cigarette smoking is estimated to be the cause of between 20 and 25% (Simons, Phillips, & Coleman, 1993) and 30% (Bartecchi, MacKenzie, & Schrier, 1994) of all cases of cervical cancer. Simons, Phillips, and Coleman (1993) examined a number of women and found that DNA damage in the cells of the cervical epithelium is significantly more common in women who smoked as compared to women who have never smoked. This damage is thought to be one factor associated with the ultimate development of cervical cancer and suggests the mechanism through which cigarette smoking contributes to the development of this disease.

There is also significant evidence to suggest that cigarette smoking is associated with accelerated calcium loss in postmenopausal women. Hopper and Seeman (1994) measured bone density in pairs of female identical twins, only one of whom smoked cigarettes. They found that the twin who smoked cigarettes tended to have a greater degree of bone loss than the nonsmoking twin following menopause, although they do not identify a mechanism through which this occurs. The authors do, however, suggest that cigarette smoking contributes to greater reabsorption of bone minerals. If this theory is correct, then the authors have identified both another negative consequence of cigarette smoking for women and the means by which smoking contributes to increased bone loss in postmenopausal women smokers.

Degrees of Risk

There is a dose-related risk of premature death from cigarette smoking. Robbins, Manson, Lee, Satterfield, and Hennekens (1994) found that male physicians who smoked less than a pack of cigarettes a day still had a significantly higher risk of both ischemic and hemorrhagic stroke than did nonsmokers; male physicians who smoked more than a pack of cigarettes a day had an even higher risk of stroke. The authors concluded that *any* cigarette use was associated with a significantly higher risk of stroke.

Many smokers believe that limiting their cigarette use will reduce their risk of cancer. However, research has shown that people who smoke only 1 to 9 cigarettes a day are still *5 times as likely* to develop lung cancer as are nonsmokers (University of California, Berkeley, 1990c); for those who smoke between 10 and 19 cigarettes a day, the risk increases to 9 times as likely. As these figures make clear, "No amount of smoking is free of risk" (University of California, Berkeley, 1990c, p. 8).

Complications for the Passive Smoker

The danger of smoking-related death is not limited to the smoker alone. Researchers estimate that "passive smoking," or inhaling the smoke from the cigarettes of others (also known as "second-hand smoke") results in the deaths of an additional 50,000 people each year in the United States (American Medical Association, 1993a). Of this number, approximately 3,000 die as a result of smoking-related lung cancer (Fontham et al., 1994). The Environmental Protection Agency (EPA) estimates that "environmental tobacco smoke" causes some 300,000 cases of various forms of respiratory disease yearly (Bartecchi, MacKenzie, & Schrier, 1994). Furthermore, second-hand smoke is thought to cause 150,000 heart attacks yearly (Associated Press, 1994b). The EPA has now classified second-hand tobacco smoke as a major carcinogen.

Evidence to support that second-hand tobacco smoke should be classified as a carcinogen is found in a recent study by a team of Greek researchers. Trichopoulos et al. (1992) examined lung tissue samples from 400 recently deceased individuals from the region of Athens, Greece. They found that nonsmokers living with cigarette smokers had "possibly precancerous" (p. 1697) changes in the lung tissue similar to the type found in recently deceased cigarette smokers. In addition, Fontham et al. (1994) examined the risk factors associated with the development of lung cancer in 653 nonsmoking women with that disease. The data were compared to 1,253 control subjects who were not exposed to tobacco smoke. The authors concluded that, overall, nonsmoking women who are exposed to second-hand smoke have a 30% greater chance of developing lung cancer than do nonsmoking women who are not exposed to tobacco smoke in their environment. The authors of both studies concluded that their research had uncovered significant evidence linking environmental tobacco smoke and lung cancer. These studies raise serious questions about the impact that cigarette smoking may have on others in the smoker's environment.

Complications from Chewing Tobacco

Many former smokers and young people who are just starting to use tobacco products believe that "smokeless" tobacco, or chewing tobacco, is safer than cigarette smoking. Contrary to popular belief, the practice of chewing tobacco is quite dangerous, producing nicotine blood levels that approximate those achieved by smoking one cigarette (Gottlieb, Pope, Rickert, & Hardin, 1993). Furthermore, individuals who chew tobacco have a fourfold greater risk for developing oral cancer than do individuals who neither chew nor smoke tobacco (Kaplan, Sadock, & Grebb, 1994). Indeed, 28 different chemical compounds capable of causing the growth of tumors have been found in "smokeless" tobacco (Bartecchi, MacKenzie, & Schrier, 1994).

Although it is not clear whether tobacco chewers have the same degree of risk for coronary artery disease that cigarette smokers do, they *do* have a greater incidence of coronary artery disease than do individuals who neither chew nor smoke tobacco. Thus, whereas tobacco chewing is often viewed as "the lesser of two evils," it is certainly not without an element of risk.

Recovery from Risk

Over time, the smoker who learns to abstain from tobacco use will enjoy a reduced risk for many of the complications caused by cigarette smoking. The risk of lung cancer decreases over a period of years; by 10 to 15 years after the last use of cigarettes, former smokers have about the same risk for developing lung cancer as nonsmokers do (Lee & D'Alonzo, 1993). Lee and D'Alonzo also found that former smokers enjoy a reduced risk of coronary artery disease, with the rate for former smokers reaching the same levels as nonsmokers in 2 to 3 years for women and 5 years for men.

Other improvements in the ex-smoker's health status include a slowing of peripheral vascular disease and improved sense of taste and smell (Lee & D'Alonzo, 1993). In addition, Grover, Gray-Donald, Joseph, Abrahamowicz, and Coupal (1994) found that former cigarette smokers as a group added between 2.5 and 4.5 years to their life expectancy when they stopped smoking. They found that cessation of cigarette use is several times as powerful a force in prolonging life as is changing one's dietary habits. Finally, as a group, heart attack sufferers who subsequently stop smoking show less cardiac impairment and lower rates of reinfarction than do those who continue to smoke after having a heart attack. Thus, there are very real benefits to giving up cigarette smoking.

The Treatment of Nicotine Addiction

Cigarette smokers who continue to smoke knowing the dangers associated with this habit often say, "I can't help myself; I'm addicted." The addiction to nicotine is so powerful that 90% of those who attempt to quit smoking in any given year ultimately fail (Benowitz & Henningfield, 1994; Sherman, 1994). Although health care workers have tried for many years to identify the factors involved in a person's successful attempt to quit smoking, they have met with little success (Kenford, Fiore, Jorenby, Smith, Wetter, & Baker, 1994). Thus, cigarette cessation programs are something of a hit-or-miss affair, in which the participants have little knowledge of what *really* works.

Smoking cessation training programs usually help between 70 and 80% of the participants to stop smoking on a short-term basis; but between 50% and 75% of those who do stop smoking go on to relapse within a year (Stevens & Hollis, 1989). That is, of those who attempt to stop smoking, approximately 65% may stop for a very few

days but only 25% to 30% will be tobacco-free a year later (Jaffe, 1989). Hughes et al. (1991) found that 65% of their experimental sample relapsed within the first month of quitting, which suggests that the first month is especially difficult for the recent ex-smoker. The reason may be that, in the first 3 to 4 weeks following cessation of cigarette smoking, the individual is especially vulnerable to smoking "cues," such as being around other smokers (Bliss, Garvey, Heinold, & Hitchcock, 1989). At such times, the individual is less likely to effectively cope with the urge to smoke and is in danger of a relapse into active cigarette smoking.

Lichtenstein and Glasgow (1992) present a model for smoking cessation in which recovery is viewed as a multistage process. This model is outlined in Table 16.1. The first stage, that of *precontemplation*, is the stage of tobacco use before the individual decides to quit smoking. During this phase, the individual has occasional, vague thoughts about quitting "one of these days." Once the smoker makes a conscious decision to give up tobacco use within the next 6 months, he or she has moved into the *contemplation* phase. When the smoker actually begins the cigarette cessation program, he or she has entered the *action* phase. Finally, after the individual has been smoke-free for 6 months, he or she begins the *maintenance* phase, during which time the individual works on remaining smoke-free. This is often a difficult task, and this period of time is associated with a high relapse rate.

As noted earlier, there seems to be an association between the frequency of cigarette smoking and the difficulty of giving up tobacco use. Cohen et al. (1989) reviewed data from 10 different research projects that involved a total of 5,000 subjects who were attempting to stop smoking.

TABLE 16.1 The Stages of Smoking Cessation

Precontemplation phase	Contemplation phase	Action phase	Maintenance phase
Smoker is not considering an attempt to stop smoking. Smoker is still actively smoking.	Smoker is now seriously thinking about trying to give up smoking within the next 6 months.	Day to stop smoking is selected. The individual initiates his or her program to stop smoking.	Having been smoke-free for 6 months, ex-smoker works to remain smoke-free.

They found that light smokers, who are defined as those who smoke less than 20 cigarettes each day, are significantly more likely to be able to stop smoking on their own than are heavy smokers. They also found that the number of previous attempts to quit smoking is not an indication of hopelessness; rather, the number of unsuccessful previous attempts is unrelated to the question of whether or not the smoker will finally be able to quit. They concluded that "most people who fail a single attempt (to quit smoking) will try again and again and eventually quit" (p. 1361).

Another factor that seems to be associated with the difficulty of attempting to quit is the smoker's *expectancies* for the nicotine withdrawal process. Tate, Stanton, Green, Schmitz, Le, and Marshall (1994) formed four subgroups from their research sample of 62 cigarette smokers. As a group, those smokers who were led to believe that they would not experience any significant distress during the nicotine withdrawal process reported significantly fewer physical or emotional complaints than did the other research groups. The authors interpreted their findings as evidence that the individual's expectations may influence how the individual interprets and responds to the symptoms experienced.

Researchers now believe that smokers who want to quit require an average of three to four attempts (Prochaska, DiClemente, & Norcross, 1992) to perhaps as many as five to seven "serious attempts" (Brunton, Henningfield, & Solberg, 1994, p. 105; Sherman, 1994) before being able to stop smoking. However, these figures reflect the *average* number of attempts. Some people will be able to quit on the first or second attempt, whereas others may require nine or ten attempts before they succeed.

Individuals who wish to give up smoking should be warned that cigarette cessation is a "dynamic process" (Cohen et al., 1989, p. 1361) in which periods of abstinence are intermixed with periods of relapse. Indeed, "the return to smoking . . . occurs so frequently that it should be thought of as a part of the process of quitting and not as a failure in quitting" (Lee & D'Alonzo, 1993, p. 39). Thus, for the ex-smoker, the struggle

against cigarette smoking is a lifelong endeavor. The individual should expect to be vulnerable to relapsing back to cigarette smoking for the rest of his or her life. To help ex-smokers in their struggle, health care workers have devised a number of different pharmacological tools to be used in the battle against cigarette smoking.

Treatment Techniques

Nicotine-containing gum was introduced as an aid to cigarette cessation in the 1980s. When the gum is chewed, the nicotine is released and slowly absorbed through the soft tissues in the mouth. The manner in which nicotine-containing gum is chewed differs from "traditional" methods. The individual must adopt a "chew-park-chew-park" system of chewing the gum (Fiore et al., 1992, p. 2691).

When used properly, about 30 minutes of chewing releases approximately 90% of the nicotine in the gum, but the gum provides a lower blood level of nicotine than that achieved by cigarette smoking. Furthermore, the use of nicotine-containing gum itself may cause such side effects as sore gums, excessive salivation, nausea, anorexia, headache, and the formation of ulcers on the gums (Lee & D'Alonzo, 1993). Also, the gum cannot be used while the individual is drinking a beverage with a high acid content, such as orange juice or coffee, because the acid blocks nicotine absorption.

Researchers disagree as to the value of nicotine-containing gum in smoking cessation programs. Some researchers believe that nicotine-containing gum is helpful (although not totally effective) in controlling both the craving for cigarettes and the irritability associated with withdrawal from cigarettes (Hughes et al., 1991). Other researchers have concluded that the success rate of nicotine-containing gum is about the same as that of a placebo, suggesting that this product is of little value in cigarette cessation programs (Fiore et al., 1992).

One reason researchers have reached different conclusions is that some studies have paired the use of the gum with intensive individual or group counseling, whereas other programs have utilized the gum alone. Research has shown that the effectiveness of nicotine-containing gum varies with the intensity of the supportive counseling the individual receives (Fiore, Smith, Jorenby, & Baker, 1994). Thus, those studies that utilized nicotine-containing gum alone or with only minimal counseling support would be less likely to find any significant effect than would programs that included an intensive counseling program.

An interesting question surrounding the use of nicotine gum is the role of individual expectations on its effects. Gottlieb, Killen, Marlatt, and Taylor (1987) conducted a study in which some subjects received nicotine-containing gum and other subjects received a placebo. Subjects who believed they received nicotine-containing gum reported fewer withdrawal symptoms, even if they actually received a placebo. Thus, the authors found that the individual's expectations as to whether they received nicotine gum seemed to play a large role in moderating their withdrawal symptoms. This study raises serious questions as to the actual effectiveness of nicotine-containing gum in cigarette cessation.

Glassman et al. (1988) explored the use of the antihypertensive drug clonidine to control the craving for nicotine. This medication has been found to be of value in the control of drug-craving in narcotics withdrawal. Glassman et al. found that more than twice as many subjects who received clonidine were able to stop smoking and remain abstinent over a 4-week span than were subjects who received a placebo.

However, in another study involving clonidine, Franks, Harp, and Bell (1989) found that clonidine produced "no statistically significant effects on quitting" (p. 3013). They suggest that earlier research studies employed small samples made up of highly motivated subjects. These individuals would be more likely to report success than would a general-practice population encountered by most physicians, if only because they were quite highly motivated to quit smoking.

In 1991, several companies introduced nico-

tine-containing transdermal patches designed to supply a constant blood level of nicotine. The theory behind the patch, which is available only by prescription, is that smokers may find it easier to break the habit of smoking if they don't actually have to smoke to obtain a moderately high blood level of nicotine. A short time, usually 2 to 8 weeks, after the individual no longer engages in the physical motions of smoking, the dosage levels of nicotine in the patches are reduced, providing a gradual taper in nicotine levels.

Researchers have found the transdermal nicotine patch to be an effective adjunct to a cigarette cessation program (Fiore, Smith, Jorenby, & Baker, 1994; Fiore et al., 1992). In two studies, Fiore et al. found that, of those individuals who had used the "patch," approximately 22% to 42% were still smoke-free 6 months after treatment, whereas only 5% to 28% of those individuals who used a placebo transdermal patch were still smoke-free 6 months after treatment. Thus, use of the transdermal nicotine patch resulted in approximately twice as many successful abstainers as a placebo patch system.

The transdermal nicotine patch is not without its drawbacks. Individuals who smoke while using the nicotine transdermal patch run the risk of nicotine toxicity and possible cardiovascular problems. Also, although the transdermal nicotine patch has been shown to reduce levels of nicotine craving, it does not totally eliminate them. Many transdermal nicotine patch users reported some degree of skin irritation under the patch. Others reported abnormal or disturbing dreams, insomnia, diarrhea, and a burning sensation in the skin surrounding the patch.

Even with the transdermal nicotine patch, a significant number of smokers return to the practice of cigarette smoking. Kenford et al. (1994) looked for factors that would predict which nicotine patch users would and which would not succeed in giving up cigarette smoking. Study participants also received group counseling. The authors found that those individuals who were able to abstain from cigarette smoking during the first two weeks of treatment—and especially during the second week—were most likely to give up their cigarette use. However, 90% of those individuals who smoked during the second week of treatment while using a transdermal nicotine patch were still smoking cigarettes 6 months later.

The results of the study by Kenford et al. (1994) are consistent with earlier findings that the first month of cigarette cessation is especially difficult for the ex-smoker. The results of this study also suggest that the transdermal nicotine patch, although useful as an adjunct to cigarette cessation programs, still is not totally effective in helping smokers quit. Indeed, there is evidence that some former smokers need to use the transdermal nicotine patches for years to abstain from cigarette use (Sherman, 1994). Although these individuals will still be obtaining nicotine in their systems, they will at least not be exposing themselves to the multitude of known or suspected toxins contained in cigarette smoke.

A nasal spray that contains nicotine has been developed for use in the control of tobacco craving. An advantage of a nasal spray is that the nicotine is rapidly absorbed through the nasal membranes, and—with the exception of some sinus irritation—there are no serious side effects from this method of nicotine administration. The spray was tested by Sutherland, Stapleton, Russell, Jarvis, Hajek, Belcher, and Feyerabend (1992). In this study, one group of volunteers received a supply of nasal spray containing nicotine, whereas another group of volunteers received a placebo spray. Both groups participated in group counseling designed to help them remain smoke-free. Only two subjects had to discontinue use of the nicotine nasal spray because of adverse side effects, a reflection of the safety of this method of nicotine replacement. The results of the study showed that heavy smokers were most likely to benefit from the use of the nasal spray. Furthermore, smokers who used the spray gained less weight than did subjects who received a placebo nasal spray. After a year, 26% of the smokers who had received the nicotine containing nasal spray had remained smoke-free, whereas only 10% of the group that received the placebo were able to remain smoke-free for a year.

The nicotine nasal spray also presents its own unique set of dangers. Blood plasma levels of nicotine obtained from the spray approach those achieved from smoking. Because of this characteristic, there is concern that users may become as dependent on the nasal spray as they were on cigarettes (Benowitz, 1992). Indeed, even Sutherland et al. (1992) found that, after 6 months, the nicotine concentrations were 75% of those found in active smokers. The authors concluded that the "systemic nicotine replacement" (p. 328) achieved through the use of the nasal spray was responsible for lower levels of nicotine craving in their sample. But it may be that the smokers' dependence on tobacco was replaced with dependence on the nasal spray.

A novel approach to the problem of smoking cessation has been the use of silver acetate to produce a disulfiramlike reaction for the smoker (Hymowitz, Feuerman, Hollander, & Frances, 1993). Chewing gum and lozenges with silver acetate have been used in Europe as a smoking cessation aid for more than a decade, although this medication is not available in the United States. When an individual who has recently used such a lozenge or gum attempts to smoke, a "noxious metallic taste" is produced (Hymowitz et al., 1993, p. 113). This obnoxious taste then causes the smoker to discard the cigarette, thus replacing the nicotine-based pharmacological reward with an aversive experience.

Silver acetate is quite dangerous, and overuse may result in *permanent* discoloration of the skin and body organs; however the authors point out that this side effect of silver acetate is quite rare and is usually seen only after "massive overuse and abuse" (Hymowitz et al., 1993, p. 113). Another drawback of silver acetate is that its effectiveness in smoking cessation has not been fully tested, although preliminary studies have had promising results.

Since it was introduced in late 1986, the antianxiety medication BuSpar (buspirone, discussed in Chapter 7) has been found to be of value in smoking cessation treatment. Subjects who receive buspirone in therapeutic dosage levels report less fatigue and anxiety while going through nicotine withdrawal. Furthermore, there is no evidence of weight gain in subjects who receive buspirone for nicotine withdrawal. The biochemical mechanism through which buspirone may counter the effects of nicotine withdrawal is not known at this time (Sussman, 1994), but this medication has proved beneficial in cigarette cessation programs.

Other agents that have been utilized in the treatment of nicotine withdrawal over the years include the tricyclic antidepressants and lobeline—a drug derived from a variety of tobacco (Lee & D'Alonzo, 1993). In spite of extensive research, however, no single substance has been proved effective in treating the symptoms of nicotine withdrawal beyond any reasonable doubt.

Although there has been a great deal of emphasis on cigarette cessation programs, perhaps as many as 95% of those smokers who quit do so without participating in a formal treatment program (Brunton, Henningfield, & Solberg, 1994; Fiore et al., 1990). For those smokers who do quit, motivation to quit smoking is "critical" (Jaffe, 1989, p. 682) to the success of their efforts. These conclusions cast some doubt as to whether extensive treatment programs for tobacco dependence are necessary. Still, formal treatment programs may be of value to heavy smokers and those at risk for tobacco-related illness.

Summary

Tobacco use was first introduced to Europe by New World explorers returning home. Once the practice of smoking or chewing tobacco reached Europe, tobacco use rapidly spread. After the introduction of the cigarette around the turn of the century, smoking became more common and soon replaced tobacco chewing as the accepted method of tobacco use.

The active psychoactive agent of tobacco, nicotine, has been found to have an addiction potential similar to that of cocaine or narcotics. A significant percentage of those who are currently addicted to nicotine will attempt to stop smoking cigarettes, but will initially be unsuccessful in doing so. Current treatment methods have been unable to achieve a significant cessation rate, and more comprehensive treatment programs, patterned after alcohol addiction treatment programs, have been suggested for nicotine addiction. To date, these treatment programs have not demonstrated a significantly improved cure rate for cigarette smoking. However, these programs may be of value for those individuals whose tobacco use has placed them at risk for tobacco-related illness.

CHAPTER SEVENTEEN

The Medical Model of Addiction

In the first section of this book, Chapters 1 through 16, we examined the various drugs of abuse, their effects, and some of the consequences that may result from their abuse. This is important information for the chemical dependency or human services professional. However, knowledge of what each drug of abuse may do does not answer two very simple yet difficult questions: Why do people use these drugs? and Why do people become addicted? In this chapter, we will explore the answers to these questions from the perspective of what has come to be known as the "medical" or "disease" model of addiction.

Why Do People Use Chemicals?[1]

At first, this question may seem rather simplistic. People use drugs because they choose to do so. The drugs of abuse are part of the environment, and every day, perhaps several times a day, each of us makes a decision whether or not to use chemicals. Admittedly, for most of us, this choice is relatively simple and may not even require conscious thought. But whether we acknowledge it or not, we are continually faced with

[1]This question refers to people who use chemicals for recreational purposes, not to those people who are addicted to chemicals.

opportunities to use recreational chemicals, and we must decide whether or not to do so.

Stop for a moment and think: Where is the nearest liquor store? If you wanted to, where could you buy some marijuana? If you are over the age of about 15, the odds are very good that you could either answer each of these questions yourself, or find somebody who could. But why didn't you go out and buy any of these chemicals on your way in to work or school this morning? Why didn't you buy a recreational drug or two on your way home last night?

The answer is that you chose not to. Your decision not to use chemicals may be made without any conscious thought, but on some level you made a choice. So, in one sense, the answer to the question of why people use the drugs of abuse is because they choose to do so. But there are a number of factors that influence this decision.

The Reward Potential

The question of why a person might use alcohol or another drug of abuse is rather complex. The novice chemical user may try one or more drugs in response to peer pressure, or in anticipation of its pleasurable effects. Researchers call this the "pharmacological potential," or the "reward potential," of the chemical or chemicals being used (Meyer, 1989a). Not surprisingly, virtually all the drugs of abuse have a high reward potential (Crowley, 1988).

Stated very simply, the drugs of abuse make the user feel good. To illustrate this point, consider that cocaine's effects have been likened to that of sexual orgasm. The "rush" from intravenously administered narcotics or cocaine has been described in similar terms. Indeed, so powerful is cocaine for some users that they prefer the drug to a human lover!

One of the basic laws of behavioral psychology is that if something either increases the individual's sense of pleasure or decreases his or her discomfort, then the person is likely to repeat that behavior. Similarly, if a certain behavior increases the individual's sense of discomfort or reduces the person's sense of pleasure, he or she is unlikely to repeat that behavior. Any immediate consequence—either reward or punishment— has a stronger impact on behavior than does delayed consequence.

When these rules of behavior are applied to substance abuse, it is clear that the immediate consequences of chemical use (the immediate pleasure) have a stronger impact on behavior than the delayed consequences (possible addiction or disease at an unspecified later date). Thus, it should not be surprising to learn that many people are tempted to keep using one or more drugs of abuse because the immediate effects are pleasurable.

Social Learning

However, many people do not find the drugs of abuse immediately pleasurable. Sometimes a user must be *taught* to both recognize the drug's effects and interpret them as pleasurable. For example, first-time marijuana users must often be taught how to smoke it and how to recognize its effects. They may even need to be told why marijuana intoxication is so pleasurable (Peele, 1985; Kandel & Raveis, 1989). A similar learning process is seen with heroin users. First-time heroin users are often taught by experienced users what effects to look for and why these drug-induced feelings are so desirable (Lingeman, 1974).

A similar learning process takes place with alcohol. It is not uncommon for the first-time drinker to become so ill after a night's drinking that he or she will swear never to drink again. However, more experienced drinkers help the novice learn how to drink and how to derive pleasure from alcohol's effects. This feedback is often informal and comes from a variety of sources: a "drinking buddy," newspaper articles, advertisements, television programs, conversations with friends and co-workers, and casual observations of others who are drinking. The outcome of this social learning process is that the novice drinker is taught how to drink and how to enjoy the experience.

Individual Expectations

Another factor that influences the individual's decision whether to use recreational chemicals is the person's expectations for that drug. One's expectations have been found to strongly influence how a drug's effects are interpreted. For example, recall that Gottlieb, Killen, Marlatt, and Taylor (1987) found that individuals who *believed* they had received nicotine-containing gum, whether they actually had or not, reported few cigarette withdrawal symptoms. The critical factor was their expectations for the gum's effects.

People in Western cultures also have a number of expectations for alcohol. Brown, Goldman, Inn, and Anderson (1980) differentiate at least six different areas in which people have preconceptions about the effects of alcohol. They found that—among other things—their subjects expected alcohol to positively enhance life experiences, magnify physical and social pleasure, and increase sexual performance. The authors also found that their subjects fully expected that moderate alcohol use would increase their social aggressiveness, make them more assertive, and reduce their tension.

These individual expectations for alcohol are formed well before the first experiment with this chemical (Smith, 1994). Furthermore, the individual's expectations for alcohol take on a powerful role in shaping later drinking behavior. After the adolescent has started to experiment with alcohol, he or she modifies the initial alcohol expectations in light of personal experience. If the adolescent found alcohol's effects to be pleasurable, the stage is set for further alcohol use (Smith, 1994).

The impact of the individual's expectations on chemical use patterns is not limited to alcohol. For example, researchers have found that the individual's expectations for LSD is one of the variables that may contribute to experiencing a "bad trip." Because novice LSD users are more likely to anticipate negative consequences from the drug than more experienced users are, their anxiety seems to set the stage for a bad trip.

Individual expectations express themselves in two different ways. First, if a person's expectations about a specific drug are extremely negative, she or he will not even experiment with that chemical. For example, if you were to suggest that someone experiment with a well-known poison such as cyanide, their response would probably be something like "Are you crazy or something?"

Second, for the individual who does choose to use drugs, her or his expectations for that drug will influence how its effects are interpreted. Through formal and informal feedback mechanisms, the individual has gained knowledge about how to use a drug, what to look for, and why these effects are desirable. Using all this information as a basis, the individual evaluates his or her chemical use to decide whether it was personally rewarding.

Cultural Influences

The decision to use or not use one or more chemicals is made within the context of the culture in which a person is a member. Each culture has evolved certain attitudes and feelings that govern the use of mood-altering chemicals (Leigh, 1985). These cultural attitudes and beliefs then form the framework within which each individual's decision about chemical use is made and provide a standard by which the individual's

chemical use is measured. The cultural guidelines specify (1) which chemicals can and cannot be used, (2) what frequency of use is permitted, and (3) what sanctions will apply if these rules are violated. The social group also provides its members information about the effects of different chemicals and why the use of these chemicals is or is not desirable.

For each person, cultural influences serve as significant determinants of drug-use patterns (Peele, 1985), and they can encourage or inhibit the actual development of addiction. Peele (1985) states:

> In cultures where use of a substance is comfortable, familiar, and socially regulated both as to style of use and appropriate time and place for such use, addiction is less likely and may be practically unknown. (p. 106)

Thus, according to Peele, it is only *when a given society fails to regulate* (1) the style of chemical use, (2) the time that the chemical may be used, or (3) the place in which that chemical can be used that chemical abuse becomes a problem. It is Peele's position that the problem of substance abuse is a result of society's failure to regulate *acceptable* substance use, not its failure to *eliminate* all drug use.

The Jewish and Italian-American cultures are excellent examples of the power of social rules to govern chemical use. In both cultures, drinking is limited mainly to religious or family celebrations. Excessive drinking is strongly discouraged, and "proper" (socially acceptable) drinking behavior is modeled by adults during religious or family activities. It is no coincidence that these two groups have relatively low rates of alcoholism.

Peele (1984) notes that Chinese-American adults also model proper drinking behavior for their children. Alcohol is neither viewed as a rite of passage into adulthood nor associated with social power. In contrast, the Irish-American culture views alcohol use far more liberally; it is considered a rite of passage and is encouraged through peer pressure. For these reasons, Peele (1984, 1985) concludes that the Irish-American subculture subsequently demonstrates higher rates of alcoholism than do Chinese-Americans.

Kunitz and Levy (1974) explored the different drinking patterns of the Navaho and Hopi Indians. These cultures co-exist in the same part of the country and share similar genetic histories. However, Navaho tribal customs accept public group drinking but consider solitary drinking a mark of deviance. For the Hopi, however, drinking is more likely to be a solitary experience; alcohol use is not tolerated within the tribe, and those who drink are shunned. These two groups living in close geographic proximity, clearly demonstrate how different social groups develop different guidelines for chemical use for its members.

In some subcultures, an individual's use of chemicals is seen as a sign of maturity, and the specific drugs being abused serve as a signpost of the individual's "growth." For example, in U.S. culture, adolescents often view drinking as a sign of entry into adulthood, almost a "rite of passage" (Leigh, 1985). Within this context, it should not be surprising to learn that the adolescent peer subculture frequently encourages repeated episodes of alcohol abuse (Swaim, Oetting, Edwards, & Beauvais, 1989).

In this section, our discussion for the most part has been limited to the use of alcohol. Alcohol is the most common recreational drug used in the United States but this isn't true for every cultural group. For example, the American Indians of the Southwest frequently ingest hallucinogenic mushrooms as part of their religious ceremonies. In the Mideast, alcohol is prohibited, but hashish is an accepted recreational drug. In both cultures, strict social rules dictate when these substances can be used, the conditions under which they can be used, and the penalties for unacceptable substance use.

The point to remember is that each culture provides its members guidance about what is acceptable or unacceptable substance use. But within each culture, there are various subgroups that may adopt the parent culture's standards only to a limited degree. For example, one social group may strictly prohibit the use of alcohol,

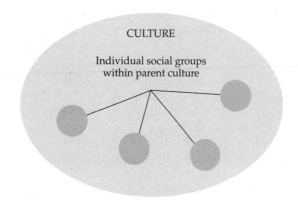

FIGURE 17.1 The relationship between individual social groups and the parent culture

another may permit alcohol use only on religious holidays, and a third may allow the rare social use of alcohol. Other social groups may utilize alcohol freely but limit the allowable level and frequency of intoxication.

Thus, even within a single culture, there will be social groups that have different standards than those of the parent culture. The relationship between different social groups and the parent culture is illustrated in Figure 17.1.

Social Feedback Mechanisms

However, there is a subtle, often overlooked, feedback mechanism that exists between the individual and his or her social group. Although an individual's behavior is shaped, at least in part, by the larger social group, individuals also help shape the behavioral expectations of the social group by choosing whom to associate with. Alcoholics (and other drug users) tend to drift toward social groups where their drinking is at least tolerated, if not actively encouraged; at the same time, addicts avoid social groups where drug use is discouraged.

Kandel and Raveis (1989) found that one important predictor of whether or not an individual would use cocaine was whether she or he had friends who also used cocaine. They also found that a given individual's cocaine use pattern was extremely similar to that of his or her friends.

Those individuals who use cocaine tend to associate with others who also use cocaine; those who avoid cocaine tend to associate with other nonusers.

In another study, Simpson, Crandall, Savage, and Pava-Krueger (1981) found that, before participation in a substance abuse treatment program, 60% of their sample of narcotics addicts spent "a lot" (p. 38) of time engaged in "street" leisure activities. Such recreational activities center on behaviors involving other addicted individuals. After the completion of treatment, only 13% of the sample continued to associate with active narcotics addicts.

Once an individual is aware of the social guidelines regarding chemical use, he or she is then faced with a choice. One option is to adopt the standards of the larger social group and associate with others who do the same. However, if the cultural standards are inconsistent with personal values and choices, the individual can seek a different social group that endorses his or her beliefs.

In terms of drug use, the individual who has tried chemicals and found them physically and psychologically rewarding must then evaluate whether there are social rewards for the drug use or social sanctions against it. If there are social rewards and the user has found the drug experience rewarding, the individual is likely to use that chemical again. If there are social sanctions against the use of that chemical, then the individual must decide how important the use of that drug is compared to membership in the social group. Then the individual must either find a way to reconcile further use of that drug while remaining in the same social group or find a social group that permits continued drug use.

Although most people do not think in these exact terms, their thinking is similar. For example, many people, if questioned, would admit to being "closet" drug users. Such people go to great trouble to hide their use of alcohol or other recreational chemicals from neighbors and friends. The person who sneaks around the neighborhood hiding empty alcohol bottles in the neighbors' trash cans is attempting to recon-

cile personal use of alcohol with social expectations. Too many empty alcohol bottles in one's own trash might lead to unpleasant questions or suspicions; it is better to hide the evidence than run the risk of discovery.

There are also those who would, if closely questioned, admit to having experimented with one or more drugs of abuse. But these individuals would also admit that, although they found the drug's effects pleasurable, they decided that further use of that drug was not possible given their social status, and they stopped using that drug. For example, many people who used marijuana and hallucinogenics during the "hippie" era of the late 1960s and early 1970s would refer to their drug use as a "phase that I was going through," that later seemed inconsistent with their growing maturity.

Unfortunately, some people find that a chemical's effects are desirable enough to encourage further abuse despite social sanctions against its use. In the service of their drug use, they drift toward social groups that encourage and support the drug use.

Personal Life Goals

Another factor that influences an individual's decision to begin or continue using chemicals is whether or not the drug use is consistent with personal long-term goals or values. This is rarely a problem with socially approved drugs such as alcohol and, to a smaller degree, tobacco. But, consider the example of a junior executive who has just won a much hoped-for promotion, only to find that the new division has a strong "no smoking" policy.

The executive may decide that giving up smoking is part of the price to pay for the promotion, and then proceed to quit smoking. In such a case, the individual has evaluated to what degree further use of tobacco is consistent with the life goal of a successful career.

However, the individual may elect to search for a new position rather than accept the restriction on smoking. In this case, the individual has decided that the cost of giving up cigarettes is

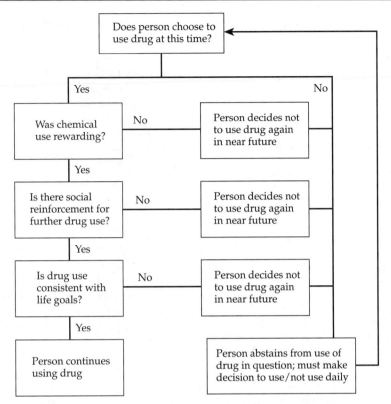

FIGURE 17.2 The chemical use decision-making process

greater than the benefits of the promotion. Just as in these hypothetical examples, people must evaluate whether or not the use of a recreational drug is consistent with their own long-term goals before making a decision to continue its use.

In summary, all the factors discussed have been found to play a role in a given individual's decision to begin to use alcohol or other drugs. A flowchart of the decision-making process is shown in Figure 17.2. However, we are discussing the individual's decision to use alcohol or drugs on a recreational basis. The factors that *initiate* chemical use are not the same factors that *maintain* chemical use (Zucker & Gomberg, 1986). Although a person may begin to use recreational chemicals for one reason, over time other forces develop that reinforce the use of these chemicals. For example, a person may

begin to use narcotic analgesics because they help him or her deal with painful memories. However, after becoming physically addicted to the narcotics, the fear of withdrawal may be a reason to continue using the drugs.

Why Do People Become Addicted to Chemicals?

No one really knows why people become addicted to drugs. Although many competing theories seem to have some validity in certain situations, a comprehensive theory of addiction has yet to be discovered. It *is* known, however, that many people experiment with recreational chemicals, and a percentage of them will become addicted.

The American Psychiatric Association's *Diagnostic and Statistical Manual of Mental Disorders,*

4th edition (or *DSM-IV*) (1994) identifies the following criteria that identify someone as addicted to recreational chemicals.

1. Preoccupation with use of the chemical between periods of use.
2. Using more of the chemical than had been anticipated.
3. The development of tolerance to the chemical in question.
4. A characteristic withdrawal syndrome from the chemical.
5. Use of the chemical to avoid or control withdrawal symptoms.
6. Repeated efforts to cut back or stop the drug use.
7. Intoxication at inappropriate times (such as at work), or when withdrawal interferes with daily functioning (such as when hangover makes person too sick to go to work).
8. A reduction in social, occupational or recreational activities in favor of further substance use.
9. Chemical use continues in spite of the individual having suffered social, emotional, or physical problems related to drug use.

Any combination of four or more of these signs identifies the individual as suffering from the "disease" of addiction. The "disease model" of substance abuse, or the "medical model" as it is also known, holds that (1) addiction is a medical disorder, just as cardiovascular disease or a hernia is; (2) there is a biological predisposition toward addiction; and (3) the disease of addiction is progressive.

The medical model of addiction may be the most difficult aspect of drug abuse to write about. Depending on which theory one is reading, virtually every one of the factors that influences recreational chemical use reviewed in this chapter has been suggested as "the" cause of drug abuse. Although substance abuse professionals often speak of the disease model of addiction, there is no single, universally accepted model. Rather, there is a group of loosely allied researchers who believe that drug addiction is the outcome of a biomedical or psychobiological

process, and so chemical dependency should be classified as a "disease."

But the disease model of chemical dependency has not been universally accepted. There are those who argue with equal fervor that alcohol and drug addiction fit the criteria for a "disease" about as well as the proverbial square peg in the round hole. It has even been suggested that the issue of whether or not addiction is a true "disease" is nothing more than a "turf battle" between the mental health and the medical professions (Goodwin & Warnock, 1991, p. 485).

At present, however, the treatment of chemical addiction in the United States is considered to fall within the realm of medicine. In this section, we will discuss the disease model of addiction and examine some of the research that proponents believe supports their belief that the compulsive use of chemicals is a true "disease."

Jellinek's Model of Alcoholism

The work of E. M. Jellinek (1952, 1960) has had a profound impact on the evolution of the medical model of addiction. Jellinek concentrated on the prototypical addiction—alcoholism. Before the American Medical Association's decision to classify alcoholism as a formal "disease" in 1956, alcoholism was viewed as a moral disorder. Alcoholics were viewed as immoral individuals both by society at large and by the majority of physicians.

Like others before him, Jellinek (1952, 1960) argued that alcoholism is actually a disease, like cancer or pneumonia. Certain characteristics of the disease, according to Jellinek, include (a) the loss of control over one's drinking, (b) a specific progression of symptoms, and (c) if left untreated, the end result of death.

In an early work on alcoholism, Jellinek (1952) suggested that addiction to alcohol progresses through four different stages. The first of these stages, which he called the *prealcoholic phase*, is marked by the individual's use of alcohol for relief from social tensions. In the prealcoholic

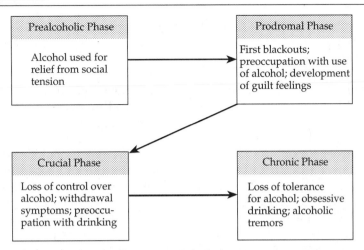

FIGURE 17.3 The four stages of alcoholism

stage, the roots of the individual's loss of control are evident. The individual no longer drinks only on a social basis but has started to drink for relief from stress and anxiety.

As the individual uses more and more alcohol, he or she enters the second phase of alcoholism, the *prodromal phase.* This second stage is marked by the development of memory blackouts, secret drinking (also known as hidden drinking), a preoccupation with alcohol use, and the individual's guilt over his or her behavior while intoxicated.

With the continued use of alcohol, the individual eventually becomes physically dependent on alcohol, a hallmark of the *crucial phase.* Other symptoms of this third stage of drinking are a loss of self-esteem, a loss of control over one's drinking, social withdrawal in favor of alcohol use, self-pity, and a neglect of proper nutrition. During this phase, the individual attempts to reassert his or her control over alcohol by entering into short periods of abstinence, only to return to the use of alcohol.

Finally, continued alcohol use leads the alcoholic into the *chronic phase.* The symptoms of the chronic phase include a deterioration in one's morals, drinking with social inferiors, the development of motor tremors, an obsession with drinking, and—for some—the use of "substitutes" when alcohol is not available (such as

rubbing alcohol). A graphic representation of these four stages of alcoholism is shown in Figure 17.3.

In 1960, Jellinek presented a theoretical model of alcoholism that was both an extension and a revision of his earlier work. According to this model, the alcoholic is unable to consistently predict in advance how much he or she will drink at any given time. Like other diseases, alcoholism has specific symptoms that include the physical, social, vocational, and emotional complications often experienced by the compulsive drinker (Jellinek, 1960). As before, Jellinek claims that alcoholism has a progressive course that, if not arrested, ultimately results in the individual's death.

However, in his 1960 model, Jellinek went further than he had previously by attempting to classify different patterns of addictive drinking. As Dr. William Carpenter had in 1850, Jellinek viewed alcoholism as a disease that could be expressed in a number of different forms, or styles, of drinking (Lender, 1981). Unlike Dr. Carpenter, who thought that there were three types of alcoholics, Jellinek identified five subforms of alcoholism. Jellinek used the first five letters of the Greek alphabet to identify the most common forms of alcoholism, although he also admitted that other subtypes of alcoholism were possible in different parts of the world. Thus, although Jellinek's model was culture-specific, it allowed for the possibility of forms of alcohol use other than those found in the United States.

The first of Jellinek's (1960) subtypes of alcoholics is the *alpha* drinker, who is psychologically dependent on alcohol but does not suffer from any of the physical complications caused by chronic alcohol use. According to Jellinek, alpha drinkers can abstain from alcohol use for short periods of time, but only if necessary. An example of the alpha drinker might be the businessman who "needs" a martini or two before dinner to unwind from the day's troubles.

As noted above, Jellinek (1960) did not view the alpha drinker as physically dependent on alcohol. Furthermore, Jellinek did not believe that the alpha pattern of drinking is automatically progressive. Indeed, he believed this drinking pattern is quite stable for an extended period of time, as in the case of a businessman who has two (and only two!) martinis after work every day for fifteen years.

If the alpha drinking pattern were to escalate into another form of alcoholism, Jellinek believed it would evolve into what he termed the *gamma* form of alcoholism. The gamma pattern of alcoholism will be discussed in more detail later, but the point to remember here is that Jellinek (1960) viewed the alpha form of alcoholism as relatively stable, only rarely progressing to more serious forms of alcohol use.

Jellinek (1960) also classified some drinkers as *beta* alcoholics. The beta drinking pattern is very similar to the alpha pattern of drinking, but the beta drinker has developed physical complications in addition to the psychological dependency on alcohol. The beta alcoholic may demonstrate medical symptoms of chronic alcohol use, such as alcoholic gastritis and cirrhosis of the liver, both of which develop only after extended periods of alcohol use. If the beta alcoholic progressed, it would also be to the gamma form of drinking, according to Jellinek.

The *delta* alcoholic demonstrates physical dependence on alcohol, including alcohol tolerance, "craving" when he or she cannot drink, and a loss of control over alcohol. But the delta

alcoholic would show few or no physical complications that could be traced to alcohol use. In contrast, the gamma alcoholic has physical withdrawal symptoms, alcohol "craving," physical dependence on alcohol, and various medical complications caused by alcohol use. The gamma alcoholic also demonstrates a progressive loss of control over alcohol use, according to Jellinek (1960). As noted before, both the alpha and, less frequently, beta patterns could progress to the gamma pattern of alcohol use over time.

Finally, the *epsilon* alcoholic may best be classified as the "binge" drinker. This form of alcoholism is least frequently encountered in the United States, according to Jellinek (1960), where the alpha and the gamma drinking patterns are most common. Jellinek mentioned other cultural-related patterns of drinking (such as "fiesta drinking") that are worthy of study, but may not be true forms of alcoholism.

Jellinek's (1960) model of alcoholism offers a number of advantages to physicians. First, it provides a diagnostic framework within which physicians can classify different patterns of drinking. This is in contrast to the restrictive dichotomous view in which the patient is either alcoholic or not. Second, prior to Jellinek's (1960) work, alcoholism was viewed as a moral weakness. His model of alcoholism as a physical disease made it worthy of study and of "unprejudiced access" (Vaillant, 1990, p. 5) to medical treatment.

Since Jellinek (1960) proposed his model of alcoholism, several research studies have attempted to determine the model's validity. For example, Schuckit, Smith, Anthenelli, and Irwin (1993) examined the drinking patterns of 636 males hospitalized for alcoholism. The authors found that, although there was remarkable variation in the specific problems encountered by the subjects, there was clear evidence of a progression in the severity of alcohol-related problems. Furthermore, by their late twenties, just under 75% of the sample had started to engage in morning alcohol use and experience alcohol-related job problems. By their mid-thirties, many of the men in the study started to experience alcohol-related health problems. On the basis of their study, Schuckit et al. concluded that, although the specific symptoms encountered were different than those reported by Jellinek (1960), there was evidence of "a general progression of alcohol-related life problems" as a result of chronic alcohol use (p. 790, italics in original omitted). Thus, this study supports Jellinek's theory that alcoholism is a progressive disorder that results in more serious complications over time.

Although Jellinek's (1952, 1960) model was introduced as only a theoretical model of alcoholism, it has become the standard model for alcoholism in the United States. Jellinek's model has also been used without significant modification since the time that it was introduced. Although developed as a theory for alcoholism, this model has also been applied to virtually every other pattern of drug abuse. Yet, as we will discuss in Chapter 18, there are serious flaws in the Jellinek model.

The Genetic Inheritance Theories

In the years that have passed since Jellinek's work, researchers have started to explore the genetics of alcoholism and other forms of drug addiction. Researchers have long been aware that alcoholism seems to run in families. But it has only been in the past 50 years that researchers have had the tools necessary to explore the genetics of alcoholism. Proponents of the disease model of addiction often point to these studies as evidence that alcoholism (and, by extension, the other forms of addiction) are actually biomedical disorders.

One of the most extensive research studies exploring the genetics of alcoholism was conducted by Cloninger, Gohman, and Sigvardsson (1981). They used adoption records of some 3,000 individuals from Sweden, where extensive records are kept on all parties in adoption cases. The researchers found that children of alcoholic parents were likely to grow up to be alcoholic themselves, even in cases where the children were reared by nonalcoholic adoptive parents almost from birth.

The authors also found that the children who grew up to be alcoholic essentially fell into two groups. The first subgroup was made up of children of alcoholics who themselves developed alcohol-use disorders. During young adulthood, these individuals drank in moderation, but later in life their drinking progressed to the point where they could be classified as alcoholic. Even so, Cloninger, Gohman, and Sigvardsson found that these individuals generally functioned well within society and only rarely demonstrated antisocial behaviors. These individuals have come to be known as "Type 1" alcoholics (Goodwin & Warnock, 1991).

Cloninger, Gohman, and Sigvardsson (1981) also found a strong environmental impact on this group. For example, for children of alcoholic parents who were adopted in infancy by a middle-class family, the probability of becoming alcoholic in adulthood was no greater than chance. Although this risk is still markedly higher than what one finds in the general population, it is still lower than the risk for children of alcoholics who are raised by poor parents; the chances are greater that these children will grow up to be alcoholics. These findings suggest a strong environmental influence on the evolution of alcoholism despite genetic inheritance.

According to Cloninger, Gohman, and Sigvardsson, the second, smaller group of alcoholics were more violent alcoholics and were all males. These individuals, who are now known as "Type 2" alcoholics (Goodwin & Warnock, 1991), tended to be involved in criminal behaviors. A male child born to a "violent" alcoholic ran almost a 20% chance of himself becoming alcoholic, no matter what the social status of the adoptive parents. This suggests a strong genetic influence for this subgroup of alcoholics.

Over the past 50 years, a virtual flood of research has appeared in which various theories have proposed that alcoholics (or other addicts) are somehow different than nonaddicts. The range of this research is far too extensive to discuss in this chapter, but the general theme of this pool of research is that alcoholics metabolize alcohol differently and at different sites than nonalcoholics do, and that alcoholics react differently than nonalcoholics do to the effects of the drug.

The general thrust of these research articles is that there is a biological difference between the alcoholic and nonalcoholic. Blum et al., (1990) explored the possibility that a specific gene, known as the *dopamine D2 receptor gene,* was involved in the predisposition toward alcoholism.

Dopamine is one of the neurotransmitters affected by alcohol, and researchers have identified two different subtypes of receptors in the brain that respond to dopamine—the D_1 and D_2 receptors. Blum et al. examined samples of brain tissue from 70 cadavers for their research, half of which were from known alcoholics, and half from nonalcoholics. The authors found that 77% of the alcoholics but only 28% of the nonalcoholics possessed the dopamine D_2 receptor gene. This discovery suggests to Blum et al. that there is a genetic basis for alcohol use.

In an extension of the original research, Noble, Blum, Ritchie, Montgomery, and Sheridan (1991) compared tissue samples from the brains of 33 known alcoholics and a matched group of 33 nonalcoholic controls. On the basis of their "blind" study of the genetic makeup of the tissue samples,[2] the authors concluded that there is strong evidence of a genetic foundation for severe alcoholism involving the D_2 dopamine receptor. As we will discuss in Chapter 18, however, these studies have been challenged by other researchers.

Marc Schuckit (1994) took a different approach to try to identify biological predictors to alcoholism. In the 1980s, he tested 227 men and found that 40% of the sons of alcoholics but only 10% of the sons of nonalcoholics were "low responders" to a standard dose of alcohol. "Low responders" are those who are not as strongly affected by the alcohol as are individuals in the control group. Ten years later, the author con-

tacted 223 of the original sample of men who were raised by alcoholic parents. Of the men who had an abnormally small response to the initial alcohol challenge test, 56% had become alcoholic. Of the men who did not demonstrate an abnormally low physiological response when originally tested, only 14% had become alcoholic. Schuckit suggests that an abnormally low response to a moderate dose of alcohol may indicate that the individual is relatively insensitive to the effects of alcohol, which in turn may contribute to a tendency to drink more often and to consume more alcohol per session.

As we will discuss in the next chapter, although this study does seem to reveal some significant differences between those who do and those who do not become alcoholic, it still does not provide a final answer to the question of what biochemical factors predict the later development of alcoholism. Current clinical research hints that such a difference does exist, but no *unequivocal* biochemical or biophysical difference has been identified.

The Personality Predisposition Theories

Many researchers believe that substance abuse can be traced back to the individual's personality or to some form of psychological defect within the person. Indeed, many researchers have come to believe that there are personality patterns that predict subsequent chemical use. To the psychoanalytic therapist, addiction is "the behavioral manifestation of psychic imbalance arising from frustration, deprivation and emotional pain" (Smith, 1990, p. 62). This definition is consistent with the work of Karen Horney (1964), who views substance abuse as a reflection of emotional pain. According to Horney, the individual attempts to "narcotize" (p. 45) anxiety experienced through the use of chemicals. Khantzian (1985) suggests that some people are drawn to the narcotics because these drugs help control internal feelings of rage and aggression. Others seem to be drawn to cocaine in their attempt to

[2]In a "blind" research study, the data are examined, without knowing whether any given piece of data is from the research sample or from the control sample.

relieve feelings of depression (Kandel & Raveis, 1989).

Certainly, there is evidence to suggest that individuals who abuse chemicals have suffered significant psychological trauma in their lives. Estimates of those female alcoholics who had either been neglected or sexually abused range from 40% to 70% (Coleman, 1988b). Fossum and Mason (1986) report an even higher figure, noting that in some adolescent chemical dependency treatment centers 75% of their female clients report having been sexually abused. Clinical evidence also strongly suggests that sexual or physical abuse by parents or significant others can leave deep emotional scars on a child. In adult life, these battered children may turn to drugs to help them deal with the emotional pain of having been physically, emotionally, and/or sexually abused (Kaufman, 1989).

Bradshaw (1988a) proposes that *all* compulsive behavior, including the compulsive use of chemicals, reflects the individual's attempt to escape the shame experienced in the family of origin. In response to the shame and pain of growing up in his family, Bradshaw (1988a) states, "I felt sane only when I was drunk" (p. 89). However, when people compulsively use one—and only one—method of escaping from the experience of shame, they become addicted to that system of control. Furthermore, the control of psychological pain through any form of compulsive behavior is effective for only a short period of time. Although "compulsive behaviors may help us temporarily avoid feelings or problems, they don't really stop the pain" (Beattie, 1989, p. 14). Eventually, the individual is faced with the problem of how to cope with this pain time and time again.

In a series of research projects attempting to identify a preexisting "alcoholic personality" (Hoffman, Loper, & Kammeier, 1974; Loper, Kammeier, & Hoffman, 1973), researchers examined the Minnesota Multiphasic Personality Inventory (MMPI) profiles of 38 males who had taken the MMPI while they were students in college. These scores were then compared with MMPI profiles obtained from these same individuals, after their admission to a chemical dependency treatment program. The profiles did reveal a tendency toward impulsive behavior but did not reveal any other sign of significant pathology. In spite of these findings, the authors concluded that there do exist personality patterns that predate the development of alcoholism and that can be measured by such personality instruments as the MMPI.

When Weiss, Mirin, Griffin, and Michael (1988) explored the psychiatric diagnosis of 149 cocaine abusers admitted to a private hospital from 1982 to 1986, they found a shift in the personality types of those abusing cocaine. They discovered that cocaine abusers were less likely to have mood disorders but were more likely to suffer from personality disorders, especially the antisocial personality disorder. Weiss et al. concluded that current cocaine users are unlikely to be attempting to self-medicate depressive feelings—as may have been true in the late 1970s and early 1980s—and that current cocaine users are more likely to have a personality disorder than were cocaine users in the past two decades.

Franklin (1987) also believes that there is a psychological predisposition toward narcotics abuse. Perhaps, the author suggests, the addict suffers from an ongoing depressive disorder that predisposes him or her to use narcotics. Furthermore, before the individual began to use narcotics, the feelings of depression may have been accepted as a normal emotional state. After being introduced to drugs, however, the individual may discover that distress is not "normal" and that there is a chemical escape from the continuous emotional pain. The narcotics provide the individual with at least the illusion of control over the depression the individual has known throughout life. However, the illusion of "control" ultimately comes to dominate the individual's life, and the person becomes addicted to narcotics.

Alcohol is occasionally utilized in an attempt to self-medicate depression. However, as we discussed in Chapter 4, research suggests that a primary depressive disorder is found in only a minority of the cases of chronic alcohol dependence.

The research into whether there exist certain personality characteristics that predispose one toward alcoholism or other forms of chemical abuse is quite suggestive. There do appear to be certain personality traits associated with chemical use or dependency. However, it is difficult to determine whether these personality traits precede the development of the drug dependency or are a result of frequent chemical use. To date, no clearly identified causal factor has been found, and research into possible personality factors that may predispose one toward alcohol or substance abuse continues.

Summary

The "medical" or "disease" model of addiction has come to play an important role in the treatment of substance abuse in the United States. Based on the work of E. M. Jellinek, the "disease" model of alcoholism has come to be applied to virtually every other form of substance abuse as well. Jellinek viewed alcoholism as a progressive disorder, with specific stages. Contrary to popular opinion at the time, Jellinek suggested that the alcoholic was not a social failure but someone who suffered from a disease that would, if not treated, result in his or her death. In time, the field of medicine came to accept this new viewpoint, and alcoholism came to be viewed as a medical disorder.

Since the early work of Jellinek, other researchers have attempted to identify a specific biophysical dysfunction that forms the basis for the addictive disorders. Most recently, drawing on medicine's growing understanding of human genetics, scientists have attempted to identify the genetic basis for alcoholism and the other forms of drug addiction. However, to date, the exact biochemical or genetic factors that predisposes one to become addicted have not been identified.

Are People Predestined to Become Addicts?

Over the past century, researchers approached the problem of alcohol and substance abuse from a number of different perspectives. As we discussed in the last chapter, some believe that individuals who abuse chemicals do so because of a biological or personality predisposition. As such, these theories are often said to reflect a "disease" model of chemical abuse. The individual is thought to abuse alcohol or drugs because of a personality or genetic flaw beyond their control. In a sense, the individual is viewed as predestined to abuse chemicals by his or her biological or psychological heritage.

The second school of thought maintains that there are no biological or personality traits that predispose an individual to abuse chemicals; rather, much of what we believe to be true about substance abuse is based on the false assumption that addiction is a "disease." In this chapter, some of the reactions against the "disease" model of substance abuse will be examined.

Challenges to the Disease Model of Addiction

The concept of "disease" is viewed from the framework of medicine as practiced in the United States. There are often subtle (and sometimes not so subtle) philosophical differences between how the medical community in the United States views disease and how disease is viewed in other parts of the world. Thus, to understand illness, one needs to understand the diagnostic system—the "yardstick," so to speak—by which disease is measured.

Within the framework of U.S. medical practice, one component of a "disease" is that it has a biophysical foundation. In infectious diseases, this is the bacterium, virus, or fungus that invades the host organism. Another class of diseases are those that are caused by a genetic disorder, which results in the abnormal growth or functioning of an organism. In a third class of diseases, the optimum function of the organism is disrupted by acquired trauma. In each case, however, the disease process disrupts the optimal functioning of an organism in one way or another.

As noted in previous chapters, some believe that there is a genetic "loading" for alcoholism, although the exact nature of predisposition has not been clearly identified (Goodwin & Warnock, 1991). The case for a genetic predisposition to other forms of addiction is even weaker. But, it is argued, if one assumes that a genetic predisposition exists for alcoholism, such a predisposition must exist for all forms of addiction. If it is true that there is a genetic predisposition for addictive behaviors, then substance abuse can be said to be a "disease." However, there are those who challenge the medical model of the addictions.

Reaction to the Jellinek Model

As we discussed in Chapter 17, the "Jellinek" model has become *the* model of the addictions. However, in the 30 years since the model was first advanced, a number of flaws have come to light. First, Jellinek based his work on surveys that were mailed out to members of Alcoholics Anonymous; but of the many hundreds of surveys mailed out, only 98 responses were received. Thus, although Jellinek received a response from only a minority of those individuals contacted, it was on this data that he based his comprehensive theory of alcoholism.

As we will discuss in the chapter on AA, members of this organization are self-selected, and there is little evidence that members of AA are representative of alcoholics in general. Furthermore, Jellinek assumed that those individuals who responded to his survey did not differ from those who failed to return the questionnaire. However, the two groups are different in at least one significant characteristic: one group agreed to participate in the study whereas the other did not. If there is one major difference between groups, there may be other significant differences as well. Still, Jellinek built a model of alcoholism for all alcoholics generalized from his limited sample. Since its introduction, his model has been used as the basis for planning treatment programs for untold thousands of alcoholics who have entered treatment.

The Jellinek model also failed to take into account that drinking patterns often change over time (Vaillant, 1983). Even Schuckit et al. (1993), who concluded on the basis of their research that there was a progression in the severity of alcohol-related problems over time for the chronic drinker, acknowledged that alcoholics tend to alternate between periods of abusive and nonabusive drinking. Thus, the steady, heavy drinker may, in response to internal or external pressure, cut back to the occasional social use of alcohol. Similarly, the rare social drinker may, in a period of stress, drink to excess day after day for a period of time and then return to a pattern of only occasional alcohol use.

Jellinek's (1960) theory that alcoholism is a progressive disorder has become gospel for many substance abuse counselors and has been elaborated on in endless counseling sessions. Indeed, for many years, it was part of the foundation on which the medical model of alcoholism rested. Yet researchers disagree as to whether alcoholism is *automatically* progressive (Skog & Duckert, 1993). At best, the progression of alcohol-related symptoms suggested by Jellinek is found in only a minority (25% to 30%) of cases (Toneatto, Sobell, Sobell, & Leo, 1991). The Joint Committee of the National Council on Alcoholism and Drug Dependence as much as admitted this in its current definition of alcoholism, which states that alcoholism is "often [but not automatically] progressive" (Morse & Flavin, 1992, p. 1013).

Jellinek's theory also assumes that alcoholics have lost control over their drinking, but research has failed to corroborate this characteristic (Skog & Duckert, 1993). Rather, research suggests that alcoholics tend to regulate their drinking to achieve a desired emotional state (Peele, 1989). At best, the alcoholic may demonstrate *inconsistent* control over his or her drinking, and at different times the alcoholic consumes different amounts of alcohol (Toneatto et al., 1991; Vaillant, 1990). But there is no evidence to support the concept of loss of control as suggested by the Jellinek model.

To be fair, Jellinek (1960) did not claim his model was the perfect theory of alcoholism. Rather, he presented it as a preliminary theory of a hitherto unrecognized disease. Nevertheless, and in spite of its flaws, the Jellinek model has become "virtually gospel in the field of alcohol studies" (Lender, 1981, p. 25) and in the treatment of other forms of drug addiction. Certainly, Jellinek (1960) did not intend his model to be applied to forms of chemical dependency other than alcoholism. Thus, one of the cornerstones of the medical model of addiction appears to be seriously flawed; but it is on this flawed foundation that many current treatment techniques are based.

The Genetic Inheritance Theories

As we have seen, several studies have suggested a possible genetic predisposition toward addiction. However, in spite of continued research, the nature and impact of this genetic loading remain unclear. For example, Cloninger, Gohman, and Sigvardsson's (1981) work (see Chapter 17) is often used by proponents of the medical model to support the contention that there is a biological predisposition for alcoholism. Although the original intent of their investigation was to explore the genetics of alcoholism, the authors were surprised to find evidence suggesting a strong environmental impact as well. They discovered that even in cases where the child's genetic inheritance seems to predispose that child to alcoholism, if that child is adopted by a middle-class family in infancy, his or her chances of actually being alcoholic in adulthood are no greater than chance. However, if the child is adopted into a poor family, the chances are greater that this child will grow up to be an alcoholic. These findings suggest a strong environmental influence on the evolution of alcoholism, in spite of an individual's genetic inheritance for "Type 1" alcoholism.

Type 1 alcoholism, also called *milieu-limited alcoholism,* was the most common form of alcoholism Cloninger, Gohman, and Sigvardsson encountered. The "typical" Type 1 alcoholic, who could be either male or female, engaged in non-problematic alcohol use until around the age of 25. In the average case, the individual did not begin to drink to excess until after the age of 25. Furthermore, even when the individual's drinking became a problem, it was often not recognized and usually went untreated (Cloninger, Gohman, & Sigvardsson, 1981).

The second, smaller group of alcoholics found by Cloninger, Gohman, and Sigvardsson were the more violent alcoholics and were often involved in criminal behaviors. Alcoholics in this group, who are generally all male, were classi-

fied as "Type 2" alcoholics. This subgroup is often called *male-limited alcoholism.* The adopted male offspring of a "violent" alcoholic ran almost a 20% chance of himself becoming alcoholic, regardless of the social status of the adoptive parents.

However, here again the statistics are misleading. For, although almost 20% of the male children born to a "violent alcoholic" themselves become alcoholic, more than 80% do not follow this pattern. This suggests that additional factors, such as environmental forces, may play a role in the evolution of alcoholism for Type 2 alcoholics.

Murray, Clifford, and Gurling (1983) compared identical and fraternal twins on the assumption that identical twins, who are by definition genetically the same, would demonstrate different rates of alcoholism than the fraternal twins. However, the authors failed to find such an anticipated similarity, casting doubt on the hypothesis that alcoholism is purely a genetically mediated disorder.

Pickens, Svikis, McGue, Lykken, Heston, and Clayton (1991) attempted to isolate the impact of genetic inheritance on the development of alcoholism for pairs of both male and female twins. They concluded that "the influence of genetic factors appears to be somewhat weaker than the influence of shared environmental factors, especially for female subjects" (p. 25). However, this conclusion was contradicted by Kender, Heath, Neale, Kessler, and Eves (1992), who examined the drinking patterns of over 1,000 pairs of female twins and reached several conclusions.

First, the authors concluded that environmental influences are indeed a significant factor in the development of alcoholism in women, and these environmental factors account for 40% to 50% of the inheritability of alcoholism. However, what is equally important, the authors concluded that 50% to 60% of the liability for the development of alcoholism in the women studied was the result of genetic inheritance. The authors thus concluded that genetic inheritance is a major factor in the development of alcoholism. Current research thus suggests that both a biological predisposition toward alcoholism and environmental factors are involved in the development of alcohol use patterns. However, researchers have yet to determine the exact role that each plays in the evolution of addictive alcohol use. At this time, about all that can be said is that in the case of identical twins, where one twin is alcoholic, the concordance rate for alcoholism in both twins is only 58% (Schuckit, 1987).

These findings are suggestive. If alcoholism were mediated only by the individual's genetic inheritance, then you would expect that identical twins would have a concordance rate of nearly 100%, since they are the same genetically. Clearly, while there is a possible genetic component to alcoholism, there is also evidence that environmental factors play a strong role in its development. Schuckit (1987) suggests that some of these environmental factors include an unstable home environment in the early years, a father with a relatively low-status occupation, and an extended neonatal hospital stay for the infant who would later grow up to become an alcoholic. However, this remains only a theory.

The Dopamine D$_2$ Connection

In Chapter 17, we discussed the theory that a specific gene, which controls the development of the dopamine D$_2$ receptor within the brain, is a cause of alcoholism (Blum et al., 1990; Noble, Blum, Ritchie, Montgomery, & Sheridan, 1991). This line of research, while suggestive of a possible biological foundation for alcoholism, has not been supported by subsequent research (Bolos, Dean, Lucas-Derse, Ramsburg, Brown, & Goldman, 1991; Parsian & Cloninger, 1991).

For example, Bolos et al. (1991) used a different, more extensive methodology than did Blum et al. (1990), subtyping their subjects according to the age of onset of alcoholism, severity of alcoholism, whether or not the subject qualified for a diagnosis of antisocial personality disorder, and family history. The authors concluded that there was no evidence of a "widespread association between the D$_2$ receptor gene and alcoholism" (p. 3160).

Parsian et al. (1991) also explored the genetics of alcoholism and concluded that no "specific gene influencing the risk or expression of alcoholism has been identified" (p. 655), although they admit that several possible biological factors were uncovered. After an extensive research project that is far too complicated to discuss in detail in this text, Parsian et al. concluded that their results "cast doubt on the D$_2$ receptor locus having a major and direct causative role in most cases of alcoholism" (p. 662). In other words, their results suggest that the D$_2$ dopamine receptor gene is not the biological foundation for alcoholism.

Uhl, Persico, and Smith (1992) reviewed the current literature on the D$_2$ dopamine receptor gene and its possible association with alcoholism. They concluded that although this line of research seems to identify at least one genetic factor for alcoholism, the existing research studies failed to utilize a random sample of alcohol users and control subjects. Thus, it is possible that differences in the genetic makeup of various ethnic groups—or some other, undiscovered, variable—might result in the apparent association between the D$_2$ dopamine receptor gene and alcoholism.

Even if the dopamine D$_2$ connection does play some role in the biochemistry of addiction,

> [k]nowing that drug dependence has a neurochemical basis does not tell us why some people but not others use drugs regularly and heavily, why they use them in some circumstances and not others, and why different people prefer different drugs. (*Harvard Medical School Mental Health Letter*, 1992a, p. 2)

Further research into the role of the D$_2$ receptor gene and the genetics of alcoholism itself continues. At present, the theory that the D$_2$ receptor gene plays a role in the development of alcoholism has been challenged by Gelernter, Goldman, and Risch (1993), who concluded that "Based on all we know about the genetics of alcoholism, it would seem that a single gene is unlikely to be in itself responsible for a large proportion of illness" (p. 1673). But that is exactly what proponents of the dopamine D_2 theory were looking for: a single gene that could account for alcoholism. Although Helernter, Goldman, and Risch acknowledge that the initial studies were suggestive, each of the earlier studies that had discovered a relationship between the dopamine D_2 receptor gene and alcoholism was flawed in some way.

In Chapter 17, we briefly reviewed the results of Schuckit's (1994) study in which he reexamined 223 men that he had tested a decade earlier. At the time of his first test, he found that 40% of the men who had been raised by alcoholic parents but only 10% of the control group demonstrated an abnormally low physical response to a standard dose of an alcoholic beverage. A decade later, 56% of the men who had the abnormally low physiological response to alcohol had progressed to the point of alcoholism . However, in Schuckit's study, only a minority of the men who had been raised by an alcoholic parent demonstrated an abnormally low physiological response to the alcohol challenge test. Thus, Schuckit's figures[1] suggest that only 91 of the experimental group of 227 men had this abnormal response. Furthermore, a full decade later, only 56% of these 91 men (or just 62 men of the original sample of 227 men) had progressed to alcoholism. So although Schuckit's (1994) study suggests possible biochemical mechanisms through which alcoholism might develop, Schuckit does not seem to have identified the biochemical basis for alcohol dependence.

Other Challenges to the Disease Model of Addiction

No matter how you look at it, addiction remains a very curious "disease." Even Vaillant (1983), who has long been a champion of the disease model of alcoholism, concedes that, to make alcoholism fit into the disease model, it had to be "shoehorned" in (p. 4). Furthermore, even if al-

coholism is a disease, "both its etiology and its treatment are largely social" (Vaillant, 1983, p. 4).

Rodgers (1994) has even suggested the possibility that what we call "addictions" are actually a misapplication of existing neurobiological reward systems. According to this view, evolution allowed for the development of a "reward system" in animals to reinforce behaviors that contribute to survival, such as eating, reproducing, and drinking water. Unfortunately, this reward system is sometimes fooled by chemicals like alcohol, opiates, and cocaine into operating when these survival-centered activities are not in progress. This reward is not intentional, according to this view. Rather, by coincidence, some substances happen to be able to trigger the reward system in human brains, just as, by coincidence, some chemicals happen to be poisonous. Thus, "The inescapable fact is that nature gave us the ability to become hooked because the brain has clearly evolved a reward system, just as it has a pain system" (S. Childers, as quoted in Rodgers, 1994, p. 34). In other words, we all hold the potential to become addicted because we are all biologically "wired" with a reward system. However, at this point, we do not understand the exact reason why some people are more easily trapped by this reward system than are others.

The concept of addiction simply does not fit easily into the medical model. Dreger (1986) comments that alcoholism is a rather unusual "disease," in that drinking is "promoted by every Madison Avenue technique and by every type of peer pressure one can imagine. No other disease is thus promoted" (p. 322). Dreger raises an interesting point: If addiction is indeed a disease, why is the use of the offending agent, in this case alcohol, promoted through commercial means?

Individual Responsibility

Modern medicine "always gives the credit to the disease rather than the person" (B. Siegel, 1989, p. 12), and this is certainly true for the addictive disorders (Peele, 1989; Tavris, 1990). For example, Pratt (1990) suggests that "Activation of the disease of addiction, once an individual is ex-

[1]The data provided in Schuckit's (1994) study were used to calculate these figures. Where necessary, the figures were rounded off.

posed to activating agents, is genetically prede-termined" (p. 18). From this perspective, once the individual has been exposed to the "activating agents," he or she ceases to exist except as a genetically preprogrammed disease process! This is another, rather extreme, example of the medical model's tendency to credit the disease rather than the person.

Dole and Nyswander (1965) contend that even a single dose of narcotics forever changes the brain structure of the narcotics addict, making him or her crave further narcotics use (Dole, 1988). In fact, the whole concept on which methadone maintenance is based is the belief that narcotics are so powerful that just a single dose takes away all of the individual's power of self-determination. If narcotics are so incredibly powerful then one must account for the thousands of patients who receive doses of narcotics for extended periods of time to control pain without developing a "craving" for narcotics. Furthermore, patients who receive even massive doses of narcotic analgesics for the control of pain do not report a sense of euphoria (Rodgers, 1994). And many individuals "chip" (occasionally use) narcotics for years, without ever becoming addicted to these drugs. This seems to cast some doubt on Dole and Nyswander's theory that exposure to narcotic analgesics causes changes in the brain that predispose an individual to use these chemicals again.

Another example of the manner in which the medical model devalues the individual's power is Blum and Payne's (1991) contention that alcohol causes an "irresistible craving" (p. 237). Yet, alcoholics readily agree that they can resist the craving for alcohol if the reward for doing so is high enough. Many alcoholics successfully resist the desire to drink for weeks, months, years, or even decades, casting doubt on the concept of an "irresistible" craving for alcohol.

Although relapses occur, it seems that it is not so much a matter of "irresistible craving" that causes a return to chemicals as it is a combination of other factors. Indeed, Rodgers (1994) suggests that, for some addicts, the rush they feel when

they return to the substance use can only be felt after first going through withdrawal.

Once a person has been diagnosed as having a certain disease, he or she is expected to take certain steps toward recovery. According to the medical model, the "proper way to do this is through following the advice of experts (e.g., doctors) in solving the problem" (Maisto & Connors, 1988, p. 425). Unfortunately, as we noted in Chapter 1, physicians are not required to be trained in either the identification or the treatment of addiction. The medical model of addiction thus lacks internal consistency. Although medicine claims that addiction is a "disease," it does not routinely train its practitioners in how to treat this ailment.

Problems in Defining the Addictive Disorders

At this point, there is no standard definition of what constitutes an addiction. The most common form of chemical dependency, alcoholism, has been called simply a "bad habit" (Szasz, 1972, p. 84), and addiction itself has been described as "a bad habit that is especially difficult to change" (*Harvard Medical School Mental Health Letter*, 1992b, p. 2). Admittedly, it is up to the individual to try to overcome bad habits, but this does not make them "diseases"; "if we choose to call bad habits 'diseases', there is no limit to what we may define as a disease" (Szasz, 1972, p. 84). Twenty years after Szasz's warning, Leo (1990) confirms that "As addictions have been converted into diseases (alcoholism), bad habits have been upgraded and transformed into addictions (yesterday's hard-to-break smoking habit is today's nicotine addiction)" (p. 16).

Leo contends that the outcome of this transformation has been the birth of a multitude of "pseudo ailments" (p. 16) through which people have been able to avoid responsibility for a variety of socially unacceptable behaviors. Indeed, so pervasive has this process become that Leo calls the current era the "golden age of exoneration" (p. 16). As Ehrenreich (1992) observes, one of the benefits of modern medicine is that although we may not "have a cure for every disease, alas, there's no reason we can't have a disease for every cure" (p. 88).

Once the treatment industry established itself, other "diseases" were discovered for which AA's twelve-step model could be applied. The twelve-step model has now been adapted for more than 100 different conditions that are believed (at least by some people) to be forms of addiction (*Harvard Medical School Mental Health Letter*, 1992b). But many believe that drug abuse is a "mythical disease" (Szasz, 1988, p. 319), and they question whether there isn't a better way of dealing with drug abuse.

Thomas Szasz (1988) argued that, essentially, drugs have no inherent value. It does not matter whether the specific drug in question is a natural agent, like morphine, or the product of human ingenuity, like fentanyl. According to Szasz, by themselves, drugs are neither good nor bad. It is the way in which the drugs are used that determines their value. In his essay, Szasz (1988) suggests that society has made an arbitrary decision to classify some drugs as "dangerous" and others as acceptable for social use. Yet the bases for these decisions are not scientific studies but "religious or political (ritual, social) considerations" (p. 316). Szasz further charges that the current "war" on drugs is really a "war on human desire" (p. 322). The problem is not so much that people use chemicals, but that people desire to use them for personal pleasure.

The Unique Nature of Addictive Disorders

In spite of all of the studies that have been conducted over the years, researchers continue to overlook a very important fact. Unlike other diseases, drug abuse and addiction require the active participation of the "victim." As Savage (1993) observes, the capacity for addiction rests with the individual, not (as so many would have us believe) with the drug itself. The addictive disorders do not force themselves on the individual in the same sense that an infection might. Alcohol or drugs do not magically appear in the

individual's bloodstream. Rather, the "victim" of addiction must go through several steps to introduce the chemical into his or her body.

Consider the case of heroin addiction. The addict must first obtain the money necessary to buy the drug. Next he or she must find somebody who is selling heroin and then actually buy some for use. The "victim" must then prepare the heroin for injection (mixing the powder with water, heating the mixture, pouring it into a syringe), find a vein to inject the drug into, and then insert the needle into the vein. Finally, after all these steps, the individual must actively inject the heroin into his or her body.

This is a rather complicated chain of events, each of which involves the active participation of someone who is then said to be a "victim" of a disease process. If it took as much time and energy to catch a cold, pneumonia, or cancer, it is doubtful that any of us would ever be sick a day in our lives!

Another, indirect, challenge to the disease model of alcoholism comes from Viktor Frankl (1978), a psychiatrist interested in psychosis. Psychosis is another disorder in which there appears to be a strong genetic component, as is the case with drug addiction. Frankl (1978) describes psychosis as

> a matter of the bodily system's biochemistry. However, what the patient makes of his psychosis is entirely the property of his human personality. The psychosis that afflicts him is biochemical, but how he reacts to it, what he invests in it, the content with which he fills it—all this is his personal creation, the human work into which he has molded his suffering. (p. 60)

Thus, in Frankl's opinion, the individual retains responsibility and the power of choice in the face of a genetically influenced disorder.

The same might be said of chemical addiction. Evidence suggests a possible biological predisposition toward alcoholism, a "matter of the bodily system's biochemistry," in Frankl's (1978) words. However, the individual's reaction to the addiction, what he or she invests in the addiction, how he or she fills the addictive void within, are all the personal creation of the addict. Thus, the individual retains responsibility for personal behavior, even if he or she has a "disease" such as addiction (Vaillant, 1983, 1990).

In the past 50 years, proponents of the medical model of alcoholism have attempted to identify the biological foundation for abusive drinking. Over the years, there has been a virtual flood of research articles, many of which have announced that the authors of one study or another have found that alcoholics either seem to metabolize alcohol differently than nonalcoholics or seem to be relatively insensitive (or, depending on the research study, more sensitive) to the effects of alcohol as compared to nonalcoholics. Proponents of the medical model of addiction often point to these studies as evidence of a biological predisposition toward alcoholism.

However, despite the fact that it is more than a decade old, Nathan's (1980) observation continues to ring true for researchers in the field of addiction: "no differences have been found in the rate of metabolism, route of metabolism, site of metabolism, or susceptibility to the effects of drugs, between people who become addicts and those who do not" (p. 243). Thus, at this point, the disease model of addiction as it now stands does not appear to provide the ultimate answer to the question of why people become addicted to drugs of abuse.

The Disease Model as Theory

Treadway (1990) suggests that the disease model can provide "a useful metaphor or refrain for many clients" (p. 42) to help them understand their compulsion. But he warns that mental health professionals become rather "uncomfortable when it is presented as scientific fact." But proponents of the disease model of addiction tend to speak of it not as a theoretical model but as an established fact. Furthermore, proponents of the disease model defend it from *all* criticism. Indeed, many seem to have adopted a "cultlike" philosophy, in which those who disagree with

the disease model are viewed as unenlightened savages. It is not uncommon for those who question the disease model to be met with comments such as "If you really understood alcoholism, you would see that it is a disease," or "Obviously, you do not really understand alcoholism."

An unfortunate tendency within science is that, once a certain theoretical viewpoint has become established, proponents of that position work to protect that theory from both internal and external criticism (Astrachan & Tischler, 1984). This process can clearly be seen in the disease model of addiction. In the current atmosphere, legitimate debate over strengths and weaknesses of the different models of addiction is discouraged. There is only one "true" path to enlightenment, according to proponents of the disease model, and its wisdom should not be questioned.

The tendency for proponents of the disease model to turn a deaf ear to other viewpoints is exacerbated by the fact that the disease model has become "big politics and big business" in the United States (Fingarette, 1988, p. 64). This model of addiction has formed the basis of a massive "treatment" industry into which many billions of dollars and thousands of years of labor have been invested. Thus, the medical model has taken on a life of its own.

What is surprising is not that the disease model exists but that it has become so politically successful. The treatment methods currently in use for addiction have not changed significantly in 40 years (Rodgers, 1994). Imagine the uproar that would result if a physician were found using the technology of 40 years ago to treat a disorder such as cancer or cardiovascular disease. Yet, in the field of substance abuse treatment, treatment methods have remained static for the past two generations.

There is also strong evidence that current treatment methods for the addictions are possibly less effective than doing nothing at all (Peele, 1989). Even such a strong proponent of the medical model as the psychiatrist George Vaillant (1983) concludes that there is no significant difference in "recovery" rates between those who are treated for alcoholism and those who are not. A number of other studies have reached similar conclusions. However, proponents of the medical model are hardly likely to go to insurance companies or the public and admit they were wrong or that their methods do not work. Rather, as Peele (1989) points out, when the treatment of an addictive disorder is unsuccessful, the blame is put on the patient. He or she "did not want to quit" or "was still in denial" or any of a thousand other excuses. But the blame is never placed on the "disease" model, despite all the evidence that it has not been successful in the treatment of the addictive disorders.

Summary of the Reaction to the Disease Model of Addiction

A welcome breath of fresh air is offered by the chief of the Molecular Neurobiology Laboratory of the National Institute on Drug Abuse, Dr. George Uhl (Uhl, Persico, & Smith, 1992), who suggests that addiction rests on a foundation of 30% genetic predisposition and 70% environmental factors. He suggests that, even when the genetic predisposition is present, if the environment does not support drug use addiction would not occur. Unfortunately, many researchers in the field of addiction continue to claim that chemical abuse and addiction are exclusively brought about by either environmental factors or biological predisposition.

Although the data currently available seem to point to a biological factor to substance abuse, researchers have not been able to identify the specific environmental factor, nutritional deficit, or genetic pattern that brings about addiction. In their summary of the current state of the research on a biological predisposition, Goodwin and Warnock (1991) state that, although alcoholism is known to run in certain families, "We do not believe that alcoholism definitely has been shown to be genetic" (p. 485). Similarly, the University of California at Berkeley (1990d) concluded that, in spite of significant efforts to identify a personality or biological predisposition toward addiction, "there's no proof that

anyone is chemically, genetically or psychologically doomed" (p. 2). Even if there is a genetic basis for alcoholism, Crabbe and Goldman (1993) contend that "there is little likelihood of finding a single gene that determines whether a person will be alcoholic or not"; indeed, "the most important genes related to alcoholism may be those that interact—each exerting small, less distinct influences" (p. 302) on the evolution of behavior. Even then, the authors suggest, various environmental forces also play a role in shaping the individual's behavior.

Thus, although the disease model of chemical dependency has dominated the treatment of substance abuse in the United States, it is not without its critics. Not surprisingly, in light of this criticism, the medical model of addiction has not found wide acceptance outside the United States and (to a lesser degree), Canada.

Personality Predisposition Theories of Addiction

Personality factors have long been thought to play a role in the development of addiction (Butcher, 1988; Jenike, 1991). There are a number of variations on this "predisposing personality" theme. For example, Tarter (1988) notes that the personality characteristics of the antisocial personality disorder and certain neurotic traits may increase the risk of subsequent addiction. Along these same lines, Jenike (1989) identifies a history of antisocial behavior as one factor that predicted whether U.S. American servicemen who had used opiates while in Vietnam would continue using narcotics after returning home.

The predisposing personality position is strongly deterministic and seeks to find factors that may predict a vulnerability toward addiction. However, such theoretical models do not allow for more than a general statement that such personality characteristics might increase the long-term risk that a person will become addicted.

In Chapter 17, we discussed a series of research projects that tried to identify a preexisting "alcoholic personality" (Hoffman, Loper, & Kammeier, 1974; Loper, Kammeier, & Hoffman, 1973) by comparing the MMPI profiles of 38 known males who had taken the MMPI while they were in college to their MMPI profiles following admission to a chemical dependency treatment program. Recall that the authors concluded that the profiles did reveal a tendency toward impulsive behavior on the part of the students but failed to reveal any other sign of significant pathology. Still, the authors concluded that there are personality patterns that predate the development of alcoholism that can be measured by such personality instruments as the MMPI.

What these researchers did not attempt to answer, however, was how many students who displayed the predisposing characteristics when they took the MMPI in college never subsequently became addicted to chemicals. Thus, it is not known whether the personality patterns found by the authors were a significant indicator of future addiction for the majority of the alcoholics studied, or only a pattern that was, by coincidence, common to those who were addicted to alcohol.

In spite of a spirited search for the so-called "alcoholic personality" that has gone on for the past 50 years, such a personality pattern remains elusive at best (Schuckit, Klein, Twitchell, & Smith, 1994; Miller & Kurtz, 1994). But the belief persists that (1) alcoholics are developmentally immature, (2) the experience of growing up in a disturbed family helps shape the personality growth of the future alcoholic, and (3) alcoholics tend to overuse ego defense mechanisms such as denial. Despite the lack of evidence supporting these beliefs, much of what is called "treatment" in the United States is based on these assumptions.

How did the myth of the "alcoholic personality" evolve? Nathan (1988) postulates that the characteristics of the so-called "addictive personality" found by earlier researchers may reflect a misdiagnosis, a confusion of the antisocial personality disorder with a prealcoholic person-

ality pattern. Admittedly there is a distinct tendency for those diagnosed as having an antisocial personality disorder (APD) to utilize chemicals (Schuckit et al., 1994). Indeed, it has been suggested that substance abuse may be an unrecognized aspect of the APD (Peele, 1989) because society tends to separate antisocial behavior from chemical use. For example,

> [t]hose arrested for drunk driving frequently also have arrest records for traffic violations when they aren't drunk. . . . In other words, people who get drunk and go out on the road are frequently the same people who drive recklessly when they're sober. (Peele, 1989, p. 154. Italics in original omitted)

However, in U.S. society, as soon as an individual commits a criminal act while under the influence of chemicals, that person's behavior is viewed as being controlled by the chemical, no matter what that individual might have done when not under the influence of drugs.

As we will discuss in Chapter 27, "The Process of Intervention," the line between where the addictive disorders end and where the personality disorders begin has become blurred. In part, this is because the so-called "alcoholic personality" shares many behavioral traits with the personality disorders, especially the antisocial personality disorder.[2]

Bean-Bayog (1988) considered the available evidence and postulated that the so-called "alcoholic personality" is a result of the impact of chronic alcoholism on the personality pattern, not a precondition of the addiction. Thus, the alcoholic personality characteristics are a result of the disease process, not a contributing factor to the development of the disease.

According to Bean-Bayog (1988), much of the research conducted to date on identified addicts has been based on the mistaken assumption that the personality characteristics precede the addiction when in fact they are part of the addictive

[2]However, as Schuckit et al. (1994) point out, alcoholism and antisocial personality disorder are two separate disorders.

process. It would be as if researchers had thought for years that the pain of a broken leg caused the injury to the bone, rather than that the pain was a signal of a broken limb.

Thus, there is little conclusive evidence that there exist personality characteristics that predispose the individual to addiction. However, the study of the whole area of personality growth and development—not to mention the study of those forces that initially shape and later maintain addiction—is still so poorly defined that we cannot resolve this issue with certainty.

The Misuse of the Medical Model

Unfortunately, the disease model of alcoholism has been misused, or "misapplied," to the point where "Judges, legislators, and bureaucrats . . . can now with clear consciences get the intractable social problems caused by heavy drinkers off their agenda by compelling or persuading these unmanageable people to go elsewhere—that is, to get 'treatment'" (Fingarette, 1988, p. 66).

Indeed, it has been suggested that the "war on drugs" that began in the early 1980s evolved as a politically inspired program to control those individuals who were defined by conservative Republicans as social deviants (Humphreys & Rappaport, 1993). According to Humphreys and Rappaport, the war on drugs essentially served the Reagan administration as a "way to redefine American social control policies in order to further political aims" (p. 896). They claim that, by shifting the emphasis of social control away from the community mental health center movement and toward the war on drugs, justification was also found for a rapid and possibly radical expansion of the government's police powers and the use of military force in foreign countries (such as the invasion of Panama).

This disturbing article raises serious questions as to the degree to which the social problem of chemical abuse and the medical model of addiction were used as an excuse to further a political party's agenda. Certainly, the problem

of drivers who operate motor vehicles while intoxicated presents a very real problem of social deviance. However, one must question the wisdom of sending the chronic offender to "treatment" time and time again when his or her acts warrant incarceration. As Peele (1989) has argued, incarceration may help bring about a greater behavior change in these people than would repeated exposure to short-term treatment programs.

In an ideal world, we would know when treatment should be offered as an alternative to incarceration, and when incarceration should be imposed on the chronic offender. Unfortunately, all too often, the courts fail to consider this issue before sending the offender to "treatment" once more.

The Final Common Pathway Theory of Addiction

As should be evident by now, there have been strong challenges to the medical model of substance abuse. In their review of the genetics of alcoholism, Crabbe and Goldman (1993) conclude that "there are many factors associated with whether a person becomes an alcoholic, one of which is genetics" (p. 297, italics in original omitted). At the same time, the psychosocial models of drug use have also been challenged as being too narrow in scope, and unable to account for the phenomenon of drug addiction.

But there is another viewpoint to consider, one called the *final common pathway* theory of chemical dependency. The final common pathway is a nontheory in the sense that this view of addiction is not supported by any single group or profession. The final common pathway theory holds that there is an element of truth in all the theories of drug addiction, but none alone is able to account for the phenomenon of drug abuse.

From the final common pathway perspective, addiction is the endpoint, not the starting point, a unique pattern of growth. The "causes" of an addictive disorder vary from individual to individual, and may include social forces, psychological conditioning, an attempt to come to terms with internal pain, a spiritual shortcoming, or some combination of other factors. The proponents of this position admit that there may be a genetic predisposition toward substance abuse, but they are also willing to accept that there may not be.

In the final analysis, the final common pathway model of addiction views alcoholism as a common endpoint that can be reached by any number of different paths. In one case, environmental forces may predispose the individual toward substance abuse; in another case, environmental forces may actually serve to reduce the individual's risk of becoming addicted to chemicals (Crabbe & Goldman, 1993). Rather than view alcoholism (and, by extension, the other forms of drug addiction) as simply the result of genetic forces, the professional must develop a comprehensive overview of the patient to answer the question, What caused this individual to become addicted to chemicals?

This, then, is the core element of addiction according to the final common pathway theory of addiction: addiction is the common endpoint for each individual who suffers from the compulsion to use chemicals. To treat the addiction, the chemical dependency counselor must identify the forces that both brought about and continue to support the individual's addiction to chemicals. With this understanding, the chemical dependency counselor can establish a treatment program that will help the individual achieve and maintain sobriety.

Summary

Although the medical model of drug dependency has dominated the treatment industry in the United States, this model is not without its critics. For each study that purports to identify a biophysical basis for alcoholism or other forms of addiction, there are other studies that fail to document such a difference. For each study that claims to have isolated personality characteristics that seem to predispose one toward addiction, there are other studies that either fail to assign these characteristics predictive value or find that the characteristic in question is a result of the addiction, not a precursor to it.

It was suggested that the medical model of addiction is a metaphor through which people may better understand their problem behavior. However, the medical model of addiction is a theoretical model—one that has not been proved, and one that does not easily fit into the concept of "disease" as the U.S. medical community understands the term. Indeed, it has been suggested that drugs themselves are valueless; it is the use to which people put the chemicals that determines whether they are good or bad.

Addiction as a Disease of the Human Spirit

To some, addiction is a disease of the "spirit." The concept of alcoholism as a spiritual disorder forms the basis of the Alcoholics Anonymous program (Miller & Kurtz, 1994). From this perspective, understanding the reality of addiction is ultimately to understand something of human nature. Unfortunately, modern society, especially Western medicine, tends to disparage matters of the spirit. When the subject is brought up, the "enlightened" person turns away as if embarrassed by the need to discuss something so primitive.

The word "spirit" is derived from the Latin *spiritus,* which means the divine living force within each of us. In us, life is aware of itself as apart from nature (Fromm, 1956). However, with this "self-awareness" comes the painful understanding that each of us is forever isolated from our fellow humankind. Fromm considers this awareness of our basic isolation as comparable to being in an "unbearable prison" (1956, p. 7), in which are found the roots of anxiety and shame. "The awareness of human separation," wrote Fromm, "without reunion by love—is the source of shame. It is at the same time the source of guilt and anxiety" (p. 8).

A flower, bird, or tree cannot help but be what its nature ordains: a flower, bird, or tree. A bird does not think about being a bird or what kind of a bird it might become. The tree does not think about "being" a tree. Each behaves according to its nature to become a specific kind of bird or tree. But humans possess the twin gifts of self-awareness and self-determination. We may, within certain limits, be aware of ourselves and decide our fate. These gifts, however, carry a price. Fromm (1956, 1968) viewed the awareness of our fundamental aloneness as the price that we have to pay for the power of self-determination. In gaining self-awareness, we have come to know loneliness. It is only through the giving of "self" to another through love that Fromm (1956, 1968) envisions us able to transcend this isolation to become part of a greater whole.

Merton (1978) holds a similar view of the nature of human existence. Merton clearly understands that one cannot seek happiness through the compulsive use of chemicals; "there can never be happiness in compulsion" (1978, p. 3). Rather, happiness can be achieved through love shared openly and honestly with others. Martin Buber (1970) takes an even more extreme view, holding that it is only through our relationships that our life has definition. Each person stands "in relation" to another, and the degree of relation—the relationship—is defined by how much of the "self" one offers to another and is received in return.

At this point, you may question what relevance this material has to a text on chemical dependency. The answer is found in the observation that the early members of Alcoholics

Anonymous came to view alcoholism (and, by extension, the other forms of addiction) as a "disease" not only of the body but also of the spirit. In so doing, they transformed themselves from helpless victims of alcoholism into active participants in the healing process of sobriety.

Out of this struggle, the early members of Alcoholics Anonymous came to share an intimate knowledge of the nature of addiction. They came to view addiction not as a phenomenon to be dispassionately studied but as an elusive enemy that held each member's life in its hands. The early members of AA struggled not to find the smallest common element that might "cause" addiction but to understand and share in the healing process of sobriety. In so doing, the early pioneers of AA came to understand that recovery is a spiritual process through which the individual recovers the spiritual unity that cannot be found through chemicals.

Self-help groups such as Alcoholics Anonymous and Narcotics Anonymous[1] do not postulate any specific theory of how chemical addiction comes about. As Herman (1988) notes, unlike either medical or mental health professionals, "12-Step programs do not dwell on the causes of addiction" (p. 52). Rather, any person whose chemical use interferes with his or her life is assumed to have an addiction problem. To AA's founders, the need to attend AA was self-evident; either you were addicted to alcohol or you were not.

Addiction itself was viewed as a spiritual flaw. The drugs do not bring about addiction; the individual comes to abuse or be addicted to drugs because of what he or she believes and holds to be important (Peele, 1989). Such spiritual flaws are not uncommon and usually pass unnoticed in the average person. But for the addict, his or her spiritual foundation is such that chemical use is deemed acceptable, appropriate, and desirable.

According to Peele (1989), this spiritual flaw

is expressed in people's tendency to try to escape responsibility for their lives. Personal suffering is, in a sense, a way of owning responsibility for one's life and an inescapable fact of life. If we are alive, we will encounter problems and suffering. But some of us

> will go to quite extraordinary lengths to avoid our problems and the suffering they cause, proceeding far afield from all that is clearly good and sensible in order to find an easy way out, building the most elaborate fantasies in which to live, sometimes to the total exclusion of reality. (Peck, 1978, p. 17)

In this the addict is not unique, for it is often difficult to accept the pain and suffering that life offers to us. We all must come to terms with personal responsibility and with the pain of our existence. But the addict chooses a different path from the average person's. Addiction can be viewed as an outcome of a process through which the individual comes to utilize chemicals to avoid recognition and acceptance of life's problems. The chemicals come to lead the individual away from the problems of daily life in return for the promise of comfort and relief.

Diseases of the Mind, Diseases of the Spirit: The Mind/Body Question

As B. Siegel (1986) and many others have observed, modern medicine has come to enforce an artificial dichotomy between the individual's "mind" and "body." As a result of this dichotomy, modern medicine has become rather mechanical, with the physician treating "symptoms" or "diseases" rather than the patient as a whole (Cousins, 1989; B. Siegel, 1989).

In a sense, the modern physician can be said to be a very highly skilled technician who often fails to appreciate the unique person who is now in the role of a patient. Diseases of the body are viewed as within the realm of physical medicine, whereas diseases of the mind fall in the province of the psychological sciences. Diseases of the human spirit, according to this view, are the specialty of clergy (Reiser, 1984).

---

[1] Although there are many similarities between AA and NA, these are separate programs. On occasion, they may cooperate on certain matters, but each is independent of the other.

The problem is that the patient is not exclusively a "spiritual being" or a "psychosocial being" or a "physical being" but is a unified whole. Thus, when a person abuses chemicals, the drugs affect that person "physically, emotionally, socially, and spiritually" (Adams, 1988, p. 20). Unfortunately, society has difficulty accepting that a disease of the spirit, such as addiction, is just as real as a disease of the physical body.

But humans are spiritual beings, and self-help programs such as AA and NA view addiction to chemicals as a spiritual illness. Their success in helping people achieve and maintain sobriety suggests that there is some validity to this claim. However, society still adheres to the artificial mind/body dichotomy, struggling to come to terms with the disease of addiction, which is neither totally a physical illness nor exclusively one of the mind.

The Growth of Addiction: The Circle Narrows

In speaking of the role of alcohol in the alcoholic's life, Brown (1985) notes that, as the disease of alcoholism progresses, the alcoholic comes to center his or her life around the use of the chemical. Indeed, alcohol may be viewed as the "axis" (Brown, 1985, p. 79) around which the alcoholic's life revolves. Alcohol comes to assume a role of "central importance" (p. 78) both for the alcoholic and the alcoholic's family. Peele (1989) argues that one reason alcohol or drugs is able to assume a role of central importance in the individual's life is because the person's value system tolerates chemical use as an acceptable behavior.

It is difficult for those who have never been addicted to chemicals to understand the importance addicts attach to their drug of choice. The addicted person is preoccupied with chemical use and will protect his or her source of chemicals. It is not uncommon for cocaine addicts to admit that, if forced to choose, they would choose cocaine over friends, lovers, or even family.

The grim truth is that the active addict is, in a sense, morally insane. The drug has come to take on a role of central importance in the addict's life over other people and other commitments. Addicts, in a very real sense "never seem to outgrow the self-centeredness of the child" (*The Triangle of Self-Obsession*, 1983, p. 1). As stated in the book *Narcotics Anonymous* (1982),

> Before coming to the fellowship of N.A., we could not manage our own lives. We could not live and enjoy life as other people do. We had to have something different and we thought we found it in drugs. We placed their use ahead of the welfare of our families, our wives, husbands, and our children. We had to have drugs at all costs. (p. 11, italics in original omitted)

Kaufmann, in his elegant introduction to Buber's (1970) text, spoke of those whose all-consuming interest is themselves. They care of nothing outside of that little portion of the universe known as "self." In this sense, chemical addiction might be viewed as a form of self-love, or perhaps as a perversion of self-love. It is through the use of chemicals that people seek to cheat themselves of the experience of reality, replacing it with the distorted desires of the "self."

It is difficult for the nonaddicted person to understand the importance the addicted person attaches to further drug use. To say that the addict demonstrates an ongoing preoccupation with chemical use is something of an understatement. The addicted person may also demonstrate an exaggerated concern about maintaining a supply of the drug and may avoid those who might prevent further drug use. For example, an alcoholic who, with six or seven cases of beer in storage in the basement, goes out to buy six more cases "just in case" is clearly preoccupied with maintaining an "adequate" supply.

Addicts tend to view other people —when their existence is recognized at all—as either aids or impediments to their own drug use. Nothing is allowed to come between the individual and his or her drug. It is for this reason that recovering addicts speak of their still addicted counterparts as morally insane.

The Circle of Addiction: The Addict's Priorities

The authors of *Narcotics Anonymous* conclude that addiction is a disease composed of three elements: (1) a compulsive use of chemicals, (2) an obsession with further chemical use, and (3) a total self-centeredness on the part of the individual. It is this total self-centeredness—the spiritual illness that causes the person to demand "what I want when I want it!"—that makes the individual vulnerable to addiction.

As the disease of addiction progresses, the individual comes to center his or her life around continued use of the chemical. But for the addict to admit this obsession would be to accept the reality of personal addiction. So, people who are addicted to chemicals begin to use the defense mechanisms of denial, rationalization, projection and/or minimization to justify their increasingly narrow range of interests both to themselves and to significant others.

To support his or her addiction, the individual must renounce more and more of the "self" in favor of new beliefs and behaviors that make it possible to continue to use chemicals. This is the spiritual illness of addiction, as the individual comes to believe that "nothing should come between me and my drug use!" No price is too high nor any behavior unthinkable if it allows for further drug use. This, as Peele (1989) points out, is a value judgment the individual makes.

As the economic, personal, and social cost of continued drug use mount, the individual often lies, cheats, and steals to maintain the addiction. Addicted persons have been known to sell prized possessions, steal money from trust accounts, misdirect medications prescribed for patients, and deny their feelings for family members, all to continue their drug use.

Some addicts examine the cost demanded of their drug use and turn away from chemicals,

with or without formal treatment. But others accept the cost willingly. Many addicts go to great pains to hide the evidence of their drug addiction; more than one "hidden" alcoholic has ultimately confessed to "taking the dog for a walk" at night to hide empty bottles in neighbor's trash cans. Addicts have been known to hide drug supplies under rocks in the countryside, behind books in the living room, under the sink in the kitchen, behind the headboard of the bed, and in a multitude of other places, all to maintain the illusion that they are not using chemicals.

Even addicts themselves are confused as to what brought this change in personality. When you ask addicts why they use chemicals, they are often unable to give a reason. At the same time, addicts are likely to envy and be mystified by the average person's ability to say "no" to chemical use. They simply do not know why they started or why they continue to use the drugs. They are, in a very real sense, spiritually blind.

As the addiction comes to control more and more of the individual's life, greater and greater effort must be expended to maintain the illusion of normalcy. Gallagher (1986) relates how one physician, addicted to the synthetic narcotic fentanyl, ultimately bought drugs from the street because it was no longer possible to divert enough drugs from hospital sources to maintain his drug habit. When the telltale scars from repeated injections of street drugs began to form, this physician intentionally burned himself on the arm with a spoon to hide the scars.

The addict also finds that significant effort must be invested to maintain the addiction. More than one cocaine or heroin addict has turned to prostitution to finance his or her habit. Everything is sacrificed to obtain and maintain what the addict perceives as an "adequate" supply of chemicals.

To combat the deception inherent in addiction, both AA and NA place heavy emphasis on the issue of honesty. Drug dependency hides behind a wall of deception, and honesty is the way to break through this deception and bring addicts face to face with their addiction.

Some Games of Addiction

For several reasons, individuals who are addicted to drugs often seek out sources of legitimate pharmaceuticals, either as their primary source of chemicals or to supplement their drug supply. First, as Goldman (1991) observes, pharmaceuticals can be purchased legally if there is a legitimate medical need for the medication. Second, pharmaceuticals are medication of a known product at a known potency level. The drug user does not have to worry about low potency, impurities, or misrepresentation. Third, pharmaceuticals are much less expensive than street drugs. For example, the pharmaceutical analgesic hydromorphone costs about $1 per tablet at a pharmacy; on the street, each tablet can sell for as much as $45 to $100 (Goldman, 1991). Thus, there is great demand on the street for pharmaceutical medications. To manipulate physicians into prescribing desired medications, addicts are likely to "use ploys such as outrage, tears, accusations of abandonment, abject pleading, promises of cooperation, and seduction" (Jenike, 1991, p. 7).

One favorite manipulative "scam" is for the addict (or accomplice) to visit the hospital emergency room (Klass, 1989) or physician's office with either a real or a simulated illness in an attempt to obtain desired medications. Sometimes they complain of "kidney stones" or that they need relief from some other painful condition. Sometimes addicts complain of bleeding from the alimentary or respiratory tracts (Cunnien, 1988).

When asked for a urine sample, which would show traces of blood if the person suffered from a real kidney stone, addicts have been found secretly pricking their finger with needles to squeeze a few drops of blood into the urine. Another common practice is for the addict to insert foreign objects such as darning needles into the urethra to irritate the urethral lining. This will cause a small amount of bleeding from the injured tissues, thus providing a sample of bloody urine.

Addicts play many "games" to obtain a pre-scription for narcotics from a sympathetic doctor. Addicts have been known to go to an emergency room with a broken bone, have the bone "set," and go home with a prescription for a narcotic analgesic. Once at home, the addict (or the accomplice) removes the cast and then visits another hospital emergency room to have another cast applied and to receive yet another prescription for a narcotic analgesic. In a large city, this process may be repeated ten times or more (Goldman, 1991).

Some addicts have been known to keep detailed records on computer, outlining physicians consulted, pharmacies used, and dates of the last visit so the addict does not visit the same facility too often and raise suspicion that he or she is actually manipulating to get medications (Goldman, 1991). It is also not unusual for addicts to study medical textbooks to learn what symptoms to fake and how to provide a convincing presentation of these symptoms to health care professionals. For example, Salloway, Southwick, and Sadowsky (1990) describe the case of a 39-year-old narcotics addict and Vietnam War veteran who simulated the symptoms of a posttraumatic stress disorder allegedly triggered by an industrial accident. Ultimately, it was discovered that the patient's presenting story was simply an elaborate manipulation designed to obtain narcotics and shelter.

Addicts have been known to have "conned" their psychiatrist into keeping their supply of cocaine for them. Although professing an interest in therapy, the addicts' real purpose is to use the therapist to provide a safe "stash" for their drugs. They thus avoid the fear of being caught by the police or having their drugs stolen by other addicts.

The only price addicts have to pay for this deception is to show up a few days a week, confess their latest transgression of having purchased more cocaine, then reluctantly allow the therapist to take possession of all but the immediate day's supply of the drug as an incentive to come back. The drug supply is then "safe" and the therapist believes that he or she has outmanipulated the addict into staying in therapy.

What the therapist may not realize is that he or she is now at risk of being charged with possession of a controlled substance. The addict could even deny any knowledge of the cocaine being there in the first place. The therapist could then quite possibly face criminal charges, while the addict looks for another place to "stash" the drugs.

Dealing with the Games of Addiction

A friend of mine who worked in a maximum security penitentiary for men was warned by older, more experienced corrections workers not to try to "out-con a con." It's nearly impossible to out-manipulate an individual whose entire life centers on the ability to manipulate others. As my friend was advised, "You should remember that, while you are home, watching the evening news, or going out to see a movie, these people have been working on perfecting their 'game.' It is their game, their rules, and in a sense their whole life."

This is also a good rule to keep in mind when working with the addicted person. Addiction is a lifestyle that, to a large degree, involves the manipulation of others into supporting the addiction. This is not to say that addicts cannot "change their spots" if necessary—at least for a short time. This is especially true early in the addiction process or during the early stages of treatment.

Addicts often go "on the wagon" for a few days or even a few weeks to prove both to themselves and to others that they can "still control it." Unfortunately, by attempting to "prove" their control, addicts actually demonstrate their *lack* of control over the chemicals. They may, as Stuart (1980) observed, be able to give up the drug for a period of time if the reward is large enough. However, as the addiction progresses, it takes more and more to motivate the addict to give up the drug, even for a short time. Often, even "a short time" becomes too long.

There is no limit to the manipulations that addicts will use to try to support their addiction. Vernon Johnson (1980) spoke at length of how

the addict will even use compliance as a defense against treatment. Overt compliance can be, and often is, utilized as a defense against accepting one's own spiritual, emotional, and physical deficits. In Johnson's (1980) experience, compliance is marked by a subtle defiance, almost as if the addict is "only going through the motions" to avoid further confrontation. In the struggle to avoid facing the reality of the addiction, the addict uses a small piece of the truth as a defense against having to accept the whole truth.

Honesty as Part of the Recovery Process

The author of *Narcotics Anonymous* (1982) warned that the addict's progression toward accepting that he or she is addicted is not easy. Indeed, self-deception is part of the price addicts pay for their addiction, according to NA. As stated in the "big book," "Only in desperation did we ask ourselves, 'Could it be the drugs?' " (pp. 1–2).

Addicts often speak with pride about how they have been more or less drug-free for various periods of time. The list of "reasons" for becoming drug-free is virtually endless. One person may be drug-free because his or her spouse threatened divorce if the drug use continued (but the addict secretly longs to return to chemical use and will if he or she can find a way to do so). Another person is drug-free because his or her probation officer has a reputation for sending people to prison if their urine sample (drawn under strict supervision) is positive for chemicals (but the addict is counting the days until probation is over, and may secretly use the drug if he or she can get away with it). But in each instance, the person is drug-free only because of an external threat, and once the threat is removed, the individual usually drifts back to chemicals. It is simply impossible for one person to provide the motivation for another person to remain drug-free forever. However, as Peele (1989) points out, the individual must choose to avoid further drug use if he or she is to achieve or maintain sobriety. Personal choice, or commitment to sobriety, is a necessary ingredient to recovery.

Many addicts in treatment simply switch addictions to give the appearance of being drug-free. It is not uncommon for an opiate addict in a methadone maintenance program to use alcohol, marijuana, or cocaine. The methadone does not block the euphoric effects of these drugs as it does the euphoria of narcotics. Thus, the addict can maintain the appearance of complete cooperation, appearing each day to take his or her methadone without protest, while freely using cocaine, marijuana, or alcohol.

In a very real sense, the addicted person has lost touch with reality. Over time, those who are addicted to chemicals come to share many common personality traits. As we have seen, there is some question whether this personality type—the so-called addicted personality—predates addiction or evolves as a result of the addiction (Bean-Bayog, 1988; Nathan, 1988). However, this chicken-or-the-egg question does not alter the fact that, for addicts, their addiction always comes first, and their lives are centered around chemical use.

Many addicts will go without food for days on end, but few will willingly go without using chemicals for even a short period of time. Cocaine addicts admit they would give up sexual relations to continue using cocaine. Just as the alcoholic will often sleep with an "eye opener" (an alcoholic drink) already mixed by the side of the bed, addicts speak of having a "rig" (a hypodermic needle) loaded and ready for use, so they can inject the drug even before they get out of bed in the morning.

Many physicians firmly believe that their patients have no reason to lie to them. One physician went so far as to boast that he knew that a certain patient did not have prescriptions from other doctors because the patient "told me so!" Chemical dependency professionals need to keep in mind at all times these twin realities: (1) for the person who is addicted, the chemical comes first, and (2) the addicted person centers his or her life around the chemical. To lose sight of these facts is to run the danger of being trapped in the addict's web of lies, half-truths and manipulations.

Recovering addicts openly speak of how manipulative they were, and will often admit that they were their own worst enemy. As they move along the road to recovery, addicts come to recognize that they also deceived themselves as part of the addiction process. One inmate said, "Before I can run a game on somebody else, I have to believe it myself." As the addiction progresses, addicts do not question their perception, but come to believe what they need to believe, to maintain the addiction.

It is for this reason that self-help groups such as Alcoholics Anonymous and Narcotics Anonymous place such heavy emphasis on honesty. Recovering addicts recognize that honesty is their own defense against the self-deception they used in the past to support their addiction.

False Pride: The Disease of the Spirit

In the final analysis, every addiction is a disease of the spirit. Edmeades (1987) relates a story about Carl Jung treated an American, Rowland H., for alcoholism in 1931. Immediately after treatment, Rowland H. relapsed, but Jung would not accept him back into analysis. Rowland's only hope of recovery, according to Jung, lay in a spiritual awakening, which he later found through a religious group.

Carl Jung thought of alcoholism (and by implication all forms of addiction) as a disease of the spirit (Peluso & Peluso, 1988). AA's *Twelve Steps and Twelve Traditions* (1981) describes addiction as a sickness of the soul. In support of this perspective, Kandel and Raveis (1989) found that a "lack of religiosity" (p. 113) was a significant predictor of continued use of cocaine or marijuana for young adults having previous experience with these drugs. The reverse of this is also true: Peluso and Peluso (1988) report that for addicts who achieve sobriety, a spiritual awakening appears to be an essential element of their recovery.

In speaking with addicts, one is impressed by how much the addict has suffered. It is almost as if one could trace a path from the emotional trauma to the addiction. Yet the addict's spirit is not crushed at birth, nor does the trauma that precedes addiction come about overnight. The individual's spirit comes to be diseased over time, as the addict-to-be comes to lose his or her way in life.

According to Fromm (1968), "we all start out with hope, faith and fortitude" (p. 20). However, the assorted insults of life often join forces to bring about disappointment and a loss of faith, and the individual comes to feel an empty void within. Graham (1988) claims that this is a turning point; if something is not found to fill the addict's "empty heart, he will fill his stomach with artificial stimulants and sedatives" (p. 14). Poland presents an excellent example of this process, where many of the country's "no future" generation—young adults whose futures have been throttled by years of economic hardship and martial law—have turned to heroin to ease their pain (Ross, 1991).

Few of us escape this moment of ultimate disappointment or ultimate awareness (Fromm, 1968). It is at this moment that many choose to "reduce their demands to what they can get and do not dream of that which seems to be out of their reach" (Fromm, 1968, p. 21). The Narcotics Anonymous pamphlet *The Triangle of Self-Obsession* (1983) observes that, for most, this process is a natural part of growing up. But the person who is in danger of addiction refuses to reduce those demands. The addict-to-be comes to demand "What I want, when I want it!" Addicts say, "[we] refuse to accept that we will not be given everything. We become self-obsessed; our wants and needs become demands. We reach a point where contentment and fulfillment are impossible" (*The Triangle of Self-Obsession*, 1983, p. 1).

People feel despair when they view themselves as powerless. Existentialists speak of the realization of ultimate powerlessness as awareness of one's nonexistence. In this sense, some people come to feel the utter futility of their existence. When a person faces the ultimate experience of powerlessness, a choice must be made: either accept one's true place in the universe or distort one's perceptions to maintain the illusion of being more than what one actually is.

It is only by accepting one's true place in the universe and the pain and suffering that life may offer that one is capable of any degree of spiritual growth (Peck, 1978). Many who reach the point of ultimate disappointment choose to turn away from reality, for it does not offer them what they think they are entitled to. In so doing, these people become somewhat grandiose and exhibit the characteristic false pride so frequently encountered in addiction.

It is impossible to maintain the illusion of being more than what one is without an increasingly large investment of time, energy, and emotional resources. Merton (1961) suggests that it is the lack of true humility that allows despair to grow within. Humility implies an honest, realistic view of self-worth. Despair rests on a foundation of a distorted view of one's place in the universe. This despair grows with each passing day, as reality threatens time and again to force on the individual an awareness of the ultimate measure of his or her existence.

In time, external supports are necessary to maintain this false pride. Brown (1985) points out that alcohol is able to offer the individual an illusion of control over his or her feelings. This is a common characteristic of every drug of abuse. If life does not provide the pleasure one feels entitled to, at least this comfort and pleasure may be found in a drug. Drugs offer freedom from life's pain and misery—at least for a while.

When faced with this unwanted awareness of their true place in the universe, addicts must increasingly distort their perceptions to maintain the illusion of superiority. In this fight to avoid the pain of reality, the chemical injects the ability to seemingly choose one's feelings at will. What the individual often does not realize until after the seeds of addiction have been planted is that the chemical offers an illusion only. There is no substance to the self-selected feelings brought about by the chemical, only a mockery of peace. The deeper feelings made possible through the acceptance of one's lot in life seem to be a mystery to the addicted person. "How can you be happy?" they ask; "You are nothing like me! You don't use!"

Humility is the honest acceptance of one's place in the universe (Merton, 1961). This includes the honest and open acceptance of one's strengths and one's weaknesses. When individuals become aware of the reality of their existence, they may either accept their lot in life or choose to struggle against existence itself.

To struggle against this acceptance is, in effect, to place oneself above all else and to say "Not as it is, but as I want it!" It is a cry against the ultimate knowledge of being lost that Fromm (1968) spoke of. This despair is often so all-inclusive that the "self" seems unable to withstand its attack; addicts have described this despair as an empty, black void within. As Graham (1988) notes, addicts then attempt to fill this void with the chemicals they find around them. If false pride is a sickness of the soul (*Twelve Steps and Twelve Traditions*, 1981), chemical use might be viewed as a reaction against the ultimate despair of encountering one's lot in life—the false sense of being that says "Not as it is, but as I want it!" in response to one's discovery of personal powerlessness.

Many have come to view substance abuse as essentially seeking to join with a higher power. But in place of the spiritual struggle that Peck (1978, 1993) speaks of as necessary to achieve inner peace, the addict tries to take a shortcut through the use of chemicals. Thus, May (1988) views addiction as sidetracking "our deepest, truest desire for love and goodness" (p. 14). Drugs come to dominate the individual's life until at last the person believes that he or she cannot live without them. Further spiritual growth is impossible if chemical use is the first priority.

In the process of sidetracking the drive for truth and spiritual growth, the addict develops a sense of false pride that is expressed as a form

of narcissism. The clinical phenomenon of narcissism is itself a reaction against perceived worthlessness, loss of control, and emotional pain so intense that it almost seems physical (Millon, 1981). According to Millon (1981), people with a narcissistic personality view their own self-worth in such a way that "they rarely question whether it is valid" (p. 167) and they tend to "place few restraints on either their fantasies or rationalizations, and their imagination is left to run free."

Although addicts are not usually true narcissistic personalities, they have significant narcissistic traits. Narcissism, or false pride, is based on the lack of humility, a point Merton (1961) explores at length. Addicts come to distort their perceptions not only of "self" but also of others in the service of their pride. People whose entire life centers on themselves "imagine that they can only find themselves by asserting their own desires and ambitions and appetites in a struggle with the rest of the world" (Merton, 1961, p. 47).

Here are the seeds of addiction. The chemicals of choice allow users to assert their own desires and ambitions over everyone else's. Brown (1985) speaks at length of the illusion of control over one's feelings that alcohol gives an individual, and May (1988) speaks of how chemical addiction reflects a misguided attempt to achieve complete control over one's life. The drugs of abuse give users a dangerous illusion of control over the external world. They believe they are asserting their will over others, but in reality they are losing their will to the chemical.

Addicts often speak with pride of the horrors they have suffered in the service of their addiction. In the process of "euphoric recall," addicts selectively recall only the pleasant aspects of their drug use (Gorski, 1993). More than one addict, for example, has expounded on the quasisexual thrill experienced through cocaine or heroin, in the process dismissing the fact that this drug cost the addict a spouse, family, and tens of thousands of dollars.

There is a name for the distorted view of oneself and of one's world that comes about with chronic chemical use. It is called the insanity of addiction.

Denial, Projection, Rationalization, and Minimization: The "Four Musketeers" of Addiction

The traditional view of addiction is that all human behavior, including the addictive use of chemicals, rests on a foundation of characteristic psychological defenses. In the case of chemical dependency, the defense mechanisms involved are denial, projection, and rationalization. These defense mechanisms, like all psychological defenses, are thought to operate unconsciously in both the intrapersonal and interpersonal spheres. They exist to protect the individual from the conscious awareness of anxiety.

Often without knowing it, the addict employs these defense mechanisms to avoid recognizing their addiction. Once the reality of the addiction is recognized, there is an implicit social expectation to deal with that addiction. Thus, to understand addiction, one must also understand each of these characteristic defense mechanisms.

Denial

Denial is traditionally viewed as a characteristic defense of the addict. Kaplan and Sadock (1990) define *denial* as "a disregard for a disturbing reality" (p. 20). In this sense, denial functions as a form of "Catch-22" for the addicted person. First, it prevents the person from being aware of the danger signs of the growing addiction and so blocks the awareness of anxiety. But while avoiding the experience of anxiety, the individual is also avoiding coming to terms with his or her addiction. Thus, denial is a form of self-deception used to help the individual avoid anxiety and emotional distress (Shader, 1994).

A person in denial has selective perception. The Alcoholics Anonymous program (to be discussed in more detail in a later chapter) calls this selective perception "tunnel vision." Furthermore, it is interesting to note that Perry and

Cooper (1989) identify denial as a rather immature defense mechanism usually found in a person who is experiencing significant internal and interpersonal distress.

Projection

The second of the psychological defense mechanisms commonly found in addiction is that of *projection,* defined by Kaplan and Sadock (1990) as the process through which "what is emotionally unacceptable in oneself is unconsciously rejected and attributed to others" (p. 20). Johnson (1980) defines projection somewhat differently, noting that the act of projection is the act of "unloading self-hatred onto others" (p. 31, italics in original omitted).

At times, projection is expressed through misinterpreting the motives or intentions of others (Kaplan & Sadock, 1990). Young children often exclaim, "See what you made me do?" when they have misbehaved; this is an expression of projection. Addicts often do this as well, blaming their addiction or other unacceptable aspects of their behavior onto others.

Rationalization

The defense mechanism of *rationalization* is defined by Kaplan and Sadock (1990) as the process through which "an individual attempts to justify feelings, motives, or behavior that otherwise would be unreasonable, illogical or intolerable" (p. 20). In a later work, the authors also noted that rationalization may express itself through the individual's "invention of a convincing fallacy" (1991, p. 184) through which their behavior may seemingly be justified. Addicts use rationalization when they blame their addiction on their spouse or family or on their medical problems (one 72-year-old alcoholic blamed his drinking on the fact that he had pneumonia when he was 12). Anyone who has ever worked with an addicted person will recognize that rationalization is one of the most important defensive devices the addict uses.

Minimization

The defense mechanism of *minimization* operates in a different manner than the three we have just discussed. In a sense, minimization is like the defense mechanism of rationalization, but it is more specific. Addicts who use minimization as a defense will actively try to give the impression that their drug use is less than it actually is.

The alcoholic, for example, might drink out of an oversized container—perhaps the size of three or four regular glasses—and then admit to having "only three drinks a night!" The addict may claim to "only use once a day" and hope that whoever is doing the interview does not think to ask whether a "day" means 24 hours or just when it is light outside. Another trick is for the addict to describe time spent in treatment or jail as "straight time," overlooking the fact that they were simply unable to get drugs.

All these defense mechanisms operate automatically and quite unconsciously to protect the individual from the painful awareness of the addiction. Sometimes these defenses seem quite farfetched. For example, there is the rationalization, offered to this author by a number of different addicts, that marijuana use does not constitute addiction because marijuana is "an herb," and thus a natural substance; you can only, or so the rationalization goes, become addicted to artificial chemicals like alcohol, amphetamines, or heroin. Another popular rationalization is that it is "better to be an alcoholic than a needle freak . . . after all, alcohol is legal." More than one addict has denied his or her addiction, despite compelling evidence to the contrary, through the use of one or more of these common defense mechanisms.

Alternative Views of the Defense Mechanisms

Although the traditional view of substance abuse in the United States has been that the four defense mechanisms presented are traditionally found in cases of chemical dependency, this view is not universally accepted. There is a small, increasingly vocal minority that offers alternative frameworks within which substance abuse professionals might view the defense mechanisms encountered in their work with addicted individuals.

Stanton Peele, as noted earlier, has been a vocal critic of the medical model of chemical dependency. In *Diseasing of America* (1989) he spoke at length of how treatment centers often interpret the individual's refusal to admit to his or her addiction as a confirmation that the individual *is* addicted; the individual is automatically assumed to be "in denial" of his or her chemical abuse problem. However, according to Peele, a second possibility all too often overlooked by treatment center staff is that the individual really *isn't* addicted. The individual's refusal to admit to being addicted may be a reflection of reality, and not an expression of denial. This possibility underscores the need for an accurate assessment of the client's substance use patterns to determine whether there is or is not a need for active intervention or treatment.

Miller and Rollnick (1991) offer a theory that radically departs from the belief that addicts typically utilize denial as a major defense against the admission of being "sick." The authors suggest that, as a group, alcoholics do not use denial more frequently than any other average group. Rather, the authors suggest that a combination of two factors makes it *appear* that addicts frequently employ defense mechanisms in the service of their dependency. First, the authors suggest that the process of selective perception by treatment center staff makes it appear that addicts frequently use defense mechanisms, pointing to the phenomenon known as the "illusion of correlation" to support this theory. According to the illusion of correlation, humans tend to remember information that confirms their preconceptions and forget or overlook information that fails to meet their conceptual model. Substance abuse professionals would be more likely to remember clients who *did* use defense mechanisms because that is what they were trained to expect.

Second, Miller and Rollnick (1991) suggest that, when substance abuse rehabilitation professionals utilize the wrong treatment approach for the client's unique stage of growth, the resulting conflict is interpreted as evidence of denial, projection, minimization, or rationalization. On the basis of their work with addicts, Berg and Miller (1992) also found that "denial" was attributed to clients who received the wrong treatment approach. Thus, both teams of clinicians concluded that defense mechanisms such as "denial" may be not a reflection of a pathological condition but the result of the wrong intervention.

Summary

Many human service professionals who have had limited contact with addicts tend to have a distorted view of the nature of drug addiction. Having heard the term *disease* applied to chemical dependency, the inexperienced human service worker may think in terms of more traditional illnesses and may be rudely surprised at the deception that is inherent in drug addiction.

Although chemical dependency is a disease, it is a disease like no other. As noted in an earlier chapter, it is a disease that requires the active participation of the "victim." Self-help groups such as AA and NA view addiction as a disease of the spirit, and they offer a spiritual program to help their members achieve and maintain sobriety.

In a sense, addiction is a form of insanity. The insanity of addiction rests on the psychological defense mechanisms of rationalization, denial, and projection. These three defense mechanisms, along with minimization, shield the addict from an awareness of the reality of the addiction until the disease has progressed quite far. To combat this deception, Alcoholics Anonymous emphasizes honesty, both with self and with others, as the central feature of its program.

CHAPTER TWENTY

Chemicals and the Neonate: The Consequences of Drug Use During Pregnancy

The problem of maternal drug abuse during pregnancy is actually part of a more inclusive danger: that of maternal exposure to *any* chemical during pregnancy. Physicians have long been aware that a multitude of different chemical compounds can cross the placenta and enter the fetal circulatory system. Unfortunately, many of these chemicals can cause great harm to the developing fetus.

And the effects of chemical exposure for the mother will be far different than those for the developing fetus (Chasnoff, 1988). First, the fetus lacks the fully developed liver and excretory systems of the mother. Second, pregnancy is a time of rapid fetal growth, when many organ systems are developing. Anything that disrupts the process of fetal growth may prevent or distort the development of these organ systems, which will have lifelong consequences for the child.

Thus, maternal drug use during pregnancy can have dangerous consequences for the developing fetus. Virtually every drug of abuse is able to cross the placenta and enter the fetal circulation (Behnke & Eyler, 1993). Although medical science has long been aware of this fact, little attention has been paid to the implications of maternal drug abuse on fetal growth and development (Chasnoff & Schnoll, 1987). Even today, more than a generation after the latest "war on drugs" began, virtually nothing is known about either the short- or long-term consequences of maternal drug abuse on the developing fetus (Chasnoff, 1991a; Zuckerman & Bresnahan, 1991).

The possible impact of maternal chemical use on fetal development would not be an issue if it were a rare phenomenon. Unfortunately, this is not the case. In the United States, illicit drug use is thought to be a complicating factor in approximately 24% of all pregnancies (Bays, 1992), and in some parts of the country, up to *38%* of all pregnant women admit to the use of, or test positive for, one or more recreational drugs (*Alcoholism & Drug Abuse Week*, 1990b). Given that the fetus is uniquely vulnerable to environmental influences during the prenatal period of rapid growth, the potential danger of maternal chemical use during pregnancy is readily apparent.

A Note of Caution

It is very difficult to identify the effects of a given chemical on fetal growth and development. There are thousands of different factors that influence both fetal growth and maternal health. The possibility of maternal illness during pregnancy, polychemical exposure, genetic predisposition toward various medical problems, and the woman's state of health prior to pregnancy are but a few of the factors that must be considered in studying the effects of chemical use on fetal growth and development.

For example, consider the case of a woman

who suffered from a kidney disease *before* she became pregnant and failed to receive adequate prenatal care because of limited financial resources. Should her child's small size at birth be attributed to her cigarette smoking, her mother's poor health, the lack of prenatal care, a poor diet (a common consequence of poverty), or to a familial tendency to give birth to smaller children? These are all factors that must be considered in attempting to identify the effects of maternal drug use on the growing fetus.

The Scope of the Problem

There is significant evidence to suggest that recreational drug use during pregnancy is associated with such complications as preterm labor, early separation of the placenta, fetal growth retardation, and any of a number of congenital abnormalities. At its most extreme, if the mother is addicted at the time of delivery, the child will share the mother's addiction. In the United States, more than 1,000 children a day are born to mothers who are addicted to chemicals (Byrne, 1989a). But, even if the child is not addicted at the time of birth, maternal drug use during pregnancy might interfere with the normal development of various organ systems. For example, Dominguez, Vila-Coro, Aguirre, Slipis, and Bohan (1991) concluded that exposure to recreational drugs during pregnancy is one cause of subsequent brain and vision abnormalities in children.

The medical care of children who were exposed prenatally to recreational drugs is an expensive affair. Chasnoff (1991a) estimates that the median cost of care for children born to mothers who had used illicit chemicals during pregnancy was between $1,100 and $4,100 higher than for children whose mothers did not use illicit chemicals while pregnant. Considering that between 350,000 and 739,000 children are exposed to illicit chemicals before birth (Chasnoff, 1991a), there is a potential expenditure of between $385 million and $3 billion in

additional medical costs each year for treatment of drug-related neonatal health problems.

When these children reach school age, they will require further specialized services that are an additional expense for society. Barden (1991) notes, for example, that whereas the average educational cost for a child is approximately $3,000 a year, the cost of the special education classes often required by children born addicted to drugs may be as high as $15,000 a year per child. This expense is in addition to the extra medical costs, costs for social services, and so on that these children often require.

Fetal Alcohol Syndrome

Researchers believe that 35% to 75% of women who are pregnant consume alcohol at least once during their pregnancy (Behnke & Eyler, 1993). When an expectant mother drinks, the alcohol quickly crosses the placenta into the fetal bloodstream. The blood alcohol level of the fetus reaches the same level as the mother's in only 15 minutes (Rose, 1988). Thus, the fetus is often an unwilling participant in the mother's alcohol use. And if the mother has been drinking shortly before giving birth, the smell of alcohol can be detected on the newborn's breath (Rose, 1988).

It has only been in the past 25 years that researchers have discovered that pregnant women who drink on a regular basis run the risk of causing alcohol-induced birth defects in their children, a condition known as the *fetal alcohol syndrome* (or FAS). Nobody knows how much or how often a pregnant woman must drink before there is a risk of FAS developing. But there is a known association between maternal alcohol use during pregnancy and developmental abnormalities in the fetus.

The full prevalence of alcohol-related birth defects is not known (Cordero, 1990). Youngstrom (1992) reports that 1 child in 700 to 750 suffers from FAS; Spohr, Willms, and Steinhausen (1993) estimate 1 to 2 cases of FAS for every 1,000 children. But these statistics only reflect the proportion of children with FAS to the total number of live births. To alcoholic mothers, perhaps between 2.5% (Gottlieb, 1994) and 6% (Charness, Simon, & Greenberg, 1989) of the children born will have FAS.

Fetal alcohol syndrome is thought to be the most severe end of a continuum of disabilities brought on by maternal alcohol use during pregnancy (Streissguth, Aase, Clarren, Randels, LaDue, & Smith, 1991). Infants who demonstrate some, but not all, the symptoms of FAS, a condition known as *fetal alcohol effects* (or FAE) (Streissguth et al., 1991; Charness, Simon, & Greenberg, 1989). Perhaps another 3 to 5 children of every 1,000 suffer from fetal alcohol effects (Spohr, Willms, & Steinhausen, 1993).

Two different factors seem to play a role in determining whether the child will develop FAS (Charness, Simon, & Greenberg, 1989): (1) whether the mother drinks heavily during all or only part of her pregnancy, and (2) the genetic vulnerability of the fetus to maternal alcohol use. If the mother drinks heavily throughout pregnancy and the fetus is especially vulnerable to the effects of the alcohol in the mother's system, there is a very real danger that the child will be born with fetal alcohol syndrome.

Characteristics of Fetal Alcohol Syndrome

Infants who suffer from the full fetal alcohol syndrome usually have a lower than normal birth weight, a characteristic pattern of facial abnormalities, and often a smaller brain size at birth. In later life, children with FAS often demonstrate behavioral problems such as hyperactivity, a short attention span, impulsiveness, inattentiveness, poor coordination, and numerous other developmental delays (Committee on Substance Abuse and Committee on Children With Disabilities, 1993; Gilbertson & Weinberg, 1992; Charness, Simon, & Greenberg, 1989).

Children with FAS also exhibit slower growth patterns following birth and are more likely to be retarded. Indeed, maternal alcohol use during pregnancy is thought to be the leading cause of

mental retardation in the United States (Charness, Simon, & Greenberg, 1989; Streissguth et al., 1991). It is also the only cause of birth defects that is totally preventable (Beasley, 1987).

As a group, children with FAS usually fall in the mild to moderately retarded range following birth, with an average IQ of 68 (Chasnoff, 1988).[1] However, some 40% of children with FAS have measured IQs of above 70, a score that is often used to determine which children qualify for special services (Streissguth et al., 1991). This is not to say that these children have not suffered from the mother's use of alcohol during pregnancy; rather, they do not qualify for special support services because their measured IQ happens to be higher than the cut-off score of 70 typically used to determine who qualifies for remedial services.

Research findings to date suggest that there is no "safe" dose of alcohol during pregnancy (Committee on Substance Abuse and Committee on Children With Disabilities, 1993). Maternal alcohol use during the first trimester of pregnancy is especially dangerous, as the fetus seems to be extremely sensitive to the effects of alcohol during this stage of development (Chasnoff, 1988). However, Gottlieb (1994) suggests that alcohol use at *any* point in pregnancy should be avoided.

Unfortunately, even when children who suffer from FAS are identified at birth, they may never achieve normal growth or intelligence, even with the best possible intervention program (Spohr, Willms, & Steinhausen, 1993; Mirin, Weiss, & Greenfield, 1991). For example, Aase (1994) states that children with "classic" (p. 5) FAS grow at only 60% of the normal rate for height and 33% of the normal rate for weight gain. One study found that only 6% of those students with FAS could function without special help in regular school classes (Streissguth et al., 1991). These researchers found that the aver-

[1] An IQ of 68 falls in the mildly retarded range of intellectual function. The average IQ is 100, with a standard deviation of 15 points.

age reading level for adolescent and adult FAS victims was the fourth grade, and the average arithmetic skill level for their sample was the second grade.

For FAS children, "major psychosocial problems and lifelong adjustment problems were characteristic of most of these patients" (Streissguth et al., 1991, pp. 1965–1966). Surprisingly, the low birth-weight characteristic of FAS seems to at least partially resolve itself by adolescence. However, "none of these [adolescent or young adult] patients were known to be independent in terms of both housing and income" (p. 1966) at the time of the study. These findings underscore the lifelong impact of maternal alcohol use during pregnancy on the child.

Breast-Feeding and Alcohol Use

Animal research suggests that, even if the mother does not drink during pregnancy, if she drinks during the period of time that she is breast-feeding, the infant may absorb alcohol through the mother's milk (Little, Anderson, Ervin, Worthington-Roberts, & Clarren, 1989). Little et al. (1989) found a direct relationship between the level of exposure to alcohol through the mother's milk and developmental delays in the infant. Furthermore, the more the mother drinks while she is breast-feeding, the greater the developmental delay in the infant.

Maternal alcohol use by the woman who is breast-feeding her child may also interfere with the normal development of the child's immune system (Gilbertson & Weinberg, 1992). These results strongly suggest that alcohol use during breast-feeding is a risk factor for the infant and should be avoided.

Cocaine Use During Pregnancy

As recently as 1982, some medical textbooks claimed that maternal cocaine use did not have a harmful effect on the fetus (Revkin, 1989). The wave of cocaine abuse and addiction in the United States during the late 1970s and early 1980s found health care professionals unprepared to deal with the large numbers of women in their childbearing years who began to abuse cocaine.

In the 1980s and early 1990s, estimates of the number of cocaine-using pregnant women varied. At one point, approximately 15% to 17% of *all* cocaine users were women of childbearing age (Weathers, Crane, Sauvain, & Blackhurst, 1993; Peters & Theorell, 1991). In the United States alone, estimates of the number of infants exposed to cocaine in utero ranged from 158,000 (Mayes, Granger, Frank, Schottenfeld, & Bornstein, 1993) to 720,000 (Dumas, 1992) cases each year. In some communities, fully 31% of the children born tested positive for cocaine at birth (Weathers et al., 1993).

Although marijuana is the most commonly abused illicit chemical in the United States, in some communities cocaine actually replaced marijuana as the illicit chemical most commonly abused by pregnant women[2] (Ney, Dooley, Keith, Chasnoff, & Socol, 1990; American Academy of Family Physicians, 1990b). The possible consequences of maternal cocaine use frightened medical professionals, but only limited research data on the effects of fetal cocaine exposure was available in the early to mid-1980s.[3] Medical researchers, fearing the worst, began to speak of an epidemic of cocaine-disabled children and struggled to understand what effects, if any, maternal cocaine use might have on the developing fetus.

Identifying Cocaine-Induced Neonatal Developmental Problems

Medical researchers have had great difficulty determining the effects of maternal cocaine use on the developing fetus. The first problem is

[2]The classification of illicit chemicals does not include alcohol or tobacco, because these chemicals can be legally purchased.

[3]Unfortunately, there is not much more available to medical researchers now.

identifying infants who have been exposed to cocaine at some point in their prenatal development. In adults, blood or urine toxicology tests detect cocaine for only 24 to 48 hours following the drug use. However, the newborn child's liver is still quite immature and is unable to produce normal amounts of *pseudocholinesterase,* the enzyme that biotransforms cocaine (Peters & Theorell, 1991; House, 1990). Thus, the newborn child requires longer to metabolize and excrete any cocaine in the body. Research has shown that the metabolites of cocaine require 4 to 6 days to be eliminated from the body of newborn children (Levy & Rutter, 1992). However, even the prolonged period necessary for cocaine biotransformation and excretion in the newborn allows urine and blood toxicology tests to detect only *recent* maternal cocaine use (Volpe, 1995). It is difficult to determine the effects of maternal cocaine use on the developing fetus, when it can be detected only in the few days prior to giving birth.[4]

Another complicating factor is that many of the fetal developmental problems initially attributed to maternal cocaine abuse could be caused by other factors. Such noncocaine factors include maternal lifestyle, lack of prenatal care, concurrent use of drugs other than cocaine, and poor maternal nutritional habits. For example, in a provocative study, Racine, Joyce, and Anderson (1993) propose that at least some of the complications seen in children born to cocaine-abusing mothers may not be from the drug use but from poor prenatal care instead. Racine, Joyce, and Anderson compared birth records of children born to cocaine-using mothers who had seen a doctor at least four times during pregnancy with those of children born to cocaine-using mothers who had not received even this limited prenatal care. They found significant improvements in the birth weight of children born to mothers who

had seen a doctor at least four times during pregnancy, even if the mothers used cocaine during her pregnancy.

Prenatal medical examinations are a routine precaution during pregnancy, with an emphasis placed on preventive medical care for the woman and her unborn child. Yet Sexson (1994) found that, for many cocaine-abusing pregnant women, the first medical treatment received was when they went to the hospital at the start of labor. Thus, it could be that a lack of proper prenatal medical care may actually have caused some of the fetal growth problems that medical researchers initially attributed to maternal cocaine abuse.

Concurrent use of other chemicals and cocaine is an additional confounding factor. Sexson (1994) found that fully 50% of the women were using cocaine were also using alcohol during their pregnancy. As we discussed in the last section, alcohol is a known risk factor for abnormal fetal development. Also, an unknown (but significant) percentage of cocaine-abusing mothers also smoke cigarettes, a practice known to have a negative effect on prenatal growth and development, and many cocaine-abusing mothers also engage in polydrug use. Sexson also found a high incidence of sexually transmitted diseases (STDs) among women who used cocaine during pregnancy. Many pathogens that cause STDs are able to disrupt normal fetal development as well as cause damage to the mother's body. Given that all these factors have the potential to influence fetal growth and development, it is difficult, if not impossible, to isolate the effects of maternal cocaine use from the effects of other known maternal risk factors.

The Professional Bias

As researchers struggled to understand the effects that prenatal cocaine exposure may have on both the mother and the developing fetus, an unspoken anticocaine bias developed in many professional journals. Articles that found ad-

[4]Volpe (1995) suggests that it may be possible to detect evidence of maternal cocaine use through traces of cocaine found in the infant's *hair* if the mother had used cocaine in the last two trimesters of pregnancy. However, this procedure is not in general use and remains controversial.

verse effects from maternal cocaine use were more likely to be published than were articles that failed to document a negative impact (Volpe, 1995; Raskin, 1994). The average health care worker, unaware of this bias, assumed that maternal cocaine abuse was indeed the cause of the numerous birth defects attributed to it.

Horror stories began to spread suggesting that maternal cocaine abuse was responsible for a wide range of abnormalities, including: spontaneous abortions, early separation of the placenta, poor fetal growth and possible low birth weight, small head size at birth, fetal urinary tract abnormalities, fetal skull abnormalities, possible strokes (for both mother and fetus), fetal cardiac system abnormalities, fetal kidney malformations, structural abnormalities in the fetal brain, and damage to the fetal small intestine. Maternal cocaine use during pregnancy was thought to be one reason many women are unable to carry their babies to term. In some U.S. communities, as many as 17% of the women who experienced preterm labor were found to have measurable amounts of cocaine in their urine (Ney et al., 1990; Cordero, 1990). Some physicians went so far as to advocate routine urine toxicology testing for any woman who experiences preterm labor (Peters & Theorell, 1991).

Now that the cocaine use epidemic of the 1970s and 1980s is over, researchers are able to examine the effects maternal cocaine use may have on fetal development in more detail. Surprisingly, physicians have concluded that the "great majority of cocaine-exposed pregnancies did not result in fetal structural abnormalities" (Behnke & Eyler, 1993, p. 1366). Indeed, in spite of the popular image painted by the mass media in the late 1980s and early 1990s, there is no "typical" cocaine-baby syndrome (Sexson, 1994; Day & Richardson, 1994). Medical researchers have found "no consistent pattern of congenital abnormalities . . . and no increased incidence of malformations" (Behnke & Eyler, 1993, p. 1365) in children born to cocaine-using mothers.

To illustrate the contradictory pattern of research findings, consider that some researchers found evidence suggesting that children born to mothers who used cocaine during pregnancy are more likely to suffer "crib death" ("Sudden Infant Death Syndrome," or SIDS). Perhaps as many as 15% of the infants whose mothers used cocaine during pregnancy were found to suffer from SIDS, a potentially fatal condition that is seen in only three-tenths of 1% of those children whose mothers do not use cocaine during pregnancy (Peters & Theorell, 1991). Other studies, however, have failed to find this association (Plessinger & Woods, 1993; Weathers et al., 1993). If an increased risk of SIDS is a consequence of maternal cocaine use during pregnancy, one would expect it to be repeatedly shown in research studies that examined the subject.

Researchers now question whether children born to mothers who used cocaine during pregnancy are more likely to suffer from SIDS. For example, Kandall, Gaines, Habel, Davidson, and Jessop (1993) found only a *slightly* higher incidence of SIDS in children whose mothers had used cocaine during pregnancy. Thus, until research answers the question one way or another, maternal cocaine use during pregnancy must be considered a *potential but not proven* factor in the possible development of SIDS. The use of cocaine during pregnancy should be avoided, to be sure, but medical researchers are still divided on the question of whether maternal cocaine abuse predisposes the baby to SIDS following birth.

This leaves us with the question of how maternal cocaine use during pregnancy may affect fetal development. After decades of study, we still do not know. Research into the effects of maternal cocaine use on fetal brain development has only recently been started, and the results will not be known for many years (Day & Richardson, 1994). However, on the basis of animal research and what we do know about the clinical effects of cocaine on the user's body, we can make an educated guess as to some of the ways cocaine might disrupt fetal development.

For example, animal research has demonstrated that cocaine use by the mother results in constriction of the blood vessels in the placenta and uterine bed, which reduces the blood flow to the fetus for a period of time. The reduction in uterine blood flow is postulated to be one possible cause of poor intrauterine growth for the fetus of cocaine-using mothers. This is also thought to be the mechanism by which maternal cocaine abuse during pregnancy can result in premature labor and birth in humans (Behnke & Eyler, 1993; Plessinger & Woods, 1993; Glantz & Woods, 1993; Chasnoff, 1991b). Cocaine is suspected of being able to cause strong contractions in the uterus, which may, in turn, initiate labor. Indeed, Sexson (1994) reports that many street addicts believe that cocaine is capable of bringing on a late-stage abortion, and there is reason to suspect that some women use cocaine for this purpose.

Cocaine's vasoconstrictive effects may also be the mechanism by which maternal cocaine abuse results in injury to the developing bowel of the fetus (Cotton, 1994; Plessinger & Woods, 1993). Animal research suggests that maternal cocaine use causes damage to the mesenteric artery, which provides blood to the intestines. An alternative hypothesis is that cocaine is able to cause a reduction in blood flow to "nonvital" (Plessinger & Woods, 1993, p. 271) organ systems of the developing fetus, including the intestines. In either case, maternal cocaine use is a suspected cause of damage to the intestines of the developing fetus in humans.

Some evidence also suggests that infants born to mothers who use cocaine during pregnancy may suffer from small strokes prior to birth (Volpe, 1995; Levy & Rutter, 1992; Chasnoff, 1988). These small strokes are thought to result from rapid changes in the mother's blood pressure brought on by her cocaine use, and are similar in nature to those occasionally seen in adults who use cocaine. Chasnoff (1988) also notes that there is evidence that cocaine use during pregnancy may also result in cardiac and central nervous system abnormalities in the fetus.

The danger of CNS developmental abnormal-ities for the fetus is hardly insignificant. Research has shown that more than one-third of the infants who are exposed to cocaine during pregnancy have structural abnormalities of the brain that can be detected by computer tomographic scans (CAT scans) or ultrasound examination (Plessinger & Woods, 1993; Behnke & Eyler, 1993; Zuckerman & Bresnahan, 1991). One research study found that 6% of cocaine-exposed infants showed evidence of having had at least one cerebral infarction (Volpe, 1995).

In addition, "crack" has been implicated as a significant cause of child neglect, for several different reasons. First, children who are born addicted to cocaine often have poor interactive skills during the first weeks of life, during which time the all-important "bonding" with the mother should be taking place. As a result of poor bonding, the mother is not as invested in her child and may interact with the child less than she normally would. Preoccupation with cocaine addiction may also cause parents to service their addiction at the expense of their child's care (Byrne, 1989a; Revkin, 1989).

Researchers have affirmed that, when the expectant mother uses cocaine, at least some of the cocaine crosses the placenta and enters the fetal blood. However, animal research raises the question of the *amount* of cocaine that may enter the fetal circulation. In some animal species, the placenta may be able to metabolize limited amounts of cocaine before it enters the fetal circulatory system. If true, this limits the transfer of cocaine to the fetus from the mother's blood (Plessinger & Woods, 1993). However, these findings are based on animal research, and there is no clinical evidence at this point to suggest that the human placenta shares this characteristic.

Fortunately, it now appears that only a minority of those children born to women who used cocaine during pregnancy suffered any long-lasting problems. Although maternal cocaine use during pregnancy should not be encouraged, there is evidence to suggest that the initial reports of potential harm to the fetus may have misrepresented the scope of the problem. The question of how dangerous cocaine abuse during pregnancy might be for the fetus and the mother remains to be answered.

Breast-Feeding and Cocaine Use

Because cocaine is highly lipid soluble, it can be stored in breast milk and passed on to the infant through breast-feeding (Peters & Theorell, 1991; Revkin, 1989). But the level of cocaine exposure for the child may be far higher than it is for the mother. Research has shown that cocaine levels in maternal milk may be *8 times* as high as the level of cocaine in the mother's blood (Revkin, 1989). If the cocaine-using mother breast-feeds her infant, the child may be exposed to extremely high levels of cocaine.

Narcotics Use During Pregnancy

Most of the 125,000 estimated female intravenous drug users in the United States abuse narcotics at least occasionally (Hoegerman & Schnoll, 1991). As do a large number of other chemicals, the narcotics cross the placenta and enter the bloodstream of the fetus. It is estimated that between 1 and 21% of expectant mothers will use a narcotic analgesic at least once during pregnancy (Behnke & Eyler, 1993). In other words, approximately 300,000 children are exposed to narcotics in utero each year in the United States (Glantz & Woods, 1993). Most of these women use narcotic pharmaceuticals for limited periods under a physician's supervision for medical reasons.

But after cocaine, heroin is the most commonly abused illicit drug by expectant mothers, accounting for almost 25% of all cases of fetal exposure to illegal drugs (American Academy of Family Physicians, 1990b). Each year in the United States, some 9,000 (Glantz & Woods, 1993) to 10,000 (Zuckerman & Bresnahan, 1991) children are born to women who are addicted to narcotics.

Unfortunately, many early symptoms of pregnancy—feelings of fatigue, nausea, vomiting, pelvic cramps, and hot sweats—may be interpreted as early withdrawal symptoms, rather than possible pregnancy (Levy & Rutter, 1992). Even physicians experienced in the treatment of narcotics addiction find it difficult to diagnose pregnancy in narcotics-addicted women. All too often, rather than seek prenatal care, the woman tries to self-medicate what she believes is withdrawal by using even higher doses of narcotics. The fetus is thereby exposed to significant levels of narcotic analgesics (and the chemicals that are used to "cut" street narcotics) by a woman who is not even aware that she is pregnant.

Narcotics abuse during pregnancy carries a number of serious consequences for both the mother and the developing child. In addition to the dangers associated with narcotics abuse alone, the pregnant woman who abuses opioids runs the risk of septic thrombophlebitis, postpartum hemorrhage, depression, gestational diabetes, eclampsia, and death.

Other physical complications associated with narcotic abuse during pregnancy include stillbirth, breech presentation during childbirth, placental insufficiency, spontaneous abortions, premature delivery, neonatal meconium aspiration syndrome (which may be fatal), neonatal infections acquired through the mother, low birth weight, and neonatal narcotic addiction (Glantz & Woods, 1993; Levy & Rutter, 1992; Hoegerman & Schnoll, 1991; Chasnoff, 1988). In addition, children born to women who are addicted to narcotics have a 2 to 3 times higher risk of suffering from SIDS than do children whose mothers have never used illicit chemicals (Kandall et al., 1993). Volpe (1995) suggests that the risk of SIDS increases with the severity of the infant's withdrawal from narcotics.

Because chronic narcotics use during pregnancy results in a state of chronic exposure to opiates for the fetus, these infants are physically dependent on narcotics at birth. Within 24 to 72 hours after birth, the infant, no longer able to absorb drugs from the mother's blood, begins to go through drug withdrawal. Depending on the specific narcotic(s) being abused by the mother, the withdrawal process for the newborn may last for weeks or even months (Volpe, 1995; Levy & Rutter, 1992; Hoegerman & Schnoll, 1991).

Symptoms of neonatal narcotic withdrawal include muscle tremors; hyperactivity; hyperirritability; a unique, high-pitched cry; frantic efforts to find comfort; sleep problems; vomiting; loose stools; increased deep muscle reflexes; frequent yawning; sneezing; seizures; increased sweating; dehydration; constant sucking movements; fever; and rapid breathing (Anand & Arnold, 1994). In the past, neonatal narcotics withdrawal resulted in almost a 90% mortality rate (Mirin, Weiss, & Greenfield, 1991). In response to increased medical awareness of the special needs of the addicted infant and improved withdrawal programs, the mortality rate for these children has dropped significantly in recent years (Mirin, Weiss, & Greenfield, 1991).

Surprisingly, in light of the dangers of maternal narcotics abuse to the fetus, it is not recommended that the mother be withdrawn from opioids during pregnancy. Hoegerman and Schnoll (1991) warn that, except in extreme circumstances, the dangers associated with maternal narcotics withdrawal during pregnancy outweigh the potential for harm to the developing fetus. The authors recognize that infants born to mothers who are addicted to narcotics present special needs and require specialized care to survive the first few days of life and beyond. But they cite evidence suggesting that maternal narcotics withdrawal during pregnancy may result in extreme stress for the fetus, possibly resulting in fetal death. Instead, it is recommended that the mother be maintained on methadone during pregnancy. Following delivery, both the mother and child can then be detoxified through the use of methadone (Miller, 1994; Hoegerman & Schnoll, 1991).

Breast-Feeding and Narcotics Use

The narcotics user who is breast-feeding her child will pass some of the drug on to the infant through the milk (Lourwood & Riedlinger, 1989). Although the effects of a single dose of narcotics have only a minimal impact on the child, prolonged use of narcotics may cause the child to become sleepy, eat poorly, and possibly develop respiratory depression.

Because the infant has "immature liver metabolizing functions" (Lourwood & Riedlinger, 1989, p. 85), there is a danger that narcotics will accumulate in the child's body if the mother is using a narcotic analgesic during breast-feeding. Indeed, the baby who is breast-fed by an opiate-abusing mother may actually obtain sufficient amounts of narcotics through breast milk to remain addicted (Zuckerman & Bresnahan, 1991).

Marijuana Use During Pregnancy

Some researchers believe that marijuana is the most commonly abused illicit substance by women of childbearing age (Day & Richardson, 1991). In the United States alone, up to 6 million women of childbearing age use marijuana on a regular basis (Bays, 1990). Still, relatively little is known about the effects of marijuana use on either the pregnant mother or the fetus (Dreher, Nugent, & Hudgins, 1994; Day & Richardson, 1991). Research into the possible effects of maternal marijuana use on fetal growth and development often provides conflicting or inconclusive results, and researchers have yet to uncover a consistent pattern of marijuana-induced effects on the developing fetus. For example, Nahas (1986) concludes that marijuana use during pregnancy may contribute to "intrauterine growth retardation, poor weight gain, prolonged labor, and behavioral abnormalities in the newborn" (p. 83), but other researchers (Behnke & Eyler, 1993; Day & Richardson, 1991) found conflicting evidence. Thus, it is not clear at this time whether marijuana use during pregnancy has an effect on fetal growth.

Roffman and George (1988) report that several research studies have found significant evidence that marijuana use by the pregnant woman may result in developmental problems such as lowered birth weight and possible CNS abnormalities for the fetus. According to Bays (1990), women who use marijuana at least once a month during pregnancy have a higher risk of premature delivery and low birth-weight babies, and their children tend to be smaller than normal for their gestational age.

On the other hand, Dreher, Nugent, and Hudgins (1994) examined 24 babies born in rural Jamaica, where heavy marijuana use is common. These 24 infants were known to have been exposed to marijuana, and their development was contrasted with 20 infants who were not exposed to marijuana. The authors failed to find *any* developmental differences in the two groups that could be attributed to maternal marijuana use. Indeed, where the authors *did* observe differences between the two groups of infants, it was possible to attribute these differences to the mother's social status. Compared to the mothers who did not use marijuana, marijuana-using mothers lived in households with a greater number of adults and fewer children, which allowed more care to be given to the newborn.

Although these studies are suggestive, there is too little known about either the short-term or long-term effects of maternal marijuana use during pregnancy to allow researchers to reach any definite conclusions (Day & Richardson, 1991). Furthermore, it is not possible at the present time to isolate the effects of maternal marijuana use from the effects of poor nutrition, maternal use of other drugs, poor prenatal care, or poor maternal health. However, given the lifelong consequences for the child if maternal marijuana use does have an impact on the fetus, marijuana use during pregnancy should be discouraged.

Breast-Feeding and Marijuana Use

THC, the active agent of marijuana, passes into human milk and is passed on to the infant during breast-feeding. Breast-feeding by mothers who smoke marijuana is thought to result in slower motor development for the child in the first year of life (*Pediatrics for Parents*, 1990; Frank, Bauch-

ner, Zuckerman, & Fried, 1992). Admittedly, this conclusion is based on a preliminary study, but it does suggest a potential hazard that should be avoided, if at all possible.

Benzodiazepine Use During Pregnancy

There is some question as to whether women who are pregnant should use any of the benzodiazepines, especially during the first trimester of pregnancy. In the 1970s, clinical reports surfaced suggesting that the benzodiazepines may contribute to the formation of cleft palates in children, although this conclusion has not been supported by further research (Miller, 1994). Miller (1994) suggests that "If there is a link between diazepam and oral clefts, it is a weak one" (p. 69). However, the prudence of benzodiazepine use during pregnancy is still being challenged. For example, Laegreid, Ragnar, Nils, Hagberg, Wahlstrom, and Abrahamsson (1990) concluded that there is sufficient evidence of benzodiazepine-induced damage to the developing fetus that these drugs should be used only with extreme caution by pregnant women.

Although Miller (1994) found that only 0.4% of the children born to mothers who had used benzodiazepines during pregnancy suffered from facial development problems—and that most of these could be corrected through surgery—the author also found that animal research does suggest *possible* neurological changes in offspring exposed to benzodiazepines prenatally. Thus, until further research can determine whether there is potential danger to the fetus, the benefits of benzodiazepine use should be weighed against the potential for harm before these drugs are used during pregnancy.

Breast-Feeding and Benzodiazepine Use

Because the benzodiazepines are found in the nursing mother's milk, Graedon (1980) suggests that nursing mothers also not use benzodiazepines. Lourwood and Riedlinger (1989) point out that these drugs are metabolized mainly by the liver, an organ that is not fully developed in the infant. They thus conclude that nursing mothers should not use any of the benzodiazepines.

Buspirone and Disulfiram Use During Pregnancy

Buspirone has not been studied in sufficient detail to determine whether it holds potential for harm to the human fetus (Miller, 1994). Animal research on rats found an increased risk for stillbirth when buspirone is used at high dosage levels, but there does not appear to be any effect on the speed with which newborn rats were able to learn, their level of motor activity, or their emotional development.

Animal research on disulfiram suggests that the combination of alcohol with disulfiram is potentially dangerous for the fetus, and so it is not recommended for use in pregnant women (Miller, 1994). Furthermore, animal research suggests that a metabolite of disulfiram, diethyl-dithiocarbamate, may bind to lead and allow this metal to cross the blood-brain barrier and reach the central nervous system. Lead is a known toxin that can cause neurological disorders and mental retardation. There is a need for further research into this potential danger to determine whether disulfiram use may contribute to higher lead levels in humans.

Cigarette Use During Pregnancy

Between 25 and 40% of pregnant women smoke cigarettes (Behnke & Eyler, 1993). Unfortunately, the mother's use of cigarettes is a risk factor for the fetal developmental problems. In fact, the possibility exists that maternal cigarette use during pregnancy might be *worse than maternal cocaine use* in terms of fetal development (Cotton, 1994).

Medical researchers have long known that children born to mothers who smoke during pregnancy are likely to be underweight at birth;

the American Medical Association (AMA) (1993a) estimates that 20% to 30% of the problem of low birth-weight children can be traced to tobacco use. Furthermore, nicotine use during pregnancy seems to be associated with premature labor and delivery and stillbirth. According to American Medical Association (1933a), pregnant women who smoke have a 30% higher risk of stillbirth, and there is a 26% higher risk of infant death within the first few days after birth. Women who smoke or are exposed to cigarette smoke during pregnancy are more likely to suffer spontaneous abortion, decreased blood flow to the uterus, and vaginal bleeding (Lee & D'Alonzo, 1993).

There is also evidence (Olds, Henderson, & Tatelbaum, 1994) that maternal cigarette smoking during pregnancy may contribute to neurological problems for the developing fetus and for subsequent cognitive developmental problems for the child. In their study, the authors found that children born to mothers who smoked 10 or more cigarettes a day during pregnancy scored an average of 4.35 points lower on a standardized intelligence test at ages 3 to 4 than did children born to nonsmoking mothers. The authors concluded that the observed effects were due to maternal cigarette use during pregnancy. Day and Richardson (1994) also report that there is evidence of a link between cigarette smoking and such neurodevelopmental problems as impulsiveness and attention deficits, although it is not clear what role cigarette smoking plays in the development of these problems.

Over-the-Counter Analgesic Use During Pregnancy

Aspirin

Women who are or suspect that they may be pregnant should not use aspirin except under the supervision of a physician (Shannon, Wilson, & Stang, 1992). Aspirin has been implicated as a cause of low birth weight in babies born to women who used it during pregnancy. There is also evidence suggesting that aspirin may be a cause of stillbirth and increased risk of perinatal mortality (United States Pharmacopeial Convention, 1990).

Briggs, Freeman, and Yaffe (1986) explored the impact of maternal aspirin use on both the fetus and the infant whose mother was breast-feeding. The authors report that the use of aspirin by the mother during pregnancy might produce "anemia, antepartum and/or postpartum hemorrhage, prolonged gestation and prolonged labor" (p. 26a). They also found aspirin to be implicated in a significantly higher risk of perinatal mortality and retardation of intrauterine growth when used at high doses by pregnant women. The authors also caution that maternal use of aspirin in the week before delivery may interfere with the newborn's ability to form blood clots. The United States Pharmacopeial Convention (1990) went even further, warning that women should not use aspirin in the last two weeks of pregnancy. Aspirin has been found to cross the placenta, and research suggests that maternal aspirin use during pregnancy may produce higher levels of aspirin in the fetus than in the mother (Briggs, Freeman, & Yaffe, 1986).

Chasnoff (1988) points out that, because the liver of the fetus is not fully developed, it is often difficult to predict the fate of any drug in the fetus' body. And because the fetus often lacks the highly developed renal function of the mother, it is difficult for the fetus to excrete a drug even if the drug could be metabolized into an excretable form. These factors make it difficult to predict the impact of any drug on the fetus.

Briggs, Freeman, and Yaffe (1986) further observe that many "hidden" forms of aspirin are also consumed during pregnancy. According to Chasnoff (1988), between 50 and 60% of women use some form of analgesic during their pregnancy. Such a large number of women using various chemicals under poorly controlled conditions makes it quite difficult to assess the impact of aspirin use on the fetus or the nursing mother (Briggs, Freeman, & Yaffe, 1986). However, Briggs, Freeman, and Yaffe warn that preg-

nant women should not use aspirin or products that contain aspirin on the grounds that the benefit-to-risk ratio of such drug use has not been established.

Breast-Feeding and Aspirin Use

Although there have been no proven problems in women who breast-feed their children, the use of aspirin in women who choose to breast-feed is not recommended (United States Pharmacopeial Convention, 1990; Briggs, Freeman, & Yaffe, 1986). Lourwood and Riedlinger (1989) also suggest that mothers on "high continuing doses" (p. 84) of aspirin should not breast-feed, but they did not warn against occasional use of aspirin.

Acetaminophen

Acetaminophen has been found to be "safe for short-term use" at recommended dosage levels by pregnant women (Briggs, Freeman, & Yaffe, 1986, p. 2a). Although there have been no reports of serious problems in women who have used acetaminophen during pregnancy, Briggs, Freeman, and Yaffe note that the death of one infant from kidney disease shortly after birth was attributed to the mother's continuous use of acetaminophen at high dosage levels during pregnancy. However, there is a need for further research into the effects of this analgesic during pregnancy.

Breast-Feeding and Acetaminophen Use

Although acetaminophen is excreted in low concentrations in the mother's milk, Briggs, Freeman, and Yaffe (1986) found no evidence suggesting that this has any adverse effect on the infant. However, Lourwood and Riedlinger (1989) note that acetaminophen is metabolized mainly by the liver, which is still quite immature in the newborn child. They recommend that the mother who breast-feeds during the immediate postpartum period not use this drug. However, they did not warn against the occasional use of acetaminophen by women who are breast-feeding their children after the postpartum period.

Ibuprofen

It is not recommended that ibuprofen be used during pregnancy. When used at therapeutic dosage levels, this drug has not been found to cause congenital birth defects (Briggs, Freeman, & Yaffe, 1986), but similar drugs have been known to inhibit labor, prolong pregnancy, and possibly cause other problems for the developing child.

Breast-Feeding and Ibuprofen Use

Research suggests that ibuprofen does not enter human milk in significant quantities when used at normal dosage levels (Briggs, Freeman, & Yaffe, 1986). It is thus considered "compatible with breast feeding" (p. 217i). Indeed, Lourwood and Riedlinger (1989) report that ibuprofen is "felt to be the safest" of the nonsteroidal anti-inflammatory drugs for women who are breast-feeding.

Inhalant Use During Pregnancy

Virtually nothing is known about the effects of the various inhalants on the developing fetus. Although only a small percentage of those who experiment with inhalants go on to abuse these chemicals on a chronic basis, more than 50% of those persons who chronically abuse inhalants are women "in their prime childbearing years" (Pearson, Hoyme, Seaver, & Rimsza, 1994, p. 211). It is thus safe to assume that some children are being exposed to one or more of the inhalants during gestation.

Researchers have only just started to study the effects of toluene inhalation on the developing fetus. Toluene is found in many forms of paint and solvents and is known to cross the placenta into the fetal circulation when the mother inhales

its fumes. In adults, about 50% of the toluene inhaled is biotransformed into hippuric acid, and the remainder is excreted unchanged (Pearson et al., 1994), but neither the fetus nor the newborn child has the ability to metabolize toluene. There is thus some question as to whether the effects of toluene exposure for the fetus or newborn are the same as they are for the adult who inhales toluene fumes.

To attempt to answer this question, Pearson et al. (1994) examined 18 infants who were exposed to toluene through maternal paint sniffing during pregnancy. They found several similarities between the effects of toluene and the effects of alcohol on the developing fetus. They found that, as with FAS, toluene exposure during pregnancy may cause a wide range of problems including premature birth, craniofacial abnormalities (such as abnormal ears, thin upper lip, small nose), abnormal muscle tone, renal abnormalities, developmental delays, abnormal hair patterns, and retarded physical growth. To explain the similarities between the effects of toluene abuse and alcohol abuse on the developing fetus, the authors hypothesize that toluene and alcohol may both result in a state of maternal toxicity. This state of maternal toxicity may, in turn, contribute to the fetal malformations. Although this research is only preliminary, it does suggest that toluene exposure during pregnancy may have lifelong consequences for the developing fetus. Until proved otherwise, it would be safe to assume that maternal abuse of the other inhalants would have similar destructive effects on the growing fetus.

Blood Infections Acquired During Pregnancy

Women who abuse injected drugs, such as the narcotics or cocaine, and then share intravenous needles, run the risk of contracting any of a number of infections from other addicts. If a pregnant woman becomes infected, her fetus may be exposed to the same infection. Indeed, children born of mothers who use intravenously administered drugs may develop any of the blood infections commonly found in addicted persons.

It is quite possible for the fetus to acquire AIDS through the mother's blood. Pope and Morin (1990) report that, in New York City, 2% of the babies have HIV antibodies in their blood at the time of birth. Almost one-third of the children born to a woman infected with HIV will themselves be infected with the virus (Glantz & Woods, 1993). Unfortunately, it is not possible to determine which children are infected with HIV at the time of birth; only 30% to 50% of the children who test positive for HIV at birth are actually infected (Revkin, 1989). The other 50% to 70% are "false positives" caused by maternal antibodies that normally circulate in the blood of the fetus before delivery.

These antibodies from the mother's blood may remain in the child's system for up to a year following delivery (McCutchan, 1990). During this time, the mother will not know whether she has a healthy child or a child infected with HIV. This uncertainty makes it difficult for the mother to "bond" with the child because she does not know whether the child will survive.

The transmission of blood-born infections from mother to child often is not thought of as a common problem. Yet in some populations, a significant percentage of the children born have been exposed to one or more infections as a result of the mother's use of intravenous drugs. These children are indeed hidden victims of drug addiction.

Summary

In the past decade, the first steps have been taken toward understanding how drug addiction affects a woman's life. Some evidence suggests that women come to use chemicals for different reasons than men and that they support their addiction through different means. In spite of this evidence, relatively little research has been done on the problem of drug dependency in women.

Infants born to women who have used chemicals of abuse during pregnancy represent a special subpopulation. These children are often born addicted to the drugs the mother used during pregnancy. In many cases, the mother's chemical use during pregnancy causes physical complications for the child, which may include stroke, retardation, low birth weight, and a number of other drug-specific complications. The over-the-counter analgesics present a special area of risk, as the effects of these medications on fetal growth and development are not well understood. However, available research suggests that the OTC analgesics should be used with caution by pregnant or nursing women. Finally, the developing fetus is also at risk of contracting blood infections from the pregnant woman who shares hypodermic needles with other addicts.

CHAPTER TWENTY-ONE

Hidden Faces of Addiction

There are many faces to chemical dependency, and many of these images are familiar to us all. An example is the stereotypical "skid row" alcoholic, drinking a bottle of cheap wine wrapped in a brown paper bag. Another popular image is that of the young male heroin addict with a belt wrapped around his arm, pushing a needle into a vein. A popular stereotype of the chemically addicted woman is that of the "fallen" woman, who is immoral, often a poor parent, and certainly not from the middle or upper social classes.

Unfortunately, as Schneiderman (1990) observes, popular stereotypes of the addict are usually quite persistent and grossly inaccurate. Furthermore, popular stereotypes serve to limit our vision. If the addicted person deviates from our expectations, we may not recognize the chemical dependency hiding behind the social facade. For example, how many of us would expect to meet a white, middle-class, well-groomed heroin addict at work? How many people would recognize the benzodiazepine-dependency behind the smiling face of a day care worker? The purpose of this chapter is to explore some of the hidden faces of chemical dependency to demonstrate the many forms that substance abuse can take.

Women and Addiction: An Often Unrecognized Problem

In the not too distant past, women who were addicted to alcohol or ingredients in "patent medicines" (like opiates and cocaine) outnumbered the men by a factor of 2:1 (Lawson, 1994). As we discussed in earlier chapters, the problem of addiction to chemicals contained in patent medicines was one of the major forces behind the Pure Food and Drug Act of 1906 and subsequent similar laws. Following passage of the Pure Food and Drug Act, the problem of addiction gradually declined, until by the 1950s and early 1960s it was but a footnote in U.S. history. The upsurge in chemical use that began in the 1960s generated a great deal of interest in the impact that chemical use has on the individual. However, although health care professionals have struggled to understand the problem of substance abuse, "the drug literature in general has paid relatively little attention to women" (Griffin, Weiss, Mirin, & Lang, 1989, p. 122; Lawson, 1994; Blume, 1994).

Indeed, the traditional picture of women and chemical abuse is that "only 'bad' women get hooked, that they must be poor or sexually available or weak and stupid" (Lawson, 1994, p. 138).

Unfortunately, the problem of drug addiction among women has only recently received much professional attention (Gossop, Griffiths, & Strang, 1994; Brady, Grice, Dustan, & Randall, 1993). Thus, only now are health care professionals starting to explore whether the popular stereotypes of women addicts are true or not.

Although drug abuse and addiction are common problems among women, the substance abusing woman rarely fits the popular stereotype of a person with a chemical use problem (Lawson, 1994; Joyce, 1989). The woman who is an alcohol or drug addict is not the "fallen woman." She is a person who, like countless thousands of others, has developed a substance abuse or dependency problem.

The Research Bias

Unfortunately, there has been a longstanding bias against research into the problem of drug abuse by women. As a result, much of what we *think* we know about addiction in women is based on the treatment of men. There has been very little research into the possibility that women might offer unique needs, or unique challenges, in the rehabilitation setting. While researchers have learned a lot in the past 15 years, a great deal remains to be discovered about the evolution of substance abuse in women and whether there are significant differences between the needs of male and female addicts.

Statement of the Problem

Currently, it is believed that fully 40% of those who are chemically dependent are women (Lawson, 1994; Anderson, 1993). In spite of the awareness that women make up such a large percentage of the addicted population, researchers have only recently started to understand that there are both obvious and subtle differences in substance use patterns between men and women.

Women appear to be underserved in the area of treatment, both in terms of the number of treatment programs designed to meet their needs, "and of quality of service" by those treatment programs that do exist (Levers & Hawes, 1990, p. 528). For example, while treatment program directors would dispute this claim, fewer than one-third of the treatment programs surveyed were found to have specialized treatment components for women (Wilsnack, 1991). Anderson (1993) arrived at an even more depressing figure, stating that only 10% of the treatment programs in the United States are designed with a woman's special needs in mind, yet 25% of those admitted for alcoholism treatment are women (*Alcoholism & Drug Abuse Week*, 1994a).

Obviously, these are inadequate resources to meet the need of female addicts. This situation is so dismal that Levy and Rutter (1992) maintain that the treatment industry as a whole has failed to meet the needs of women who are addicted to drugs. Certainly, the treatment industry is inadequately servicing women who both are addicted to chemicals and have children (Raskin, 1994).

Gender Differences in Addiction

There are significant differences between men and women in the way that addiction evolves. For example, addicted women enter the rehabilitation system by different routes than do addicted men (Weisner & Schmidt, 1992). Alcohol-addicted women are far more likely than alcoholic men are to suffer from a primary depression (Blume, 1994). Thus, women tend to drift toward mental health counseling, whereas men seek substance abuse treatment, suggesting that there are different treatment "pathways" for the different sexes (Weisner & Schmidt, 1992).

Women who enter the workforce are thought to be two to three times as likely to develop problems with alcohol as are women who do not work outside the home (Kruzicki, 1987). However, addiction is more difficult to detect in the working woman (Pape, 1988). Many women in the workforce are working below their potential capacity, often in low-status, high-frustration positions. Thus, their chemical use is less likely to interfere with their job performance than is true for men (Kruzicki, 1987), making it more difficult to identify women who are abusing drugs or alcohol.

Also, the threat of loss of employment if the addict does not seek treatment is not as effective for women as for men. Many women do not work outside of the home (Kruzicki, 1987), and of those who do, the majority work only to supplement their husband's income. Therefore, it is often easier for a woman to simply quit her job than give in to a threatened loss of employment if she does not seek treatment (Pape, 1988).

Within the past generation, researchers have discovered that women usually obtain their drug of choice in different ways than men do. Unlike male addicts, many female addicts obtain the drugs from their own physician. Indeed, it has been suggested that sedatives and "diet pills" have become "women's drugs" (Peluso & Peluso, 1988, p. 10). Because these women legally obtain their drugs by prescription through the local pharmacy, their drug use has "been rendered invisible" (Peluso & Peluso, 1988, p. 9).

Gender Differences in Drugs' Effects

As medical researchers learn more about the effects of various drugs on men and women, they are starting to uncover significant differences in how each gender responds to different chemicals. Not surprisingly, there are also differences in how men and women react when they use one or more of the popular drugs of abuse.

Narcotics

Griffin et al. (1989) found that female narcotics addicts are likely to have started using opiates at a significantly older age than their male counterparts. But, as a general rule, women who are addicted to narcotics have a history of heavier drug use than male addicts do. At the same time, Griffin et al. found that women addicted to narcotics are approximately the same age as men at the time of their first admission into drug treatment.

On the other hand, Gossop, Griffiths, and Strang (1994) found that, in England, male narcotics addicts are more likely to inject their drug, whereas their female counterparts are more likely to inhale narcotic powder. Female addicts are also more likely to be involved in a sexual relationship with another drug user than are male narcotics addicts. Finally, just under 50% of the female narcotics addicts studied had received drugs as a present from a sexual partner. These findings suggest that narcotics addiction follows a different course for women than it does for men.

Cocaine

Research has also revealed that cocaine use patterns differ between men and women. For example, although women make up approximately 50% of those addicted to cocaine (Lawson, 1994), Griffin et al. (1989) found that female cocaine abusers start drug use at an earlier age than do male cocaine abusers.

Furthermore, the authors found that the typical female cocaine addict is significantly younger at the time of her first admission to a drug treatment program than her male counterpart. The authors also found that male and female cocaine addicts are introduced to the drug in different ways. Again, these findings suggest that cocaine abuse follows a different course for each sex. In spite of this evidence, research into narcotic and cocaine addiction has failed to address the different impact chemicals have on women as compared to men.

Alcohol

There are a number of differences between men and women who drink. First, male and female social drinkers have a different physical response to the alcohol that they consume. The typical woman who drinks on a casual, social basis produces only about half the enzyme gastric alcohol dehydrogenase in her stomach as a man does (for a further discussion of this enzyme, see Chapter 4) (Hennessey, 1992). Furthermore, a woman's blood alcohol level after consuming a given amount of alcohol is higher than a man's who consumes the same amount.

As a general rule, female alcoholics tend to experience physical complications at an earlier point in their drinking history than do male alcoholics. For example, the average length of time for a female alcoholic to develop cirrhosis of the liver is only about 13 years, whereas it may take the typical male alcoholic 22 years to develop the same disorder (Blume, 1994; Hennessey, 1992). For women, there is a known association between alcohol abuse and infertility, miscarriage, amenorrhea, uterine bleeding, dysmenorrhea, osteoporosis, and possibly breast cancer (Cyr & Moulton, 1993; Hennessey, 1992).

However, Beckman (1993) found a positive side, observing that "Women are often first to recognize their drinking problem, while men are more likely to have confrontations, especially with authorities, that bring them involuntarily into contact with treatment caregivers" (p. 236). Thus, according to Beckman, women are more accepting of the treatment process. (However, the author also notes that there are greater social barriers for women who wish to use such resources as AA.)

There is significant evidence to suggest that, when women first enter treatment for alcoholism, their addiction is more severe than what one would expect from their drinking history (Weisner & Schmidt, 1992). It also appears that women are starting to drink alcohol at an earlier age and in far greater quantities than did their older counterparts (Weisner & Schmidt, 1992). Unfortunately, Blume (1994) found that "there is evidence that the alcoholic beverage industry has targeted women as a 'growth market', with advertising designed to make drinking more acceptable to women and to change their drinking patterns" (p. 9). Thus, there is a danger that alcohol-related health and social problems may become issues for a larger percentage of women than has been true in the past.

Until recently, society has hesitated to recognize the problem of drug addiction in women because of the important role women play in society (Peluso & Peluso, 1988). Hopefully, in spite of the new forms of advertising aimed at making alcohol use more attractive to women, society will learn to face the problem of drug addiction in both men and women with openness, with compassion, and with the treatment resources to help the chemically dependent woman.

Addiction and the Elderly

It is difficult for health care professionals to accept the reality that drug addiction is a problem for the elderly, just as it is for younger age groups. The problem of alcohol or drug abuse in the elderly has been described as "staggering" (Liberto, Oslin & Ruskin, 1992, p. 975), and health care researchers now believe that alcohol or drug abuse is the second most common disorder affecting the elderly (Szwabo, 1993). Problem drinking is found in between 5 and 12% of men and 1 and 2% of women in their 60s (Blake, 1990; Hurt, Finlayson, Morse, & Davis, 1988). Some 15% to 20% of older adults abuse chemicals other than alcohol (Szwabo, 1993). Researchers estimate that between *12 and 14%* of older people hospitalized for any reason have a significant problem with alcohol, and that between 5 and 15% (Dunne, 1994; Vandeputte, 1989) and 49% (Blake, 1990) of elderly patients who seek medical treatment for one reason or another also have an alcohol- or drug-related problem.

Adams, Yuan, Barboriak, and Rimm (1993) examined discharge diagnosis statistics across the United States and found that between 19 and 77 of every 10,000 elderly patients admitted to acute care hospitals had an alcohol use disorder. As a comparison, the authors also found that the number of elderly patients being treated for myocardial infarction was between 17 and 44 per 10,000. Thus, the rates of hospital admissions for alcohol-related health problems in the elderly are "similar to those for myocardial infarction" (p. 1224), and may even exceed them.

Elderly widowers also have very high rates of alcohol dependence, with a rate of 105 alcoholic widowers per 1,000 population (Zimberg, 1978). However, even this figure, which translates into 10% of the subgroup of the elderly who have lost their wives, does not give a true picture of the problem of addiction in the elderly. Dunlop, Manghelli, and Tolson (1989) suggest that a staggering 25% of the elderly may be suffering from alcohol-related problems.

According to Abrams and Alexopoulos (1987), "more than 20 percent of patients over 65 years old admitted to a psychiatric hospital in one year could be considered drug dependent" (p. 1286). Hurt et al. (1988) also found a significant chemical dependency problem among the elderly, noting that some 10% of the patients admitted to a chemical dependency treatment unit were over the age of 65. If these figures are accurate, then alcoholism, alcohol abuse, and drug abuse are serious problems for the elderly.

The Consequences of Alcohol and Drug Addiction in the Elderly

Alcohol abuse and addiction in the older individual may either complicate the treatment of other diseases or even cause new medical problems that may become life threatening (Vandeputte, 1989). Because they are more vulnerable to the negative effects of alcohol, older drinkers are more likely to experience medical complications as a result of their drinking than are younger adults (Dunne, 1994; Rains, 1990; Hurt et al., 1988). Alcohol use by the elderly may either influence or cause such medical problems as myopathy, cerebrovascular disease, gastritis, diarrhea, pancreatitis, cardiomyopathy, and various sleep disorders (Liberto, Oslin, & Ruskin, 1992). Other disorders include hypertension, diminished resistance to infections, peripheral muscle weakness, electrolyte and metabolic disturbances, and orthostatic hypotension (a drop in blood pressure upon standing up) (Szwabo, 1993).

Unfortunately, few elderly alcoholics receive treatment for their alcohol or drug addiction (Vandeputte, 1989). As a result, medical costs increase for both the individual, and society.

The Forms of Chemical Abuse in the Elderly

Surprisingly, many older alcoholics have never demonstrated earlier problem drinking. This phenomenon has been termed "late onset alcoholism" by Hurt et al. (1988) or as "reactive alcoholics" by Peluso and Peluso (1989). Perhaps as many as 30% to 50% of the elderly alcoholic population actually began to have problems with alcohol in either middle or late life (Liberto, Oslin, & Ruskin, 1992).

Zimberg (1978) classifies older alcoholics into three subgroups: (1) those who develop drinking problems only late in life; (2) those who have a history of intermittent problem drinking over the years but who develop a more chronic alcohol problem only in late adulthood; and (3) those whose alcohol problems start in young adulthood and continue into the later years. Zimberg further classifies the second and third groups together in a category called "early-onset" (p. 240) alcoholism. This subgroup is thought to include about two-thirds of the older alcoholics. Those who demonstrate alcohol problems only in the later phases of life are said to have "late-onset" (p. 240) alcoholism and are thought to make up about one-third of the elderly alcoholic population.

Abrams and Alexopoulos (1987) found several forms of drug misuse in the elderly, including (1) intentional overuse of a medication, (2) intentional underuse of a medication, (3) erratic use of a prescribed medication, or (4) unintentional misuse by failing to provide the physician a complete drug history, including use of over-the-counter medications. The intentional misuse of prescribed medications was the largest category of drug abuse in the elderly (Abrams & Alexopoulos, 1987). However, the authors found that the elderly are far more likely to engage in *under*utilization as opposed to *over*utilization of prescription medications, mainly for financial reasons.

Detecting Chemical Abuse in the Elderly

Alcoholism is less likely to be detected in the elderly than in other age groups for a number of reasons (Dunne, 1994; Rains, 1990; Anderson, 1989b). First, traditional symptoms of excessive drinking, such as the number of drinks consumed, are poor indicators of alcoholism in the elderly. Research has shown that "Three beers at age 60 may have the same effect as 12 at age 21" (Anderson, 1989b, p. 7ex). But, unfortunately, the "impairments in social and occupational functioning attributable to alcoholism in younger people are not as obvious" in the elderly (Abrams & Alexopoulos, 1987, p. 1285). Alcohol-related problems such as blackouts, financial difficulties, and job losses in an older population are often attributed not to the individual's drinking but to medical or age-related psychosocial problems (Szwabo, 1993). For example, alcohol's effects on the individual's cognitive abilities mimic those changes associated with normal aging. Even trained physicians find it difficult to differentiate between late-onset Korsakoff's syndrome and different forms of senile dementia such as Alzheimer's disease (Anderson, 1989b; Blake, 1990; Rains, 1990).

At the same time, because of the physical effects of aging, older alcoholics are less able to withstand the physical impact of drinking (Blake, 1990; Rains, 1990). For example, even social drinking is thought to be associated with cognitive deterioration in the elderly (Abrams & Alexopoulos, 1987; Rains, 1990).

Another factor that makes it difficult to detect alcoholism in the elderly is that older alcoholics rarely announce their plans in advance (Peluso & Peluso, 1989; Vandeputte, 1989). Imagine the shock in the family if grandmother or grandfather were to announce at the dinner table that "I'm going out tonight and get wasted!" In addition, the elderly are more likely to be steady drinkers than binge drinkers, and their alcohol consumption is more likely to be private than

public. They rarely get into situations in which their drinking is obvious, such as bar-room fights, and alcohol-related blackouts are often attributed to nonalcohol-related medical problems (Peluso and Peluso, 1989).

Finally, family and friends may feel ashamed, hurt, or guilty and so may hesitate to report the addicted person's problem (Peluso & Peluso, 1989; Vandeputte, 1989). For this reason, many elderly addicts never receive treatment.

Depression in older individuals could be secondary to the use of alcohol or drugs. Unfortunately, this possibility is often overlooked by mental health professionals (Szwabo, 1993; Vandeputte, 1989). As a result, the depressed older patient may unintentionally receive the wrong treatment by health care workers who are unaware of the cause of the depression.

As a group, the elderly are especially vulnerable to alcohol-induced drug interactions. The elderly make up 12% of the population and use 40% of all prescription and OTC medications (Szwabo, 1993). Furthermore, as a group, the elderly require more time to metabolize many drugs. Between 7 and 10% of those over the age of 55 have an alcohol abuse problem that places them at risk for alcohol-drug interactions, but few health care providers search for alcohol use in the elderly. All too often, the result is potentially deadly combinations of medications and alcohol (Peluso & Peluso, 1989).

The Treatment of the Older Alcoholic

Unfortunately, only a minority of elderly persons with a drug or alcohol problem are currently receiving help for that problem. Addiction in the elderly is underrecognized, underreported, and undertreated. In addition, the older alcoholic or drug abusing patient presents special treatment needs rarely found in younger addicts. Yet few treatment programs are geared to meet the needs of the older drug or alcohol abusing patient (Szwabo, 1993).

To meet these special treatment needs, Dunlop, Manghelli, and Tolson (1989) recommend that treatment programs for the elderly include the following components.

1. A primary prevention program to warn about the dangers of using alcohol as a coping mechanism for life's problems.
2. An outreach program to identify and serve older alcoholics who might be overlooked by more traditional treatment services.
3. Detoxification services personnel trained and experienced in working with the elderly, who frequently require longer detoxification periods than younger addicted persons.
4. Protective environments for the elderly, or structured living environments that allow the individual to take part in treatment while being protected from the temptation of further alcohol or drug use.
5. Primary treatment programs for those who could benefit from either inpatient or outpatient short-term primary treatment programs.
6. Aftercare programs to help the older alcoholic make the transition from primary care to independent living.
7. Long-term residential care for those who suffer from severe medical or psychiatric complications from alcoholism.
8. Access to social work support services.

Older alcoholics or drug abusers may require weeks or even months to fully detoxify from alcohol or drugs (Anderson, 1989b). Rains (1990) suggests that older alcoholics may require up to 18 months of abstinence to fully recover from the effects of drinking. Thus, the standard 21- to 28-day inpatient treatment program may fail to meet the needs of an elderly client who would hardly have completed the detoxification process before being discharged as "cured." Older adults may also require help in building a non-alcoholic support structure to enable them to break the bonds of their drinking behavior (Anderson, 1989b).

Treatment professionals must help older addicts deal with more than just their chemical addiction. For example, in addition to their drinking problem, older alcoholics are also experiencing age-specific stressors such as retirement, bereavement, loneliness, and the effects of physical illness (Dunlop, Manghelli, & Tolson, 1989; Zimberg, 1978).

On the bright side, however, is evidence suggesting that the elderly respond better to treatment than do younger alcoholics (Blake, 1990; Rains, 1990; Abrams & Alexopoulos, 1987). Group therapy approaches that include a problem-solving and social-support component are thought to be useful in working with older alcoholics, especially if such programs include Alcoholics Anonymous (Rains, 1990; Dunlop, Manghelli, & Tolson, 1989; Zimberg, 1978).

To be effective, treatment programs that work with older clients must address their special needs (Vandeputte, 1989; Dunlop, Manghelli, & Tolson, 1989). In addition to requiring longer detoxification periods, the older client often has a slower physical and mental pace than younger individuals, presents a range of sensory deficits, and very often dislikes the profanity commonly used by younger individuals in treatment (Dunlop, Manghelli, & Tolson, 1989). Unless these special needs are addressed, the individual is unlikely to be motivated to participate in treatment. However, when their needs are met, the elderly alcoholic often responds well to treatment and learns to utilize available resources to remain sober.

The Homosexual Substance Abuser

The homosexual male or the lesbian woman constitute another "hidden minority" (Fassinger, 1991, p. 157) within U.S. society. Estimates of the percentage of the population that is gay vary, with high estimates suggesting that 20% of the male population has had a homosexual experience, and between 1 and 6% of the male population has had a homosexual encounter in the last year (Seidman & Rieder, 1994). Society's response to individuals who have adopted a nontraditional form of sexuality has frequently been less than supportive, and many gay and lesbian individuals feel ostracized by a culture that neither understands nor encourages a homosexual lifestyle. Thus, the homosexual may live on the fringes of society.

Within the gay community, the "gay bar" assumes a role of central importance where homosexuals can socialize without fear of ridicule or harassment (Paul, Stall, & Bloomfield, 1991). The bar also plays a role for both gays and lesbians in discovering their sexuality. Although the homosexual bar thus may serve a useful function, its central importance within the gay community may contribute to alcohol or drug problems.

Research suggests that there is a significantly higher alcoholism rate for gay men and lesbian women than for the general population. Indeed, it has been estimated that 25% to 35% of the homosexual population meets the formal diagnostic criteria for alcoholism or drug dependency (Klinger & Cabaj, 1993). And, as a group, lesbians have higher rates of substance abuse than do nongay women of the same age (Klinger & Cabaj, 1993; Browning, Reynolds, & Dworkin, 1991).

There are a number of reasons for this association between homosexuality and alcohol abuse. Some individuals who are uncomfortable with their sexual orientation or who may anticipate rejection once their sexual preference is known may use alcohol or drugs to assuage feelings of shame or guilt (Paul, Stall, & Bloomfield, 1991). Paul, Stall, and Bloomfield found that individuals who experienced negative feelings surrounding their sexual orientation tended to use alcohol to reduce internal tension. Also, as noted above, the homosexual bar plays an important role within the gay community, often providing the only safe environment within which the individual can explore his or her sexuality.

However, it has been suggested that research samples drawn from the gay bar scene may have *inflated* estimates of alcoholism among the gay and lesbian population (Friedman & Downey, 1994). Many researchers have used the gay bar as a place to recruit potential subjects. Because the bar serves a large number of homosexual clients, it offers the researcher a chance to reach a large number of potential volunteers at once. However, statistically, those people who are most likely to frequent the bar are also more likely to have alcohol or drug problems. Therefore, individuals who were not alcohol or drug users would be underrepresented in a research sample drawn from a homosexual "bar" population.

Because of this bias, it is unfortunately impossible to determine the prevalence of alcohol and drug use problems among the gay and lesbian population (Friedman & Downey, 1994). There is also little research into the special health care needs of the gay or lesbian client, and virtually no research into what treatment methods are effective for the substance abusing homosexual. However, given estimates that gays and lesbians make up 10% to 15% of the population (Fassinger, 1991) and the estimate that approximately one-third of homosexuals abuse chemicals, a significant percentage of those in treatment for substance abuse problems live a nontraditional lifestyle.

However, the vast majority of substance abuse professionals believe that their training for meeting the needs of gay and lesbian clients was only "fair" at best. Indeed, in almost 40% of the cases, substance abuse counselors received no formal training in how to work effectively with homosexuals (Hellman, Stanton, Lee, Tytun, & Vachon, 1989). Only a small number of specialized treatment programs for homosexuals exist, and these programs are usually located in major metropolitan areas (Hellman et al., 1989).

Although there is a growing trend for specialized AA groups oriented toward the needs of gay and lesbian members (Paul, Stall, & Bloomfield, 1991), these groups are not widespread. There is thus a significant need for substance abuse counselors to become aware of the special treatment needs presented by a gay or lesbian client and to receive the training necessary to meet these needs effectively.

Substance Abuse and the Disabled

Very little research has been conducted in the area of substance use patterns among the disabled (Tyas & Rush, 1993). Nelipovich and Buss (1991) suggest that, in the United States, between 15 and 30% of the 33 to 45 million people with disabilities abuse alcohol or drugs. This rate is between 1.5 and 3 times higher than that found in the general population.

Nelipovich and Buss (1991) reviewed the treatment resources for the physically disabled available in Wisconsin and concluded that "as a group, this is a highly underserved population" (p. 344). Rather than being identified as a special-needs subgroup, the disabled are often "perceived as isolated occasional cases, only remembered because of the difficulty and frustration they present to the professionals trying to serve them" (p. 344). The authors call for "creativity" (p. 345) on the part of rehabilitation staff who are attempting to meet the needs of the disabled substance-abusing client.

Only a minority of treatment programs have the special resources (like wheelchair ramps) necessary for working with the disabled. Indeed, many programs would rather not serve this sub-population (Tyas & Rush, 1993), although drug *dealers* are only too happy to offer their services to the disabled. There are indications that at least some drug dealers are specifically targeting the hearing impaired, going so far as to learn sign language or recruit assistants who know sign language so they can sell drugs to the hearing impaired (Associated Press, 1993). Unfortunately, in the United States, the physically disabled form an invisible subgroup of chemical abusers, and so are hidden victims of drug abuse and addiction.

Substance Abuse and Ethnic Minorities

Virtually nothing is known about the natural history of substance abuse in the various minority groups in the United States. Franklin (1989), for example, found that, of 16,000 articles on alcoholism published between 1934 and 1974, only 11 "were specifically studies of blacks" (p. 1120), and virtually no research has been done on the subject of alcoholism and the black woman. According to Franklin, compared to white alcoholics, blacks "have a higher incidence of medical complications from alcoholism" (p. 1120), possibly as much as ten times what would be seen in a similar group of white alcoholics. Within the black community, Alcoholics Anonymous (AA) has become a significant part of the treatment and recovery process.

It should also be noted that there is virtually no research on the subject of alcohol or substance abuse among Native Americans, Chinese Americans, Japanese Americans, or Asian Americans. What little is known—or thought to be known—about alcohol or substance abuse patterns within these subgroups is based on studies involving mostly white subjects. Obviously, there is a need for research into the impact of substance use in these subgroups and into what treatment methods may be of value in working with members of each minority group.

Summary

We all have a stereotypical image of what an addict looks like. For some, this is the picture of the "skid row" alcoholic; for others, it is the picture of a heroin addict, sitting in the ruins of an abandoned building, ready to inject the drug into a vein. Although these images are based on reality, each image fails to accurately reflect the many hidden faces of addiction.

There is the grandfather who is quietly drinking himself to death, or the mother who exposes her unborn child to staggering amounts of cocaine, heroin, or alcohol. There is the working woman whose chemical addiction is hidden behind a veil of productivity or whose drug addiction is sanctioned by an unsuspecting physician, trying to relieve her depression or anxiety. There are faces of addiction so well hidden that even today they go unrecognized. As professionals, we must learn to look for and identify the hidden victims of addiction.

CHAPTER TWENTY-TWO

The Dual-Diagnosis Client: Addiction and Mental Illness

For the past decade, mental health professionals have known that alcohol or chemical abuse is a factor in at least one-third of the psychiatric problems encountered in therapy (Galanter, Castaneda, & Ferman, 1988). Substance abuse is also involved in approximately 60% of all first-time adult psychiatric admissions for inpatient treatment (Willoughby, 1984). In spite of this knowledge, mental health professionals have only an "inadequate understanding of the complex relationship between other psychiatric illnesses and substance use disorders" (Decker & Ries, 1993, p. 703). In this chapter, we will examine the problem of chemical abuse among individuals who also suffer from a mental illness.

A History of the Problem

There was a time when the problem of drug abuse or dependency among the mentally ill was all but ignored. Until quite recently, the problem of drug abuse or addiction in the mentally ill was thought to be quite rare and so was often overlooked by health care professionals, if only because they did not bother to look for it to begin with. If the client did abuse chemicals—even if openly addicted—the drug use was assumed to be secondary to the "primary" disease of mental illness. Mental health professionals were taught to believe that the substance abuse or addiction

would automatically go away when the "primary" psychiatric problem was resolved.

This view of the relationship between substance use disorders and mental illness did not begin to change until the early 1980s. Since then, health care professionals have come to understand more about the nature of mental illness and substance abuse, and they have discovered that the so-called dual-diagnosis client is not as rare as was once thought (Minkoff, 1989). Indeed, drug abuse or addiction is *seven times* as prevalent and alcohol abuse or addiction is *ten times as prevalent* among the mentally ill as in the general population (Kivlahan, Heiman, Wright, Mundt, & Shupe, 1991).

However, for all that has been discovered about the substance abuse problem among the mentally ill, much is left to learn. Mental health and substance abuse professionals have reached the point where they acknowledge that a drug abuse problem may exist among those who suffer from mental illness. However, beyond this vague acknowledgment that a problem exists, little is known about the dual-diagnosis patient population.

Definition of Dual Diagnosis

The first step in working with a dual-diagnosis client is to identify exactly what we mean when we say a client has a "dual diagnosis." The term *dual diagnosis* has been applied to a wide range of coexisting problems, including combinations of substance abuse or addiction and anorexia, bulimia, gambling, spousal abuse, and AIDS. For the purpose of this text, the term *dual diagnosis,* or *MI/CD* (mentally ill/chemically dependent) will be applied to individuals with a coexisting psychiatric disorder and substance abuse problem.

Protracted chemical use may result in the client developing any of a wide range of psychiatric syndromes, depending on the specific agents being used. The chronic cocaine user, for example, may experience a postcocaine depression of suicidal proportions, whereas the amphetamine addict may develop an amphetamine-related paranoia that closely resembles paranoid schizophrenia.

Furthermore, as you may recall from Chapter 4, there is a strong relationship between alcohol use and short-term depression, which usually resolves within a few days to a few weeks after abstinence has been achieved. However, the fact that so many drugs of abuse can cause the individual to suffer from what appears to be a psychiatric disorder illustrates how difficult it can be to accurately diagnose a drug-induced disorder (Galanter, Castaneda, & Ferman, 1988). Although drug-induced disorders are a significant problem, they are not primary psychiatric dysfunctions; rather, they are secondary to the individual's chemical use.

Dual-diagnosis clients, as noted above, are those clients who suffer from mental illness and also abuse or are addicted to chemicals. MI/CD clients form a distinct subpopulation of drug abusers or addicts. In the dual-diagnosis client, the mental illness and the substance abuse or addiction are separate, chronic disorders, each with an independent course, yet each able to influence the progression of the other (Carey, 1989).

The term *mentally ill* is itself quite vague. There are a range of different conditions, each with a different etiology, different treatments, and different possible outcomes that are lumped together under the heading of "mental illness"

(Weiss, Mirin, & Frances, 1992). The term *dual-diagnosis client,* although serving to identify a subset of substance abusers, is still only a vague term that fails to communicate much information about the client's unique strengths or needs.

For example, consider four hypothetical dual-diagnosis patients. The first patient suffers from schizophrenia and uses marijuana and alcohol. The second patient has a personality disorder and is addicted to alcohol. The third patient struggles with a phobic disorder and is addicted to benzodiazepines. The last patient suffers from a major depressive disorder and is addicted to heroin. Each of these patients would be classified as "mentally ill"; each of these patients also is abusing or addicted to chemicals. As such, each patient qualifies as a dual-diagnosis patient. Yet the treatment approach utilized in working with the depressed individual would be far different from the one used in working with the client who suffers from schizophrenia, and both would be different from the treatment approach for the personality disordered patient. And all three treatment approaches would be vastly different from one utilized in the treatment of a patient with a phobia.

Much of the literature that addresses the dual-diagnosis patient focuses on the problem of psychosis (usually schizophrenia) and substance abuse. There is virtually no information available, for example, on the phobic patient who also is abusing chemicals. There is a great deal that we still must learn about the myriad ways in which substance abuse and the various forms of mental illness may interact.

Dual-Diagnosis Clients: A Diagnostic Challenge

Dual-diagnosis clients represent a special challenge to treatment professionals (Riley, 1994), partly because the diagnosis of concurrent problems like mental illness and substance abuse is so difficult (Twerski, 1989). Often, it is not possible for the patient to achieve any degree of emotional stability or for staff to make an accurate diagnosis until the client is drug-free (Carey, 1989; Rado, 1988; Wallen & Weiner, 1989; Evans & Sullivan, 1990). Indeed, it may be necessary for the patient to be drug-free for *up to 4 to 6 weeks* before an accurate diagnosis can be made (Nathan, 1991).

To further complicate the diagnostic picture, the MI/CD client may be unable to discuss his or her chemical use because of the ongoing psychiatric problems (Kanwischer & Hundley, 1990). For example, the schizophrenic patient may be too disorganized to discuss his or her chemical use, and the phobic patient may be unwilling to give up what he or she considers to be an essential coping mechanism for his or her anxiety.

Dual-diagnosis clients may also actively attempt to hide their drug use from mental health professionals (Shaner, Khalsa, Roberts, Wilkins, Anglin, & Hsiech, 1993). They may do so because direct questions about alcohol or drug use contribute to feelings of defensiveness or shame (Pristach & Smith, 1990). Other dual-diagnosis patients may fear the loss of entitlements (such as Social Security or welfare payments) or be afraid that they will be denied access to psychiatric treatment if they admit to having a substance abuse problem (Mueser, Bellack, & Blanchard, 1992). But denial is also a trait found in people who are addicted to chemicals. Thus, some MI/CD clients deny their substance use problem for the same reasons other addicts do: they want to avoid admitting that they are addicted to chemicals.

These factors, either alone or collectively, help make the dual-diagnosis client quite difficult to identify. It is not uncommon for treatment professionals to require a period of weeks or even months in which to gather sufficient information to make an accurate diagnosis.

Why Worry About the Dual-Diagnosis Client?

Once, while talking to a psychiatrist about a specific client, a clinical psychologist mentioned his concern about the patient's alcohol use. The patient, who had been institutionalized for chronic schizophrenia for many years, visited a local bar once or twice a month for a few drinks. The psychiatric staff at the state hospital tolerated this patient's drinking while on occasional unsupervised "passes" from the campus, justifying the behavior on the grounds that the patient was an adult and drinking was one of his few remaining pleasures.

Unfortunately, research now suggests that even limited drug use by a mentally ill client may exacerbate a separate psychiatric disorder, complicating the individual's treatment for either disorder (Cohen & Levy, 1992; Evans & Sullivan, 1990; Ries & Ellingson, 1990; Rubinstein, Campbell, & Daley, 1990; Pristach & Smith, 1990; Drake, Osher, & Wallach, 1989). For example, Drake, Osher, and Wallach (1989) found that even minimal use of alcohol by schizophrenic patients—amounts clearly not abusive by traditional standards—was one factor that predicted which clients would require rehospitalization within a year. Alcohol can easily magnify feelings of depression, contributing to the client's distress. Use of chemicals by patients with psychiatric disorders often complicates the treatment of their mental illness.

Drug abuse traditionally has been viewed by mental health professionals as a negative influence on the course of the psychiatric disorder (Osher et al., 1994; Kivlahan, Heiman, Wright, Mundt, & Shupe, 1991; Rubinstein, Campbell, & Daley, 1990; Miller & Tanenbaum, 1989; Stoffelmayr, Benishek, Humphreys, Lee, & Mavis, 1989). In addition to exacerbating the psychiatric dysfunction, substance abuse by schizophrenic patients places an additional strain on the family in terms of economic investment (Clark, 1994).

In one study, Clark (1994) attempted to calculate the cash value of direct payments, time spent with the client, lost career opportunities, and stress-related illness for family members of dual-diagnosis clients. The estimated level of family assistance to dual-diagnosis clients was between $9,703 and $13,547 a year, whereas the value of family assistance to "adult children" without a chronic illness was, at most, $3,547 per year. Thus, there is a financial consequence for the family when one member has a dual disorder of mental illness and substance abuse.

Substance abuse may also contribute to family conflicts. As the family withdraws from the patient as a result of the increased level of conflict, his or her available social support base becomes smaller. Furthermore, psychiatric patients with weaker social support systems tend to require longer and more frequent periods of hospitalization. For example, psychiatric patients who abuse chemicals on a regular basis have hospitalization rates 250% higher than those individuals who rarely or never abused chemicals (Kanwischer & Hundley, 1990).

Thus, evidence suggests that drug use by a psychiatric patient complicates the treatment of the individual's psychiatric condition in a number of ways (Kay, Kalathara, & Meinzer, 1989). When one considers the level of pain experienced by the mentally ill, the cost of lost productivity, the cost of hospitalization and treatment, and then adds the financial, social, and personal cost brought on by substance abuse by the mentally ill, the need to address this problem becomes clear.

The Scope of the Problem

It has been estimated that, for the MI/CD population, the combined effects of substance abuse and mental illness has resulted in a loss of $273 billion in terms of productivity (Riley, 1994). By the end of the 20th century, this figure should stand close to $300 billion a year in lost productivity.

Researchers have found that substance abuse is at least twice as common in the mentally ill as in the general population (Brown, Ridgely, Pepper, Levine, & Ryglewicz, 1989; Regier et al., 1990). Indeed, evidence suggests that between one-third and one-half of psychiatric patients also have an alcohol or drug abuse problem (Evans & Sullivan, 1990; Regier et al., 1990;

Carey, 1989). Shaner et al. (1993) found that more than one-third of the sample of schizophrenic patients admitted to the abuse of CNS stimulants in the 6 months prior to their study.

The tendency to abuse alcohol or chemicals seems to be most frequently found in younger mentally ill clients (Drake, Osher, & Wallach, 1989), especially in young adult male psychiatric patients (Szuster, Schanbacher, & McCann, 1990). However, these findings may be misleading, because younger people are also more likely to have been exposed to a drug-using subculture than are older individuals (Kovasznay, Bromet, Schwartz, Ranganathan, Lavelle, & Brandon, 1993). Thus, it is not clear at this time whether the tendency for younger mentally ill patients to have abused chemicals reflects a specific form of psychopathology or the general tendency for youths in U.S. society to have used chemicals.

What is clear from the literature is that a significant percentage of those with some form of mental illness *have* abused chemicals. Brown et al. (1989) estimate that, in the younger mentally ill population, the "substance abuse rate approaches or exceeds 50%" (p. 566), a conclusion supported by others (Kanwischer & Hundley, 1990; Evans & Sullivan, 1990; Miller & Tanenbaum, 1989).

These clients are hidden victims of drug dependency. One reason they remain hidden is that psychiatrists are often not trained to detect substance abuse problems, especially in the mentally ill (Cohen & Levy, 1992). Furthermore, dual-diagnosis clients are heterogeneous in terms of psychiatric diagnosis, the drug(s) abused, and the impact that drug use has had on their lives (Osher & Kofoed, 1989; Kanwischer & Hundley, 1990). Lacking a pattern to look for, mental health professionals often fail to recognize the possibility that a mentally ill client may also have a substance abuse problem (Cohen & Levy, 1992; Peyser, 1989).

In a study by Ananth, Vandewater, Kamal, Brodsky, Gamal, and Miller (1989), a sample of 75 psychiatric patients, each of whom had al-

75 psychiatric patients, each of whom had already been seen and diagnosed by mental health professionals, were reevaluated after being admitted for psychiatric treatment. None of these patients had been diagnosed as having an alcohol or drug abuse problem at the time of admission. The authors found that 54 of the 75 subjects should also have received a diagnosis of either drug abuse, or drug dependence, in addition to their psychiatric diagnosis. Ten of the 54 subjects found to be using drugs were also either abusing or were addicted to alcohol, and 2 additional subjects were found to meet the diagnostic criteria for only alcohol abuse or dependence. Thus, of the 75 patients who had been admitted for psychiatric treatment, 75% also had an undiagnosed alcohol or drug abuse problem.

Unfortunately, just when mental health professionals are starting to understand the scope of the problem of MI/CD patients, "fewer and fewer clinics are accepting clients with this profile" (Rado, 1988, p. 5). And the total number of dual-diagnosis clients appears to be increasing. One possible explanation for this phenomenon is that professionals are becoming more aware of the existence of drug addiction in psychiatric patients and are identifying dual-diagnosis patients more often (Rado, 1988). Although mental health professionals are becoming aware of the need to diagnose and treat psychiatric patients with a substance use disorder, MI/CD clients are often refused treatment at either psychiatric or chemical dependency treatment centers (Cohen & Levy, 1992; Penick et al., 1990; Kofoed, Kania, Walsh, & Atkinson, 1986).

Characteristics of Dual-Diagnosis Clients

There is little agreement as to the characteristics of the MI/CD client. Until quite recently, researchers have generally centered their attention on the subpopulation of schizophrenic patients who abuse chemicals. However, researchers still disagree as to the characteristics of even this small subgroup of MI/CD patients (Cuffel, Heithoff, & Lawson, 1993).

Some believe that the dual-diagnosis patient is usually less impaired but also more suicidal, homicidal, and impulsive than general psychiatric patients (Kay, Kalathara, & Meinzer, 1989; Szuster, Schanbacher, & McCann, 1990). Others (Zisook, Heaton, Moranville, Kuck, Jernigan, & Braff, 1992; Mueser, Yarnold, & Bellack, 1992) claim that the dual-diagnosis client is less severely psychotic and more intelligent than non–drug-abusing patients with similar psychiatric conditions.

In contrast, Osher et al. (1994) conclude that the use of alcohol by dual-diagnosis clients (who are mainly schizophrenic) is

> associated with several aspects of poor adjustment including increased delusional symptoms . . . , depressive symptoms . . . , suicide . . . , disruptive behaviors . . . , assaultiveness . . . , treatment noncompliance . . . , housing instability and homelessness . . . , high rates of rehospitalization . . . , and generally poorer clinical outcomes. (p. 109)

And Stoffelmayr et al. (1989) suggest that dual-diagnosis clients may suffer from more generalized problems in living than do clients who do not suffer from both a psychiatric and chemical dependency problem. In other words, the authors view the MI/CD client as more impaired than the typical psychiatric patient.

In spite of this lack of consensus on the characteristics of the MI/CD population, some conclusions can be drawn about the dual-diagnosis patient group. First, available evidence suggests that although mental illness and chemical dependency are separate, chronic disorders, each has the power to influence the course of the other (Carey, 1989). For example, psychiatric patients who abuse alcohol are more likely to be rehospitalized following their stabilization in an inpatient treatment center (Osher et al., 1994; Lyons & McGovern, 1989; Drake, Osher, & Wallach, 1989). The reverse is also true: psychiatric clients who also have substance use disorders seem to have more trouble staying sober.

Second, in general terms, dual-diagnosis clients are extremely vulnerable to the effects of chemicals (Brown et al., 1989; Drake, Osher, & Wallach, 1989). Although recreational chemical use does not *cause* the mental illness, the biological vulnerabilities that resulted in the mental illness seem to indicate that the MI/CD client is especially vulnerable to the effects of recreational chemical use.

This conclusion is consistent with Drake and Wallach's (1993) finding that individuals with severe mental illness are only rarely able to use chemicals such as alcohol on a social or recreational basis. The authors found that, for MI/CD clients, "nonproblematic drinking often becomes an alcohol use disorder . . . over the long term" (p. 781). Although there is little research into moderate drinking among individuals with severe mental illness, Drake and Wallach found that only 5% of two different samples were able to continue to engage in nonproblematic drinking over time.

MI/CD clients also tend to be "binge" users rather than steady users of recreational substances (Riley, 1994). And it has been suggested that, as a group, dual-diagnosis clients are at high risk for suicide (Mueser, Bellack, & Blanchard, 1992; Ries & Ellingson, 1990). They also tend to be more manipulative than traditional psychiatric patients (Mueser, Bellack, & Blanchard, 1992; Kay, Kalathara, & Meinzer, 1989), a trait that contributes to the perception that MI/CD clients are difficult to work with.

Psychopathology and Drug of Choice

One popular theory is that MI/CD patients are attempting to "self-medicate" emotional pain through chemical use. That is, they use chemicals in an attempt to treat, or at least control, the symptoms of their psychiatric condition.

Studies such as the one conducted by Test, Wallisch, Allness, and Ripp (1990) support this hypothesis. They found that alcohol was the most frequently abused chemical in their sample, followed by marijuana. When asked why they used the chemical(s) that they did, the drug-abusing schizophrenic patients reported that their drug of choice helped them deal with feelings of anxiety, insomnia, boredom, depression, and the side effects of prescribed antipsychotic medications.

But this research has not been replicated in other studies. For example, Kivlahan et al. (1991) found that 71% of their sample of 60 volunteers being treated at an outpatient community support program for schizophrenia would qualify for a diagnosis of a "substance abuse disorder" at some point in their lives. Surprisingly, the authors found that marijuana, not alcohol, was the most frequently abused drug for their sample population. Eighty-eight percent of their sample used marijuana at least occasionally; other drugs being abused were amphetamines (used by 30% of their sample at some point), alcohol (22%), hallucinogenics (18%), and cocaine and narcotics (both used by 13% of the total sample at some point).

The conflicting results of these two investigations may be explained by the results obtained by Cuffel, Heithoff, and Lawson (1993). They examined the drug use patterns of 231 individuals who were diagnosed as suffering from schizophrenia and found that individuals in their sample tended to follow one of three different substance abuse patterns. First were those individuals who did not abuse chemicals, a group that made up 54% of the total sample. The second group consisted of individuals with schizophrenia, who tended to abuse alcohol, marijuana, or both; this subgroup made up 31% of the sample. Last were those individuals who suffered from schizophrenia and were "polysubstance" abusers, a group that made up only 14% of the overall sample.

Cuffel, Heithoff, and Lawson (1993) found that, although individuals with schizophrenia most commonly abuse alcohol, and/or marijuana, there is no apparent relationship between drug of choice and psychiatric diagnosis. The authors did find a weak statistical association between depressive symptoms and substance abuse, but not between schizophrenia and substance abuse patterns. This study suggests that there may not be any specific relationship between form of psychiatric illness and the individual's drug of choice.

In a pair of unrelated studies, Mueser, Yarnold, and Bellack (1992) and Kovasznay et al. (1993) also failed to find any significant pattern between the drugs abused and the patient's diagnosis. Mueser, Yarnold, and Bellack (1992) did find a weak trend for patients with a diagnosis of bipolar affective disorder (once called "manic-depressive psychosis") to abuse alcohol. However, they failed to find other consistent trends for drug use among the mentally ill patients they studied.

Dunn, Paolo, Ryan, and Van Fleet (1993) found that *over 41%* of the dual-diagnosis patients sampled may also have some form of dissociative disorder. The dissociative disorders are marked by episodes in which the individual loses touch with reality. In its most extreme form, the individual develops more than one personality, a condition known as *multiple personality disorder* (or MPD). However, most patients who suffer from a dissociative disorder do not develop MPD, although they do have episodes in which they "disconnect" from reality.

There appears to be a relationship between patients with dissociative disorders and substance abuse (Kolodner & Frances, 1993; Dunn et al., 1993). Although the diagnosis of a dissociative disorder is quite complex, Kolodner and Frances (1993) offer two diagnostic indicators for the patient with coexisting substance abuse and dissociative disorders. First, unlike "regular" patients who are addicted to chemicals, patients with dissociative disorders do not feel better after completing the detoxification stage of treatment. Rather, patients with dissociative disorders tend to experience significant levels of emotional pain after detoxification from chemicals. Kolodner and Frances (1993) also suggest that patients who suffer from dissociative disorders relapse at times of "relative comfort and

clinical stability" (p. 1042). This is in contrast to "regular" substance abusing patients, who are thought to relapse when under stress (see Chapter 27). The authors suggest that these situations may alert the clinician to the possibility that the patient suffers from a dissociative disorder, which can then be addressed in treatment.

As mentioned earlier, the most serious form of a dissociative disorder is the multiple personality disorder. Perhaps one-third of those who suffer from MPD are thought to also abuse chemicals (Putnam, 1989). These individuals gravitate toward CNS depressants and alcohol, although stimulants are also frequently abused. Hallucinogenics did not seem to be a popular drug of abuse for this subgroup, possibly because of the nature of MPD (Putnam, 1989). The exact reason chemicals are so popular with those who suffer from MPD is not clear, but these clients may be using chemicals in an attempt to medicate their internal distress (Putnam, 1989).

The obsessive-compulsive disorder (OCD) is the fourth most common psychiatric disorder found in the United States, affecting approximately 2.5% of the general population and perhaps as many as 10% of substance abusers (Falls-Stewart & Lucente, 1994). These figures suggest that individuals who suffer from OCD may be overrepresented in the substance abusing population, although it is not clear whether this is because patients with this disorder attempt to self-medicate through illicit drug use.

An alternative to the self-medication hypothesis is offered by Mueser, Bellack, and Blanchard (1992), who suggest that drug availability is the factor that most strongly influences the pattern of chemical use, not the specific form of psychiatric illness. This is the reason alcohol is the most popular drug of abuse for schizophrenic patients who admit to using drugs: it is the most easily available, frequently abused chemical in U.S. society (Mueser, Bellack, & Blanchard, 1992; Test, Wallisch, Allness, & Ripp, 1990). If this theory is correct, then limited availability may be the reason that Test et al. (1990) found marijuana to be the second most commonly abused drug; it may also explain why only about 3% of their sample admitted to using cocaine.

The results of these studies suggest that mentally ill patients who do use chemicals tend to abuse the full range of substances, and the self-medication hypothesis has received only limited support. However, studies exploring the issue of what kinds of drugs are most often abused by MI/CD clients have consistently failed to correlate drug use patterns within the MI/CD population with community trends. The possibility exists that the individual's drug of choice may be influenced both by the presenting psychiatric disorder and by the availability of specific drugs.

Problems in Working with Dual-Diagnosis Clients

The first step for substance abuse specialists who work with MI/CD clients is to examine their own attitudes toward psychopharmacology. For example, recovering addicts are often uncomfortable with patients' use of medications to control their psychiatric disorder, believing that any use of drugs serves only to substitute one addiction for another, despite the legitimate function of prescribed medications. Recovering addicts may also feel uncomfortable around individuals who use prescribed medications (Riley, 1994; Fariello & Scheidt, 1989; Evans & Sullivan, 1990; Penick et al., 1990). If substance abuse professionals are unable to accept the use of prescribed psychotropic medications, they should not work with MI/CD clients.

The outlook for dual-diagnosis clients has traditionally been thought to be quite poor. One of the problems most commonly encountered in working with dual-diagnosis clients is that the treatment philosophies of substance abuse counselors and mental health professionals often conflict (Carey, 1989; Osher & Kofoed, 1989; Wallen & Weiner, 1989; Howland, 1990). In addition, dual-diagnosis clients often (1) are unable to recognize that substance abuse is a personal problem, (2) cannot see the relationship between their chemical use and the problems they encounter,

or (3) cannot accept abstinence as a viable treatment goal. These factors may bring about a significant degree of confusion and frustration for both the client and the treatment professionals.

Kofoed et al. (1986) note that more severe levels of psychopathology have been associated with an unfavorable outcome for substance abusers, in part because "coexisting thought or affective disorders may exacerbate denial of substance abuse" (p. 1209). Denial of substance abuse is a significant problem in the dual-diagnosis client, which contributes to the difficulty of working with such clients.

Although the process of denial is a characteristic of the dual-diagnosis client, the added dimension of a psychiatric disorder will cause the client's denial of his or her drug addiction to express itself in different ways. In many cases, the dual-diagnosis client focuses almost exclusively on his or her psychiatric disorder in chemical dependency treatment to avoid confronting the substance abuse problem. Once the psychiatric condition is controlled, such a client is likely to self-terminate (drop out of) treatment.

This is the process of "interchangeable" or "free floating" denial, in which the client tells the mental health professional that most of the client's problems are drug-related, while telling the substance abuse counselor that most problems are caused by mental illness. Thus the client uses one disorder as a shield against intervention for the other disorder. For example (see Chapter 4), individuals who suffer from multiple personality disorder often attribute their loss of memory (experienced when one personality is forced out of consciousness and another takes over) to the use of chemicals. This is far less threatening to the individual than the acceptance of mental illness.

The mentally ill, chemically dependent client is often a "crisis user" of medical and chemical dependency services (Rubinstein, Campbell, & Daley, 1990, p. 99) frequently dropping out of treatment after the crisis has been stabilized or passed. Thus, treatment staff find it hard to become motivated to invest a lot of time and energy into working with MI/CD clients. To complicate the problem of treatment dropout, chemical dependency professionals often view dual-diagnosis patients as primarily psychiatric patients, whereas mental health professionals often view MI/CD clients as primarily substance abuse cases.

As Layne (1990) suggests, this state of affairs evolved out of the "political" (p. 176) atmosphere in which the treatment of substance abuse cases became separated from traditional psychiatric care. This division in treatment philosophy is clearly seen in the case of the dual-diagnosis client. When the MI/CD client does come into contact with a treatment center, the staff frequently views the patient as "not our problem" and refers the patient elsewhere. All too often, the outcome of this refusal-to-treat philosophy is that clients are bounced like ping-pong balls between psychiatric and chemical dependency treatment programs (Osher & Kofoed, 1989; Wallen & Weiner, 1989).

Dual-diagnosis patients frequently present behavioral challenges that make them unattractive to many chemical dependency treatment programs. At the same time, traditional psychiatric hospitals often refuse to accept these individuals until the chemical dependency issues have been addressed (Fariello & Scheidt, 1989; Penick et al., 1990). Unfortunately, staff psychiatrists in traditional psychiatric hospitals usually lack training and experience working with addicts (Riley, 1994; Howland, 1990). So, when such patients are admitted to a psychiatric facility, they may receive potentially addictive substances as part of their psychiatric care, innocently prescribed by a psychiatrist who is more experienced in working with "traditional" clients.

The MI/CD Client and Medication Compliance

To further complicate matters, medication noncompliance is a significant problem with dual-diagnosis clients (Drake & Wallach, 1989). Dual-diagnosis clients may not only refuse to take prescribed medications, they may also continue to use drugs of abuse even after admission to inpatient psychiatric treatment (Alterman, Erdlen, La Porte, & Erdlen, 1982).

Psychiatric patients often abuse drugs in an attempt at self-medication (Caton, Gralnick, Bender, & Simon, 1989; Rubinstein, Campbell, & Daley, 1990). This may be because they mistrust the prescribed medication (Evans & Sullivan, 1990) or because some psychiatric medications have a significant abuse potential of their own. For example, it is not uncommon for patients to abuse anticholinergic medications, which are often prescribed to help control the side effects of the prescribed antipsychotic agents. The anticholinergics may potentiate the effects of alcohol or the amphetamines (Land, Pinsky, & Salzman, 1991), and the "buzz" they can bring is often substituted for the effects of other chemicals when supplies run short.

To combat this poor medication compliance, Fariello and Scheidt (1989) recommend using long-term injectable phenothiazines rather than the more traditional short-term preparations to control the thought disorder and agitation often found in dual-diagnosis clients. As we will discuss later, frequent urine toxicology screenings will also verify medication compliance or noncompliance in the dual-diagnosis client.

Hatfield (1989) provides a graphic description of the internal world of schizophrenic patients, noting that these individuals "suffer high levels of stress and anxiety as they struggle to negotiate between the world as others know it and the world of their inner reality" (p. 1142). Considering the pain and suffering inherent in many forms of mental illness, it is understandable that mentally ill individuals often strive to maintain external structure and predictability to cope with their lack of internal structure and predictability.

Self-administered drugs are one way to substitute external structure and predictability for internal chaos, because the chemicals provide an illusion of control over one's feelings (Brown, 1985). Even if the drugs cause the schizophrenic patient to experience additional hallucinations, at least the individual has the illusion of controlling these hallucinations by deciding whether or not to take the chemical. This is an important consideration for those whose internal lives seem out of control because of their mental illness.

Treatment for Dual-Diagnosis Clients

Although it is becoming apparent that dual-diagnosis clients require specialized treatment programs to meet their needs, few such programs exist (Howland, 1990). The traditional approach has been to address the client's mental illness first and then, after psychiatric stabilization has been achieved, to begin to explore the client's chemical use pattern (Rado, 1988).

The decision of whether to treat the psychiatric condition or the drug dependency first is often quite arbitrary (Howland, 1990; Kofoed et al., 1986). Indeed, there is little research data to support either choice (Evans & Sullivan, 1990; Osher & Kofoed, 1989). Layne (1990) suggests treating both disorders concurrently, a possible alternative to the either/or approach utilized by other treatment centers.

A basic requirement of any treatment program for dual-diagnosis clients is a team approach, in which the different treatment philosophies of psychiatric and chemical dependency professionals can be synthesized into a unified whole and applied to each client (Riley, 1994; Osher & Kofoed, 1989; Evans & Sullivan, 1990).

Chemical detoxification is a necessary first step in treating a dual-diagnosis client (Layne, 1990; Wallen & Weiner, 1989). This requires psychiatric support from professionals who are knowledgeable in both psychiatry and chemical dependency (Evans & Sullivan, 1990). Once detoxification has been achieved, the treatment team can identify which problems are a result of the client's chemical use and which are manifestations of the client's psychiatric disorder. Then the team can decide in what order the problems need to be addressed.

As part of the evaluation process, urine toxicology screening should be conducted. There are two advantages to using urine toxicology screens at the time of admission for the dual-diagnosis client. First, when properly supervised, urine samples may yield information on what illicit chemicals the client has been using in the recent past. This information is of value during the diagnostic process. Second, urine toxicology screens can verify whether the client has taken the prescribed medications.

The Treatment Setting

The general psychiatric unit is usually unsuited to meet the needs of the dual-diagnosis client (Kofoed & Keys, 1988; Howland, 1990). Kofoed and Keys (1988) suggest that psychiatric units may be improved if treatment goals are limited to (1) detoxification from drugs of abuse, (2) psychiatric stabilization, and, (3) persuasion of the client to enter chemical dependency treatment. The clinician must be patient, often waiting years until conditions are right to finally persuade a dual-diagnosis client to enter treatment.

The ideal program for a dual-diagnosis client would have facilities for working with both psychiatric and addicted clients. This would allow the dual-diagnosis patient to be shifted from one program to another as his or her needs change during treatment. Osher and Kofoed (1989) propose a unified treatment team that has this flexibility of treatment approaches. Dual-diagnosis patients can be treated on either an outpatient (Kofoed et al., 1986) or inpatient (Pursch, 1987) basis, depending on the client's needs and the available resources. However, in more difficult cases, long-term inpatient treatment may be the only option for effectively working with the MI/CD client (Caton, Gralnick, Bender, & Simon, 1989).

The Stages of Treatment

The dual-diagnosis client usually comes to the attention of mental health or chemical dependency professionals as a result of repeated hospitalizations, legal problems, psychiatric decompensation, or eviction from his or her apartment (Fariello & Scheidt, 1989; Rubinstein, Campbell, & Daley, 1990). In fact, Durell, Lechtenberg, Corse, and Frances (1993) point out that a crisis "can provide the motivation for overcoming addiction" (p. 428). The therapist may be able to use a crisis in the client's life to help him or her face the reality of the addiction.

Lehman, Myers, and Corty (1989) identify the first phase of treatment as "acute treatment and stabilization" (p. 1020); Minkoff (1989) terms this phase *acute stabilization*. During this phase of treatment, the client's psychiatric condition is stabilized and detoxification is carried out. The possibility of a dual diagnosis is also considered by the clinician during this phase of evaluation and treatment. If the symptoms of a psychiatric disorder completely clear during detoxification, then the client is probably not a dual-diagnosis patient (Layne, 1990). If the symptoms persist after detoxification, then it is more likely that the client is a dual-diagnosis patient (Lehman, Myers, & Corty, 1989). In either case, during this phase of treatment staff should focus on helping the individual understand the relationship between the crisis and his or her untreated problem(s).

The goal of the treatment process during this phase should be that of breaking "the cycle of substance abuse, noncompliance, decompensation, and rehospitalization once the patient is sober and psychiatrically stable" (Fariello & Scheidt, 1989, p. 1066). This process may include introducing money management programs, presenting psychoeducational materials or lectures, and offering social support. It is during this phase of treatment that staff attempt to break through the denial that surrounds both the individual's mental illness and his or her addiction. Both Osher and Kofoed (1989) and Minkoff (1989) call this phase of treatment *engagement*, and Layne (1990) calls it *early engagement*. The goal during this phase of treatment is for the professional staff to strive to establish a therapeutic relationship, arrive at an accurate diagnosis, and convince the client that treatment has something to offer. Staff members should at-

tempt to work with family members or legal representatives during this period if it becomes necessary to bring the client into treatment on an involuntary basis.

In their work with dual-diagnosis clients, Kofoed and Keys (1988) concluded that peer group therapy offered "a more acceptable source of support and confrontation than is usually available . . . on a general psychiatric ward" (p. 1209). Group therapy can be an important element in working with the dual-diagnosis client, although such groups should be held in the psychiatric unit, rather than in the substance abuse unit (Kofoed & Keys, 1988; Layne, 1990).

Lehman, Myers, and Corty (1989) term the second phase of treatment *maintenance and rehabilitation*. In this phase, the clinician works toward the goal of preventing a recurrence of both the chemical abuse and the psychiatric disorder, the process Fariello and Scheidt (1989) call *breaking the cycle of addiction*. Osher and Kofoed (1989) call this phase of treatment *persuasion*. During this phase, treatment staff attempt to convince the client to accept the need for abstinence. According to Kofoed and Keys (1988), the therapeutic goals of this phase of treatment are to persuade clients to accept the reality of their drug dependency and to persuade clients to seek continued treatment.

The third phase of treatment, that of *active treatment* (Osher & Kofoed, 1989), attempts to help the client learn "the attitudes and skills necessary to remain sober" (p. 1027). Many of the same techniques utilized in general drug addiction treatment groups are useful in working with dual-diagnosis clients. In particular, Osher and Kofoed (1989) argue against lower treatment expectations or the acceptance of relapse as inevitable for dual-diagnosis clients. Layne (1990) suggests that treatment staff may need to teach the client specific life skills to learn to function in society without the use of abusable drugs, in spite of ongoing delusions.

However, the very nature of the client population offers unique challenges and requires modification of techniques used in traditional chemical dependency work. It has been suggested that, when confrontation is utilized with dual-diagnosis clients who are in treatment, it should be less intense than the confrontation used with traditional personality disordered clients (Riley, 1994; Penick et al., 1990; Carey, 1989).

As do nonpsychiatric addicts, dual-diagnosis clients use denial as a major defense. The danger is that once the psychiatric condition is controlled, the client's drug-related defenses again begin to operate (Kofoed & Keys, 1988). Dual-diagnosis clients often express a belief that, once their psychiatric symptoms are controlled, they are no longer in danger of being addicted to chemicals. These clients are often unable to see the relationship between their chemical abuse and the psychiatric symptoms they experience.

For such a client, dropping out of treatment is the ultimate expression of denial. Another form of denial, one that is also frequently found in traditional clients, is evident when the client informs the drug rehabilitation specialist that he or she has discontinued all drug or alcohol use. In effect, the client tries to "tell the counselor what he wants to hear" to avoid confrontation.

Another problem for dual-diagnosis clients is that they are often unable to utilize traditional support systems such as Alcoholics Anonymous or Narcotics Anonymous because they feel out of place in such self-help meetings (Fariello & Scheidt, 1989; Wallen & Weiner, 1989), a problem that should be addressed by treatment professionals (Layne, 1990). Instead, a group of peers is more effective in working with the dual-diagnosis client (Kofoed & Keys, 1988). In such a group, other members who may have once dropped out of treatment after their own psychiatric disorder was controlled can share their experiences with the group. The group provides an avenue through which clients can share their experiences with even limited recreational drug use and discuss the need for the support of a twelve-step group (Fariello & Scheidt, 1989; Kofoed & Keys, 1988; Rado, 1988). When the group is effective, dual-diagnosis clients are less likely to be rehospitalized (Kofoed & Keys, 1988) and function better in society.

Summary

The dual-diagnosis client presents a difficult challenge to mental health and chemical dependency professionals. Many of the syndromes that can result from chronic chemical use are virtually indistinguishable from organic or psychiatric problems. This makes it very difficult to arrive at an accurate diagnosis. Furthermore, MI/CD clients often use defense mechanisms, such as an interchangeable system of denial, which further complicates the diagnostic process.

Dual-diagnosis clients are also difficult to work with in the rehabilitation setting. When they are in treatment, dual-diagnosis clients often talk about their psychiatric problem with drug addiction counselors and talk about their drug abuse with mental health professionals. Because of these characteristics, it is necessary to modify some of the traditional treatment methods used with the chemically dependent client. For example, the degree of confrontation used in working with a personality disordered client is far too strong for working with a dual-diagnosis client. However, gentle confrontation will often work with the mentally ill and drug dependent client who is not personality disordered.

CHAPTER TWENTY-THREE

Substance Abuse by Children and Adolescents

The pharmacological revolution of the 1950s and 1960s did not cause the problem of child and adolescent substance abuse; it only gave children and adolescents a wider range of chemicals that could be abused. Indeed, the problem of substance abuse by children and adolescents has been with us for a long time; during the early 1800s, alcoholism was rampant among the youth of England (Wheeler & Malmquist, 1987).

The social changes that took place in the late 1800s and the early 1900s may have helped drive child and adolescent alcohol use underground. But there has always been a small percentage of children and adolescents who use chemicals for recreational purposes. Even as recently as 50 years ago, just under 50% of the adolescents entering high school had already used alcohol at least once (Takanishi, 1993).

Two different forces combined in the 1950s and 1960s to contribute to a new wave of child and adolescent substance abuse. First, there was a pharmacological "revolution," in which large numbers of new pharmaceuticals were introduced each year. Many of these drugs had significant abuse potential, a characteristic that, combined with the youth "rebellion" of the 1960s and early 1970s, made them attractive to children and adolescents. Second, the use of chemicals was accepted as a legitimate part of the rebellion against traditional views. These two forces helped focus social attention on the problem of child and adolescent substance use in the last 20 years. However the problem of child and adolescent substance use is not a new one: it has just taken on a new form.

Child and Adolescent Drug Use Patterns

Surprisingly, in spite of all that has been written about child and adolescent substance use in the past generation, very little is actually known about the problem (Kaminer, 1994; Evans & Sullivan, 1990). Researchers are only now starting to identify the characteristics that distinguish who will abstain from recreational drug use during childhood and adolescence, who will only use chemicals as part of a phase of experimentation, and who will go on to develop a problem with drug abuse and addiction.

Because mental health professionals are only now starting to understand the problem, there is still much to be discovered. For example, there is virtually no research into possible chemical use patterns by children (Newcomb & Bentler, 1989). This lack of information makes it difficult to determine what the implications of drug use during childhood might be for the individual's subsequent growth and development.

Furthermore, the lack of information makes it extremely difficult to identify criteria by which to classify normal and abnormal chemical use by children. Is chemical use in childhood automatically a cause for concern, or are there patterns of experimental chemical use that one might expect to see in childhood? What chemicals will children use most often? The truth is that nobody really knows the answers to these questions.

The research into teenage drug use patterns is also quite limited (Kaminer, 1991; Evans & Sullivan, 1990; Newcomb & Bentler, 1989). Much of what is known about adolescent drug use patterns is based on studies that used students as research subjects. Because between 15 and 30% of adolescents drop out of school before graduating (Eccles et al., 1993), little is known about how representative data from school-based populations are of overall adolescent drug use patterns.

This lack of data makes it quite difficult to determine current drug abuse trends. The absence of a comprehensive database also makes it difficult to identify forces that motivate the adolescent to begin to use chemicals or to determine when chemical use is just part of a normal phase of experimentation. Mental health workers have little information about when adolescent chemical use may indicate a serious problem, nor do they know much about the impact drug use might have on the adolescent's emotional adjustment.

A third factor that contributes to the confusion surrounding child and adolescent drug use is that there is a tendency to equate virtually *any* chemical use as a sign of a serious drug abuse problem (Newcomb & Bentler, 1989; Peele, 1989). Not only does this viewpoint add to the confusion about what exactly constitutes "drug abuse" by an adolescent, it also overlooks the fact that, for many adolescents, limited episodes of chemical use may reflect only a phase of experimentation or exploration (Shedler & Block, 1990).

Finally, drug use patterns among children and adolescents often show rapid fluctuation and variation. Some of the variables that influence adolescent drug use trends include geographic location, peer groups, and current drug use "trends." Inhalant abuse is one drug use fad that rapidly waxes and wanes in a given geographic area.

The Scope of the Problem

Childhood Chemical Abuse

In terms of chemical use patterns, virtually nothing is known about drug use by children. One interesting finding by Johnston, O'Malley, and Bachman (1994) is that, by the time they were in the eighth grade (approximately 13 years old), fully 67% of the students surveyed had used alcohol at least once. In England, 80% of 13-year-old students surveyed reported they had ingested a "proper drink" (Swadi, 1993, p. 341) at least once.

Statistically, the average age of the first drink is between 12 and 13 years (Novello & Shosky, 1992). Boys tend to begin drinking earlier than girls, with an average age for the first drink of alcohol being 11.9 years for boys and 12.7 years for girls (Rogers, Harris, & Jarmuskewicz, 1987). Thus, by the time they reach adolescence, most children have had at least limited experience with alcohol use. Fortunately, in spite of isolated reports of alcohol abuse problems in children as young as 11 years of age, problem drinking seems to be quite rare in preadolescents (Rogers, Harris, & Jarmuskewicz, 1987).

But alcohol is not the only recreational chemical that children or adolescents are likely to experiment with. There is strong evidence that many children use inhalants as their first mood-altering chemical (Newcomb & Bentler, 1989). As we discussed in Chapter 11, adolescent inhalant abuse is a serious problem. Some 19% of eighth graders surveyed in 1993 had used an inhalant at least once (Johnston, O'Malley, & Bachman, 1994).

Fortunately, inhalant abuse is usually a phase. Most adolescents engage in rare, episodic use inhalants over a 1- to 2-year period, after which most abandon the use of inhalants. But in about one-third of the cases, the individual "graduates" to more traditional forms of drug abuse

(Brunswick, 1989). Thus, for some children, inhalants serve as a "gateway" chemical that leads to other forms of drug abuse. Marijuana is another possible gateway substance suggested by Millman and Beeder (1994).

Kandel, Yamaguchi, and Chen (1992) examined the "gateway" theory of drug use by interviewing 1,160 subjects between the ages of 15 and 35. The authors found that, for these individuals, substance use progressed through the use of legal substances (alcohol, cigarettes) to marijuana, and from there to other "hard" drugs. Thus, there is evidence of a progression from the "gateway" chemicals to other, more serious, forms of chemical use. When viewed in this light, adolescent inhalant abuse may suggest that the individual is potentially "at risk" for more serious forms of chemical abuse later in life.

Adolescent Chemical Abuse

The available research suggests that adolescent drug use peaked sometime around the year 1981, slowly declined for about a decade, and now may be gradually increasing again (Johnston, O'Malley, & Bachman, 1994; Edwards, 1993). Not surprisingly, adolescent drug use patterns tend to mirror those of the society in which they live (Callahan, 1993). In a society where alcohol is the most popular recreational chemical, alcohol is by far the most popular chemical of choice for adolescents (Johnston, O'Malley, & Bachman, 1993, 1994).

The percentage of high school seniors who have experimented with alcohol has remained fairly stable over the past several years. For example, slightly under 90% of the class of 1990 had used alcohol at least once (Novello & Shosky, 1992; Johnston, O'Malley, & Bachman, 1993). Eighty-eight percent of the seniors from the class of 1992 and 87% of the seniors of the class of 1993 admitted to having used alcohol at least once (Johnston, O'Malley, & Bachman, 1994). Thus, with a small degree of variation, approximately 90% of graduating high school seniors will have used alcohol at least once.

Although this statistic is frightening in itself,

there is evidence to suggest that a sizable percentage of high school seniors use alcohol fairly heavily. Some 28% of the class of 1992 were estimated to have consumed 5 or more drinks at least once in the 2 weeks preceding the survey (Johnston, O'Malley, & Bachman, 1993). Fortunately, although a majority of adolescents experiment with alcohol, the heaviest alcohol use (5 or more drinks at a time at least once a week) was confined to just 500,000 students (Novello & Shosky, 1992).

The most popular form of alcohol for the adolescents surveyed is beer, although wine "coolers" are increasing in popularity (Novello & Shosky, 1992). Few adolescents seem to be drawn to "hard" liquor. Indeed, so rare is adolescent use of "hard" liquor that even occasional experimentation with vodka, gin, whiskey, or bourbon should be considered a sign of an alcohol abuse problem (Rogers, Harris, & Jarmuskewicz, 1987).

Although many parents worry about possible alcohol use by their adolescent children, they are poor sources of information about their teenager's use of this chemical. Parents tend to underestimate their teenager's alcohol consumption by a factor of at least 10 to 1 (Rogers, Harris, & Jarmuskewicz, 1987; Zarek, Hawkins, & Rogers, 1987).

Alcohol is not the only recreational chemical used by adolescents. By the time of graduation, 44% of the seniors from the class of 1991 and 43% of the seniors from the class of 1993 admitted to the use of an illicit chemical at least once (Johnston, O'Malley, & Bachman, 1994). Marijuana was the most frequently used illicit chemical, and by the time of graduation, 37% of the seniors in the class of 1991 and 35% of the seniors of the class of 1993 admitted to having used marijuana at least once. However, for eighth graders, inhalants have replaced marijuana as the most frequently used mood-altering chemical, according to Johnston, O'Malley, and Bachman. This suggests that adolescent drug use patterns may be changing.

A small percentage of adolescents have used hallucinogenics (Gold, Schuchard, & Gleaton,

1994). In their survey of 522,000 high school ju-
niors and seniors, Gold, Schuchard, and Gleaton
found that 5.3% of the students surveyed in 1993
admitted to having used hallucinogens at least
once, up from 4.9% the previous year. Johnston,
O'Malley, and Bachman (1994) offer an even
higher percentage, reporting that 10.9% of the
seniors surveyed admitted to having used a hallucinogenic substance other than LSD at least
once, and 7.4% had done so in the preceding
year.

There is evidence to suggest that LSD is also
growing in popularity among adolescents. Ten
percent of the seniors from the class of 1993 who
participated in the survey admitted to having
used LSD at least once, as compared with 8.6%
of the seniors from the class of 1992 and 8.8% of
the seniors in the class of 1991 (Johnston,
O'Malley, & Bachman, 1994).

Thus, after declining for several years, there is
evidence that adolescent drug use is again on the
rise, based on surveys of school students. Unfortunately, adolescent drug use surveys do not
give us the whole picture. These surveys frequently focus on the greatest concentration of
adolescents—those who are still in school. However, as Oetting and Beauvais (1990) point out,
there may be a self-selection process at work in
the schools. For example, adolescents who use
"hard" drugs on a regular basis are often those
students who ultimately drop out of school and
so would not be included in school-based surveys.

It is known that children who encounter academic problems in the middle to late elementary
school grades are more likely to engage in alcohol or drug abuse than are those students who
achieve high grades (Board of Trustees, 1991).
Those adolescents who are not interested in academic achievement are more likely to turn to
chemicals and are also at "high risk" for dropping out of school. Thus, surveys of adolescent
drug use patterns based on student responses
may underestimate chemical use patterns.

Another shortcoming of U.S. national surveys
is that regional variations may exist in terms of
the drug(s) of choice or patterns of use that may

not be reflected in the surveys (Oetting &
Beauvais, 1990). For example, Moncher, Holden,
and Trimble (1990) concluded that adolescent
Native Americans were two to three times as
likely to be "at least moderately involved with
alcohol" (p. 408) as were non–Native American
urban adolescents. But in most school districts,
Native American students are only a small minority of the student body. It is only in school
districts with a large proportion of Native American students that this ethnic variation in substance abuse rates would be detected. Thus,
national drug use patterns among adolescents
may or may not reflect local adolescent substance abuse behavior patterns.

Tobacco Use by Children and Adolescents

Cigarettes and other tobacco products occupy a
unique place in U.S. society. Although known to
be addictive and terribly destructive, these substances can be legally purchased by adults. Unfortunately, nicotine use and addiction are
problems that are not limited to adults.

Within the past few years, there has been
growing concern over the use of tobacco products by adolescents. The use of tobacco during
childhood or adolescence is not just a passing
phase for many individuals. Researchers have
discovered that the roots of nicotine addiction
may lie in childhood or adolescence. For example, by the age of 12, fully one-half of the
schoolchildren in Canada have already experimented with cigarette smoking (Walker, 1993).

As a general rule, adolescents tend to underestimate the addictive potential of nicotine
(Benowitz & Henningfield, 1994). According to
Benowitz and Henningfield, few adolescents
plan to smoke for the rest of their lives; rather,
they start out with the intention of quitting in a
few years. As we discussed in Chapter 15, however, once a person is addicted to nicotine, it is
quite difficult to quit. There is thus reason for
concern given that each day in the United States
an estimated 3,000 children or adolescents *begin*
to smoke (Mondi, Hooten, & Peterzell, 1994).
Furthermore, the *average* age at which smok-

ers begin to smoke is thought to be 14.5 years (Roberts & Watson, 1994). At this age, an individual is unlikely to understand the consequences of his or her tobacco use or that he or she risks developing an addiction to nicotine. An estimated 90% (Pierce et al., 1991) of adult cigarette smokers began to smoke before the age of 21. MacKenzie, Bartecchi, and Schrier (1994b) give an even earlier age, stating that 80% to 90% of all smokers begin before age 18; indeed, 90% of cigarette smokers are already *addicted* to nicotine by the age of 20 (Walker, 1993).

Johnston, O'Malley, and Bachman (1994) found that, by the time of graduation from high school, 11% of the students surveyed admitted to smoking at least 10 cigarettes each day. They also found that just under 61.9% of the seniors surveyed in 1993 had used cigarettes at least once. These figures are very similar to those obtained by DiFranza and Tye (1990), who found that 18.1% of high school seniors smoke cigarettes on a daily basis. The American Heart Association estimated that 2.2 million children between the ages of 12 and 17 smoke cigarettes (Associated Press, 1994a), and Mead (1993) offers a figure of 3 million children and adolescents in the United States who either smoke or use "smokeless" tobacco products.

Some believe that it is not by accident that children and adolescents are turning to the use of cigarettes. Indeed, given the high mortality rates associated with tobacco smoking, the very "success of the tobacco industry is dependent on recruiting people who don't believe that smoking kills" (Wasman, 1991, p. 3185) to replace smokers who either stop or who die for one reason or another. To this end, it has been suggested that tobacco advertising techniques have been developed that specifically target children and adolescents (Pierce et al., 1991; DiFranza, Richards, Paulman, Wolf-Gillespie, Fletcher, Jaffe, & Murray, 1991), as well as those who are economically disadvantaged or who live in the Third World countries (Wasman, 1991).

Although this charge hasn't been proved, it is interesting to examine the sources of revenue for

tobacco companies, as DiFranza and Tye (1990) did. They concluded that "If sales to children account for 3.3% of cigarette sales, these six . . . companies share an annual $703 million in revenues and $221 million in profits from the sale of cigarettes to children" (p. 2786). These figures raise disturbing doubts about current sales and advertising tactics used to promote tobacco use, especially to children and adolescents. The authors went on to observe that many of the children or adolescents who begin to use tobacco before age 21 will go on to become addicted. This provides "an 'investment' that will pay dividends into the future" (p. 2786) in the form of new generations of smokers for tobacco companies.

Males (1992) challenged the conclusion that tobacco advertising is a major factor in adolescent cigarette smoking. He concluded that a more important factor is the fact that 75% of all teenagers who smoke had parents who also smoked. The evidence, the author concluded, points toward the fact that "teenage smoking is largely the active continuation of a childhood of passive smoking" (p. 3282).

This theory is certainly consistent with research suggesting that the transition from a nonsmoker to smoker in childhood or adolescence appears to pass through several stages (Holland & Fitzsimons, 1991): (1) a *preparatory phase,* during which attitudes accepting of cigarette smoking are formed; (2) the *initiation phase,* in which he or she will smoke for the first time; (3) the *experimentation phase,* in which the child or adolescent learns how to smoke; and (4) the *transition* to regular smoking.

Thus, the attitudes supportive of, or at least accepting of, smoking are formed in childhood before actual smoking begins. Given this fact, Holland and Fitzsimons (1991) suggest that attempts at invervention need to be aimed at children who have not started to form pro-smoking attitudes. Attempts at intervention should focus on helping children learn social skills that will enable them to resist smoking. If the adolescent reaches 16 to 18 years of age without having initiated smoking, he or she is unlikely to do so (Holland & Fitzsimons, 1991).

Why Do Adolescents Use Chemicals?

The initial factor that influences adolescent experimentation with recreational chemical use seems to be curiosity. Some adolescents begin to use chemicals in response to peer pressure (Joshi & Scott, 1988), coupled with an inability to see themselves as vulnerable to the negative effects of alcohol or the other drugs of abuse (Alexander, 1991). It is also thought that many adolescents find that chemical use offers some relief from internal discomfort, such as feelings of depression (Joshi & Scott, 1988).

For example, chemically dependent adolescents are three times as likely to be depressed as are their nonusing counterparts (Deykin, Buka, & Zeena, 1992). Indeed, so strong is the relationship between affective disorders such as anxiety or depression and substance abuse that Burke, Burke, and Rae (1994) suggest that these conditions identify adolescents who are at "high risk" (p. 454) for later drug use disorders. Thus, evidence supports the hypothesis that adolescents use chemicals to self-medicate painful feelings.

Adolescents are also thought to use chemicals in an attempt to deal with conflict (Evans & Sullivan, 1990) and stress (Rhodes & Jason, 1990). The reasons for any given individual's chemical use is often influenced by his or her emotional maturity, available intrapersonal and interpersonal resources, and available social support systems.

The evolution of child and adolescent substance use patterns and values takes place in a swirling mixture of forces that vary in intensity at different points in the individual's early years. During the childhood years, parental influence on subsequent drug use behavior is the strongest. The child accepts parental guidance on behavior but also is very aware of parental modeling behaviors (Cohen, Richardson, & La Bree, 1994; Rogers, Harris, & Jarmuskewicz,

1987). Thus, evidence suggests that parental substance use is associated with the adolescent's subsequent chemical use (Kaminer, 1991). However the relationship between parental chemical abuse and drug use by the teenager is quite complex and involves factors other than simply whether the adolescent's parents used chemicals or not.

Cohen, Richardson, and La Bree (1994) note that several factors seem to be associated with problem adolescent alcohol use, including parental modeling behaviors, parental efforts to shape behavioral standards and values, the quality of the family's affectional interactions. In their examination of the factors that might influence adolescent smoking and alcohol use behaviors, the authors found that children whose parents spent more time with them and made greater efforts to communicate with them had lower rates of alcohol and tobacco use in the months preceding the study. On the basis of their findings, the authors called for greater efforts to include the parents of children deemed "at risk" for later chemical use in any intervention program.

Some researchers believe that it is during adolescence that peer influences come to play an increasingly important role in shaping the individual's drug use pattern. Peer influences have been termed "crucial" in the development of adolescent substance use patterns (Kaminer, 1991, p. 330). According to this theory, some adolescents find that chemical use brings a form of acceptance from other drug using teens. Others find that the drugs offer some relief from internal distress, and they tend to associate with those who also use drugs. Still other adolescents find that drug use is consistent with the risk-taking, sensation-seeking lifestyle often associated with social delinquency (Kaminer, 1991).

It has also been suggested, however, that peer groups may *not* be a major factor in adolescent alcohol abuse (Bauman & Ennett, 1994; Novello & Shosky, 1992). Novello and Shosky (1992) note that, of the 10.6 million adolescents who consume alcohol, almost one-third do so when alone rather than in groups. The authors interpret this data as evidence that the theory that adolescents use chemicals in response to peer pressure must be accepted as only a theory, and that it may not be true in all cases.

Bauman and Ennett (1994) identified several factors that might distort the relationship between adolescent peer group membership and substance use patterns. One such factor was the influence of friend selection. According to the authors, individual friendship patterns evolve in part because of a congruence of substance use patterns. In other words, drug using adolescents tend to form friendships mainly with other drug using adolescents, a pattern that may cause researchers to overestimate the influence of peer groups on substance use patterns.

A second factor that can distort the apparent relationship between substance use patterns and peer group membership is the possibility of *projection* on the part of the research subjects. In other words, when asked about their friends' substance use, drug using adolescents are more likely to respond on the basis of *their own* drug use behavior, rather than on the basis of what they know about their friends' chemical use. Bauman and Ennett (1994) point out that adolescents who do not use chemicals are more likely to be judged as drug users by their drug using friends than by their nonusing friends. On the basis of their research, Bauman and Ennett (1994) suggest that the factor of adolescent peer use on substance abuse patterns has been "overestimated" (p. 820).

Admittedly, the early adolescent years appear to be a time of special vulnerability for later drug abuse. It is during this stage of life that many adolescents begin to experiment with various "gateway" chemicals that open the door to later drug abuse problems (Pentz et al., 1989). As was noted before, such "gateway" drugs include tobacco, alcohol, marijuana, and the inhalants (Brunswick, 1989). However, at present, researchers still disagree about the relative importance of family and peer group influences on the individual's subsequent chemical use patterns.

The Adolescent Abuse/Addiction Dilemma: How Much Is Too Much?

Unfortunately, because very little is known about adolescent drug use, it is quite difficult to identify the difference between experimental drug use, an early drug use problem, a chronic drug abuse problem, or drug addiction in adolescents (Wheeler & Malmquist, 1987). Also, little is known about the differences in personality characteristics between those who abstain and those who experiment with chemicals or ultimately go on to develop some form of addiction.

Newcomb and Bentler (1989) reported that social variables such as low socioeconomic status, a lack of religious commitment, low self-esteem, and disturbed families all tend to influence adolescent drug use patterns. As noted before, one psychosocial factor that has been found to have the strongest immediate influence on adolescent drug use is peer group pressure (Newcomb & Bentler, 1989; Joshi & Scott, 1988).

However, Shedler and Block (1990) report that their longitudinal study of a group of adolescents, who were studied by investigators since they were young children, suggests that certain personality traits seem to predispose the individual to abstain from either recreational chemical use or drug abuse during adolescence. The authors found that extremes of behavior (total abstinence or serious drug abuse) were found in adolescents who were most maladjusted, whereas the healthiest group were those who had occasionally experimented with chemicals.

These findings, although surprising at first glance, do make clinical sense. The emotionally healthy adolescent might experiment with recreational drug use but ultimately would have the inter- and intrapersonal skills necessary to cope with life. However, as Shedler and Block (1990) report, those adolescents who used drugs on a frequent basis demonstrated poor impulse control, a pattern of social alienation, and emotional distress, all signs that these individuals lack the emotional resources of the first group.

Further, those individuals who totally abstained from chemical use were found to be anxious, emotionally constricted, and lacking in social skills. These individuals seem to lack the self-confidence that would allow them to explore their environment, including the possibility of recreational drug use. The authors conclude that the individual's chemical use pattern (that is, abstinence, experimental drug use, or frequent drug use) could only be interpreted in light of the individual's emotional adjustment.

Steinberg (1991) agreed that adolescent chemical use and abuse must be considered in terms of the individual's developmental stage. But in his view, chemical use is not a normal part of the adolescent experience and chemical use problems in adolescence are unlikely to disappear on their own. Steinberg viewed chemical use and abuse in the early part of adolescence as indicating serious problems in the adolescent's life. However, in later adolescence, the experimental use of alcohol or drugs may not be a reflection of serious problems so much as a reflection of society's more liberal attitude toward recreational substance use.

Adolescents who engage in "problem behavior" (Robert Haggarty, quoted in Kirn, 1989, p. 3362), including substance use or abuse, might do so in response to economic problems and a rather pessimistic view of the future. Other problem behaviors included teen pregnancies and delinquency, in Haggart's opinion. Other acute stressors might include a geographic relocation, a major psychological loss, an increase in family conflict, or increased pressure to perform in school, all of which could serve as a predictor of the initial (usually transient) use of chemicals by adolescents (Mikkelsen, 1985).

The Stages of Adolescent Chemical Use

Jones (1990) postulates that there are four different stages of drug abuse for adolescents. In the first stage, called "learning the mood swing" (p. 680), the young drug user is exposed to and learns what to expect from substance use. Of

those individuals who continue to use chemicals, many will reach the second stage of drug abuse, entitled "seeking the mood swing" (p. 680). This stage is marked by a change in friendship patterns, erratic school performance, unpredictable mood swings, and manipulative behaviors in the service of continued substance abuse.

According to Jones (1990), the third stage of substance abuse is reached when the individual is preoccupied "with the mood swing" (p. 680). During this stage, nonusing friends are dropped, family fights and confrontations develop, jobs may be lost or expulsion from school may occur, lying becomes consistent, and mood-altering chemicals are used daily. Ultimately, some individuals continue to the final stage of substance use where they must use drugs just "to feel normal" (p. 680). During this stage the individual experiences physical complications from drug use, memory loss or flashback experiences, paranoia, anger, and drug or alcohol overdoses.

Jones notes that adolescents who are depressed, run away from home, or manifest school behavior problems should be evaluated for possible substance abuse problems. Adolescents who have legal problems because of substance abuse, suicidal behaviors, delinquency problems, or recurrent accidents should be believed to be abusing chemicals "until proved otherwise" (p. 680, italics in original omitted).

Adolescent Addiction

It was once thought that adolescents were unlikely to have the opportunity to use a drug(s) long enough to develop physical dependence or withdrawal symptoms when the drug is discontinued. For this reason, Morrison (1990) suggests that the first sign of a drug abuse problem in the adolescent might be a drug-related visit to the local hospital emergency room. Kaminer and Frances (1991) take a middle-of-the-road position, suggesting that adolescent drug abusers have not had the time in which to develop an extensive history of chemical use. Thus, the "traditional" abuse symptoms of tolerance, craving, and withdrawal are not commonly encountered in the adolescent drug abusing population, according to Kaminer and Frances. Further, the authors suggest that, when these symptoms of chemical dependency are encountered in the adolescent, they are usually much less severe than they are in the adult who has been abusing drugs. Thus, it is unlikely that adolescents actually become addicted to chemicals.

Other clinicians disagree. Indeed, many believe that adolescents may become addicted to alcohol and chemicals in spite of the fact that they usually have used drugs for only a short period of time. Hoffmann, Belille, and Harrison (1987) found, for example, that more than 75% of their sample of 1,000 adolescents, all of whom were in treatment at the time, reported having developed tolerance to alcohol or other drugs. Furthermore, one-third of the sample reported withdrawal symptoms. Evans and Sullivan (1990) also found adolescents who experienced withdrawal symptoms from chemicals, although they believed it was the exception rather than the rule. These observations would suggest that it is indeed possible for adolescents to use chemicals long enough to become physically addicted to them, although it is not clear whether this is a common occurrence or not.

Farrow (1990) challenged the concept of adolescent addiction, concluding that "the number of teenagers who are truly chemically dependent is less than 1% of all users" (p. 1268). Another 10% to 15% might meet the diagnostic criteria for drug or alcohol abuse, whereas 10% to 15% of all teenagers have little or no experience with either alcohol or drugs. The remainder are occasional users of alcohol or drugs who will likely adjust "their use in non-problematic ways as they grow older" (p. 1268).

The key point to remember is that there is a difference between adolescent drug *use* and adolescent drug *abuse*. Although the individual may have started to use drugs in response to social pressure, he or she will continue to use chemicals or not in response to internal emotional states (Newcomb & Bentler, 1989).

There is significant evidence indicating that the majority of adolescents who use chemicals will not go on to develop a drug dependency problem (Kaminer, 1994; Jones, 1990). Rather, one phase of development that many adolescents go through involves experimental drug use. Of those adolescents who experiment with drugs, a small percentage will go on to develop a more serious drug abuse problem. But how should treatment professionals identify those adolescents who are part of this small percentage of potential drug abusers?

Diagnosis and Treatment of Adolescent Drug Abuse

The diagnosis of adolescent drug abuse is a complicated task requiring an extensive database to document individual drug use (Wheeler & Malmquist, 1987; Evans & Sullivan, 1990). The occasional use of alcohol or marijuana at a party is not automatically a sign of a drug abuse problem (Newcomb & Bentler, 1989). It may reflect only an isolated episode of marijuana use. Thus, the treatment professional must keep in mind the possibility that the individual has not developed a drug abuse problem when evaluating an adolescent's drug use pattern.

Referrals for a chemical dependency evaluation on an adolescent come from many potential sources. The juvenile court system frequently refers an offender for an evaluation, especially when that individual was under the influence of chemicals at the time of his or her arrest. School officials may request an evaluation on a student suspected of abusing chemicals. Treatment center admissions officers frequently recommend an evaluation, although this is usually referred to in-house staff rather than to an independent professional. Some parents, especially those with "religious, restrictive families" (Farrow, 1990, p. 1268) also request an evaluation or treatment after the first known episode of alcohol or drug use.

One important point to remember in evaluating the adolescent's chemical use pattern is that the adolescent's developmental stage may preclude him or her from being able to understand the implications of drug use. Adolescents frequently feel that they are invulnerable, and they are unconcerned with understanding the long-term consequences of substance abuse. Unlike older addicts, the adolescent has not had time to "hit bottom" and may have a rather immature view of life.

Unfortunately, adolescents' simplistic outlook on life and their chemical use may be misinterpreted by treatment staff as a sign of resistance rather than emotional immaturity. Kaminer and Frances (1991) recommend taking a multidisciplinary team approach to assessment in cases of suspected adolescent substance abuse to allow accurate identification of the client's strengths, weaknesses, and adaptive style.

Even when the legitimate need for treatment is identified, several factors could interfere with the treatment process. According to Kaminer and Frances (1991), several of these factors include (1) unrealistic parental expectations for treatment, (2) hidden agendas for treatment by both the adolescent and the parents, (3) parental psychopathology, and (4) parental drug or alcohol abuse. Another factor is parental refusal to provide consent for treatment (Kaminer, 1994). Often, combinations of these problem areas are found in the family of an adolescent drug or alcohol abuser who fails to enter or complete treatment.

The Financial Incentive for Overdiagnosis

The admissions officers of many treatment centers assume that chemical use by adolescents automatically means there is a drug abuse problem present. Such treatment professionals, perhaps with an eye more on the balance sheet than on the individual's needs, frequently recommend treatment for any adolescent drug use. For example, Harold Swift, president of the world famous Hazelden Foundation, was quoted by Iggers (1990) as asking "what harm has been done?" if a teenager is mistakenly told that he or she is addicted to chemicals.

Newcomb and Bentler (1989) recognize that the treatment of chemical dependency has become a multimillion dollar industry where, on occasion, the client's needs are placed after those of the treatment center. Almost a decade after they issued their warning, the words of the authors continue to ring true:

> There is growing concern that for various reasons, not the least of which is the profit motive, treatment programs are purposefully blurring the distinction between use and abuse (any use equals abuse) and preying on the national drug hysteria to scare parents into putting their teenager in treatment with as little provocation as having a beer or smoking a joint. (p. 246)

Unfortunately, the annual bonus for the director and staff of many inpatient treatment programs is based on the average daily census (Dr. Norman Hoffmann, quoted in Turbo, 1989). Thus, there is a financial incentive for the clinical staff to keep as many beds occupied as possible. In such a situation, it is to the financial advantage of the treatment center staff to find as many cases of "addiction" as possible. One must wonder, given this situation, how much effort the treatment center staff would invest in excluding the possibility of drug abuse in an adolescent (or even an adult) being evaluated for possible admission under these circumstances.

Forcing the individual—even if "only" an adolescent—into treatment when he or she does not have a chemical addiction may have lifelong consequences (Peele, 1989). Such action may violate the individual's rights. In some states, it is illegal to force an adolescent into treatment against his or her will, even with parental permission (Evans & Sullivan, 1990).

To date, diagnostic criteria have not been developed that will allow for the accurate identification of those adolescents who are and are not addicted to chemicals. However, drug rehabilitation programs continue to

> aim . . . to convince children they are perpetually debilitated. Only after making this concession, treatment personnel contend, can children begin to make progress through life, albeit now

convinced that they can never really be whole or lead a normal existence. (Peele, 1989, pp. 103–104)

Unfortunately, there is no research into how this treatment approach will affect the individual's subsequent emotional growth. Nor is there research to determine whether there might be a negative consequence to telling the adolescent that he or she is forever an addict at such a young age, especially when the literature does not support this extreme view. What the literature *does* show is that many adolescents will repeatedly use one or more chemicals in an abusive manner, only to settle down in young adulthood to a more acceptable pattern of chemical use (Evans & Sullivan, 1990; Peele, 1989). For example, one recent study found that among identified adolescent "problem drinkers," fully 53% of the men and 70% of the women were judged not to be problem drinkers 7 years later (Zarek, Hawkins, & Rogers, 1987). Thus, the adolescent who might have abused chemicals on a regular basis may or may not go on to develop a problem with chemicals in young adulthood.

The Risks of Underdiagnosis

The diagnosis of adolescent drug or alcohol abuse is not easily made. As a general rule, adolescents do not develop the "withdrawal symptoms, hepatic changes, or gross organic brain syndromes" (Wheeler & Malmquist, 1987, p. 438) often found in adults who are addicted to alcohol or chemicals. If the assessor were to look for these "adult" symptoms of addiction in the child or adolescent, it is possible that the chemical abuse could be entirely overlooked.

However, there are also risks associated with failing to treat adolescents for whom drug use *is* a serious problem (Evans & Sullivan, 1990). First, there is evidence that protracted chemical use might interfere with the adolescent's ability to develop age-specific coping mechanisms (Kaminer, 1994). Furthermore, by the time the individual's drug use has resulted in serious physical

changes, or when he or she has acquired a blood infection such as AIDS from "dirty" needles, the individual is scarred not just for the rest of adolescence but for life. Thus, there are very serious reasons for identifying adolescents who have a chemical use problem before it is too late to avoid lifelong damage.

As researchers explored the factors associated with suicide during adolescence, they discovered that alcoholism or drug dependence is one of the factors associated with an increased risk of suicide (Callahan, 1993). The exact nature of this relationship is not clear, but researchers do know that chemical use is a factor in 70% of all adolescent suicides (Bukstein et al., 1993; Group for the Advancement of Psychiatry, 1990).

Bukstein et al. (1993) attempted to identify the factors associated with successful adolescent suicide attempts. Although no single risk factor seemed to identify those who were to ultimately take their own lives, the authors suggest that some of the factors include (1) active chemical abuse, (2) major depression, (3) thoughts of suicide within the past week, (4) a family history of suicide and/or depression, (5) legal problems, and (6) access to a handgun.

Thus, the chemical dependency treatment professional who works with adolescents must attempt to find the middle ground between the underdiagnosis, with all the dangers associated with teenage drug and alcohol abuse, and overdiagnosis, which may leave the individual with a false lifelong diagnosis of chemical dependency.

Diagnostic Criteria for Adolescent Substance Abuse

Given the forgoing arguments, are there indicators of adolescent chemical problems? Zarek, Hawkins, and Rogers (1987) identified six different criteria that act as indicators of adolescent drug abuse: (1) using chemicals to get "smashed," (2) going to parties where drugs other than alcohol are in use, (3) refusing to attend parties where drugs are not present, (4) drinking liquor (as opposed to beer or wine), (5) using marijuana, and (6) being drunk at school. The authors concluded that the adolescent who has a drug abuse problem is likely to be "enrolled in school, but is experiencing behavior problems related to school, such as being sent to the principal, or skipping classes" (p. 485).

According to Evans and Sullivan (1990), adolescents who are experiencing problems with chemical use often demonstrate many of the following problems in school: (1) tardiness, (2) absenteeism, (3) apathy, (4) sleepiness in classes, (5) moodiness, (6) negative attitude toward school, (7) change in friends, (8) loss of interest in extracurricular activities, (9) incomplete class assignments, and (10) a change in dress patterns. The authors also point out that adolescent drug use patterns are not the same as those seen in adults, as teenagers more often have "episodic, binge-like use patterns instead of gradual increases in use" (p. 117).

Evans and Sullivan (1990) also note that the adolescent who is becoming more and more preoccupied with chemical use or who demonstrates an interest in an expanding variety of chemicals might be showing the adolescent equivalent to the progression of chemical use often seen in adults. These individuals also demonstrate a loss of control, expressed through violations of personal rules about drug use (such as "I will only drink at parties"). Thus, Evans and Sullivan argue that those adolescents with drug abuse problems can be identified, and should be treated for their chemical dependency problems.

According to Newcomb and Bentler (1989), a teenager who is experiencing problems with alcohol or drugs (1) repeatedly uses chemicals, (2) uses chemicals at an inappropriate time, or (3) has legal, school, or social problems as a result of chemical use. This drug abuse problem may be either acute, episodic, or chronic, depending on how often the individual engages in drug use.

Summary

Clearly, children and adolescents are often hidden victims of drug addiction. Yet there is a serious lack of research into the problem of child or adolescent drug use and abuse. Although mental health professionals acknowledge that peer pressure and family environment influence the adolescent's chemical use pattern, the exact role that these forces (or the media) play in shaping the adolescent's behavior is still not known. There are many unanswered questions surrounding the issue of child and adolescent drug use, and in the years to come we may see significant breakthroughs in our understanding of the forces that shape chemical use beliefs and patterns of use for youths.

In the face of this dirth of clinical research, the treatment professional must steer a cautious path between the underdiagnosis and overdiagnosis of chemical dependency in the younger client. Just as surgery carried out on the individual during childhood or adolescence will have lifelong consequences, so will the traumatic experience of being forced into treatment for a problem which may or may not exist. As with surgery, the treatment professional should carefully weigh the potential benefits of treatment against the potential for harm.

Unfortunately, although treatment professionals understand that chemical use during adolescence is one factor in a wide range of emotional and physical problems that develop during this phase of life, the diagnostic criteria needed to identify adolescents who are "at risk" for subsequent problems are still evolving. Thus, treatment professionals have no firm guidelines for determining whether an adolescent is passing through a phase of experimental chemical use or has a more serious problem.

CHAPTER TWENTY-FOUR

Codependency and Enabling

For each identified addict, there are many hidden victims. Some of these people are total strangers to the addict, such as victims of drug-related burglaries or alcohol-related motor vehicle accidents. Although these episodes are disturbing, the individual victim is not usually involved in an ongoing relationship with the addicted person. The burglary accident is an isolated incident, not part of an unhealthy relationship with an addict.

As substance abuse professionals started to explore the addict's interpersonal relationships, they found some people who, although sickened by the addict's behavior, actually behave in ways that *enable* the individual to continue to abuse drugs. Researchers have found that some family members seem to be *codependent* with the addict. Codependency and enabling have become almost themes for the current generation and are the focus of this chapter.

Enabling

In the context of substance abuse, to *enable* means to *knowingly* do something that makes it possible for another person to continue to use chemicals without having to pay the natural consequences of substance abuse. In a very real sense, someone who enables an addict protects that person from the consequences of his or her behavior. Armed with the best intentions of

protecting the addicted person, the enabler becomes part of the problem, not the solution. The enabler prevents the addict from taking advantage of the many opportunities to discover firsthand the cost of his or her addiction.

A common misconception is that only family members can enable an addict. Although an enabler may be a family member, he or she could also be a co-worker, supervisor, neighbor, friend, advisor, teacher, therapist, or even drug rehabilitation worker. Any person who *knowingly* acts to protect the addicted person from the natural consequences of his or her behavior can be said to be an enabler.

In reference to alcoholism, the booklet *The Family Enablers* (Johnson Institute, 1987) defines an enabler as *any* person who "reacts to an alcoholic in such a way as to shield the alcoholic from experiencing the full impact of the harmful consequences of alcoholism" (p. 5). The same criterion can be applied to those who enable people who are addicted to other drugs of abuse. By knowingly shielding the user from the harmful consequences of her or his behavior, one enables.

An enabler does not need to be involved in an ongoing relationship with the addict in order to enable him or her. A person who refuses to provide testimony about a crime out of fear or to avoid "becoming involved" enables the perpetrator of the crime to escape. But sometimes the enabler *is* involved in an ongoing relationship with an addicted person, as in the case of co-workers. In that case, one person could be manipulated into enabling another's addiction on an ongoing basis.

Enabling Behaviors in the Workplace

It is difficult to understand the multitude of ways in which someone can enable an addict to continue the compulsive use of chemicals. Hyde (1989) relates how one operating room staff hesitated to confront a surgeon suspected of being under the influence of chemicals, either out of denial, fear of reprisal, or a desire not to become involved. These health care professionals could be called enablers of the surgeon's continued use of chemicals.

Several characteristic behaviors of the enabler in the workplace include (1) doing work for the addicted individual when that person is unable to do his or her own required work, (2) "covering" for the impaired individual's poor performance, (3) accepting excuses or making special arrangements for the impaired individual, (4) overlooking frequent absenteeism or tardiness, and (5) overlooking evidence of chemical use (Hyde, 1989). Admittedly, it is difficult to deal with an addicted person in the workplace, especially if the addict is a supervisor or administrator. To further complicate matters, the addicted person actively tries to manipulate the interpersonal environment to force others to continue to enable his or her chemical use. Not uncommonly, the alcoholic treats enablers as if they are being granted the "privilege" of taking responsibility for the addicted person's life! The temptation is for the enabler to go along with this myth, rather than confronting the addicted person and risking retaliation.

For example, when confronted by the supervisor for being late again, an employee might respond, "You are lucky that I work here in the first place!" Perhaps out of a fear of legal action or simply from overwork, the supervisor may agree that the company is indeed lucky to have the addict as an employee. The supervisor may

warn the addict not to let "it" happen again, but without taking any firm action.

Styles of Enabling

There are essentially three different subtypes of enablers, classified by certain behaviors they have in common (Ellis, McInerney, DiGiuseppe, & Yeager, 1988). The first type is the *joiner*. To try to control the addict's chemical use, the "joiner" works to support the addict's use of chemicals and may even use drugs with the addict. A classic example of a joiner is the woman who asked for marital counseling because her husband would not limit his cocaine use to the $100 a week that she set aside in the family budget for his drug use! Another all too common example of a joiner is the spouse who drinks or who uses chemicals along with the addict, in the hope of somehow controlling the addict's chemical use. It is quite common for a spouse to go to a bar with the alcoholic, hoping that the alcoholic will learn "responsible" drinking by example.

Ellis et al. identify the second type of enabler as the *messiah*. The messiah fights against the addict's chemical use but does so in such a way that the addict is never forced to experience the consequences of his or her behavior. For example, in a group session, one father of a narcotics addict admitted that he had taken out personal loans more than once to pay off his daughter's drug debts. An addict in the group who had been in recovery for some time asked why the father would do this. "After all," the addict said, "if you pay off her debts, she won't have to worry about paying them off herself." Several other group members suggested to this parent that the daughter might need to suffer some consequences on her own and "hit bottom" to come to terms with her addiction. The father was silent for a moment and then said, "Oh, I couldn't do that! She's not ready to assume responsibility for herself!"

The third type of enabler according to Ellis et al. is the *silent sufferer*. The silent sufferer seems to believe that "As long as I suffer, I *am* somebody!" In a very real sense, the silent sufferer is a martyr who lives with the addict in spite of the pain the addicted person causes—unhappy, yet unwilling to leave. It often seems that the silent sufferer finds meaning in life only through a relationship with an addict. The "silent sufferer" protects the addicted person by "always being there and pretending that nothing is wrong" (Ellis et al., 1988, p. 109). Rather than risk losing what little emotional security the addict might offer, the silent sufferer says nothing and tries not to "rock the boat." Silent sufferers keep family conflict from breaking out, and seem to act as lightning rods, drawing all the pain and suffering away from the addict to themselves.

The Relationship Between Enabling and Codependency

The key concept to remember is that an enabler *knowingly* behaves so as to protect the addict from the consequences of his or her behavior. We have probably all behaved in ways that, in retrospect, may have enabled an addict to avoid some consequence of drug use that he or she would otherwise have suffered.

This is a point that is often quite confusing to the student of addiction. Codependency and enabling may be, and often are, found in the same person. However, one can also enable an addict without being codependent on that person. *Enabling* refers to *specific behaviors*, whereas *codependency* refers to *a relationship pattern*. Thus, one can enable addiction without being codependent; but the codependent individual, because he or she is in an ongoing relationship with the addict, also frequently enables the addict. Enabling does not require an ongoing relationship. A tourist who gives a street beggar a gift of money, knowing that the beggar is likely addicted and in need of drugs, can be said to have enabled the beggar. But the tourist is hardly in a meaningful relationship with the addict. The wife who calls in to work to say that her husband is "sick," when he is actually hungover from the night before is both codependent

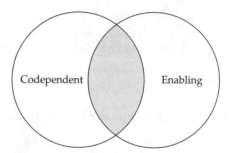

FIGURE 24.1 The overlapping relationship of codependency and enabling

and an enabler. Another example is the husband who calls to tell the probation officer that his wife cannot keep today's appointment, because she is ill. The husband knows full well that his wife had been drinking the night before and that she would fail a drug screen test and be sent to prison. This husband is both codependent and enabling his wife's continued drinking.

The issues of codependency and enabling can be thought of as "overlapping" issues that may or may not be found in the same individual. A diagram of this relationship is shown in Figure 24.1. The area of overlap between codependency and enabling represents how the codependent person may also enable the addict, an all too common occurrence. As many substance abuse rehabilitation professionals can attest to, this enabling is often carried out in the name of "love." Helping the codependent see the difference between love and enabling is often a difficult task.

Codependency

The concept of codependency has emerged in the past decade to become one of the cornerstones of rehabilitation. Surprisingly, in spite of all that has been said and written about it, there is no standard definition of codependency (Heimel, 1990; Tavris, 1990). Indeed, mental health professionals have yet to agree on as basic an issue as whether the word is hyphenated (co-dependency) or not (codependency) (Beattie, 1989).

However, even without a standard definition for the concept, many families and friends of addicted persons are aware that they have suffered, and often continue to suffer, as a result of having "a relationship with a dysfunctional person" (Beattie, 1989, p. 7).

Defining Codependency

According to Wegscheider-Cruse (1985) codependency is

> a specific condition that is characterized by preoccupation and extreme dependence (emotionally, socially, and sometimes physically) on a person or object. Eventually, this dependence ... becomes a pathological condition that affects the co-dependent in all other relationships. (p. 2)

Yet even this definition does not fully capture the flavor of codependency, and O'Brien and Gaborit (1992) offer a different definition:

> In a codependent relationship, the needs of two people are met in dysfunctional ways. The chemical dependent's need for a care taker, caused by an increasing inability to meet basic survival needs as the drug becomes increasingly intrusive ... is met by the codependent's need to control the behavior of others who have difficulty caring for themselves. (p. 129)

And in yet another definition of codependency, Gorski (1992) calls it a general term "describing a cluster of symptoms or maladaptive behavior changes associated with living in a committed relationship with either a chemically dependent person or a chronically dysfunctional person either as children or adults" (p. 15).

Although these definitions have similarities and dissimilarities, they all seek to identify different core aspects of codependency: (1) the *overinvolvement* with the dysfunctional person, (2) the *obsessive* attempts by the codependent to control the dysfunctional person's behavior, (3) the extreme tendency to use *external sources of self-worth* (approval from others, including the dysfunctional person in the relationship), and

(4) the *tendency to make personal sacrifices* in an attempt to "cure" the dysfunctional person of his or her problem behavior.

The Dynamics of Codependency

In an early paper on the subject, Beattie (1987) spoke of codependency as a process in which the individual's life has become unmanageable because he or she is involved in a committed relationship with an addict and is unable to simply walk away. Often, codependent individuals believe that somehow the addict's behavior is a reflection on them. In response to this threat to self-esteem ("*your* behavior is a reflection of *me*"), the codependent person becomes obsessed with the need to control the addict's behavior (Beattie, 1987). In so doing, the codependent assumes responsibility for decisions and events not actually under his or her control, such as the addict's drinking or drug use. More than one codependent spouse has blamed him- or herself for "causing" the alcoholic to go out on a binge after having a fight. "It's all my fault that he (or, "she") went out drinking" is a common theme for the codependent.

As we noted earlier, one symptom of codependency is a *preoccupation* (Wegscheider-Cruse, 1985) or *obsession* (Beattie, 1989) with controlling the addict's behavior. This obsession with controlling another person's behavior may extend to the point where the codependent tries to control not only the addict's substance use but all of the addict's life. An excellent example of this obsessive attempt to control the addict's behavior took place at a maximum security penitentiary for men in the Midwest. A staff psychologist received a telephone call from an elderly mother of an inmate, asking the psychologist to "make sure that the man who shares my son's cell is a good influence" on her son, because "there are a lot of bad men in that prison, and I don't want him falling in with a bad crowd!"

This woman overlooked the grim reality that her son was not in prison for singing off-key in choir practice. In fact, he had been to prison on several previous occasions for various crimes. Rather than let him live his life and try to get on with her own, this woman continued to worry about how to "cure" him of his behavior problem. She still treated him as a child, was overly involved in his life, and was quite upset at the suggestion that it might be time to let her son learn to suffer (and perhaps learn from) the consequences of his own behavior.

The Rules of Codependency

Although the codependent person often believes that he or she is going crazy, an outside observer can see certain patterns or "rules" to codependent behavior. Beattie (1989) delineates the following unspoken "rules" of codependency.

1. It's not OK for me to feel.
2. It's not OK for me to have problems.
3. It's not OK for me to have fun.
4. I'm not lovable.
5. I'm not good enough.
6. If people act bad or crazy, I'm responsible.

These rules are actively transmitted from one partner in the relationship to the other, setting the pattern for codependency. "If you weren't so unreasonable, I would never have gone out drinking last night!" is a common example of Rule 6. "You shouldn't have tried in the first place!" might enforce Rules 2, 3, 4, and 5.

Are Codependents Born or Made?

Proponents of the concept of codependency suggest that it is a *learned behavior*, often passed from one generation to another. An example of how one unhealthy generation trains another to be codependent—one that (unfortunately) is repeated time and time again—is the parent who confronts a child who wants to go to college with the taunt, "You're too dumb to go to college. The best that you can hope for is to find somebody stupid enough to marry you and take care of you!"

Scarf (1980) points out that we all tend to try to resolve "unfinished business" with our parents by re-creating these all-important early relationships in our adult lives. Frequently, especially for the individual who struggles with feelings of low self-esteem as a result of having been raised in a dysfunctional home, this means being drawn to unhealthy partners as part of the process of trying to resolve early parent/child conflicts.

In other words, we re-create our original families through our adult relationships and then attempt to resolve any unresolved conflicts through these surrogates. Depending on how healthy or unhealthy these surrogates are, this process can either be a positive one or one that traps the individual into unhealthy cycles. Heimel (1991) provides a beautiful capsule summary of this process as she describes reacting to a boyfriend's rejection with the same depression that she experienced when she was growing up:

> This is how I felt as a kid when my mother turned her back and wouldn't speak to me, when my father, my beloved father, shook his head and said, "After all we've done for you." This is how I felt when I was turning myself inside out trying to get my parents to love me, something they couldn't quite manage. (p. 42)

Because of this earlier rejection, Heimel (1991) saw herself as vulnerable to being rejected again in adulthood. She lacked sufficient self-esteem to weather the crisis of being rejected, although on one level she understood that there never was a serious relationship with the young man in question.

Children who have been exposed to physical, sexual, or emotional abuse are frequently left with significant feelings of low self-esteem. These individuals are unable to affirm the "self," possibly because they do not believe that they are valuable or capable individuals. Such victims are vulnerable to being drawn time after time to unhealthy partners in an attempt to resolve this past trauma through their current relationships. It is almost as if they are "trapped" in a never-ending cycle.

Furthermore, as the dysfunctional elements in the relationship develop, the codependent also frequently comes to feel "trapped" in the relationship. All relationships have some dysfunctional elements, but in a healthy relationship, the partners confront these unhealthy components and work on resolving them to the satisfaction of both partners. For example, one partner might express a concern to the other that their finances are getting a little tight and that perhaps they should look at cutting back on unnecessary spending for a couple of weeks. But, in the codependent relationship, the "working through" process is stalled. If one partner expresses some concern over a problem, the other partner tries to prevent the problem from being clearly identified or—if it is identified—from being resolved.

As part of an attempt to avoid displeasing the addict, the codependent restricts communications, avoiding people or topics of conversation that might displease the significant other. Eventually, a self-fulfilling cycle is established in which the codependent is afraid to say the "wrong" thing, afraid to talk to the "wrong people," and afraid to assert self-hood. The codependent is afraid to leave the relationship, believing that he or she has nobody else to turn to, yet is not happy in the relationship with the addicted individual.

Codependency and Self-Esteem

In an attempt to live up to the unspoken rules of codependency, the codependent experiences a great deal of emotional pain. The core of codependency, as viewed by Zerwekh and Michaels (1989) is "related to low self-esteem" on the part of the codependent person: "Co-dependents frequently appear normal, which in our culture is associated with a healthy ego. Nevertheless, they also describe themselves as 'dying on the inside,' which is indicative of low self-worth or esteem" (p. 111).

Lacking sufficient self-esteem to withstand the demands of the dysfunctional partner, the codependent often measures personal worth by how well he or she can take care of the addicted individual. Another way that codependents often measure self-worth is through the sacrifices they make for the addicted individual, the family, or significant others (Miller, 1988). In this way, the codependent substitutes an external measure of personal worth for the inability to generate *self*-worth.

Drug rehabilitation workers are often surprised at the amount of suffering and pain that codependent family members suffer but are confused as to why they do not do something to end the pain. There is a reward for enduring this pain. As Shapiro (1981) points out, there is a certain moral victory to be achieved through suffering at the hands of another, because suffering allows the codependent to accuse "the offender by pointing at his victim; it keeps alive in the mind's record an injustice committed, a score unsettled" (p. 115). According to Shapiro (1981), for the codependent, suffering is "a necessity, a principled act of will, from which he cannot release himself without losing his self-respect and feeling more deeply and finally defeated, humiliated, and powerless" (p. 115).

Thus, for some, the trials and suffering imposed on the codependent person become a defense against the admission of powerlessness or worthlessness. In many cases, the codependent affirms personal worth by being willing to "carry the cross" of another person's addiction or dysfunctional behavior.

Codependency and Emotional Health

There is a very real tendency for some people to *overidentify* with the codependency concept. As Beattie (quoted in Tavris, 1992, p. 194) points out, there are those who believe that codependency is "anything, and everyone is codependent." This is an extreme position that overlooks the fact that many of the same characteristics that define the codependent are also found in

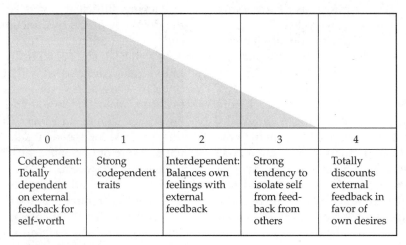

0	1	2	3	4
Codependent: Totally dependent on external feedback for self-worth	Strong codependent traits	Interdependent: Balances own feelings with external feedback	Strong tendency to isolate self from feedback from others	Totally discounts external feedback in favor of own desires

FIGURE 24.2   From codependency to isolation

healthy human relationships. Only a few "saints and hermits" (Tavris, 1990, p. 21A) fail to demonstrate at least some characteristics of the so-called codependent individual.

Even Wegscheider-Cruse and Cruse (1990), strong advocates of the codependency movement, admit that "co-dependency is an exaggeration of normal personality traits" (p. 28), which become so pronounced that the individual "becomes disabled (disease of co-dependency)" (p. 28). Codependency is thus a matter of degree.

Whereas there are some personality patterns in which the individual isolates him- or herself from interpersonal feedback, the codependent individual tends to be extremely dependent on the feedback from the significant other. The whole goal of the codependent seems to be that of winning love, approval, and acceptance from the object of his or her affection. Unable to affirm the "self," the codependent seeks to win this affirmation from the significant other.

The danger is that the significant other may withdraw even the little love and affirmation that he or she offers. The codependent becomes exquisitely sensitive to the slightest sign of disapproval or rejection from the significant other, to the point of losing touch with his or her own feelings. Thus, on one hand, there is a total sensitivity toward interpersonal feedback,

whereas on the other hand, there is a supersensitivity to this feedback.

Between these two extremes is an *interdependency* that is the hallmark of healthy relationships. The extremes between isolation and codependency are depicted in Figure 24.2. Codependency is not an all-or-nothing phenomenon. Admittedly, codependency does exist, and there are those who seem to be codependent. But *there are degrees of codependency*, just as there are degrees of isolation from interpersonal feedback. Few of us are at either extreme, and the majority of us tend to fall somewhere in the middle, exhibiting tendencies both to behave in codependent ways and to be overly isolated from feedback from others.

How to Create a Codependent

Substance abuse professionals often speak of a "cycle" of codependency that takes on a life of its own. A graphic representation of the cycle of codependency appears in Figure 24.3. Notice that there are two necessary components to the growth of codependency. The first is that one partner, the codependent, suffers from low self-esteem. If one partner *does not* suffer from low self-esteem, he or she would be able to affirm "self" and would back away from a dysfunc-

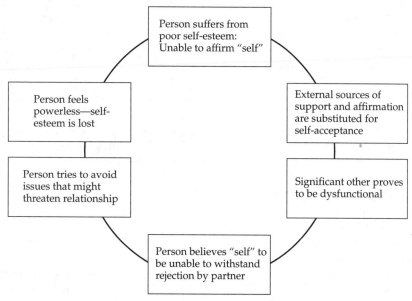

FIGURE 24.3 The cycle of codependency

tional partner—or, at the very least, find a way to cope without depending on the dysfunctional partner's approval. In this case, it is unlikely that a codependent relationship would evolve.

Second, the "significant other" must prove to be dysfunctional; if the partner were emotionally healthy, he or she would affirm the codependent. Such an atmosphere would enhance the psychological growth of the codependent, who in time would be able to affirm "self" without the need for external supports. Thus, codependency rests on an interaction between the "pathologies" (for want of a better word) of the two partners.

Opposition to the Codependency Concept

Since the time of its introduction, the reaction against the concept of codependency has been rather strong. For example, some argue that, rather than serving to "empower" the client, *the concept of codependency takes away from the individual's power.* The codependent person is told that the "disease" of codependency is progressive and that he or she can never come to

terms with the codependency unassisted (Kaminer, 1992; Tavris, 1990). Rather, it is only through an appropriate "self-help" group that the individual can face his or her codependency. The codependent is repeatedly encouraged to accept that he or she is powerless over this condition. Thus, it has been argued that the concept of codependency maintains the individual in a perpetual state of helplessness. For this reason, many critics of the codependency concept believe that self-help groups "promote dependency under the guise of recovery" (Katz & Liu, 1991, p. xii).

Kaminer (1992) suggests that, in a subtle manner, the codependency literature demands not individual growth and autonomy but conformity to a standard recipe for salvation and grace. According to the codependency model, no matter how trivial or serious the trauma, there is just one model for recovery. If the individual resists the various " insights" offered by different books on codependency, that person is automatically viewed as being in "denial" (Kaminer, 1992; Katz & Liu, 1991).

Adherents to the theory of codependency

view the condition as a universal condition. Indeed, it often seems that much of the literature on codependency strives to convince the individual that he or she is "doomed to suffer as a result of the trauma of childhood travails" (Japenga, 1991, p. 174). However, there is little research to support this position. The literature on codependency seems to discount the possibility that the individual may have successfully weathered the storm of whatever childhood trauma he or she may have suffered.

Opponents of the codependency theory point out that the literature on codependency suggests that up to 99% of all people are raised in a "dysfunctional" home, and, because of this, they *automatically* have deep emotional scars from childhood. They are "encouraged to see themselves as victims of family life rather than self-determining participants" (Kaminer, 1992, p. 13). In the codependency view, the family is nothing more than an "incubator of disease" (Kaminer, 1992, p. 12). Within this incubator, the helpless child is infected with one or more dread conditions that he or she will have to struggle with forever unless salvation is achieved through the appropriate self-help group.

Yet research suggests that even if a child is raised in a "dysfunctional" home, the child is not automatically doomed to suffer. Indeed, many—perhaps a majority—of those who are exposed to even extreme conditions in childhood find a way to adjust, survive, and fulfill their life goals (Garbarino, Dubrow, Kostelny, & Pardo, 1992). Admittedly, some children will suffer deep emotional scars as a result of childhood trauma, but children are not *automatically* doomed to suffer if their home life is less than perfect.

Evidence has been uncovered indicating that some children are able to develop a natural resilience to even extreme forms of psychological trauma (Wolin & Wolin, 1993; Werner, 1989). This natural resilience helps them weather not only the emotional storms of childhood but those of later adult life as well. Indeed, the very fact that the child's environment *is* dysfunctional might serve as an impetus to develop

positive emotional growth in many cases (Wolin & Wolin, 1993; Garbarino et al., 1992).

Another challenge to the concept of codependency is based on the theory (frequently advanced in books on the subject) that all suffering is relative. As Kaminer (1992) points out, it is hard to equate degrees of suffering. Consider two hypothetical children in two different families. Both are the oldest boys in a family of three children with an alcoholic father. In the first family, the father is a "happy" drunk, who drinks each evening after work, tells a few "funny" jokes, watches television, and falls asleep in his favorite chair. In the second family, the father drinks each evening after work and becomes violently angry, physically abusing his wife and children.

The impact that one father would have on his family would be far different from the other's. Yet, in the literature on codependency, both events are treated as equally influential. This example also underscores another criticism of the concept of codependency; the theory of codependency excuses the addicted individual from all responsibility for his or her behavior (Roehling, Koelbel, & Rutgers, 1994; Tavris, 1990). The blame is shifted from the abusive person to the spouse, sibling, parents, or even the codependent individual who "enables" this abusive, violent, or destructive behavior to continue. As Kottler (1992) observes,

[b]y subscribing to a codependency model we reinforce the idea that the client is not responsible for her behavior, that she was born or made into "a woman who loves too much," a "woman who loves men who hate women," or who has a "doormat syndrome," or any number of other euphemisms that explain the disease invading the "codependent psyche." (p. 138)

Another challenge to the concept of codependency is based on the fact that family members are judged not for their own accomplishments but on the basis of the addict's inability to abstain from chemicals. In other words, they are guilty of "addiction by association" (Katz & Liu, 1991, p. 13). The problem is not that the father is alcoholic, physically abusive, and both emotionally inappropriate and absent. Rather, the problem is that the *family* members suffer from the disease of codependency! In this manner, the disease model as applied to codependency shifts the blame from the addict to the nonaddicted individual.

Those who challenge the concept of codependency also point out that the idea of codependency is an outgrowth of the theory (popular in the 1950s) that the spouse of the alcoholic is a *co-alcoholic* (Simmons, 1991; Sher, 1991). This theory assumed that the co-alcoholic was as much in need of treatment as was the alcoholic because the co-alcoholic (1) helped to bring about the other's alcoholism, (2) continues to support it, and (3) must be quite disturbed.

In the past 40 years, the concept of the co-alcoholic has been discredited by mental health professionals. Indeed, researchers have found virtually no evidence to support the assumption that the spouse of the alcoholic has a predictable form of psychopathology (Tavris, 1992). But, some argue that the theory of co-alcoholism has apparently found new life in the codependency model. Much of what was once said about the co-alcoholic in the 1950s is repeated as "gospel truth" about the codependent of the 1990s, in spite of the fact that there is little research to support these conclusions.

Another weakness of the concept of codependency is that the term *codependent* has been modified to serve as a noun or adjective and has been given a definition that has "broadened to include anyone who has ever been involved with anyone who has ever had a problem around which a Twelve Step program has been, is being, or should be built" (Simmons, 1991, p. 26A). It is a term that ultimately fails to communicate anything meaningful about the individual. Indeed, the very nature of the defining characteristics of the "codependent" person virtually guarantees that any given individual will meet at least one of the defining "criteria" (Tavris, 1992). The term *codependent* has been applied to so many people and for so many behaviors that it is almost a secret language—a

"recoveryspeak" (Simmons, 1991, p. 26A), a form of secret handshake that might be used to bring a sense of security to people in an insane, overpowering world.

Nor is codependency limited to the world of addiction. O'Brien & Gaborit (1992) even suggest that codependency is a separate condition that may or may not actually involve a substance abusing partnership. In other words, the authors suggest that codependency is a clinical syndrome in its own right. It *may* exist in a substance abusing relationship, but that is only a coincidence. The hypothetical "disease" of codependence could also be found in a variety of nonsubstance abusing relationships, according to O'Brien and Gaborit.

Another challenge to the concept of codependency rests on its lack of firm parameters. The term appears to be vague and without foundation, and there is no consensus among professionals that the condition even exists (Roehling, Koelbel, & Rutgers, 1994). This is not to say that excessive dependency is not a clinical problem, only that *codependency* might not exist as a separate disorder. Yet the belief that there is such a thing as codependence is quite strong among some professionals.

Many of the books and articles on codependency give the impression that it rests on a foundation of "New Age sand." For example, the husband and wife team of Wegscheider-Cruse and Cruse (1990) speak knowingly of how codependency results from the "interaction between one's own manufactured 'brain chemicals'(having to do with our reinforcement center) and one's behavior that stimulates the brain to establish compulsive and addictive behavior processes" (p. 12). They go on to conclude that codependency is a disease of the brain, on the grounds that "we have a brain that gives us an excessive rush, (and) we get into self-defeating behaviors that keep the rush coming (co-dependency)" (pp. 12–13). What the authors overlook is that there is no scientific evidence to support this position. Science, to date, has failed to find evidence of "an excessive rush" (what would be a "sufficient rush"?), nor have scientists found evidence to suggest that people tend to "get into self-defeating behaviors that keep the rush coming." Indeed, such a position seems contradictory: if human beings as a race engaged in self-defeating behaviors simply for the "rush," how would we have survived long enough to become a successful species?

Thus, there is a need for balance in considering the concept of codependency. There certainly are people who experience significant hardship because of their involvement in an ongoing relationship with an addict. But not *every* person who is in such a relationship is necessarily codependent. And, according to the codependency model, the victim must somehow come to terms with his or her emotional pain while the addict remains blameless. In discussing the shortcomings of the concept of codependency, the University of California, Berkeley (1990a) concluded,

> according to adherents of this theory, families of alcoholics cannot . . . hold them responsible for the abuse. Somehow the victim must get well by

dint of pure self-analysis, meditation and prayer, without reference to the social, economic, legal and psychological forces that create dysfunctional families in the first place. (p. 7)

For many people, this is an impossible task.

Summary

In the late 1970s, substance abuse professionals were introduced to a new way of thinking about the addicted person and his or her support system. The concept of codependency was introduced as a way of explaining how members of the addict's support system behaved. However, almost from the time it was introduced, the concept of codependency has met with resistance. A number of challenges to the concept of codependency have been suggested over the years, not the least of which is that this is only a revised term for the once-popular theory that the alcoholic spouse was a co-alcoholic. Although this theory was discredited in the 1960s, some argue that it has found new life under the guise of codependency.

CHAPTER TWENTY-FIVE

Addiction and the Family

The different combinations possible between marriage, family, and addiction staggers the imagination. Many people who are or who become addicted to chemicals are married. Sometimes they marry before they begin down the road toward addiction. Sometimes one marital partner is unaware of the other's prior addiction, and suddenly the family is faced with the reality of an addicted member. An addict may choose to marry another addict, a marriage of convenience that brings with it a "using partner," an additional source of chemicals and money. Or the nonaddict might enter into marriage with full knowledge of the partner's addiction but with hopes of "saving" the addict from his or her behavior.

When an individual becomes addicted to chemicals after getting married and having children, the family is forced to come to terms with parental chemical addiction. An increasingly common pattern in these families is for the adolescent to become addicted to chemicals as well, a possibility that was discussed in Chapter 21. In this chapter, we will focus on the impact that parental substance use has on the family, and how the family learns to cope with parental drug addiction.

The problem of parental chemical use and abuse is hardly a minor one. It has been estimated that *more than 10% of the U.S. population* comes from an alcoholic home (Ackerman, 1983). Nobody knows what percentage of the population was raised in a home where the parental drug of choice was something other than alcohol. But, given the scope of the problem of illicit drug use and the fact that this social problem has existed for generations, it is safe to say that significant numbers of children have been raised in homes with some form of addiction present for many, many years.

Addiction and Marriage

Very little is known about the role chemicals play within the marital relationship. What little information is available deals almost exclusively with the "alcoholic marriage," the marriage in which one partner is alcoholic. In this type of marriage, there is often a "role reversal" (Ackerman, 1983) between the marital partners. This role reversal may eventually involve other family members as well, often spanning two or three generations. Over time, an unhealthy state of dependency evolves between the alcoholic and the other family members who have a codependent relationship with the alcoholic.

The Evolution of Marital Codependency

Bowen (1985) observes that, as a general rule, people tend to marry those who have achieved similar levels of "differentiation of self" (p. 263), which is "roughly equivalent to the concept of emotional maturity" (p. 263). A primary developmental task for the individual is to separate from his or her parents (or *individuate*) and resolve the various emotional attachments to the parents that evolved during childhood.

As we mature, our relationship patterns with our parents change. When we are young, we are completely dependent on our parents. But, as we mature, we become less and less dependent on them, until by the time of young adulthood, we are capable of dealing with life's trials on our own. This process of separating from one's parents is known as *individuation* (Bowen, 1985).

Parents can either encourage the child's emotional growth or inhibit it. Inherent in Bowen's (1985) theory is the belief that it is possible for the child to fail to learn to resolve the multiple conflicts that arise in childhood and adolescence; that is, an individual may fail to individuate. Proponents of the concept of codependency suggest that this often happens in the alcoholic home.

According to Bowen's theory, the child requires parental support and guidance during his or her emotional growth. If the parents are unable to provide the proper guidance and support because of their own emotional problems, the child may fail to make the appropriate emotional break necessary to individuate. In that case, he or she remains emotionally dependent on the parents for feedback and support. As an adult, this person views him- or herself as weak and, possibly, incomplete. This person remains dependent on external sources of feedback and support, which may be obtained from continued dependency on the parents or on a parental substitute.

In adulthood, while searching for a marital partner, we each seek to join with someone with a similar level of emotional independence (Bowen, 1985). In a union of two emotionally vulnerable individuals, each looks to the other to meet his or her dependency needs, according to Bowen. Although the marriage may offer the potential for further emotional growth for both partners, it also carries the risk inherent in emotional growth. For some, this risk is too great, and

they turn away from the other person for support to the pseudointimacy of chemicals.

Characteristics of the Alcoholic Marriage

Within the dysfunctional marriage, issues of control often become important as each person struggles to achieve some sense of order. *Conditional love* becomes an important means of control within the alcoholic marriage. Conditional love finds expression in a number of demands:

(1) You must behave in a certain way, if you want to be
    (a)   loved by me
    (b)   supported by me (and so on)
(2) If you don't meet my demands, I will
    (a)   leave you
    (b)   withdraw my love from you
    (c)   not give you money
    (d)   go out and get drunk
    (e)   abuse you physically

For the alcoholic spouse, the goal of these control "games" is to make sure that the family does not stray too far from the alcoholic fold. *Detachment* then becomes both an expression of *un*conditional love and the vehicle that transports one away from the *enmeshment* of the alcoholic home. The detached expression of love is one in which each spouse allows the other the freedom to make decisions without restriction. In working with codependent people, it is often necessary to teach them the difference between *concern* for another person and *responsibility* for that person. For example, "I might have feelings for another person, but I am not responsible for living that person's life."

It is also often necessary to help the codependent person learn appropriate interpersonal *boundaries.* The alcoholic home, resting as it does on the unstable sands of addiction, is in constant danger of being washed away. Each family member develops an unnatural involvement in the lives of the others. As part of the natural growth process that results in individuation, the child must learn to establish boundaries between "self" and "other"; but in the alcoholic home, the child learns to become *enmeshed* in the lives of others. Each person has been trained to believe that he or she is responsible for every other member of the family.

The Training of a Codependent Partner

In a very real sense, the codependent person has been "trained" to be codependent through the process of being raised in a disturbed home environment. As stated earlier, in such a situation, the individual never has the opportunity to individuate from the family of origin. Family members are frequently so enmeshed in each other's lives that personal growth is virtually impossible for everyone.

The codependent person does not learn during childhood that he or she has the right to set limits within relationships, even in the marital relationship. In many cases, the codependent person is raised to believe that violations of personal boundaries is a price to be paid for love. Codependents learn to tolerate this violation in an attempt to win the approval and love of any person who offers even the remote promise of accepting them. Sometimes, the codependent person has had his or her boundaries violated so often that he or she does not recognize appropriate limits to begin with.

Armed with these distorted perceptions of family life, the individual entering adulthood tries to find a safe, familiar environment, often without realizing that the most "familiar" environment is the one that they just escaped from! Quite often, the potential partner who most closely matches the characteristics of the home environment is another potential addict. Thus, there is an interaction of pathologies between the addicted person and the codependent person. Each gravitates toward the other and interprets the emotional response to their discovery of each other as "love."

Addicts often try to give the impression that they need somebody to take care of them. In so doing, they are looking for someone who will relieve them of some of the responsibilities of daily living so they can invest that energy into

drug use. The codependent, who frequently struggles with feelings of inadequacy, is thrilled to be needed at last. However, the addict is looking not for a partner but for a spouse who will become part of the addictive support system. Once such a person is found, the addict strives to keep the spouse in a supportive role so the addiction can be maintained.

The dance of codependency is now complete: on the one hand, there is the person who is at least potentially addicted to chemicals, who seeks as little responsibility for his or her life as possible. On the other hand, there is the codependent person who seeks to fuse with the marital partner to find the emotional strength in the partner that is lacking in the "self."

The therapeutic task in working with a codependent individual is to teach the dependent person how to detach from the addict and meet his or her own needs. This is a difficult task that requires helping the codependent person achieve the emotional independence that should have been accomplished in childhood and adolescence. The dependent person will struggle to hold on to what he or she viewed as a source of emotional security: the partner. Furthermore, premature separation may make the codependent feel useless, immobilized, and quite often hurt.

Addiction and the Family

There is actually very little information available about the effects of other forms of parental drug addiction on different members of the family constellation. What little is known addresses the issue of the impact of parental alcoholism on the family. There is much to learn about how, for example, the mother's heroin addiction might impact the emotional growth of her children.

The treatment of addiction involves the identification and ultimate modification of whatever original dysfunctional family system allowed the development and maintenance of the addiction in the first place (Bowen, 1985). In the alcoholic marriage, for example, alcoholism becomes a "secret partner," first in the marriage and then in the family. In time, this "family secret" becomes the dominating force around which the family's rules and rituals are formed (Brown, 1985).

Because of their special role in the family, parents often set the tone or themes around which the family members center their lives through the use of parental *injunctions*. In the alcoholic home, however, the parental injunctions are often (1) there is no addiction in this home, and (2) don't you dare talk about it! As noted in Chapter 24, the codependent marital relationship rests on a foundation of other "rules" (Beattie, 1989) as well.

1. It's not OK for me to feel.
2. It's not OK for me to have problems.
3. It's not OK for me to have fun.
4. I'm not lovable.
5. I'm not good enough.
6. If people act bad or crazy, I'm responsible.

All these injunctions form the emotional atmosphere in which the children are raised. It is thought that as the children grow up, they incorporate these rules into their personality, carrying the scars of childhood trauma with them into adulthood.

Being raised in an alcoholic home requires that children learn how to adapt. Indeed, the whole family must learn to adapt to meet the demands of an addicted parent (Ackerman, 1983). Unfortunately, one of the ways that the family comes to terms with parental alcoholism is to structure itself in such a way that the alcoholic parent is actually encouraged to continue drinking. Rather than forcing the alcoholic to carry out the role he or she should occupy within the family, it becomes easier just to redistribute the power and responsibilities within the family. When the family system changes to accommodate the alcoholic, other family members may find themselves holding unusually powerful positions within the new family constellation.

The process of adapting to the family's rules, values, and beliefs is a normal part of family life (Bradshaw, 1988b). However, when the family's

rules, values, and beliefs are warped by a dysfunctional parental behavior, the entire family must adapt to the unhealthy family themes. Often the family struggles to adapt to the addiction without guidance or external support, and family members come to use the same defense mechanisms characteristic of addicts: denial, rationalization, and projection.[1]

As the other family members assume responsibilities formerly held by the addict, the addict becomes less involved in family life. An older daughter may assume the responsibility for disciplining the other children, or a son may assume responsibility for making sure that the children are fed each night before they go to bed. In each case, one of the children has assumed a parental responsibility left vacant by the addict.

Thus, a paradox often exists within the alcoholic family. The family is uncomfortable with the addiction but may be quite happy with the current distribution of power and responsibility. However, if the family allows the alcoholism to continue, all the members quickly fall into the trap of becoming a part of the addict's support system, making it easier for the alcoholic to drink by "feeding into" the addict's dependency.

The ability to adapt to parental alcoholism is not without its cost, however. Such adaptation is often based on fear. According to Deutsch (quoted in Freiberg, 1991), family members in the alcoholic family constantly live "in a hypervigilant state, metaphorically walking through life on emotional eggshells, never knowing when the alcoholic will act out in an intoxicated and uncontrolled fashion" (p. 30). This fear, often in combination with guilt and real or imagined threats, may even be used by the alcoholic to control the family: "If you don't do what I want, I will go out and drink, and it will be *your* fault!"

Furthermore, within the new family constellation, different individuals may assume roles for which they are not emotionally ready. The dysfunctional home thus creates problems for

[1]The Johnson Institute (1987) uses the term *avoiding* rather than *denial*.

the emotional growth of the family members, especially the children. An example is the child who assumes the role of caretaker and then automatically assumes this same role in adulthood, seeking a spouse who needs to be taken care of. In this way, families pass the pathology from one generation to another.

It is for this reason that many professionals who work with chemical dependency view addiction as a family-centered disorder. Murray Bowen (1985), in his essay on the role of the family in the development of alcoholism, notes that "every important family member plays a part in the dysfunction of the dysfunctional member" (p. 262). When one parent is alcoholic, the other family members redistribute the parental roles to restore a sense of balance.

Without professional intervention, the dysfunctional family members are unlikely to learn or accept that it may actually be healthier to distance themselves from the addict and let the addict suffer the natural consequences of his or her behavior (Johnson Institute, 1987). Instead, the entire family assumes responsibility for the pathology of a single member, attempting to somehow "cure" the disturbed family member. In so doing, the addict is relieved of responsibility for either the addiction or its cure.

As the individual's drug use progresses, the addiction assumes a position of greater and greater importance in his or her life. Family commitments that interfere with "recreational" chemical use are dropped in favor of drug-centered activities. The son's long anticipated trip to the ball game is postponed because Dad is still too hungover from last night to be able to stand the heat and noise of the city. The long-awaited camping trip is cancelled at the last minute, because Mom went on another drinking spree last night, and is in no condition to go camping. As part of this process of family accommodation, the children stop bringing friends over to visit to avoid the embarrassment of having their friends see their addicted parent. But the family's accommodation ultimately makes it easier for the addict to continue using chemicals, knowing that he or she will not have to face co-workers,

PTA members, or their children's friends. The family "secret" is protected for another day.

The process of family accommodation to parental addiction develops over time and is often not seen clearly until after the addiction has fully developed. But the addiction does not spring into being overnight; it *evolves* over a period of time. Furthermore, the addict does not stand alone but has a family "support system" *that he or she helped mold and shape.* In turn, the family support system often functions to help them become and *remain* addicted.

The Cost of Parental Addiction

Until recently, clinicians did not understand the impact of parental alcoholism on the children's development. Current theory holds that parental alcoholism creates a disturbed home environment similar to the home where there is physical, emotional, or sexual abuse (Treadway, 1990; Miller & Hester, 1989). Thus, in theory, children raised by alcoholic parents are "at risk" for the development of various forms of psychopathology (Miller & Hester, 1989; Owings-West & Prinz, 1987). It has even been suggested that the damage caused by parental alcoholism may reach beyond the children to the *grandchildren* of the alcoholic (Stein, Newcomb, & Bentler, 1993; Beattie, 1989). Even if we limit our investigation to the immediate consequences of addiction, the suspected impact of parental substance abuse and dependency is staggering.

Owings-West and Prinz (1987) reviewed the impact of parental alcoholism on the children's psychological development. They concluded that parental alcoholism contributes to a number of behavioral problems, including conduct problems, poor academic performance, and inattentiveness. One expression of a conduct problem may be the development of an antisocial personality disorder or addictive disorder later in life (Silverman, 1989).

It is possible that some children who are raised in an alcoholic home will become "addicted" to excitement. One example is the child who engages in fire-setting (Webb, 1989). Another expression of this addiction to excitement is thought to be the development of the antisocial personality disorder (Ansevics & Doweiko, 1983). It is believed that the antisocial personality disorder is a way for the individual to come to terms with the inconsistent home environment, by helping the individual gain control of feelings of vulnerability.

As we mentioned before, children raised in alcoholic homes are frequently required to assume responsibilities far beyond their abilities or maturity. More than one young child has learned how to make sure that a parent is sleeping in such a position that he or she will not choke on vomit after a night's heavy drinking. According to Webb (1989, p. 47), children or adolescents who are raised in the alcoholic home often "spend an inordinate amount of time worrying about the safety of the whole (family) system," a responsibility that, in a healthy family, would be assumed by one or both parents. These adolescents stay awake while the alcoholic parent is out drinking, check on the safety of sleeping siblings, and develop elaborate fire escape plans that may involve returning time and time again to the burning house to rescue siblings, pets, and valuables. In response to this distorted family system, Webb (1989) suggests that many adolescents become overly mature, serious, and well-organized, all in an attempt to maintain control of their home environment.

It is Webb's (1989) position that the adolescent who is raised in an alcoholic home spends so much time and energy meeting basic survival needs that he or she does not have the opportunity to establish a firm sense of personal identity. This is not to say that *every* child raised in an alcoholic home will suffer this psychological trauma, but a greater percentage seem to experience long-lasting emotional injuries as a result of their home environment than do children raised in a more normal home.

Puig-Antich et al. (1989) conclude that the "effects of living with an alcoholic parent may precipitate very early depression in children with loaded familial aggregation for affective disorders" (p. 413). That is, they found an inter-relationship between depressive disorders and alcoholism in certain families. Although they are separate disorders, when the potential for *both* conditions are present as a result of genetic potential and environment, the children in these families are more likely to suffer from a major depressive disorder than if parental alcoholism or the potential for depression is absent.

Thus, research into the impact of parental alcoholism has revealed that children who are raised in a home where there was at least one alcoholic parent do seem to suffer some psychological harm. But the issue is not as simple as this. A number of factors shape the impact of parental alcoholism on the developing children in the family (Ackerman, 1983).

The first of these factors is the sex of the addicted parent; given the different roles each parent plays, an alcoholic mother will have a far different impact on the family than will an alcoholic father. A second factor is the length of time the alcoholic parent has actively been addicted. A third factor is the sex of the child; a daughter will be affected differently by an alcoholic father than will a son, for example (Ackerman, 1983). Fourth, the specific family constellation will play a role in how parental alcoholism will impact each individual child.

This last factor is difficult for many people to understand. To help illustrate this point, consider two different families. In the first family, the father has a 3-month relapse when the third boy in a family of 6 children is 9 years old. Contrast this child's experience with that of the oldest child in a family of 6 children whose father relapses for 3 months when the child is 9 years old. Both of these children would experience a far different family constellation than would a female only child whose father relapsed for 3 months when she was 9 years old. And all 3 children would have a far different experience in life than would the third boy in a family of 6 children whose mother was constantly drinking until he turned 14.

A final factor, as Ackerman (1983) observes, is

that it is possible for the child to escape from the brunt of the negative impact of parental addiction if he or she is able to find a *parental surrogate* (such as an uncle, neighbor, or real or imagined hero). Having a parental substitute may give the child a way to avoid the worst of the alcoholic parenting (Ackerman, 1983). (This will be discussed in a later section of this chapter.)

Adult Children of Addiction: The ACOA Movement

As we discussed earlier, many researchers believe that the effects of growing up in an alcoholic home often last beyond the individual's childhood years. Within the past generation, a large number of adults have stepped forward to claim that they were hurt by their parents' alcoholism. These individuals are known as *adult children of alcoholics* (ACOA), and an entire treatment industry has evolved to meet their perceived needs.

At this point, estimates of the number of ACOAs in the United States range from between 22 million (Collette, 1990) and 34 million adults (Mathew, Wilson, Blazer, & George, 1993). The alcoholic home shares many characteristics with other forms of dysfunctional home environments, which will leave scars on the developing child. Berkowitz and Perkins (1988) found, for example, that ACOAs are more critical of themselves and depreciate themselves more than do adult children of nonalcoholic parents. Woititz (1983), an early pioneer in the field of therapeutic intervention with ACOAs, lists a number of characteristics ACOAs have in common, some of which are (1) having to "guess" at what normal adult behavior is like, including the tendency to have trouble in intimate relationships, (2) the tendency to have difficulty following a project through from beginning to end, (3) the tendency to lie in situations where it is just as easy to tell the truth, (4) the tendency not to be able to "relax" but to always judge themselves harshly and need to always keep busy, and (5) the ten-

dency to feel uncomfortable with themselves and to constantly seek affirmation from significant others.

Hunter and Kellogg (1989) agree that ACOAs suffer from being raised in dysfunctional homes, but they argue that the traditional view of the adult child of alcoholic parents is too narrow. They claim that ACOAs often have personality characteristics *opposite* to those expected of a child raised in a dysfunctional home. For example, one characteristic thought to apply to ACOAs is that they have trouble following a project through from start to finish. Yet Hunter and Kellogg (1989) suggest that some ACOAs may actually be compulsive workaholics, who struggle to carry out a project in spite of feedback that this work is no longer necessary or that the work is actually counterproductive.

Recently, the research team of Sher, Walitzer, Wood, and Brent (1991) explored the differences between young adults raised by alcoholic parents and by nonalcoholic parents. They used a volunteer sample of college students whose parental drinking status was confirmed by extensive interviews. They report the following findings.

1. College freshmen with an alcoholic father tend to drink more and to have more symptoms of alcoholism than do freshmen who were not raised by an alcoholic father.
2. Women who were raised by an alcoholic parent or parents report a greater number of alcohol-related consequences than do their nondrinking counterparts.
3. Children of alcoholic parents have an increased risk of using not only alcohol but other drugs of abuse as well.
4. Adolescent children of alcoholic parents have more positive expectancies for alcohol than do adolescent children of nonalcoholic parents.
5. As adults, children raised by alcoholic parents tend to have higher scores on test items suggesting "behavioral undercontrol" (p. 444) than do those individuals who were not raised by alcoholic parents.

6. As college students, children raised by alcoholic parents tend to score lower on academic achievement tests than do their non-ACOA counterparts.

Although Sher et al. found a relationship between parental drinking status and the college students' adjustment and academic performance, their study failed to answer the question of what shape this assumed relationship might take. Because this study *does* suggest that parental alcoholism has a strong impact on the subsequent growth and adjustment of the children, it provides support for the theoretical model advanced by Ackerman (1983).

Drawing on data collected as a study of the prevalence of psychiatric disorders in a selected area, Mathew et al. (1993) examined the differences between the mental health of adults raised by alcoholic parents and adults who were not raised by alcoholic parents. They concluded that, as a group, "adult children of alcoholics had higher rates of dysthymia, generalized anxiety disorder, panic disorder, simple phobia, agoraphobia and social phobia than did matched comparison subjects" (p. 795).

There are other ways in which adult children of alcoholic parents have suffered in addition to developing psychiatric problems. During childhood, many children of alcoholic parents blame themselves for their parents' drinking (Freiberg, 1991), sometimes blaming themselves well into adulthood. Collette (1988, 1990), for example, describes how she blamed herself for her father's pain and was close to the point of suicide until she became involved in an ACOA self-help group. Sanders (1990) relates how he felt responsible for his father's drinking and how he "paid the price" through nights of fear and dread, listening to his father threatening to leave or arguing with his mother night after night.

Thus, a number of theoretical models have suggested that adult children of alcoholic parents will suffer from emotional distress. A number of research studies have revealed higher levels of psychiatric problems in samples of adult children of alcoholic parents, providing some support for the theoretical models advanced in the late 1970s and early 1980s. In response to this pain, many ACOA children banded together and formed self-help groups.

The Growth of ACOA Groups

Obviously, in a survey text such as this book it is not possible to examine the self-help movement for ACOAs in great detail. However, the reader should be aware of the fact that the historical growth of ACOA groups has been phenomenal. Although this movement only started in the 1970s and 1980s, there are now thought to be between 1,900 (Collette, 1990) and 4,000 (Blau, 1990) active self-help groups for ACOAs.

These numbers are a reflection of several factors, including the number of people who have been hurt by a parent's alcoholism and their desire to find peace by working through the shame and guilt that is left over from childhood (Collette, 1990).

Criticism of the ACOA Movement

The ultimate goal of the ACOA movement is to provide a self-help group format for those who believe that they were hurt by being raised in a dysfunctional environment. However, there are those who are critical of the ACOA movement or who question whether the ACOA movement can achieve its goal.

For example, Elkin (quoted in Collette, 1990), pointed out that "we all want to feel like victims" (p. 30) but that "if you identify yourself as a survivor of incest or abuse, you are making an existential and self-hypnotic statement that defines you by the most destructive thing that ever happened to you. In the short term, it's important to say it, but you can get stuck there" (p. 30).

According to Treadway (1990), another danger is that attaching a label to the adult offspring may "perpetuate the process of blaming in a new language" (p. 40). The format of the ACOA movement simply allows "adult children" to continue to blame their parents for whatever problems they may have encountered in life.

Thus, although the ACOA group may help meet the ever-present need for "a sense of community, empowerment, and spiritual renewal" (Treadway, 1990, p. 40), one must ask at what cost this sense of belonging is achieved.

Although the ACOA movement may be a tool for spiritual growth, it may also become a form of compulsive behavior for the individual. It all depends on whether the individual uses the ACOA group as a means to grow, or, as a reason to remain fixated in the past. Thus, in spite of its potential, there is a very real danger that, for some, recovery groups may themselves become an addiction (May, 1991).

The whole concept of ACOA limits the individual by keeping the focus *on the previous generation* (Peele, Brodsky, & Arnold, 1991). Admittedly, some children are raised in terrible, abusive environments. But the central thesis of the ACOA movement rests on the impact that past parental behavior (often many years past) has on the individual's *current* life problems. In a very real sense, the ACOA movement encourages individuals to define "self" on the basis of their parents' problems and choices, according to Peele, Brodsky, and Arnold.

It is possible that the ACOA movement is based on a mistaken assumption, namely that "healthy," conflict-free families really exist. Although the traditional view of the American family has been one of peace and security, the reality is far different. "Family historians," wrote Furstenberg (1990), "have been unable to identify a period in America's past when family life was untroubled" (p. 148). In other words, familial conflict has been the norm in U.S. culture, not the exception. Thus, one must question the degree to which the ACOA group movement is based on a conflict-free family model that simply has never existed.

Another criticism of the ACOA model is that it rests on an assumption that Wolin and Wolin (1993) term the *damage model*. This model holds that children raised in a dysfunctional environment will *automatically* suffer psychological harm. Claudia Black (1982), a strong proponent of the ACOA model, states that "All children are affected" (p. 27) if they are raised in an alcoholic home. It is assumed that, because some adults who grew up in a home with an alcoholic parent had certain characteristics, *all* children raised in such a home suffer emotional harm.

Yet the damage model has been challenged by research studies, such as the one by Tweed and Ryff (1991). They examined the emotional adjustment of 114 ACOAs and 127 adults from nonalcoholic families and found no clear differences in the grown children's emotional adjustment. Indeed, research reveals that many individuals are able to avoid significant emotional scars in spite of the fact that they were raised in a "dysfunctional" environment (Peele, Brodsky, & Arnold, 1991).

D'Andrea, Fisher, and Harrison (1994) administered the California Psychological Inventory (CPI) to 97 self-identified ACOA volunteers and found three different subgroups within their ACOA sample. A minority (16%) of the sample had CPI profiles suggestive of serious psychopathology. The largest subgroup, almost one-half of their sample, had a normal CPI profile.

Another study that failed to find evidence that ACOAs are different from other adults was conducted by Giunta and Compas (1994). As part of a doctoral dissertation research project under the direction of Compas, Giunta examined the responses to a questionnaire of 184 women between the ages of 25 and 35, their scores on a modified form of the Michigan Alcoholism Screening Test (MAST), and their completion of the Symptom Check List-90. No special attempt was made to identify this as a study on ACOAs; rather, the subjects were told that the study was on women's relationships. The authors conclude that there is no evidence to suggest that the adult daughters of alcohol-abusing parents are more distressed than are other adult female children. Furthermore, the authors failed to find evidence suggesting that the ACOAs in their sample were more afraid of intimacy or that all children of alcoholic parents are in need of treatment, as suggested by Claudia Black (1982).

These findings cast doubt on the damage model—the foundation of the ACOA movement—indicating instead that a more appropriate model for how children respond to the problem of having an alcoholic parent might be called the *"challenge model"* (Wolin & Wolin, 1993). This model takes into account the possibility of individual resiliency, something the damage model fails to do.

The child who is able to thrive in spite of adverse childhood conditions is said to be *resilient*. Werner (1989) studied a number of such children, who were "at risk" because of social or biological trauma but who went on to succeed in life. She found that these children seem "to be particularly adept at recruiting . . . surrogate parents when a biological parent was unavailable . . . or incapacitated" (p. 108D). This conclusion is supported by Parker, Barrett, and Hickie (1992), who found that "childhood adversity is not always associated with a poor outcome" (p. 883), especially if the child is able to form stable, supportive relationships later in life.

Indeed, the quality of subsequent interpersonal relationships may moderate or overcome the impact of poor parenting (Parker, Barrett, & Hickie, 1992; Werner, 1989). These studies provide at least partial support for Ackerman's (1983) conclusion that, if the child finds a suitable parental substitute, it is possible for the child to escape from the full consequences of parental alcoholism. At the same time, these studies seem to raise questions about the validity of the ACOA model.

Further evidence that a "dysfunctional" environment may not always have lasting consequences for the individual was provided by Garbarino et al. (1992). They examined the effects of extreme psychological trauma on children, especially children raised in the inner cities or war zones. It was found that, for a majority of these children—perhaps as many as 80%—there are no permanent scars caused by the stress of being raised in the inner city or a war zone. Indeed, for many children, the challenge of meeting the demands of living in such an environment enabled them to become stronger. However, the authors concluded that one factor was essential for the child to survive and not be

scarred by the experience of growing up in such an environment: a stable, mature relationship with at least one adult.

Another criticism of the ACOA movement is that the ACOA model rests on the unproven assumption that children raised by an alcoholic parent "manifest a unique kind of pathology" (Miller & Hester, 1989, p. 8). The limited research to date does suggest that children of alcoholic parents are more likely to experience some psychological problems, such as depression, more often than children raised in a nonalcoholic home. However, these reports are inconclusive and often fail to be replicated in follow-up studies (Goodwin & Warnock, 1991).

Thus, the research literature has failed to support some key components of the ACOA model. In their research, D'Andrea, Fisher, and Harrison (1994) found little evidence to support the theory that "adult children" of alcoholic parents share similar characteristics. Indeed, after reviewing their data, the authors concluded that "there is a danger in assuming . . . that growing up in an alcoholic home inevitably leads to dysfunction in adulthood" (p. 580).

Domenico and Windle (1993), who examined the intrapersonal and interpersonal functioning of 616 middle-aged women, also failed to find evidence that supported the theory of ACOA psychopathology. The authors compared the adjustment of women who were adult children of an alcoholic parent with that of women who were not raised by an alcoholic parent. Although they found that the ACOA women seemed to have higher levels of depression and lower levels of self-esteem, as a group the ACOA women scored in the normal range on the tests used in this study. These findings are consistent with those of Seilhamer, Jacob, and Dunn (1993), who failed to find any consistent impact, either positive or negative, of parental alcoholism on parent-child interactions.

One is left with the impression that, in the absence of hard research data, the foundation of the ACOA movement is nothing more than "assertions, generalizations and anecdotes" (University of California, Berkeley, 1990a, p. 7).

Indeed, a very real shortcoming of the ACOA literature is that it is "long on rhetoric and short on empirical data" (Levy & Rutter, 1992, p. 12). Yet, on the basis of this literature, many have labeled significant portions of society as diseased or "dysfunctional," in the jargon of the ACOA movement.

Another criticism of the ACOA movement is based on the fact that the self-help movement, of which the ACOA movement is a part, has become something of a growth industry in this country (Blau, 1990; Boyd, 1992). It has even been suggested that the publishing industry, armed with the knowledge that the majority of purchasers of self-help books are women, slant their titles and design their covers to attract the attention and activate the insecurities of women (Boyd, 1992). One could very well argue that the ACOA movement is the stepchild of the publishing industry, which then used the movement to develop a market for a new line of self-help books.

When the ACOA movement began in the early 1980s, it focused on the survivors of extreme abuse, according to Blau (1990). However, over the years, the definition of what constitutes "abuse" has become blurred to the point where the tendency to blame "parents for what they did or didn't do has become a national obsession—and big business" (Blau, 1990, p. 61; Kaminer, 1992). But because of the lack of diagnostic rigor and the vague language of the ACOA movement, virtually *96% of the population can be said to have been raised in a "dysfunctional" family* (Peele, Brodsky, & Arnold, 1991). Indeed, many of the proponents of the self-help movement quote this 96% figure, in spite of the fact that there has never been any research to support its accuracy (Hughes, 1993). Given this fact, one must wonder to what degree the characteristics identified by the proponents of the ACOA movement reflect not some form of pathology but simply the problems in living in today's society that we all experience. But now, thanks to an overabundance of self-help books, we have the "language" for which to blame our parents and grandparents for all of our life problems.

In reality, there has been very little research into the psychological dynamics of families of alcoholics or other forms of addiction (D'Andrea, Fisher, & Harrison, 1994; University of California, Berkeley, 1990a; Goodwin & Warnock, 1991; Sher, 1991). Furthermore, very little is known about what constitutes a "normal" family or the limits of unhealthy behaviors (which we all have) that may be tolerated in an otherwise "normal" family.

Blau (1990) challenges the very essense of ACOA, on the grounds that the entire concept of the "adult child" is a reflection of the "baby-boomers' " resistance to accepting that they are now adults who are themselves entering middle adulthood. Developmentally, the adults of the "baby-boomer" generation are no longer the children of their parents, at least in the same sense that they were three decades ago. They are now middle-aged adults who are discovering that they will not fulfill all the dreams of young adulthood. Perhaps, as Blau (1990) suggests, the ACOA movement is a reaction by the "baby-boomer" generation against growing older.

From this perspective, it is understandable that the ACOA movement places great emphasis on the so-called "inner child." However, the "inner child" concept is not a part of any single therapeutic theory. Rather, the theory behind the ACOA concept of the inner child is a complex blend of "[Carl] Jung, New Age mysticism, holy child mythology, pop psychology, and psychoanalytic theories about narcissism and the creation of a false self" (Kaminer, 1992, p. 17). Another challenge to the ACOA emphasis on the "inner child" is made by Hughes (1993). The pursuit of the "inner child," he writes, comes "just at the moment when Americans ought to be figuring out where their Inner *Adult* is, and how that disregarded oldster got buried under the rubble of pop psychology and short-term gratification" (p. 29, italics added for emphasis). When one stops to consider that "inner child" is based on a phase of life when the individual is developmentally, socially, psychologically, and neurologically immature, one wonders about the degree to which this construct is able to meet the demands of adult life.

The ACOA movement places great emphasis on blame. Unfortunately, as Blau (1990) points out, there is a danger that the individual will become "stuck" in blaming his or her parents for the inevitable disappointments and frustrations of adulthood. Rather than focusing on learning how to accept personal responsibility for one's decisions in life, the ACOA movement seems to "lock" the individual into a cycle of blaming his or her parents. Blau's (1990) work gives the impression that the force behind the ACOA movement is a rebellion against aging by the "baby-boomer" generation. Much as they blamed older generations for the world's problems during the Vietnam War era, the "baby-boomer" generation is still blaming their parents for their own frustration as they pass through middle adulthood.

Finally, as Levy and Rutter (1992) point out, the ACOA movement is essentially a white, middle-class invention. It is not known whether this model applies to inner-city children, whose parents may be addicted to heroin or cocaine, who may come from a single-parent family, and so on. As the authors note, children of heroin and cocaine addicts are "primarily nonwhite, minority members who live in poverty. They have no national movement . . . do not write books and make the rounds of the talk shows" (p. 5). Thus, virtually nothing is known about them. However, as the authors remind us, many children are raised by parents who are addicted to chemicals other than alcohol and in environments other than the white, middle-class world. There is no research as to whether the ACOA model applies to these other children of addiction or not.

Summary

This chapter explored the family of the addicted individual and the impact that one individual's addiction to chemicals is thought to have on the rest of the family. Unfortunately, there are few research studies that actually explore the impact of one member's alcohol or drug addiction on the other members of the family. Much of what is assumed to be true about such families is based on theory, not established fact.

The theory of codependency assumes that the codependent individual is "trained" by a series of adverse life events to become dependent on the feedback and support of others. It also assumes that family members adopt new roles as the addicted person gives up the power and responsibility that he or she would normally hold within the family. In this manner, the family comes to "accommodate," or adapt to, the individual's chemical addiction.

From the perspective of the codependency model, the individual's substance abuse is viewed as a family-centered disorder that is passed on from one generation to the next. The self-help group movement of "adult children" of alcoholics is viewed as a logical response to the pain and suffering that the family members experienced by participating in a "dysfunctional" family. However, the "adult child" concept has met with some criticism. Some health care professionals stress that the theory behind the ACOA movement places too much emphasis on past suffering at the expense of possible resilience on the part of the individual or his or her future growth. Further criticism has been made of the ACOA movement on the grounds that it automatically assumes that the individual has experienced some lasting psychological trauma as a result of parental alcoholism or drug addiction. This theory has never been tested, and thus much of the ACOA self-help movement rests on an unproven assumption. Research is needed to begin to understand how chemical addiction impacts on the growth and development of both the individual family members and the family unit.

CHAPTER TWENTY-SIX

The Assessment of Chemical Dependency

For many who are addicted to chemicals, the first step toward rehabilitation is an alcohol and drug use assessment (Donovan, 1992). Through the chemical dependency assessment, a substance abuse or mental health professional attempts to answer several interrelated questions. First, the assessor tries to determine whether the client is or is not an *abuser* of chemicals. Second, the assessor seeks to determine whether or not the client is *addicted* to chemicals. Finally, if there is evidence that the client is either an abuser of chemicals or is addicted to chemicals, the assessor attempts to provide an overview of the client's chemical use pattern and to make the appropriate referrals.

The Theory Behind Alcohol and Drug Use Assessments

As Cohen and Marcos (1989) observe, mental health professionals are increasingly being called on to distinguish those individuals "whose criminal ('bad') behavior is not necessarily attributable to being mentally ill ('mad')" (p. 677). Chemical dependency professionals are being asked to make the same determination for those thought to be addicted to chemicals. Some people come to the attention of the criminal justice system because they have committed crimes to service their addiction. Sometimes treatment is a more viable option than legal sanctions, and

it is often the task of the substance abuse professional to determine whether a given individual will benefit from treatment for a substance abuse problem.

In addressing this issue, Lewis, Dana, and Blevins (1988) warn that

> merely walking into a substance abuse treatment facility does not, in and of itself, warrant a diagnosis of "chemical dependency" or "alcoholism." Rather, clinicians must carefully evaluate the client and only then make decisions concerning diagnosis and treatment. (p. 75)

This is a timely warning for a number of reasons. First, there are those who would like to excuse their antisocial behavior by attributing it to an "illness," such as chemical dependency. The first duty of the assessor should be to establish a firm basis either for a diagnosis of chemical dependency or for not making such a diagnosis. It is only after the diagnosis has been established—*if it is established*—that the need for treatment might be considered. Treatment centers that assume that a client *must* have a problem with chemicals simply because he or she is there do not serve the client's interests, only their own. *The need for treatment must be established and well documented.*

Second, if all addicts were carbon copies of each other, there would be no need for an assessment to proceed beyond answering the question

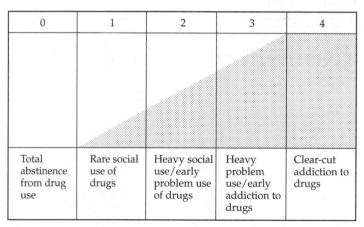

0	1	2	3	4
Total abstinence from drug use	Rare social use of drugs	Heavy social use/early problem use of drugs	Heavy problem use/early addiction to drugs	Clear-cut addiction to drugs

FIGURE 26.1 The continuum of addiction

of whether the individual is addicted. However, every person who is addicted to one or more chemicals presents the clinician with a unique combination of strengths, needs, hopes, fears, and past experiences. Given this fact, to "the extent that treatment is individualized, a careful evaluation can help to determine optimal goals and strategies" (Miller & Rollnick, 1991, p. 89).

On the basis of the information uncovered during a careful evaluation, the substance abuse rehabilitation professional can identify the appropriate goals and treatment strategies for each client. The opposite is also true; without a careful evaluation of the client's strengths, experiences, and needs, it will be difficult to identify the appropriate goals for that individual or to effectively intervene.

Chapter 1 introduced the concept of addiction as a continuum. The chart in Figure 26.1 illustrates the continuum of drug use and abuse, which ranges from total abstinence from chemicals to the stage of chronic addiction.

Quite simply, the assessment process involves a professional evaluation of where the individual being assessed might fall on the continuum. The person may, on evaluation, be found to present strong evidence of a drug dependency problem. However, it may also be determined that the client has not progressed past the stage of heavy

social use of chemicals. In some cases, the assessment process will reveal that the client is a social user of chemicals. It all depends on the client and the specific information available to the assessor.

Defining Drug Abuse and Drug Dependence

As we discussed before, two elements necessary to define an addiction to chemicals are *dependence* on the chemical and *tolerance* to the drug's effects (Kamback, 1978). As the individual's body adapts to the continuous use of one or more chemicals, there is a declining effect from the initial dosage levels. To achieve the same effect once accomplished with a relatively low dose, larger and larger doses must be used. This is tolerance.

Dependence on a chemical is diagnosed by the presence of a characteristic *withdrawal syndrome* when the drug is discontinued. The body, as it adapts to the continued presence of the drug being used, alters its normal biological activities. When the drug is discontinued, there is a period of time during which the body must again adapt—this time to the absence of the chemical. During this period of readaptation to the absence of the chemical, the individual experiences the characteristic withdrawal syndrome for that chemical.

Abel (1982), in addressing the difference between abuse and dependence, identifies four interrelated elements that are necessary for the diagnosis of addiction: (1) a compulsion to continue the drug use, (2) the development of tolerance, (3) major withdrawal symptoms following discontinued use, and (4) adverse effects from drug use for both the individual and society.

The diagnosis of chemical dependency is, unfortunately, retrospective; it is made only after the disorder is fully developed. Even after the addict reaches this point, however, one does not always clearly see all four of the elements outlined above in every case. The existence of one symptom of addiction is often taken as evidence by health care professionals that the other symptoms also exist.

When a patient goes through major withdrawal symptoms from alcohol, benzodiazepines, barbiturates, or narcotics, for example, one can safely assume that this person is also tolerant to the drug's effects, because tolerance usually occurs before the development of physical withdrawal symptoms from these chemicals. The withdrawal symptoms also imply the compulsive use of one or more drugs, as the patient had to frequently use the drug for a long period of time for physical dependency to develop. The withdrawal process also suggests that the drug has adverse effects on the individual, if only in the form of the withdrawal process itself.

The exact nature of the withdrawal syndrome will reflect the specific drugs that were used, the length of time the individual used the drugs, and whether the individual discontinued the chemical use all at once or gradually. Tolerance and dependence must *both* be present to diagnose an addiction to one or more chemicals.

However, there also is a phenomenon known as *psychological dependence* on a chemical. This is a state in which the individual habitually uses one or more drugs in an attempt to deal with anxiety or stress. The term *habituation* has also been applied to this phenomenon. In these cases, there is no *physical* adaptation to the use of the drug, in the sense that the body does not incorporate the drug into its normal function. But there is a *psychological* adaptation, in that the users come to believe that they *need* the drug. For example, an individual whose only alcohol use is a "nightcap" every night just before going to bed to "unwind" has very likely developed a psychological dependence on the alcohol to help deal with the accumulated stress and frustration of daily living. As such, this person could be said to have become habituated to alcohol.

It is the assessor's responsibility to determine whether the client's chemical use pattern should be classified as "social use," "abuse," or "addiction" to one or more drugs. This process is quite complicated, however, and involves gathering information from a wide variety of sources. In so doing, the assessor must work within the data privacy laws.

The Assessor and Data Privacy

The client *always* has a right to privacy; that is, the assessor does not automatically have access to personal information about the client. The client may refuse to answer a specific question or refuse permission for another person to reveal specific information to the assessor. The assessor must respect the client's right to control access to personal information.

Both federal and state data privacy laws often apply when working with individuals who are thought to be addicted to drugs or alcohol. If the client agrees to the assessment, he or she is then willingly providing information during the assessment process. However, the client still retains permission to refuse to answer any question. If information is required from someone other than the client, *the professional should always obtain written permission* from the client authorizing the assessor to contact specific individuals to obtain information about the client's chemical use or any other aspect of his or her life. This written permission is recorded on a form known as a *release of information authorization form.*

Occasionally, a client will refuse such permission. The client retains this right and can refuse to allow the assessor to speak with *any* other person. This refusal in itself says a great deal about how open and honest the client has been with the assessor, especially if the evaluator has explained to the client exactly what information will be requested.

One way to avoid this refusal is to have the client sit in on the collateral interview. A drawback to this solution is that the client's presence might inhibit the freedom of the collateral information source to discuss his or her perception of the client. In this case, a potentially valuable source of information about the client would be unavailable to the assessor. Thus, it is rarely productive to have the client or the client's representative sit in on collateral interviews.

When the client is being referred for an evaluation by the court system, the court often provides referral information about the client's previous legal history. The courts also often include a detailed social history of the client, which was part of the presentence investigation. If asked, the evaluator should acknowledge having read this information but should not discuss the contents of the referral information provided by the courts. Such discussions are to be avoided for two reasons. First, the purpose of the clinical interview is to assess the client's *chemical use patterns.* A discussion of what information was or was not provided by the court does nothing to further this evaluation. Second, the client or his or her attorney has access to this information through established channels. Thus, if the client wishes to review the information provided by the court, he or she may do so at another time through established legal channels.

During the clinical interview, clients occasionally ask to see the records provided by the court. Frequently, these clients are checking to see what information has been provided by the courts, in order to decide how much and what they should admit to during the interview period. This often

reflects the philosophy, "Let me know how much *you* know about me, so that I will know how 'honest' I should be!" Often a simple statement to the effect that the client can obtain a copy of the court record through established legal channels is all that is needed. Those persistent clients who demand to see their court records on the grounds that "it is about me, anyway" are to be reminded that the purpose of the interview is to explore the client's drug and alcohol use patterns, not to review court records. However, under no circumstances should the professional let the client read his or her referral records. To do so would be a violation of the data privacy laws because the referral information was released to the professional, *not* to the client.

When the final evaluation is written, the assessor should identify the source of the information summarized in the final assessment. Collateral information sources should be advised that the client, or his or her attorney, has a right to request a copy of the final report *before* the interview. It is *extremely* rare for a client to request a copy of the final report, although technically the client does have the right to do so after the proper release-of-information authorization forms have been signed.

Diagnostic Rules

Many, perhaps most, clients initially resist a diagnosis of chemical dependency (Washton, 1990). For this reason, two diagnostic rules should be followed as closely as possible in the evaluation and diagnosis of a possible drug addiction, even in special cases. If it is not possible to adhere to either one or both of these diagnostic rules, the professional making the diagnosis should identify the reason for this situation to avoid missing important information.

Rule 1: Gather Collateral Information

A fundamental aspect of chemical dependency is deception. Therefore, the individual attempting to make a diagnosis of addiction should *utilize as many sources of information as possible.* Evans and Sullivan (1990), in discussing the need for as wide a database as possible, caution, "Never, ever diagnose using information based only on the client's presentation at the time of assessment" (p. 54). Every chemical dependency professional has encountered cases in which the individual being evaluated has claimed to drink "only once a week" or "no more than a couple of beers after work." The person's spouse, however, often reports that the client is intoxicated almost every night.

To minimize the danger of deception and to develop as comprehensive a history of the individual as possible, the chemical dependency professional should use as many different sources of information as possible. Slaby, Lieb, and Tancredi (1981) recommend that such collateral information sources include the patient's family, friends, and co-workers or employer; clergy members; local law enforcement authorities; and the patient's primary care physician and psychotherapist (if any).

Obviously, time restrictions of the assessment process could prevent the use of some of these collateral resources. For example, if the assessment must be completed by the end of the week and the professional is unable to contact the client's mother, it may be necessary to write the final report without benefit of her input. Also, other people involved may simply refuse to provide any information. It is the assessor's responsibility, however, to *attempt* to contact as many of these individuals as possible and to include their views in the final evaluation report.

Rule 2: *Always* Assume Deception Until Proven Otherwise

Not all addicts automatically lie. Indeed, there is evidence to suggest that, *as a group,* alcoholics are quite accurate in their self-reports of the amount of alcohol consumed and the frequency of their alcohol use (Donovan, 1992). But, as noted earlier, the nature of addiction is deception. Sierles

(1984) found that substance abusers are one of the two groups of patients most likely to attempt to deceive assessors (individuals with a history of sociopathic behaviors comprise the other subgroup). Cunnien (1988) notes that the addict will be "persistent" (p. 25) in his or her attempts to deceive others.

At times, alcoholics minimize the amount of alcohol they admit to consuming to hide the full extent of their drinking. Opiate addicts who are admitted for detoxification, on the other hand, often exaggerate the amount of drugs they use in hopes of obtaining more drugs from the detoxification center staff. Cocaine addicts may also exaggerate their drug use, although this is not found consistently. Some cocaine addicts, rather than exaggerate their drug use, may initially deny or minimize their use of the drug.

When evaluating a person's drug use, it is not unusual for professionals to encounter a person who claims to be using a given amount of heroin or cocaine, only to later find out from friends of the client that the person has *never* used opiates or cocaine. This client is probably attempting to impress the evaluator, the courts, or drug using "friends."

Alcoholics have been known to admit to drinking "once or twice a week," until reminded that their medical problems are unlikely to have been caused by such moderate drinking levels. At this point, they sometimes admit to more frequent drinking episodes. However, even when confronted with such evidence of serious, continual alcohol use, many alcoholics have been known to deny the reality of their alcoholism.

Clients have been known to admit to "one" arrest for driving under the influence of alcohol or possession of a controlled substance. However, records provided by the court at the time of admission into treatment often reveal arrests in two or three different states for similar charges. When confronted, these clients may respond that they thought that the evaluator "only meant in *this* state" or that "since that happened outside of this state, it doesn't apply." Thus, it is clear that, to avoid the danger of deception, the assessor must utilize as many different sources of information as possible.

The Assessment Format

Although every individual is unique, there is a general assessment format that can be used when evaluating a client's known or suspected chemical addiction. This assessment format is modified as necessary to take into account the differences between individuals. For the remainder of this chapter, we will be discussing this format.

Area I: Circumstances of Referral

The first step in the diagnostic process is to examine the circumstances under which the individual is seen. For example, a patient who is in a hospital alcohol detoxification (or "detox") unit for the first time is far different from the patient who has been in the detox unit 10 times in the last 3 years. Thus, the first piece of data for the chemical dependency assessment is a review of the circumstances surrounding the individual's referral.

The manner in which the client responds to the question "What brings you here today?" can provide valuable information about how willing a participant the individual will be in the evaluation process. If the individual responds, "I don't know, they told me to come here," or "You should know, you've read the report" is obviously being less than fully cooperative. The rare client who responds "I think I have a drug problem" is demonstrating some degree of cooperativeness with the assessor. In each case, the manner in which the client identifies the circumstances surrounding his or her referral for evaluation provides the assessor valuable information.

Area II: Drug and Alcohol Use Patterns

The next step is for the evaluator to explore the individual's drug and alcohol use patterns *both past and present*. All too often, clients claim to drink "only once a week" or to have had "nothing to drink in the last six months." Treatment center staff are not surprised to find out that this drinking pattern has been the rule *only* since the person's last arrest for an alcohol-related offense.

From time to time, the assessor encounters a person who proudly claims not to have had a drink or not to have used chemicals in the past 6–12 months, or perhaps even longer. This person may neglect to report that he or she was locked up in the county jail awaiting trial during that time, or was under strict supervision after being released from jail on bail and had little or no access to chemicals. This is far different from having purposely abstained. Thus, the evaluator should explore the client's living situation to determine whether there were any environmental restrictions on the individual's drug use. Obviously, a person who is incarcerated, in treatment, or whose probation officer requires both frequent and unannounced supervised urine screens to detect drug or alcohol use has an environmental restriction imposed on him or her. In such cases, a report of having "not used drugs in 6 months" may be the literal truth but is certainly misleading.

The individual's chemical use pattern and *beliefs about his or her drug use* should then be compared with the circumstances surrounding referral. For example, the person who states that he or she does not have a problem with chemicals but has earlier admitted to being arrested for possession of a controlled substance twice in 4 years is providing two important, but quite discrepant, pieces of information. Several important areas should be explored at this point in the evaluation process. The evaluator needs to consider (1) whether the client has ever been in a treatment program for chemical dependency and (2) whether the individual's drug or alcohol use has ever resulted in legal, family, financial, social, or medical problems. The assessor also needs to consider whether the client has ever demonstrated any signs of either psychological dependency or physical addiction to drugs or alcohol.

To understand this point, one need only contrast the case of two hypothetical clients who are seen following their arrest for driving a motor vehicle while under the influence of chemicals. The first person claims (and the collateral source agrees) that he or she only drank in moderation once every few weeks. Furthermore, the background check conducted by the courts revealed that this client never had any previous legal problems of any kind. However, after receiving a long-awaited promotion, the client celebrated with some friends. The client was a rare drinker who drank heavily on this occasion and subsequently misjudged the amount of alcohol that had been consumed.

In contrast, the second client's collateral information sources suggest a more extensive chemical use pattern than the client admitted to during the interview. A background check conducted by the police at the time of the arrest revealed several prior arrests for the same offense.

In the first case, one could argue that the client simply made a mistake. Although the client was driving under the influence of alcohol, he or she had *never* done so in the past and does not fit the criteria necessary for a diagnosis of even heavy social drinking. The report to the court would outline the sources of data examined and, in this case, provide a firm foundation for the conclusion that this individual made an isolated mistake in driving after drinking.

But in the second case, the individual's drunk driving arrest was the tip of a larger problem, which was outlined in the report to the court. The assessor would detail the sources of information that support this conclusion, including information provided by family members, the client's physician, the client, the county sheriff's department, and the client's friends. The final report in this case would conclude that the client had a significant addiction problem requiring treatment in a chemical dependency treatment program.

Area III: Legal History

Part of the assessment process should include an examination of the client's legal history. This information can be based on the individual's self-report or on a review of the client's police record as provided by the court, the probation or parole officer, or other source. *It is important to identify the source of the information on which the report is based.* The client's legal history should include the following:

- charges that have been brought against the client in the past by the local authorities, and their disposition
- charges that have been brought against the client in the past by authorities in other localities, and their disposition
- the nature of current charges (if any) against the individual

There are many cases on record in which an individual was finally convicted of a misdemeanor charge for possession of less than an ounce of marijuana. However, all too often, a review of the client's police record reveals that the individual was *arrested* for a felony drug-possession charge and that the charges were reduced through plea bargaining agreements. In some states, it is possible for the charge of driving a motor vehicle under the influence of alcohol (a felony in many states) to be reduced to a misdemeanor charge, such as public intoxication, through plea bargaining.

The assessor needs to determine *both the initial charge and the ultimate disposition* by the court of these charges. The assessor should specifically inquire whether the client has had charges brought against him or her in other states or by federal authorities. Individuals may admit to *one* charge for possession of a controlled substance, only for the staff to later find out that the client has had several arrests and convictions for the same charge in other states. Or the client may admit to having been *arrested* for possession charges in other states but fail to mention that he or she had left the state before the charges were brought to trial. Many clients reason that, because they were never *convicted* of the charges, they will not have to mention them during the assessment. The fact that the charges were never proved in court because he or she was a fugitive from justice (as well as the fact that interstate flight to avoid prosecution is a possible federal offense) may well be overlooked by the client.

Military Record

One important (and often overlooked) source of information for some clients is their *military history*. Many clients report only on their civilian legal history unless specifically asked about their military legal record. Clients who may have denied any drug or alcohol legal charges whatsoever may, after questioning, admit to having been reprimanded or charged with chemical use while in the military.

The assessor must specifically inquire whether an individual has ever been in the service. If the client denies military service, it may be useful to ask *why* the client has never been in the service. Often, this question elicits a response such as "I wanted to join, but I had a felony arrest record," or "I had a DWI (driving while under the influence of alcohol) on my record and couldn't join." These responses provide valuable information to the assessor and open new areas for investigation.

If the client has been in the military, it may be important to determine whether the client's discharge status was an honorable discharge, a general discharge under honorable conditions, a general discharge under dishonorable conditions, or a dishonorable discharge. Was the client ever brought up on charges while in the service? If so, what was the disposition of these charges? Was the client ever referred for drug treatment while in the service? Was the client ever denied

a transfer or promotion because of drug or alcohol use? Finally, was the client ever transferred because of his or her drug or alcohol use?

The client's legal history should be verified, if possible, by contacting the court or probation or parole officer, especially if the client was referred for evaluation for an alcohol or drug related offense. The legal history often provides significant information about the client's lifestyle and the extent to which drug use has (or has not) resulted in conflict with social rules and expectations.

Area IV: Educational and Vocational History

The next step in the assessment process is to determine the individual's educational and vocational history. This information, which can be based on the individual's self-report, school, or employment records, provides information on the client's level of function and whether chemical use has interfered with school or work. As before, the evaluator should identify the source of this information.

For example, the client who says that she dropped out of school in the tenth grade "because I was into drugs" presents a different picture than does the client who completed a bachelor of science degree from a well-known university. The individual who has had five jobs in the last 2 years might present a far different picture than the individual who has held a series of responsible positions and was regularly promoted within the same company for the last 10 years. Thus, the assessor should attempt to determine the client's educational and vocational history to determine the educational level, potential, and the degree to which his or her chemical use has affected his or her educational or work life.

Area V: Developmental and Family History

The assessor can often uncover significant material through an examination of the client's developmental and family history. The client may reveal that his or her father was "a problem drinker" but hesitate to call that parent an alcoholic. How the client describes parental or sibling chemical use might reveal how the client thinks about his or her own chemical use. For example, the client who hesitates to call a family member an alcoholic but is comfortable with the term *a problem drinker* might be hinting that he or she is also uncomfortable with the term *alcoholic* applied to him- or herself. But the client may also have accepted the rationalization that he or she is "a problem drinker," just like the family member.

Information about either parental or sibling chemical use is important for another reason as well. As we discussed in the chapter on alcohol, there is significant evidence suggesting a genetic predisposition toward alcoholism. By extension, one might expect that future research will uncover a genetic link toward other forms of drug addiction as well.

In addition, the assessor can explore the client's attitudes about parental alcohol and drug use in the home while he or she was growing up. Did the client view this chemical use as normal? Was the client angry or ashamed about his or her parents' chemical use? Does the client view chemical use as a problem for the family or not?

Thus, it is important for the assessor to examine the possibility of either parental or sibling chemical use, both in the past or at present. Such information offers insights into the client's possible genetic inheritance, especially whether he or she may be "at risk" to develop an addiction. Furthermore, an overview of the family environment provides clues about how the client views drug or alcohol use.

Family environments differ. The client whose parents were rare social drinkers has been raised in a far different environment than the client whose parents were drug addicts. The client who reports never knowing his or her mother because she was a heroin addict who put the children up for adoption when they were little might view drugs far differently than the client who was raised to believe that hard work would see a person through troubled times and whose parents never drank.

Area VI: Psychiatric History

Chemical use often precipitates either outpatient or inpatient psychiatric treatment. A natural part of the assessment process should be to discuss with the client whether he or she has ever been treated for psychiatric problems, either as an inpatient or an outpatient. For example, clients may admit to having been hospitalized for observation because they were hallucinating, had attempted suicide, were violent, or depressed.

Perhaps months or years later, on admission to chemical dependency treatment, the client reveals that he or she was using drugs at the time of psychiatric treatment. Often, when asked, the client confesses that he or she failed to mention this drug use to the staff of the psychiatric hospital. The client may have lied to the hospital staff, or the psychiatric admissions staff simply may not have asked the appropriate questions. It is important, then, to ask whether the client has *ever* been hospitalized for psychiatric treatment, has ever had outpatient psychiatric treatment, and had revealed to the mental health professional the truth about his or her drug use.

If possible, the assessor should obtain a release-of-information form from the client and request the discharge summary from the treatment center where the client was hospitalized. The possibility that drugs contributed to the psychiatric hospitalization or outpatient treatment should be either confirmed or ruled out, if possible. This information allows the assessor to determine whether the client's drug use has resulted in psychiatric problems serious enough to require professional help.

As noted in the chapter on the CNS stimulants, it is not uncommon for chronic use of amphetamines or cocaine to cause a drug-induced psychosis that is, at least in its early stages, very similar to paranoid schizophrenia. A client who reports having spent a short time in a psychiatric hospital for a "brief psychosis" may well have developed such a drug-related problem, whether or not it was recognized as such by the hospital staff.

Area VII: Medical History

Clients who are chemically dependent will often have a history of numerous hospitalizations for the treatment of accidents or injuries that may have been drug-related. For example, one client reported having been hospitalized many times after rival drug dealers had tried to kill him. Over the years, he had accumulated an impressive assortment of knife wounds, gunshot wounds, and fractured bones from these "business transactions" that had, in his words, "gone bad." However, he had never been hospitalized for a drug overdose. An assessor who asked, "Have you ever been hospitalized because of a drug overdose?" would never learn the details of these hospitalizations, because the client viewed them as "business transactions," not a result of personal drug use. On a similar note, alcoholics who drive while under the influence of alcohol are often hospitalized following "accidents" that may or may not be alcohol-related.

The assessor should inquire about periods of hospitalization *for any reason* and explore whether or not these were drug-related. A client who is hospitalized following an automobile accident may contract hepatitis B (a liver infection transmitted through the blood) through a blood transfusion. If that accident was caused by the person's drinking, then indirectly this client may be said to have contracted hepatitis B as an indirect result of his or her drinking.

The client who admits to the use of intravenous drugs and is hospitalized for the treatment of endocarditis, an infection of the heart valves, may have shared needles with other addicts. Or, the infection may have developed from malnutrition after a protracted period of drug use. It is up to the assessor to try to determine whether the person's chemical use was a causal agent in the client's hospitalization at any point. Such infor-

mation often helps the assessor gain a better understanding of the client's chemical use and its consequences.

Area VIII: Previous Treatment History

In working with a person who may be addicted to chemicals, it is helpful for the evaluator to determine whether the client has ever been in a treatment program for chemical dependency. This information, which may be based on the client's self-report or on information provided by the court system, sheds light on the client's past and on the client's potential to benefit from treatment.

The person who has been hospitalized three times for a heart condition and who continues to deny having any heart problems is denying the reality of his or her condition. The same is true for the client who says that she does not think she has a problem with chemicals but who has been in drug treatment three times; she may not have accepted the reality of her drug addiction. The problem then becomes one of making a recommendation for the client in light of his or her previous treatment history and current status.

The assessor should pay attention to the discharge status from previous treatment programs and to the period of time after treatment that the person maintained sobriety. Clients often claim to have been sober for months but fail to mention that they were in treatment (or in jail!) during this time. Clients may admit that they started to use drugs shortly after they were discharged, if not before. Unfortunately, the situation of a client who reports using chemicals on the way home following treatment is well known to chemical dependency treatment professionals.

A client who admits to having used chemicals during previous treatment is providing valuable information about his or her possible attitude toward the current treatment exposure as well. This client would have a different prognosis than would a client who had maintained total sobriety for 3 years following the last treatment exposure and then relapsed. Clients should be asked *when they entered treatment, how long were they there,* and *when they started to use chemicals following treatment.*

The Clinical Interview

The clinical interview forms the cornerstone of the chemical dependency assessment. Information from the client should include data on the client's previous chemical use. But because the client may either consciously or unconsciously distort the information he or she provides, other sources of data should also be used in the evaluation of a person suspected to be addicted to chemicals.

The first part of the interview process is an introduction by the assessor. The assessor explains that questions will be asked about the client's possible chemical use patterns and that *specific* responses are most helpful. The assessor also explains that although many of these questions may have been asked by others in the past, this information is important. The client is then asked whether he or she has any questions, after which the interview will begin.

The assessor should attempt to review the diagnostic criteria for chemical dependency outlined by the American Psychiatric Association's (1994) *Diagnostic and Statistical Manual of Mental Disorders* (4th edition), also known as the *DSM-IV*. This manual provides a framework within which to diagnose chemical dependency.

Many of the questions utilized in the clinical interview are designed to explore the same piece of information from different perspectives. For example, at one point in the interview process the client might be asked, "In the *average* week, how many nights would you say that you use drugs or alcohol?" At a later point in the interview the client might be asked, "How much would you say, on the average, that you spend for drugs or alcohol in a week?"

The purpose of this redundancy is not to "trap" the client so much as provide different perspectives on the client's chemical use pattern. A client who claims to use alcohol one or two nights a week might admit to spending $50 each

week on chemicals. When asked how it could cost $50 a week if the client only drinks once or twice weekly, the client might explain that he or she drinks at a bar and often buys drinks for friends. This information reveals more about the client's chemical use pattern, helping the assessor better understand the client.

Other Sources of Information

Medical Test Data

Unfortunately, laboratory test data is of only limited value in the assessment of a person who is suspected of being addicted to chemicals. There are no blood or urine tests specific for alcohol or drug addiction that a physician could use for general screening purposes. It has been suggested that elevations in certain blood tests, such as liver function tests, might serve as "alerting factors" (Hoeksema & de Bock, 1993, p. 268) for possible alcohol dependence. However, in general, blood and urine tests are not suitable for providing conclusive proof that a person is (or, is not) abusing one or more chemicals.

Thus, laboratory test data provide but one piece of information, suggesting that the patient may or may not be abusing one or more chemicals. However, medical test data and medical professionals are able to provide important hints about a person's chemical use status. For example, if a patient's personal physician had warned him or her about alcohol-related liver damage 3 years earlier, the problems caused by the patient's alcohol use date back at least that far. And if a client who claims never to have used marijuana tests positive for THC on a supervised blood or urine toxicology test, the patient was probably using marijuana in addition to whatever drugs of abuse he or she admits to using. Thus, medical tests or the patient's physician can often

- confirm the presence of certain chemicals in the client's blood or urine samples

- identify the *amount* of certain chemicals present in a person's blood or urine sample
- determine whether the drug levels in the blood or urine sample have increased (suggesting further drug use), remained the same (which also might suggest further drug use), declined (suggesting no further drug use since the last test)
- offer hints as to how long the patient has been using chemicals

The detection of chemical use by laboratory testing is a very technical art involving many different variables (Verebey & Turner, 1991). Furthermore, both blood and urine toxicology testing involves an element of intrusiveness; urine toxicology testing involves, at the very least, an invasion of privacy, and the process of obtaining a blood sample for toxicology screening is physically invasive (Cone, 1993).

However, medical test data is quite useful in some situations. It is not uncommon, for example, for a client who was involved in an automobile accident to claim to have had "only two beers" when he or she started to drive. A blood alcohol (or BAL) test conducted within an hour of the accident may reveal that the client's BAL was far higher than what would be achieved from "only" two beers. Clients who test negative for marijuana on one occasion may very well test positive only a few days later. Subsequent inquiry will often reveal that he or she used drugs sometime after the first test, thinking that he or she was "safe" and would not be tested for drugs again for a long time. Such drug use would be detected by *frequent* and *unannounced* urine tests, which are *closely supervised* to detect illicit drug use.[1]

Thus, medical test data are often a valuable source of objective information about a client's drug use. A client may appear sleepy from lack of sleep or from using drugs or alcohol in the past few hours. The laboratory test data can often make this determination. The assessor should always attempt to utilize medical test information whenever possible to further establish a foundation for the diagnosis of chemical dependency.

Psychological Test Data

A number of psychological tests can either directly or indirectly be of use in the diagnosis of chemical dependency. Many assessment tools available today are paper-and-pencil tests, filled out either by the client (and as such are known as *self-report* instruments) or by the assessor as he or she asks questions of the person being evaluated. Self-report instruments offer the advantages of being inexpensive and usually inoffensive to the client (Stuart, 1980).

One of the most popular assessment instruments is the Michigan Alcoholism Screening Test (or MAST) (Selzer, 1971). This test is composed of 24 questions that can be answered either "yes" or "no," depending on whether the item applies to the respondent. Test items are weighted with a value of 1, 2, or in some cases 5 points. A score of 8 points or more suggests alcoholism. The effectiveness of this test has been demonstrated in clinical literature (Miller, 1976), but this test addresses *only* alcoholism (Lewis, Dana, & Blevins, 1988) and thus is of limited value in cases where the person uses other chemicals.

An interview format for alcoholism that is growing in popularity is the CAGE questionnaire (Ewing, 1984). CAGE is an acronym for the four questions that make up the questionnaire:

1. Have you ever felt you ought to CUT DOWN on your drinking?
2. Have people ANNOYED you by criticizing your drinking?
3. Have you ever felt bad or GUILTY about your drinking?
4. Have you ever had a drink first thing in the

[1]Cone (1993) spoke at length about using saliva for toxicology tests to determine whether the client has been using an illicit chemical. Unfortunately, although this technique is neither intrusive nor invasive in the same way that blood and urine toxicology tests might be, the tools to conduct such saliva tests are not widely available. Furthermore, the effectiveness of such tests has not been adequately proved. Still, this technology might be useful in the years to come.

morning to steady your nerves or to get rid of a hangover (EYE-OPENER)?

A "yes" response to any one of these four questions suggests the need for a detailed inquiry by the assessor. The CAGE questionnaire has an 80% to 90% accuracy rate in detecting alcoholism when a client answers "yes" to two or more of these questions.

Other assessment tools are available as well. In their work, Roffman and George (1988) provide examples of a self-report instrument used in the evaluation of marijuana use patterns. Washton, Stone, and Hendrickson (1988) discuss the use of the Cocaine Abuse Assessment Profile in their essay on the evaluation of cocaine users. These tests, although useful, are of limited value in the assessment of polydrug users.

The original MMPI was introduced 50 years ago. In 1965, the MacAndrew Alcoholism Scale (also known as the Mac scale) was introduced after an item analysis suggested that alcoholics tended to answer 49 of the 566 items of the MMPI differently than nonalcoholics did. A cutoff score of 24 items out of 49 answered in the "scorable" direction correctly identified 82% of the alcoholic and nonalcoholic clients in a sample of 400 male psychiatric patients (Graham, 1990). Subsequent research has suggested, however, that this scale might measure a general tendency toward addiction, rather than the specific behavior of alcoholism (Graham, 1990).

After 7 years of research, an updated version of the MMPI, the Minnesota Multiphasic Personality Inventory-2 (or MMPI-2) was introduced in 1989. The Mac scale was modified slightly but was retained essentially in its original form. However, since the time of its introduction, research has revealed that black clients tend to score higher on the Mac scale than do white clients. Furthermore, clients who are extroverted, exhibitionistic, or assertive, or who experience "blackouts" for *any* reason or enjoy risk-taking behaviors, all tend to score higher on the Mac scale, even if they are not addicted (Graham, 1990).

Although the Mac scale was designed to de-

tect alcoholics, Otto, Lang, Megargee, and Rosenblatt (1989), working with the original MMPI, discovered that alcoholics might be able to "conceal their drinking problems even when the relatively subtle special alcohol scales of the MMPI are applied" (p. 7). Thus, it is possible to obtain either "false positive" or "false negative" results from the MMPI Mac scale. Until it's proved otherwise, counselors should assume that the revised Mac scale on the MMPI-2 shares this same weakness with the original Mac scale.

Unlike many other assessment tools, the MMPI offers the additional advantage of having five built-in "truth" scales. These scales offer insight into how truthful the individual taking the test may have been and are discussed in more detail by Graham (1990). A major disadvantage of the MMPI is that it is possible for the individual taking the test to "intentionally diminish . . . the level of pathology evident in overall MMPI profiles" (Otto et al., 1989, p. 7). Furthermore, in spite of the built-in truth scales, individuals who want to project an image of themselves as being well adjusted may still accomplish their goal and reduce measured levels of distress.

Overall, a major disadvantage of paper-and-pencil tests is that they are best suited to clients who are unlikely to "fake" (the technical term is *positively dissimulate*) answers on the test in order to appear less disturbed (Evans & Sullivan, 1990). A common problem, well known to chemical dependency professionals, is that these instruments are subject to the same problems of denial, distortion, and outright misrepresentation often encountered in the clinical interview.

Clients have been known to initially deny the use of a chemical only to subsequently test positive for the drug on a urine toxicology test conducted at the time of admission. Clients have also been known to overestimate or underestimate either the amount or the frequency of their drug use. Such distortion may be unintentional, as in a case where the person simply forgets an episode of chemical use, or it may be quite deliberate.

Roffman and George (1988) point out that distortion in self-report inventories can occur if the client does not know how potent the drug or drugs were. How did the drug or drugs interfere with the individual's ability to evaluate the drug's effects? A client may honestly believe that he or she was only mildly intoxicated, whereas an outside observer may believe that the client was "dead drunk."

One technique that may be useful in the detection of intentional dissimulation is to review the test results not only with the client but with the client's spouse or significant other also present. Often, the spouse or significant other contradicts the client's response to one or more test items, providing valuable new data for the assessment process. For example, on the Michigan Alcoholism Screening Test (MAST), clients often answer "no" when asked whether they had ever been involved in an alcohol-related accident. Suppose one client's wife brings up "that time when you drove off the road into the ditch a couple of years ago." When the client points out that the police had ruled the cause of the accident to be ice on the road, the wife may respond, "But you told me that you had been drinking earlier that night."

Another technique, one I frequently use, is to administer the same test or ask the same questions twice during the assessment process. For example, the Michigan Alcoholism Screening Test may be administered during the initial interview and again at the follow-up interview a week or so later. If there are significant discrepancies, they are explored with the client to determine the reason.

Clients have been known to score as many as 13 points on the initial administration of the MAST, a score well above the cutoff score necessary to suggest alcoholism. At follow-up a week later the same clients may score only 9 points, which, although lower, is still above the cutoff score necessary to suggest alcoholism. The difference in test scores suggests some degree of deception on the clients' part. When a client's test is later reviewed with the spouse present, several other items may be found to apply to the client, suggesting a final score of perhaps 24 points.

Thus, psychological test data can often pro-vide valuable insights into the client's personality pattern and his or her chemical use. Many such tests require a trained professional to administer them and interpret their results to the client. However, when used properly, psychological test data can add an important dimension to the diagnostic process.

Outcome of the Assessment Process

At the end of the assessment, the chemical dependency professional should be in a position to state his or her opinion as to whether the client (1) is addicted to one or more chemicals, (2) is a serious abuser of one or more chemicals, or (3) does not seem to have a problem with chemicals. Based on this assessment, the professional should then be able to decide whether treatment is necessary and make some recommendations as to the disposition of the client's case. Figure 26.2 is a flowchart outlining the assessment process.

Obviously, if the client is found to be addicted to one or more chemicals, a recommendation that he or she enter treatment would be appropriate. Such a treatment recommendation may be for inpatient or for outpatient treatment, depending on the client's needs. However, if the client is found to be only an abuser of chemicals, the decision must be made whether to recommend chemical dependency treatment or not. Other recommendations might include participation in self-help groups such as Alcoholics Anonymous or Narcotics Anonymous or a referral to a mental health center for evaluation and treatment.

However, it is possible that the client will be found not to present a drug abuse or addiction problem but still be in need of professional support. A referral for marital counseling, for example, might be made if there is evidence of a marital problem in a client who does not seem to be addicted to chemicals. The assessor can still make an appropriate referral, even if he or she has not found evidence of addiction.

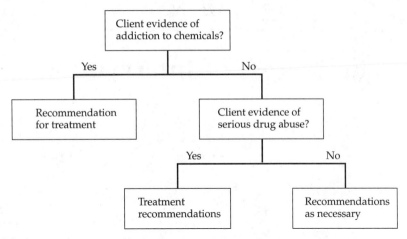

FIGURE 26.2 A flowchart of the assessment process

Summary

The assessment process should include information from a number of sources if it is to provide the most comprehensive picture of the client's chemical use pattern possible. Information from the client is collected during one or more clinical interviews, through which the assessor attempts to obtain accurate data on the individual's chemical use. Information should also be obtained from collateral sources whenever possible, as such collateral information may be more revealing than the client's self-report.

Information from medical personnel in a position to evaluate the client's physical status can often prove valuable in understanding a client and the role that drugs have played in his or her life. Finally, psychological test data may reveal much about the client's personality profile and drug use patterns. However, psychological test data suffer from the drawback that they are easily manipulated by a client who wishes to dissimulate.

The outcome of the assessment process should be a formal report in which the evidence supporting the conclusion that the client is or is not chemically dependent is outlined. Recommendations for further treatment may be made at this time, even if the client is found not to be addicted to chemicals.

CHAPTER TWENTY-SEVEN

The Process of Intervention

Vernon Johnson (1980) notes that alcoholics, like all addicts, are "not in touch with reality"; however, they are "capable of accepting some useful portion of reality, *if that reality is presented in forms they can receive*" (p. 49, italics in original). The first step in treatment is to attempt to break through their system of denial to get them to recognize and accept the fact that they are in need of help. This is done through the process of *intervention.*

It is not easy to obtain a commitment from an addict to enter *and remain in* a treatment program. More than one addicted person has entered treatment one day and left shortly afterward, having satisfied the stipulation of parents, judges, or family to enter a treatment program. "After all," many seem to reason, "nobody said anything about my *staying* there, did they?"

Addicts often openly admit that they are addicted to chemicals not because of a desire to achieve or maintain sobriety but because this admission offers an excuse to *continue* to use chemicals. The addict enters into a circular pattern of logic, an elaborate rationalization, by which the word *addicted* comes to mean *hopelessly addicted*. Because they are "hopelessly addicted," at least in their own estimation, they give themselves permission to continue using chemicals.

This is a bizzare justification for chemical use that overlooks the fact that addiction is a treatable disease. The first part of treatment is con-

vincing the person that he or she is indeed addicted and in need of help for the drug dependency that has come to dominate his or her life. This awareness, and the commitment to enter into treatment, is often achieved through the intervention process.

A Definition of Intervention

It was once thought that addicts had to "hit bottom," as it is called in AA, before they could accept the need for help. "Bottom" is the point where the individual has to admit utter and total defeat. Vernon Johnson (1980), a pioneer in the intervention process, challenges this belief, suggesting that the addict could learn to accept the reality of his or her addiction *if this information were presented in language that he or she could understand.*

Because of the physical and emotional damage that uncontrolled addiction can cause, Johnson (1980) advocates *early intervention* in cases of drug addiction. In a later work, he identifies intervention as

[a] process by which the harmful, progressive and destructive effects of chemical dependency are interrupted and the chemically dependent person is helped to stop using mood-altering chemicals, and to develop new, healthier ways of coping with his or her needs and problems. (Johnson Institute, 1987, p. 61)

Twerski (1983), who also advocates early intervention in cases of drug addiction, defines intervention as "a collective, guided effort by the significant persons in the patient's environment to precipitate a crisis through confrontation, and thereby to remove the patient's defensive obstructions to recovery" (p. 1028). Rothenberg (1988), who explored the legal ramifications of intervention, notes that the intervention process for alcoholism consists of "talking to the alcoholic, confronting his or her denials, and breaking down defenses so as to secure agreement to seek treatment" (p. 22).

Each of these three definitions contains various components of the intervention process. Intervention is an *organized* effort on the part of (1) *significant others* in the addict's environment to (2) *break through the wall of denial, rationalization, and projection* by which the addict seeks to protect his or her addiction; the purpose of this collective effort, which is (3) *usually supervised* by a chemical dependency professional is to (4) secure an agreement to *immediately* seek treatment.

Characteristics of the Intervention Process

A significant characteristic of intervention is that *there is no malice in the intervention process.* It is not a session to allow people to vent pent-up frustration. Rather, the intervention process is a "profound act of caring" (Johnson, 1986, p. 65) through which significant others in the addict's social circle break the rule of silence surrounding the addiction. Each person confronts the addicted person with specific evidence that he or she has lost control of drug use in language that the addict can understand.

The participants also express their desire for the addict to seek professional help for the drug problem (Williams, 1989). In the process, each member affirms concern for the addict but offers hard data showing how the addicted person is no longer in control of his or her life. The collective hope is that those involved will be able to break through the addict's system of denial and

that the addict will accept the need for help. This is the central theme around which an intervention session is planned.

According to Johnson (Johnson Institute, 1987), effective intervention sessions are *planned in advance* and repeatedly *rehearsed* by the individual participants to ensure that the information presented is appropriate for an intervention session. Williams (1989) agrees on the need for a rehearsal session, warning that participants should be informed that the goal of intervention

> is not . . . that persons "admit" to being addicted, or that they have behaved in a manner that has caused others pain, or that they were wrong, or even that they were under the influence of a drug (including, of course, alcohol) in any given situation. Diagnosing chemical dependency is not part of an intervention. The goal is to elicit an agreement from the person to be evaluated for possible chemical dependency and to follow the resulting recommendations. (p. 99)

Thus, the goal of intervention is not to get the individual to admit that he or she has a problem with chemicals but to convince the individual of the need to immediately be evaluated and, if treatment is recommended, to follow through with this recommendation.

The Mechanics of Intervention

As noted, the intervention process is *planned* and should be rehearsed beforehand by the participants. It should involve *every* person in the addict's life who has something to add, including the addict's spouse, siblings, children, friends, supervisor, employer, minister, coworker, or others. Johnson (Johnson Institute, 1987) suggests that the supervisor be included because the addict often uses his or her perception of job performance as an excuse not to listen to the others in the intervention project. Each individual is advised to bring forward *specific incidents* in which the addict's behavior, especially the chemical use, interfered with his or her life in some manner.

Individually confronting an addicted person is difficult at best and in most cases is an exercise in futility (Johnson Institute, 1987). Any person who has tried to talk to an addicted person will attest that the addict will deny, rationalize, threaten, or simply avoid any confrontation that threatens her or his continued drug use. The spouse who questions whether the alcoholic was physically able to drive the car home last night may be met with the response "No, but my friend Joe drove the car home for me, then walked home after he parked the car in the driveway." However, if Joe is *also* present, he could confront the alcoholic about how he did *not* drive the car home last night, or any other night for that matter.

Before the group is brought together for an intervention session, it is unlikely that anyone checked out the isolated lies, rationalizations, or episodes of denial. The addict's denial, projection, and rationalization often crumble when confronted with all the significant people in his or her environment. This is why a collective intervention session is most powerful in working with the addict.

Twerski (1983) observes that it is common for the person for whom the intervention session was called to make promises to change his or her behavior. Although these promises may be made either in good faith or simply as a means of avoiding further confrontation, the fact remains that, because the disease of addiction "responds to treatment and not to manipulation, it is unlikely that any of these promises will work, and the counselor must recommend treatment as the optimum course" (Twerski, 1983, p. 1029).

If the person refuses to acknowledge the addiction or acknowledges it but refuses to enter treatment, each participant in the intervention session should be prepared to detach from the addict. This is *not* an attempt to manipulate the addict through empty threats. Rather, each person should be willing to follow through with a specific action to help themselves begin to detach from the addict should he or she refuse to enter treatment. For example, if the employer or supervisor has decided that the company can no longer tolerate the addict's behavior, then as

soon as it is his or her turn to speak at the intervention session, he or she needs to clearly state that if the addict does not seek treatment, employment will be terminated. If the addict then refuses treatment, the employer or supervisor should follow through with this action.

Family members should also have thought about and discussed possible options through which they can begin to detach from the addict. This should be done before the intervention session. During the rehearsal, each participant should practice informing the addicted person what he or she will do if the addict does not accept treatment. If the addicted person refuses treatment (possibly by leaving the session before it ends), each person should follow through with the alternative plan.

Again, there should be no malice in this action. There is a very real danger that, without proper guidance, the intervention session may become little more than a weapon used by some family members to control the behavior of another (Claunch, 1994). The participants in the intervention process should not engage in threats or force the addicted person into treatment. Although having the addicted person see and accept the need for treatment is one goal of the intervention process, it is not the only one. An even more important goal of the intervention process is for participants to begin to break the conspiracy of silence that surrounds the addict (Claunch, 1994).

In the intervention process, each participant learns that he or she has the right to *choose* how he or she will respond if the addict chooses to continue to use chemicals. The addicted person is still able to exercise his or her own freedom of choice by either accepting the need for treatment or not. But now the involuntary "support system" composed of friends and family members will not be as secure; people will be talking to each other and drawing strength from each other. Although having the addict either accept the need for treatment or gain a clear understanding of the consequences of not going into treatment is one goal of the intervention session, an equally important goal is that everyone in the family be *heard* when voicing his or her concern (Claunch, 1994).

Family Intervention

Family intervention is a specialized intervention process in which *every* concerned family member gathers together under the supervision of a trained professional and plans a joint confrontation of the individual. The purpose of the family intervention session, like that of all other forms of intervention, is to break through the addict's denial, allow the family members to voice their concerns, and possibly obtain a commitment from the addict to enter treatment. The focus is on the individual's drug using behaviors and on the concern that the participants have for the addict.

An advantage of the family intervention session is that, through confrontation, family members can begin to "detach" from the addict. The conspiracy of silence that existed within the family is broken, and family members may begin to communicate more openly and more effectively. Meyer (1988) describes the intervention process as an "opportunity for healing" (p. 7) for this reason. The participants in the intervention session can both express their love and concern for the addicted person and at the same time reject the addict's drug-centered behaviors.

The family intervention process allows the various members of the addict's social circle to come forward, compare notes, and express their concern for the individual's lifestyle. Sometimes, the family members, friends, employers, or whoever is involved in the intervention process will write down detailed lists of specific incidents. The information that is reviewed during the intervention session should be highly specific to avoid as much confusion as possible. Sometimes, family members will bring in a personal diary to use as a reference in the intervention session. One advantage of the written notes is that they help to focus the individual on the specific information that he or she wishes to bring to the intervention session.

During the rehearsal, the professional who coordinates the intervention session decides who will present information and in what order. As much as possible, this planned sequence is followed during the intervention session itself. The participants do not threaten the addict. Rather, they present specific concerns and information that highlights the need for the addicted person to enter treatment. Johnson (1980) provides a good overview of the intervention process.

An Example of a Family Intervention Session

In this hypothetical intervention session, the central character is a patient named Jim. Also involved are his parents, two sisters, and a chemical dependency counselor. The intervention session is held at Jim's parents' home, where Jim has been living. During the early part of the session, Jim asserts that he never drinks to the point of passing out. He also claims that, he always drinks at home so that he won't be out on the roads while intoxicated. For these reasons, he does not believe that his drinking is as bad as everybody says it is and he sees no reason everybody should be so concerned.

Jim's sister Sara also lives at home with their parents. She immediately points out that, just 3 weeks ago, Jim had run out of vodka early in the evening after having four or five mixed drinks. She relates that Jim had driven to the liquor store to buy a new bottle or two. Sara states that she is not calling Jim a liar but that she *knows* he had driven a car after drinking on this occasion. She was concerned about the possibility that he might have an accident and still feels uncomfortable about this incident. She is afraid that he might do it again and that next time he might not be so lucky as to make it back home again in one piece.

Jim's mother then speaks. She points out that she found her son unconscious on the living room floor twice in the past month. She gives the exact dates of these occurrences and describes her discontent at seeing Jim passed out on the floor, surrounded by empty beer bottles. She picked up the empty bottles to keep them from being broken by accident and covered Jim up with a blanket. But she also is concerned and believes that her son is drinking more than he thinks.

As Jim's mother finishes, his sister Gloria presents her information and concerns. She states that she had to ask Jim to leave her house last week, which was news to the rest of the family. She took this step, she explained, because Jim was intoxicated, loud, and abusive toward his nephew. She points out that everyone who was present, including her son's friend who happened to be visiting at the time, smelled the alcohol on his breath and was repulsed by his behavior. Gloria concludes by stating that Jim is no longer welcome in her home unless he goes through treatment.

At this point, the chemical dependency counselor tells Jim that his behavior was not so different from that of thousands of other addicts. The counselor also explains that at this point in the intervention session many addicts promise to cut back or totally eliminate the drug use, a prediction that catches Jim by surprise because he was about to do the same. His protests and promises die in his throat before he even opens his mouth.

Before Jim can think of something else to say, the counselor points out that Jim shows every sign of having a significant alcohol problem. The counselor lists the symptoms of alcohol addiction one by one, pointing out how Jim's family has identified different symptoms of addiction in their presentations. "So now," the counselor concludes, "we have reached a point where you must make a decision. Will you accept help for your alcohol problem?"

If Jim says "yes," family members will explain that they have contacted the admissions officer of two or three nearby treatment centers that have agreed to hold a bed for him until after the intervention session has ended. Jim will be given a choice of which treatment center to enter and will be told that travel arrangements have been taken care of. His luggage is packed in the car and, if he wishes, the family will escort him to treatment as a show of support.

If Jim says "no," the family members then will confront him about the steps they are prepared to take to separate from his addiction. His parents may inform him that they have arranged for a restraining order from the court and present him with papers informing him that he will be arrested if he comes within a quarter of a mile of his parents' home. Other family members might then inform Jim that, until he seeks professional assistance for his drinking, he is not welcome in their homes either. If his employer is present, Jim may be told that his job is no longer there for him if he does not enter treatment.

Jim will be told that, no matter what he may think, these steps are not being taken as punishment. Each person will inform him that, because of his drug addiction, they find it necessary to detach from him until he chooses to get his life in order. Each person will affirm his or her concern for Jim but will also start the process of no longer protecting Jim from his addiction.

These decisions have all been made in advance of the intervention session. Which option the participants take rests largely on Jim's response to the question, Will you accept help for your alcohol problem? Through the process of intervention, the family members have been helped to identify boundaries—the limits they can enforce for their own well-being (Claunch, 1994).

Intervention and Other Forms of Chemical Addiction

The Johnson Institute (1987) has addressed the issue of intervention when the person's drug-of-choice is not alcohol but any of a wide range of other chemicals. The same techniques used in alcoholism also apply to cases involving cocaine, benzodiazepines, marijuana, amphetamines, or virtually any other drug of abuse. Significant others gather, discuss the problem, and review their data about the addict's behavior. Practice intervention sessions are held, and the problems are addressed during the practice sessions as they are uncovered.

Finally, when everything is ready, the formal intervention session with the addicted person is held. The addict may need to be tricked into attending the intervention session, but there is no malice in the attempt to help the addict see how serious his or her drug addiction has become. Rather, there is a calm, caring review of the facts by person after person until the addict is unable to defend against the realization that he or she is addicted to chemicals and in need of professional help.

Arrangements are made in advance for the individual's admission into treatment. This may be accomplished by a simple telephone call to the admissions officer of the treatment center. The caller can explain the situation and ask if the center would be willing to accept the target person as a client. Usually, the treatment center staff will want to carry out its own chemical dependency evaluation to confirm that the person is an appropriate referral to treatment. But most treatment centers should be more than willing to consider a referral from a family intervention project.

The Ethics of Intervention

As humane as the goal of intervention is, questions have been raised concerning the ethics of this practice. Rothenberg (1988) notes that there is some question as to whether it is necessary to validate the diagnosis of chemical dependency before an attempt at intervention is made. In other words, should there be an independent verification of the diagnosis of drug addiction before an attempt at intervention is carried out? If there is not, what are the legal sanctions that can be brought against a chemical dependency professional who, in good faith, supervises an attempt at intervention? This question becomes very important in light of the fact that some families will attempt to use the intervention process as a weapon they can employ to control the behavior of a wayward individual (Claunch, 1994). To avoid this potential danger, the wise treatment professional may want to indepen-

dently confirm the diagnosis before allowing the intervention process to proceed.

Furthermore, the question of whether chemical dependency professionals involved in an intervention project should tell the client that he or she is free to leave at any time has not been answered (Rothenberg, 1988). There is a possibility that current intervention methods are in violation of either state or federal law. Failing to inform the client that he or she is free to leave might be interpreted as a violation of the laws against kidnapping or unlawful detention.

Rothenberg's (1988) warning raises some interesting questions for the chemical dependency professional in both the moral and legal areas. In future years, the courts may rule that the professional is legally obligated to inform the client that he or she is free to leave the intervention session at any time. Furthermore, the courts may rule that the professional can make no move to hold the client either by physical force, or by threats, should he or she express a desire to leave. Or the courts may rule that intervention is a legitimate treatment technique when used by trained professionals. No legal precedent for this area has been established at this time. Therefore, chemical dependency professionals are advised to consult with an attorney to discuss the specific laws that may apply in their area of practice.

Legal Intervention

Sometimes intervention comes in a much simpler form: through the courts. An individual may be arrested for driving while under the influence of alcohol (a DWI, as it is called in some states), for possession of a controlled substance, or for some other drug-related charge. The judge may offer an alternative to incarceration: *either* you successfully complete a drug treatment program, *or* you will be incarcerated.

The exact length of time spent in jail depends on the specific nature of the charge brought against the person. However, either/or treatment situations are unique in that individuals are offered a choice. They may elect to spend time in jail or to accept the treatment option. In so doing, they are not *ordered* into treatment; rather, they have made the choice to enter treatment. The individual always has the choice of incarceration, if he or she does not believe that treatment is necessary.

"Either/or" treatment admissions are easier to work with than voluntary admissions to treatment. Indeed, court-sponsored intervention is a powerful incentive to treatment (Moylan, 1990). The very fact that there is a legal hold on the person means that the person is much less likely to leave treatment when his or her denial system is confronted. Also, the very fact that the person was admitted on an either/or basis is information that can be used to confront the individual about the nature of his or her addiction problem. After all, it is difficult for the person who has just been arrested for a second or third drug-related charge to deny that chemicals are a problem for them, although this has been known to happen.

Collins and Allison (1983) reviewed the treatment programs of some 2,200 addicts who were "legally induced to seek treatment" (p. 1145) and found that those who chose treatment as an alternative to incarceration did as well in treatment as those who were there voluntarily. Furthermore, those who were in treatment at the court's invitation were more likely to stay in treatment longer than were those who had no restrictions placed on them. The authors concluded that

> the use of legal threat to pressure individuals into drug treatment is a valid approach for dealing with drug abusers and their undesirable behaviors. Legal threat apparently helps keep these individuals constructively involved in treatment and does not adversely affect long-term treatment goals. (p. 1148)

According to E. Matuschka (1985), "Treatment which carried a coercive element has been shown to have a higher cure ratio than treatment without a coercive element" (p. 209). Thus, those who accept treatment as an alternative to incar-

ceration seem to do better than individuals who enter treatment on a voluntary basis (Collins & Allison, 1983; E. Matuschka, 1985). It seems that legal intervention is a viable alternative for some who would not accept the need for treatment if left to their own devices.

Peele (1989), on the other hand, views such either/or referrals as intrusive and counterproductive. He points out that individuals convicted of driving a motor vehicle while under the influence of chemicals respond better to legal sanctions (such as jail or probation) than to being forced into treatment. Peele (1989) argues strongly that the individual should be held responsible for his or her actions, *including the initial decision to use chemicals,* and that chemical use or abuse does not excuse individuals from responsibility for their behavior.

Treatment or Incarceration: When Is Treatment Appropriate?

As noted earlier, the courts may offer the person convicted of a drug-related charge the opportunity to enter into a drug treatment program rather than go to jail or prison. Although many individuals have utilized this "last chance" to begin serious work on their recovery from drug addiction, many others use "treatment" to avoid jail or prison.

The opportunity to participate in a treatment program should not be substituted for incarceration when incarceration is deserved. Unfortunately, all too often the individual is offered the opportunity to enter treatment without an examination of his or her motivation. For example, one must question the motive of the alleged drug "pusher" who is arrested with several pounds of a controlled substance and who enters "treatment" before going to court. Similarly, one should question the motive of a person arrested for the fifth time while driving under the influence of chemicals who enters "treatment" on the advice of his or her attorney before going to court. Some chronic drinkers are quite open about the fact that they plan to continue to drink and that their only motivation for entering "treatment" is to avoid the legal consequences brought on by their alcohol use. "I'm here because my attorney said that it would look good in court" is a common refrain heard by treatment center staff.

Chemical dependency treatment professionals frequently encounter individuals who "suddenly remember" having to go to court for a drug-related charge. This sudden revelation is often made within the first or second week of admission. The treatment center staff is then placed in the uncomfortable position of having to allow the client to leave treatment briefly to go to court, secure in the knowledge that they have been used by the addict against the courts. Some addicts have openly boasted that they entered "treatment" in order to make a better impression on the judge and jury.

Another example of the way in which "treatment" is abused is the person who enters treatment to stop his or her personal use of chemicals while openly admitting that he or she plans to continue to sell drugs to others. How seriously is the individual going to participate in the treatment program, and how cost-effective will treatment be under these circumstances? Unfortunately, this is a question that the courts often do not ask. It is easier for the overworked legal system to accept "treatment" as an option without an examination of whether or not it is likely to be effective in helping the individual come to terms with his or her drug use.

A physician who indiscriminately prescribes antibiotics for every patient who comes into the office would quickly be brought up on charges of incompetence. The decision to utilize one medication or another is not one that should be taken lightly. Obviously, the physician must weigh the potential benefits of each different approach to the patient's problems against the anticipated risk for each possible treatment method. The same is true for chemical dependency treatment. Although the option of treatment in place of incarceration should certainly be considered by the courts, it must be remembered at all times that the treatment program is *not* the answer to every drug-related problem.

In identifying when treatment is most appropriate, the professional should keep in mind that *treatment should never stand between the individual and the natural consequences of his or her behavior.*

Other Forms of Intervention

Another form of "either/or" situation arises when an addict's spouse or employer sets down the law; "*Either* you stop drinking, *or* I will (leave you, fire you). Often, the physician is the person who establishes the either/or situation by threatening to file commitment papers on the addict unless he or she enters treatment. One individual, in treatment shortly after his wife had filed for divorce, said simply, "I didn't think that she meant it . . . I guess she did!"

Adelman and Weiss (1989) found that "employees coerced into treatment by their employers had better treatment outcomes than employees who volunteered for treatment" for alcoholism (p. 515). The authors concluded that treatment programs that utilize such "constructive coercion" (p. 515) may actually be more effective in working with alcohol addicts than programs that do not encourage the use of this method of intervention.

This is not to say that the intervention process will meet with success or even that a court-ordered treatment exposure will result in a commitment to recovery. As noted earlier, the alcoholic may reach a point where he or she will sacrifice just about everything to support the addiction. In this sense, alcoholism is not very different from the other forms of chemical addiction. There are cases known where the addicted person accepted the loss of job, family, and spouse as part of the price to be paid for addiction.

Court-Ordered Involuntary Commitment

In some states, it is possible for people to be committed to treatment against their will if the courts have sufficient evidence to believe that they are in imminent danger of harming themselves or others. "Harm to self" might include neglect, and more than one alcoholic who fell asleep in the snow while walking home has been surprised to learn that this constitutes a danger to "self."

The exact provisions of a court-ordered commitment vary from state to state, and some states have no provision for such commitments. Obviously, chemical dependency professionals in each state must consult with an attorney to review the exact legal statutes that apply. However, one should be aware that the laws of many states allow for the courts to intervene, should the person's chemical use put his or her life or the life of others in danger.

Occasionally, the individual enters treatment on a voluntary basis. As Johnson (Johnson Institute, 1987) observes, although this does occasionally happen, it is unusual. It is more common for addicts to continue to use chemicals if they can do so without having to pay one or more consequences. It is for this reason that external pressure of some kind—be it family, legal, medical, or professional—is often necessary to help the addicted person see the need to enter treatment.

Summary

The intervention process is an organized effort on the part of significant others in the addicted person's social environment to break through the wall of defenses that protect the individual from the realization that his or her life is out of control. Intervention projects are usually supervised by a substance abuse rehabilitation professional and are held with the goal of securing an agreement for the individual to immediately enter treatment. However, the individual retains the right to choose whether or not to enter treatment. Participants in the intervention project must be prepared for either choice and have alternate plans in hand if the addict does not accept the need for treatment.

The individual also retains certain rights during the intervention process itself. Indeed, the individual cannot be detained if he or she expresses the wish to leave the intervention session. The question of when legal sanctions should be imposed or when treatment should be substituted for these legal sanctions is not always easy to answer, and needs to be examined for each case.

CHAPTER TWENTY-EIGHT

The Treatment of Chemical Dependency

Over the past decade, there has been considerable discussion both in the professional journals and by the media on the merits and disadvantages of treatment for substance abusers. Unfortunately, this debate may give the impression that there is a single, standard treatment format for individuals who are abusing or are addicted to recreational chemicals. The truth is that there are many different forms of treatment, each with its own group of followers.

In this chapter, we will explore some of the basic elements of substance abuse treatment. The specific components of treatment may vary from one program to another. For example, a treatment program that specializes in working with alcoholic businessmen would have little use for a methadone maintenance component. Yet, there are also many common elements to the treatment process, which is the focus of this chapter.

Characteristics of the Substance Abuse Rehabilitation Professional

For every form of substance abuse rehabilitation, there is one individual who is designated as the primary contact person for the recovering addict. To effectively help persons with substance use disorders, the helper should possess certain characteristics. One of the most important characteristics of the counselor is that he or she have no pressing personal issues. Individuals who are dealing with chemical dependency or psychological issues of their own should be discouraged from actively working with recovering addicts, at least until they have resolved their own problems. If the counselor is preoccupied with personal problems, including those of chemical addiction, he or she is unlikely to be able to help the client advance further in terms of personal growth.

In his work on the characteristics of the effective mental health counselor, Rogers (1961) outlined a number of characteristics that he thought are essential:

- warmth
- dependability
- consistency
- the ability to care for and respect the client
- the ability to be separate from the client (that is, the ability not to try to "live through" a client)
- the ability not to be perceived as a threat by the client
- the ability to free oneself from the urge to judge or evaluate the client
- the ability to see the client as a person capable of growth

These characteristics are also found in the person who has strong interpersonal relationship skills. Adelman and Weiss (1989) examined the personality attributes of successful treatment staff members at an alcoholism treatment center and concluded that those staff members who possessed the highest level of interpersonal skills were best equipped to help their clients. The authors based their conclusions on a study they designed in which the treatment outcome of clients of alcoholism counselors with low interpersonal skills were compared with those of counselors who had high interpersonal skills. The authors found that clients of low-skill counselors were twice as likely to relapse as were clients whose counselors had high interpersonal skill levels. Although Adelman and Weiss (1989) do not use the same terms Rogers (1961) does, the implication is clear that the most effective counselor is one who is well adjusted and accepting of others.

One point that needs to be clarified is that *these characteristics do not mean that the chemical dependency professional should be permissive!* Human service professionals occasionally confuse permissiveness with interpersonal warmth. Just as it is possible to be too confrontational, it is also possible to be too permissive. *Caring for clients does not mean protecting them from the consequences of their behavior.*

Confrontation and Other Treatment Techniques

For a number of years, substance abuse rehabilitators in the United States have used a "hard-hitting, directive, exhortational style" (Miller, Genefield, & Tonigan, 1993, p. 455) that serves to overwhelm the addict's defenses. Confrontation is a central feature of this treatment approach and, in theory, is used to help the client begin to understand the reality of his or her addiction or the need for treatment (Twerski, 1983).

Admittedly, the *appropriate* use of confrontation can be quite useful in working with some clients, but there is no evidence that confrontation is effective in the treatment of alcoholism (Hester, 1994). Indeed, *inappropriate* confrontation might even be counterproductive when

used with addicted individuals; *empathy* for the client is a more useful tool (Miller, Genefield, & Tonigan, 1993). Indeed, the research carried out by Miller, Genefield, and Tonigan (1993) indicates that, as the therapist's level of confrontation increases, the client's level of resistance also increases.

Miller, Genefield, and Tonigan suggest that a "supportive-reflective" (1993, p. 455) style of therapy is more effective than confrontation in working with substance abusing clients. Thus, there appears to be little evidence to support the extensive use of confrontation as a treatment technique (Miller, Genefield, & Tonigan, 1993; Miller & Rollnick, 1991; Lewis, Dana, & Blevins, 1988). To work effectively with an addicted person, the professional needs *all* the counseling skills outlined by Rogers (1961), not just the ability to confront others.

The Minnesota Model of Chemical Dependency Treatment

It is something of an understatement to say that what has come to be called the "Minnesota Model" of chemical dependency treatment has been a success. First designed in the 1950s by Dr. Dan Anderson, the Minnesota Model has long served as one of the major treatment formats in the fight against alcoholism and drug abuse.

To earn money to finish his college education, Dr. Anderson worked as an attendant at the state hospital in Willmar, Minnesota (Larson, 1982), returning there after graduation to work as a recreational therapist. He was assigned to work with the alcoholics, the least desirable position at that time.

Anderson was influenced by the work of Mr. Ralph Rossen, who was later to become the Minnesota state commissioner of health. At the same time, the growing influence of Alcoholics Anonymous was used by Dan Anderson and a staff psychologist by the name of Dr. Jean Rossi as a means of understanding and working with alcoholics. They were supported in this approach by the medical director of the hospital, Dr. Nelson Bradley (Larson, 1982). Coming from different professions, each person contributed a different perspective on the alcoholic's needs and addiction. To this team was added the Reverend John Keller, who had been sent to Willmar State Hospital to learn about alcoholism in 1955. The staff then had "knowledge of medicine, psychology, AA and theology together under one roof to develop a new and innovative alcohol treatment program" (Larson, 1982, p. 35).

This new treatment approach, since called the Minnesota Model, was originally designed to work with dependency on alcohol (*Alcoholism & Drug Abuse Week,* 1990a). Since its introduction, it has also been used as a model for the treatment of other forms of chemical addiction. The Minnesota Model utilizes a *treatment team* composed of chemical dependency counselors familiar with AA, psychologists, physicians, nurses, recreational therapists, and clergy, all of whom work with the client during his or her treatment program.

The first stage of the Minnesota Model treatment approach, the *evaluation* phase, involves each member of the treatment team meeting with the client to assess the client's needs from the professional's area of expertise. Each professional then makes recommendations for the client's treatment plan.

In the second stage, the stage of *goal setting,* the professionals meet as a team to discuss the areas they believe should be the focus of treatment. This meeting is chaired by the individual who will ultimately be responsible for the execution of the treatment process. This person is usually the chemical dependency counselor, who will function as the client's case manager. Each assessment and recommendation is reviewed and discussed by the treatment team. The members then select those recommendations that they agree are most appropriate in helping the client achieve and maintain sobriety.

The client, the parole or probation officer, and possibly interested family members also participate in the treatment plan meeting. Both the client and family members are free to recom-

mend additional areas of concern or to suggest specific goals they would have included in the treatment plan. The case manager reviews the treatment goals that were identified as being of value to the client and discusses the rationale for these recommendations.

On the basis of this meeting, the case manager and client enter the third stage of the treatment process, *developing a formal treatment plan.* The treatment plan that emerges is multimodal and offers a wide variety of potential treatment goals and recommendations. It identifies specific problem areas, behavioral objectives, methods by which one can measure progress toward these objectives, and a target date for each goal. The treatment plan will be discussed in more detail in the next section of this chapter, but a flowchart of the treatment plan process is presented in Figure 28.1.

The strength of the Minnesota Model of treatment lies in its redundancy and its multimember concept. The information provided by the client is reviewed by many different professionals, each of whom may, on the basis of his or her training, identify a potential treatment problem that others may have overlooked. This allows for the greatest possible evaluation of the client's needs, strengths, and priorities.

Another advantage of the Minnesota Model is that it allows different professionals to work together in the rehabilitation of the client. The team, with the combined training and experience of its individual members, offers a wider range of services than any single chemical dependency counselor ever could. In addition to multidisciplinary intake evaluations, each professional on the treatment team can work with the client *if that client presents special needs.*

Thus, the chemical dependency counselor does not need to try to be a "jack of all trades." Rather, if the client presents a need that one staff member cannot fulfill, a referral to another member of the team for specialized treatment can be made. This feature has helped make the Minnesota Model one of the dominant treatment program models in the field of chemical dependency rehabilitation.

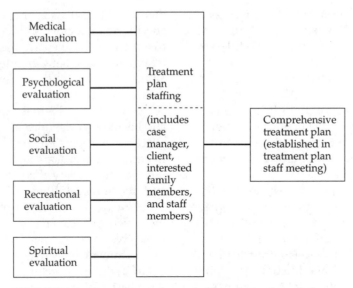

FIGURE 28.1 Flowchart of the evolution of a treatment plan

The Treatment Plan

No matter what treatment approach the therapist elects to utilize, he or she should develop a *treatment plan* with the client. The treatment plan is "the foundation for success" (Lewis, Dana, & Blevins, 1988, p. 118) of the treatment process. It is a highly specific form, which in some states might be viewed as a legal document. Different treatment centers tend to use different formats, depending on the specific licensure requirements and the treatment methods being utilized.

However, all treatment plans share several similarities. First, the treatment plan provides a brief summary of the problem that brought the client into treatment. A second section provides a brief summary of the client's physical and emotional state of health. A third section contains the individual's input into the treatment process. The next section is the heart of the treatment plan; this is where the specific goals of treatment are identified. The discharge criteria follow, listing the steps that must be accomplished to discharge the client from treatment. Finally, there is a brief summary of the steps that will be part of the client's *aftercare* program.

The heart of the treatment plan, as noted

above, is where the specific treatment goals are outlined. This section of the treatment plan is often labeled "Treatment Goals." Treatment goals should include (1) a *problem statement*, or brief statement of the problem, (2) *long-term goals*, (3) *short-term objectives*, (4) *measurement criteria*, and (5) a *target date*.

The *problem statement* is a short statement, usually only a sentence or two, that identifies a *specific problem* to address in treatment. The *long-term goal* is the ultimate objective, and as such it is a general statement of a hoped-for outcome. The long-term goal statement is also usually only one or two sentences in length. The *short-term objective* is *a very specific behavior that can be measured*. The objective statement is usually between one and three sentences long and identifies the measurement criteria by which both the client and staff will assess the client's progress toward this objective. Finally, the *target date* is usually a simple sentence that identifies a specific date by which this goal will be achieved.

An example of a treatment goal for a 24-year-old male polydrug addict (cocaine, alcohol, marijuana, and occasionally benzodiazepines) who has used chemicals daily for the last 27 months might appear as follows:

Problem: Client has used chemicals daily for at least the past two years and has been unable to abstain from drug use on his own.

Long-Term Goal: That the client achieve and maintain sobriety.

Short-Term Objective: That the client not use mood-altering chemicals while in treatment.

Method of Measurement: Random supervised urine toxicology screens to detect possible drug use.

Target Date: Scheduled discharge date.

The typical treatment plan may identify as many as five or six different problem areas. Each of these goals can be modified as the treatment program progresses, and each provides a yardstick of the client's progress. Obviously, if the client is not making progress on *any* of the goals, it is time to question whether the client is serious about treatment.

Criticism of the Minnesota Model

The Minnesota Model has been challenged for a number of reasons. First, the model was designed to work with cases of alcoholism. There is no research available to support its application to other forms of substance addiction, yet the Minnesota Model has been utilized in the treatment of virtually every known form of substance abuse (*Alcoholism & Drug Abuse Week,* 1990a).

When it was first developed, the client's length of stay at Willmar State Hospital was often arbitrarily set at 28 days. However, little research data supports the need for a 28-day inpatient treatment stay (Turbo, 1989). Unfortunately, the 28-day treatment program has become something of an industry standard both for Minnesota Model programs (Turbo, 1989) and as a guide for insurance reimbursement (Berg & Dubin, 1990). In their review of the cost-effectiveness of various treatment methods, Holder, Longabaugh, Miller, and Rubonis (1991) decided that there is insufficient evidence to conclude

that the Minnesota Model itself is an effective treatment approach for alcoholics.

Other Treatment Formats for Chemical Dependency

In recent years, health care professionals and mental health care workers have developed a number of different treatment approaches to alcoholism rehabilitation that differ from the Minnesota Model. The guiding philosophy of these different treatment programs is often quite different than that of the Minnesota Model. Although it is not possible to do full justice to each treatment philosophy, we will briefly examine some of the more promising treatment models that have emerged in the past two decades.

Detoxification Programs

There is some controversy as to whether detoxification by itself can be called "treatment." However, because many chemical dependency programs offer detoxification services—either as part of their regular treatment program or as a separate component—it will be classified as a form of minimal treatment for the purpose of this text. But one should keep in mind that there are few treatment professionals who advocate detoxification as the *only* treatment method to be used in the rehabilitation of the addict.

Chemical detoxification programs should meet the standards of state and federal licensing boards. The detoxification process should be carried out under the supervision of a physician who has both training and experience in this area. Each withdrawal candidate should be evaluated by a trained physician to determine whether an inpatient or outpatient detoxification program best meets the client's needs (Miller, Frances, & Holmes, 1988).

Detoxification from many chemicals of abuse is so dangerous that it should *only* be attempted on an inpatient basis. Drugs that may require inpatient detoxification include alcohol, barbiturates, and benzodiazepines. As we discussed in earlier chapters, withdrawal from such drugs may precipitate life-threatening seizures. Because of this danger, inpatient detoxification programs should have adequate facilities for the medical support of clients, including on-duty medical personnel (nurses and physicians), appropriate support medications (such as anticonvulsants), and equipment to administer them.

But for many drugs of abuse, outpatient detoxification is a viable treatment option. Outpatient detoxification requires daily follow-up by the detoxification staff to check the patient's progress and compliance with treatment (Miller, Frances, & Holmes, 1988). Patients being withdrawn from drugs should be closely monitored to detect signs of drug overdose or seizures and to verify medication compliance (Miller, Frances, & Holmes, 1988). Unfortunately, it is not uncommon for addicts to "help out" the withdrawal process by taking additional drugs when they are supposedly being withdrawn from chemicals.

In theory, "detox" programs may serve as a funnel through which individuals in need of substance abuse treatment can be directed toward the most appropriate rehabilitation program; in practice, this can be difficult to achieve. When detox is separate from the rehabilitation program, many patients admitted for detoxification fail to "graduate" to treatment (Miller & Rollnick, 1991). Thus, it seems best if detoxification is carried out at facilities with substance abuse rehabilitation programs, so that treatment staff can begin to work with the patient while he or she is still in the process of withdrawing from chemicals.

The "detox" program is vulnerable to abuse in a number of ways. Some addicts go through detoxification dozens or even hundreds of times to give themselves a place to live (Whitman, Friedman, & Thomas, 1990). Other individuals "check into detox" to give themselves a place to hide from drug debts or the police. It is also not uncommon for narcotics addicts to seek admission to a detox program when they are unable to obtain drugs. Sometimes they want to lower their daily drug requirement to a level they can more easily afford.

Narcotics Withdrawal

Programs that specialize in the treatment of narcotic addiction often offer controlled withdrawal from opiates. Occasionally, a hospital offers narcotic withdrawal programs even if it offers no long-term treatment for narcotic addicts. The detoxification component in each center tends to be very much the same as that offered in other treatment centers. (The actual mechanics of narcotics detoxification will be discussed in Chapter 31.)

Videotape and Self-Confrontation

Many programs include videotaping clients while they are under the influence of chemicals, to allow them to see their own behavior while intoxicated. The goal of this procedure, according to Holder et al. (1991), is to allow the drinker's own drunk behavior to illustrate the need for treatment. After the individual has recovered from the acute effects of drinking, he or she is forced to watch the videotape. Unfortunately, there is no evidence to suggest that this brief treatment approach is effective.

Acupuncture

Acupuncture is a form of "alternative medicine" that is occasionally applied to the treatment of the addictive disorders. Treatment professionals still disagree as to how acupuncture works. Small sterile needles are inserted into specific locations on the individual's body in an attempt to treat the patient's condition. At this time, there is limited evidence that this treatment technique is effective in the rehabilitation of substance abusers (Holder et al., 1991).

Family and Marital Therapy

Many treatment programs include a family or marital therapy component. According to Williams (1989), the addict's defense system and those of the family tend to be *inter*reinforcing; family members develop defense mechanisms that reinforce those of the addicted person. Within a family systems approach, it becomes necessary to modify the role that the drug use behavior plays in the family. The family system as a whole needs to be modified, a process often best carried out during the intervention session (Williams, 1989). Otherwise, the family as a unit will resist any change in the alcoholic's behavior.

In their review of the cost-effectiveness of various treatment methods for alcoholism, Holder et al. (1991) conclude that marital therapy is potentially useful and effective as a treatment approach. Unfortunately, there are many theoretical models of family therapy, and it has rapidly become a specialized area of expertise with a vast field of literature of its own (Bowen, 1985). Thus, special training is necessary for the counselor to effectively work with families. Also, as we discussed in Chapter 24, some of the reasons family therapy is thought to be effective in the treatment of substance abuse have been challenged. Thus, family and marital counseling is not the ultimate answer to the problem of how to help the drug addicted individual.

It is beyond the scope of this chapter to provide a comprehensive overview of the fields of marital and family therapy in general or even the specialized application of marital therapy to the treatment of addiction. However, the chemical dependency professional should be aware that these are specialized areas of training.

Group Therapy Approaches

Yalom (1985) believes that group therapy offers a number of advantages over individual therapy. First, therapy groups allow one professional to work with a number of different individuals at once. Second, group members can learn from each other and offer each other feedback. Finally, because of the nature of the therapy group, each individual can find within the group members a reflection of his or her family of origin, allowing

each person to work through problems from earlier stages of growth.

Therapy groups are frequently the primary treatment approach offered in chemical dependency treatment programs. Although individual sessions may be needed for special problems too sensitive to discuss in a group situation, the client is usually encouraged to bring his or her concerns to group. Groups can meet every other day, daily, or more often than once a day, depending on the pace of the program.

Unfortunately, there is limited evidence that group psychotherapy approaches are at all effective in the rehabilitation of substance abusers (Holder et al., 1991). According to Stanton Peele (1989), the harsh confrontational style groups commonly employed in therapeutic communities have been ineffective in working with recovering addicts. Peele suggests that therapy groups focus on helping the recovering addict learn effective coping skills, such as behavioral response training and stress management techniques.

Assertiveness/Social Skills Training

Lewis, Dana, and Blevins (1988) found special assertiveness training groups to be useful in building self-esteem and self-confidence in interpersonal relationships, which individuals addicted to chemicals often lack. In addition to assertiveness training, many other social skills can be taught to the recovering addict. Fortunately, assertiveness and social skills training have proved to be quite effective in the rehabilitation of alcoholics (Holder et al., 1991).

Self-Help Groups

The best known self-help group is Alcoholics Anonymous, which is discussed in detail in Chapter 32. However, brief mention of self-help groups such as AA should be made at this time. It has been argued that AA is actually a form of treatment (Tobin, 1992), but whether it is or not is a philosophical question, and the answer depends on the individual's beliefs.

Participation in a self-help group such as AA

is often a required component of both inpatient and outpatient treatment programs. Many community AA or NA groups have extended an invitation to local treatment programs to allow their clients to participate in scheduled meetings. If the treatment program is large enough, an on-campus AA or NA meeting may also be scheduled, limited to clients in treatment.

There are a number of advantages to AA or NA involvement for clients in treatment. Both AA and NA are potentially chemical-free support groups for new members. As such, both AA and NA offer opportunities for members to model drug-free interpersonal interactions. Each group also offers the opportunity for the new member to develop a drug-free support system to use in times of crisis following treatment. Members in the AA or NA group may, in speaking of their own problems, offer the newcomer insight into his or her own problems and suggest possible solutions based on their own experience.

However, Peele (1989) points out that many people recover without joining either AA or NA, raising questions about whether or not the individual *must* participate in such a self-help group. At this point, it seems best if the treatment program does have some provision for self-help group participation. But there is no evidence that mandatory participation in AA or NA is of value (Holder et al., 1991).

Biofeedback Training

A number of treatment plans advocate the use of biofeedback training as an aid to the treatment of addictive disorders. The technique of biofeedback involves monitoring select body functions, such as skin temperature or muscle tension, and providing information to the individual as to how his or her body is reacting. Depending on the parameter selected (such as muscle tension of a certain muscle group, skin temperature, or brain-wave patterns) and the training provided, the individual is thought to be able to learn how to modify his or her body function at will. This skill, in turn, is thought to allow the individual

to learn how to change these body functions in a desired direction, such as to relax without the use of drugs.

Peniston and Kulkosky (1990) attempted to teach a small number of patients in an alcoholic treatment program to change the frequency with which their brain could produce two specific electrical patterns, known as *alpha* and *theta* waves. These patterns of electrical activity in the brain are thought to reflect the individual's process of relaxation and stress-coping responses. The authors found that their sample had significant changes on standard psychological tests used to measure the personality pattern of the respondent and that these changes continued over an extended follow-up period. The authors suggest that biofeedback training, especially alpha and theta brain-wave training, might offer a new and possibly more effective treatment approach for working with the chronic alcoholic.

Ochs (1992) examined the application of biofeedback training techniques to the treatment of addictive disorders and concluded that the term *biofeedback training* for the addictions is a bit misleading. Different clinicians employ a wide range of techniques, and a wide range of body functions are employed for biofeedback training. Yet, in spite of the variations in treatment techniques, Ochs found that biofeedback training for the treatment of addictive disorders does seem to have value, especially when biofeedback is integrated into a larger treatment format designed to address social, economic, vocational, psychological, and familial problems.

Harm Reduction Model

The *harm reduction* (HR) model of substance abuse rehabilitation is quite different from the Minnesota Model, the criminal justice model of substance abuse intervention, or the other models of treatment discussed in this chapter. Most treatment models are based on a "zero tolerance" of chemical use (Marlatt, 1994), which does not accept the possibility of *any* chemical use by the individual.

However, the harm reduction model has a

different focus: limiting the amount of damage caused by chemical(s) until the individual achieves total abstinence. The use of nicotine skin patches and nicotine gum are examples of the HR philosophy (Marlatt, 1994), in that they reduce the individual's risk of negative consequences from cigarette smoking. From this perspective, formal detoxification from chemicals in a medical setting might also be viewed as a form of harm reduction by protecting the individual from many of the dangers of withdrawal during detoxification.

Another example of the HR philosophy are the "needle exchange" programs in place in several cities in the United States. Because the virus that causes AIDS is often transmitted through contaminated intravenous needles (see Chapter 30), some cities allow addicts to exchange "dirty" needles for new, uncontaminated ones. This way, the transmission of the virus that causes AIDS is slowed or perhaps even stopped.

Although the HR model is somewhat controversial, it does seem to offer an alternative to the less tolerant Minnesota Model or criminal justice models.

Aftercare

Aftercare involves those elements of treatment that will be carried out after the individual has been discharged from treatment. If, for example, the person entered into individual psychotherapy to address an issue uncovered in treatment, it is entirely likely that this therapy will continue long after the individual is discharged from the inpatient rehabilitation program. Individual therapy on a once-a-week basis with a psychotherapist would then become a part of the aftercare program.

Downing (1990) concludes that an effective aftercare program should (1) address the chem-

ical dependency issues identified in treatment, (2) address mistaken beliefs and interpersonal conflicts that might contribute to relapse, (3) help the individual establish what Downing (1990) terms "the habit of sobriety" (p. 22), (4) help the individual make the necessary changes in his or her lifestyle to maintain sobriety, and (5) "Serve as a monitor of sobriety" (p. 22).

Participation in AA or NA may also be part of an aftercare program. A medical problem that requires ongoing medical supervision and support should be a part of the aftercare program, as well as aftercare placement in a transitional living facility, such as a halfway house. If the individual presents any special needs, these should also be included as specialized elements of the aftercare program.

The aftercare program is designed and carried out on the assumption that treatment does not end with the individual's discharge from a formal treatment program. Rather, treatment is the first part of a recovery program that (hopefully) continues for the rest of the individual's life. The aftercare component of the treatment plan addresses those issues that need attention following the individual's discharge from the rehabilitation program.

Summary

In this chapter we described the Minnesota Model of treatment, one of the primary treatment models found in the United States. We also explored the concept of a *comprehensive treatment plan*, the heart of the treatment process. We discussed various treatment models that have recently emerged, and we examined assertiveness training, biofeedback, and the role of marital and family therapy as components of a larger treatment program.

CHAPTER TWENTY-NINE

Treatment Formats for Chemical Dependency Rehabilitation

The question of whether substance abuse treatment is effective no longer sparks the fierce debate among health professionals it once did. It is generally accepted that treatment is cost-effective. For example, treatment has been found to be *seven times as effective* in reducing cocaine use as law enforcement activities (Scheer, 1994b; *Minneapolis Star-Tribune*, 1994).

Instead, the current debate centers on the relative merits of *outpatient* versus *inpatient* formats (Youngstrom, 1990b). This debate, although spirited, remains without resolution. In this chapter, we will review some of the characteristics of an average outpatient treatment program and the typical inpatient program, as well as some of the issues that have been raised about their relative advantages and disadvantages.

Outpatient Treatment Programs

Outpatient treatment programs for addiction are many and varied. For example, the "DWI school" is designed for the individual who is arrested for the first time while driving under the influence of chemicals. The DWI school is an outpatient psychoeducational approach for first-time offenders, who are assumed to have simply made a mistake by driving under the influence of chemicals but who do not seem to be addicted to drugs. The whole thrust of the DWI school is to help the individual understand the dangers inherent in driving while under the influence of chemicals, in hopes that he or she will learn from the mistake.

Outpatient chemical dependency treatment is best defined as a formal treatment program that (1) involves one or more professionals trained to work with individuals who are addicted to chemicals, (2) is designed specifically to work with the addicted person to help him or her achieve and maintain sobriety, (3) will utilize family, marital, individual, and/or group therapy to help the addicted person come to terms with his or her problems, and (4) does so on an outpatient basis.

Components of Outpatient Treatment Programs

Outpatient treatment programs utilize many of the components of treatment discussed in the previous chapter. Such programs usually adopt individual and group therapy formats, and possibly marital and family therapy, for working with the addicted person. Most such programs follow a twelve-step philosophy patterned after Alcoholics Anonymous. The individual is expected to attend regular self-help group meetings as part of the treatment format.

The individual's treatment program is usually coordinated by a certified chemical dependency counselor (sometimes called an "addictions" or "substance abuse" counselor). A formal treatment program is established, review sessions are scheduled on a regular basis, and the client's progress toward the goals established is monitored by staff.

The general approach of both individual and group therapy is to work through the addicted person's system of denial, combined with counseling to help the client learn how to face the problems of daily living *without* the use of chemicals. This is accomplished, in part, through psychoeducational lectures presenting factual information about the disease of chemical addiction and its treatment.

Referrals to vocational counseling centers or community mental health centers for individual, family, or marital counseling are made as necessary. Some programs provide weekly or monthly "family nights," where family members are encouraged to participate and discuss their concerns. Other programs feature a "family group" orientation, where couples participate together on a day-to-day basis. In such a format, the spouse of the addicted person sits in on the group sessions and participates as an equal in the group therapy.

Whatever the general approach, the goal of any outpatient treatment program is to enhance the highest level of functioning while providing support for the alcoholic. Some programs require that the detoxification phase of treatment be carried out either at a detoxification center or in a general hospital. However, the individual is generally expected to have stopped all chemical use before starting any treatment program.

Abstinence from alcohol, as well as from any other drug use, is expected. Many treatment programs either require the use of Antabuse or perform random urine tests to detect alcohol or drug use by the patient. One advantage of using random urine samples for toxicology screening is that the staff can determine whether there is evidence of Antabuse in the urine sample, indicating whether the individual is taking the Antabuse as prescribed.

The goal of outpatient treatment is to allow the individual the opportunity to live at home, continue to work and continue to engage in family activities while participating in a rehabilitation program designed to help the client achieve and maintain sobriety (Youngstrom, 1990b). This approach is helpful for some, although research suggests a high dropout rate for outpatient treatment programs.

Advantages of Outpatient Treatment

There is an obvious cost advantage inherent in outpatient treatment as compared to inpatient treatment. A 28-day inpatient treatment program might cost between $7,000 and $30,000, depending on the daily fee for each specific treatment setting (Turbo, 1989; *Alcoholism & Drug Abuse Week*, 1990a). In contrast, a 6-month outpatient treatment program might cost as little as $1,000 (Turbo, 1989).

Surprisingly, although inpatient treatment initially costs more, because of available insurance coverage, many clients actually pay *less* for inpatient treatment than for outpatient treatment. Outpatient treatment programs traditionally are not reimbursed at the same rate as the more expensive inpatient substance abuse program by health insurance carriers. This factor often fuels a tendency for health care providers to recommend inpatient over outpatient treatment programs (Berg & Dubin, 1990).

Another advantage of the outpatient format is that the patient does not have to be removed from his or her environment. Unlike inpatient treatment programs, there is no community reorientation period needed after outpatient treatment (Youngstrom, 1990b; Bonstedt, Ulrich, Dolinar, & Johnson, 1984).

Nace (1987) suggests that the "ideal" outpatient treatment program would last a full year. This, in itself, is an advantage over inpatient treatment programs, which tend to be shorter in duration. A treatment program of a year's duration would offer long-term follow-up for the crucial first year of sobriety, a time when the individual is likely to relapse. The patient who knows that he or she will be subjected to random urine toxicology screening as part of a year-long outpatient program may be less likely to use drugs.

Berg and Dubin (1990) outline an intensive outpatient treatment program that is divided into four phases. Each of the first three phases—intensive, intermediate, and moderate treatment—is designed to last for two weeks. However, the authors note, any given individual's placement is determined by "the severity of the patient's addiction, progress in treatment, financial resources, and ability to attend the program" (p. 1175). The final phase of treatment, the extended phase, involves an aftercare meeting once a week for an indefinite period of time.

Because outpatient treatment programs generally last longer than inpatient programs, Lewis, Dana, and Blevins (1988) believe that this format offers the counselor a longer period of time to help the client achieve the goals outlined in his or her treatment plan. The client also has an extended period of time in which to practice and perfect new behaviors that will support sobriety.

Outpatient treatment programs offer yet another advantage over inpatient treatment programs: flexibility (Turbo, 1989). Treatment participation can be through an *outpatient day treatment* program, where treatment activities are scheduled during normal working hours, or through an *outpatient evening treatment* program. Finally, outpatient treatment programs offer the client the opportunity to practice sobriety while still living in the community.

Drawbacks of Outpatient Treatment

Although statistical research has found no significant difference in the percentage of outpatient treatment program "graduates" who remain sober as opposed to those who complete inpatient treatment programs for drug addiction, this is not to say that outpatient treatment is as effective as inpatient treatment. Rather, inpatient treatment programs tend to deal more effectively with a different class of client than do outpatient treatment programs, making comparisons difficult.

Outpatient treatment programs occasionally have difficulty with clients whose detoxification from chemicals is quite complicated. Berg and Dubin (1990) conclude, however, that only approximately 10% of those individuals going through alcohol withdrawal require hospitalization. In contrast, Dumas (1992) suggests that individuals who smoke cocaine will require inpatient hospitalization, at least at first, to "interrupt the compulsive pattern of drug use, and to treat the . . . drug-induced medical and psychiatric problems" (p. 907). Thus, outpatient detoxification from chemicals is not always an option for the patient.

The outpatient treatment program does not offer the same degree of structure and support found in an effective inpatient drug addiction program. Furthermore, outpatient treatment programs offer less control over the client's environment. They are thus of limited value for patients who require a great deal of support during the early stages of sobriety. Although outpatient treatment of substance abuse seems to work for many clients, it does not appear to be the ultimate answer to the problem of chemical dependency.

Inpatient Treatment Programs

The inpatient treatment program might best be defined as a residential treatment facility where the client lives while he or she participates in treatment. Such programs usually deal with the hard-core, seriously ill, or "difficult" patient—individuals for whom outpatient treatment either has not been successful or has been ruled out because of the severity of the person's chemical use.

Residential treatment programs have evolved to provide the greatest degree of support and help possible. Inpatient treatment is also "the most restrictive, structured, and protective of treatment settings" (Klar, 1987, p. 340). It combines the greatest potential for positive change with high financial cost and the possibility of branding the patient for life (Klar, 1987). Therefore, the decision to utilize inpatient treatment is one that should not be made lightly.

Often, the inpatient treatment program provides detoxification services as part of the treatment program, and there is rapid access to medical support services for the seriously ill patient. Such programs are usually found in a hospital setting. Other forms of inpatient treatment might not provide the same degree of medical support but are found in *therapeutic communities*, in a *halfway house* setting, or in nonhospital-based inpatient rehabilitation centers.

Varieties of Inpatient Treatment

Detoxification Programs

As we mentioned in Chapter 28, many chemical dependency programs offer general detoxification services either as part of the regular treatment program or as a separate component of treatment. Such detoxification programs should meet the standards of state licensing boards and should be carried out under the supervision of a physician who has both training and experience in this area.

Detoxification is not, in itself, a treatment for chemical dependency (Miller & Hester, 1986; National Academy of Sciences, 1990). Research has shown that simple detoxification from chemicals usually fails to bring about a major change in drug use behavior. Rather, detoxification is a necessary prelude to the treatment process. Detoxification can be carried out as part of a hospital-based service or at a regional "crisis center," but in either case the main emphasis is on medically supervised detoxification from chemicals. These centers have, for the most part, replaced the "drunk tank" once so common in county jails.

Although detoxification from chemicals is often carried out on an inpatient basis, there are those who question the need for inpatient detoxification from drugs on a routine basis (*Alcoholism & Drug Abuse Week*, 1990a; Berg & Dubin, 1990). It has been argued, for example, that only a minority of alcoholics actually require inpatient detoxification; other patients, perhaps a majority, could safely be detoxified from alcohol in a community setting (Miller & Hester, 1986; Berg & Dubin, 1990). Miller, Frances, and Holmes (1988) advocate that each patient in withdrawal be evaluated by a trained physician to determine whether inpatient or outpatient detoxification is necessary.

The National Academy of Sciences (1990) evaluated the merits of inpatient versus outpatient detoxification from chemicals and concluded that, on purely technical grounds, detoxification does not automatically require inpatient hospitalization. What the National Academy of Sciences termed *ambulatory detox* (p. 175) would result in a significant savings over the cost of inpatient detoxification without any apparent reduction in the effectiveness of the withdrawal process. Furthermore, if an individual patient proves unable to complete detoxification on an outpatient basis, he or she can always be admitted to an inpatient detoxification center after the less restrictive outpatient detoxification process has been shown not to work.

As noted in Chapter 28, outpatient detoxification requires daily follow-up from the detoxification staff to monitor the patient's progress and compliance with the withdrawal process (Miller, Frances, & Holmes, 1988). Patients being withdrawn from drugs should be closely monitored by staff to detect signs of drug overdose or seizures (Miller, Frances, & Holmes, 1988). Also, the chemical dependency professional should constantly be aware that detoxification services can be abused by addicted persons.

Therapeutic Communities

There is no generally recognized model of the therapeutic community (TC) (DeLeon, 1994; National Academy of Sciences, 1990). Rather, there are a multitude of programs that differ in recommended length of stay, client-to-staff ratio, and staff composition. In general, however, the "traditional" TC can be viewed as a program whose guiding philosophy is that drug abuse is a deviant behavior, reflecting impeded personality development or chronic deficits in social, educational, and economic skills. : ... The principal aim of the TC is a global change in life-style: abstinence from illicit substances, elimination of antisocial activity, development of employability, and prosocial attitudes. (DeLeon, 1994, p. 392)

"Traditional" TC programs usually require a commitment of between 1 and 3 years (DeLeon, 1994, 1989), although some programs have a minimal commitment of only 6 months. The extended length of stay is considered necessary because the TC approach views drug abuse as a disorder of the *whole* person. To change the drug using behavior, it is necessary to change the whole person, a process that takes time. Such long-term residential treatment programs are thought to be quite effective with individuals whose addiction is complicated by an antisocial personality disorder, or what *Alcoholism & Drug Abuse Week* (1990a) calls "social pathology" (p. 3).

When the TC movement began, it focused mainly on those addicted to opiates—at least, in the United States. However, this is no longer true. The majority of the clients in today's TCs were using chemicals other than opiates prior to their admission to treatment (DeLeon, 1994).

Ellis et al. (1988) suggest that one reason the TC is so effective is its utilization of a single therapeutic model. Such consistency is of value when working with the antisocial personality (Ansevics & Doweiko, 1983). Unfortunately, the TC model is followed by only a minority of treatment programs. It has been reported (DeLeon, 1989) that, of the estimated 500 drug-free residential treatment programs in this country, less than 25% follow the therapeutic community model.

DeLeon (1989) identifies a central tenet of the TC model as "its perspective of drug abuse as a *whole person* disorder" (p. 177, italics in original). Other characteristics of the TC include social and physical isolation, a structured living environment, a firm system of rewards and punishments, an emphasis on self-examination, and the

confession of past wrongdoing. Clients are expected to work, either outside the TC in an approved job or as part of the TC support staff. Many TCs offer some potential mobility from the status of client to that of a paraprofessional staff member (National Academy of Sciences, 1990).

Although many TCs utilize the services of mental health professionals, many paraprofessional staff members are former clients of TCs. The theory is that only a person "who has been there" can understand the addict. Such paraprofessional counselors are thought to be effective in breaking through the client's denial and manipulation, as other addicts will have had similar experiences they can call on in working with the newcomer.

The TC might offer an extended family for the individual, a "family" that the recovering addict may be encouraged never to leave. Indeed, according to Lewis, Dana, and Blevins (1988), the original members of Synanon (one of the early therapeutic communities) were expected to remain there on a permanent basis.

As a group, TCs suffer from significant dropout rates. The first 15 days is an especially difficult period for many clients; during this period, the "dropout" rate is highest (*The Addiction Letter*, 1989b). DeLeon (1994) suggests that 30% to 40% of those admitted to a TC will drop out in the first 30 days. Furthermore, over the course of treatment, a significant percentage of those who do not leave on their own are asked to leave or are discharged from treatment for various rule infractions (Gelman, Underwood, King, Hager, & Gordon, 1990). Ultimately, only 15% to 25% of those admitted to TCs actually graduate (DeLeon, 1994; The National Academy of Sciences, 1990). The recovery rates of those who drop out of TCs in the earliest phases of treatment "basically cannot be distinguished from those . . . individuals who did not enter any treatment modality" (The National Academy of Sciences, 1990, p. 167).

There is a great deal of controversy surrounding TCs. Some caution that the therapeutic community might not be a positive step for the individual (Ausabel, 1983). Many of these programs use methods such as ego stripping and unquestioned submission to the rules of the program. Lewis, Dana, and Blevins (1988) point out that the social isolation inherent in the TC prevents the client from going out into the community to try new social skills. The harsh confrontation and high relapse rates often found in the TC has also drawn criticism from Lewis, Dana, and Blevins (1988).

However, others note that the TC has been effective in some cases in which traditional treatment methods have been of limited value. (DeLeon, 1989, 1994; Peele, 1989; Yablonsky, 1967). Peele (1989) found that the TC functions best when it strives to help the individual learn social skills and values inconsistent with drug using behaviors. The journal *Alcoholism & Drug Abuse Week* (1990a) concluded in its review of the therapeutic community concept that such programs are quite effective, with as much as 80% of patients completing the program remaining drug-free, and the National Academy of Sciences (1990) concludes that those who remain in the program the longest are most likely to achieve a sober lifestyle.

Hospital-Based Inpatient Treatment

Traditional inpatient drug rehabilitation is often carried out either in a center that specializes in chemical dependency treatment or in a traditional hospital setting as part of a specialized drug treatment unit. Many of these programs utilize the "Minnesota Model," which was explored in detail in the previous chapter. There is no standard treatment program under the Minnesota Model; rather, it offers a great deal of flexibility to accommodate the various needs of different individuals. Residential treatment programs usually place strong emphasis on a twelve-step philosophy and utilize individual and group therapy extensively.

Inpatient rehabilitation programs, especially those in a hospital setting, often include a detoxification component. Adelman and Weiss (1989) report that medically supervised withdrawal

from alcohol dependency results in higher patient retention rates, improving the patient's chances of achieving and retaining sobriety. Whether part of a hospital or not, inpatient treatment programs utilize a variety of different treatment methods and draw on the varied skills of the different members of the treatment team to best help the client.

The client's length of stay in treatment depends on several different factors. Among them are the client's motivation and the community resources available to help him or her stay sober.

Inpatient Treatment: Is There a Legitimate Need?

A decade ago, Miller and Hester (1986) noted that "the relative merits of residential treatment are less than clear" (p. 794). Today, Chick (1993) notes that, for treating alcoholics, "The advantages of inpatient versus outpatient care . . . have been difficult to show" (p. 1374). Yet, in spite of such statements, outpatient treatment programs are still viewed by many as inferior to treatment carried out in an inpatient setting.

After a review of some 16 research studies, Miller and Hester (1986) concluded that there is no significant difference between inpatient and outpatient alcoholism rehabilitation programs on various measures of patient improvement. The authors explored the *length* of inpatient treatment as one possible variable affecting treatment outcome, but they found no statistically significant improvement for longer-term treatment programs as compared with programs of shorter duration. The authors did admit that their data suggests that inpatient treatment is possibly more advantageous for long-term addicts. However, posttreatment aftercare programs were found to play a more significant role in ultimate success or failure than the specific form of treatment utilized (Miller & Hester, 1986). Although they are strong critics of inpatient treatment, Miller and Hester (1989)

do not advocate the abolition of residential treatment. There may be subpopulations for whom more intensive treatment is justifiable. From the limited matching data available at present, it appears that intensive treatment may be better for severely addicted and socially unstable individuals. (p. 1246)

In response to Miller and Hester's original (1986) work, Adelman and Weiss (1989) conducted their own research into the merits of inpatient treatment. They report that 77% of those alcoholics treated for alcoholism eventually require some form of inpatient treatment. The authors also found that treatment programs in "medically oriented facilities" (p. 516) have lower dropout rates than do treatment programs in nonmedical centers. Furthermore, patients discharged after short inpatient treatment programs tend to relapse more frequently than do those who remain in treatment longer.

It has been suggested that, in most cases, "aggressive outpatient treatment" (Bonstedt et al., 1984, p. 1039) of alcoholism is more cost-effective than inpatient treatment programs. Bonstedt et al. also point out that "the majority of alcoholics do not have to be hospitalized each time they present for treatment" (p. 1039). The issue of whether a prior history of chemical dependency treatment automatically excludes outpatient treatment is thus still disputed among professionals.

Recently, Walsh et al. (1991) randomly assigned 227 workers at a large factory known to be abusing alcohol to one of three treatment programs: compulsory attendance at Alcoholics Anonymous, compulsory inpatient treatment, or a choice between these two alternatives. The authors were surprised to find that although the referral to compulsory AA meetings *initially* was more cost-effective, inpatient treatment resulted in higher abstinence rates in the long run.

The Advantages of Inpatient Treatment

Although the case for outpatient treatment programs is a strong one, there are certain advantages to inpatient treatment programs. These advantages make the inpatient treatment the method of choice in some cases, especially the more advanced cases of addiction. Inpatient rehabilitation programs offer *more comprehensive treatment programming* than is possible in an outpatient treatment setting (Klar, 1987). This is an advantage in cases of advanced drug dependency because the addicted individual has often centered his or her life around the chemical for such a long period of time that he or she will be unable to utilize a less restrictive treatment approach.

Inpatient treatment programs offer the advantage of almost total control over the client's environment (Berg & Dubin, 1990). For clients accustomed to a drug-centered lifestyle, the concept of a drug-free way of life is often quite foreign. Inpatient treatment programs offer the advantage of a structured environment where individual and group therapy sessions, meals, recreational opportunities, self-help group meetings, and spiritual counseling are all scheduled for the client.

Clients often report that they have not been eating on a regular basis prior to entering treatment. An inpatient rehabilitation setting allows staff to monitor and treat dietary disorders that may have been caused by the individual's addicted lifestyle. Supplementary vitamins or dietary supplements are often beneficial in such cases, and inpatient treatment allows staff to closely monitor the client's recovery from the physical effects of addiction.

Many clients attend their first Alcoholics Anonymous meeting while in an inpatient setting. In some cases, the client affirms that he or she would never have attended AA or NA meetings if not required to by treatment staff. Adelman and Weiss (1989) contend that participation in Alcoholics Anonymous is an essential component of an effective inpatient treatment program.

Another advantage of inpatient treatment is that it can provide *around-the-clock support during the earliest stages of sobriety*. It is not unusual to find a client sitting up at two o'clock in the morning, talking about personal problems with the staff member on duty. Nor is it uncommon to find a client still up at 3 o'clock in the morning pacing through the earliest stages of withdrawal. When such a client is asked what he or she would do if he or she were not in treatment, the most common answer is that "I would go out and score some drugs!"[1]

Because these clients are in treatment, they are able to draw on the support services of the staff on duty to help them through the pain and discomfort of withdrawal. This support might be in the form of a sympathetic ear or the administration of previously prescribed medications to ease the client's discomfort. Staff members may offer suggestions to help the client through the trials of withdrawal, such as to walk around the ward or have something to eat. In other words, staff will "be there" for the client.

Inpatient treatment programs offer the additional advantage of *close supervision of clients.* Addicted clients often live alone or lack close interpersonal support. In such cases, a medical emergency could go undetected for hours or days. In an inpatient treatment setting, medical emergencies can be detected quickly and the appropriate action taken.

The close supervision by staff members also helps discourage further drug use. Clients, especially those with a long-standing drug problem, are often tempted to "help out" with the detoxification process by taking a few additional drugs or drinks during withdrawal. Narcotic addicts have been known to inject drugs that they brought into treatment with them, and alcoholics have been known to take a drink or two from a bottle that was thoughtfully packed away in some hidden corner of a suitcase.

Some inpatient treatment centers search the client's belongings on admission. Other programs use the "honor system," in which other clients confront the individual using chemicals in treatment. Most inpatient treatment centers use urine toxicology screenings to detect illicit drug use during treatment. The close supervision inherent in an inpatient treatment setting provides the opportunity for staff members to

request a urine sample *immediately*, should they suspect drug use by clients.

According to Nace (1987), inpatient treatment is of value in cases where outpatient treatment has become a "revolving door" for the individual. Inpatient settings are also of value in cases in which the individual has experienced repeated crisis situations while in outpatient treatment, has had several aborted attempts to utilize outpatient treatment, or has been unable to establish an effective therapeutic alliance in a less restrictive setting. Individuals who must be treated for multiple problems (physical and psychiatric) while being treated for drug addiction also benefit from inpatient treatment (Nace, 1987).

How to Decide on a Treatment Setting

Whether to utilize inpatient or outpatient treatment for a client is perhaps one of the most important decisions that a treatment professional will make (Washton, Stone, & Hendrickson, 1988). It is often a difficult decision as well. In recent years, questions have been raised as to whether inpatient treatment of chemical dependency is inherently better than outpatient treatment programs.

Outpatient treatment programs offer several advantages over inpatient programs. As we have mentioned, it is usually less expensive to participate in an outpatient treatment program than to enter an inpatient treatment program. A sad, rarely discussed, fact is that the restrictions on funding will play a role in deciding which treatment options are available for the individual. The person whose insurance will pay for only outpatient treatment will have financial restrictions placed on his or her treatment options.

The Group for the Advancement of Psychiatry (1990) offers the following criteria to use to determine which treatment program is best suited for a client: (1) whether the client's condition is associated with significant medical or psychiatric conditions or complications, (2) severity of actual or anticipated withdrawal from the drugs being used, (3) multiple failed attempts at

---

[1]The word *score* usually is interpreted to mean "buy" or "obtain."

outpatient treatment, (4) the client's social support systems, and (5) the severity of the client's addiction and possibility of polysubstance abuse. Outpatient rehabilitation is best suited to clients who have not had an extensive prior treatment history (Nace, 1987). The individual's motivation for treatment and the need for inpatient detoxification from chemicals should be considered in the decision whether to recommend inpatient or outpatient treatment. Another factor that should be considered is the patient's overall medical condition. Finally, the individual's psychiatric status, and availability of social support should be evaluated when considering outpatient treatment (Nace, 1987; Group for the Advancement of Psychiatry, 1990). Obviously, a deeply depressed individual who is recovering from an extended period of cocaine use might benefit more from the greater support offered by an inpatient treatment program, at least during the initial recovery period when the depression is most severe.

Washton, Stone, and Hendrickson (1988) also identify several criteria by which the need for inpatient treatment for drug dependency can be evaluated (some of the factors are the same as those listed above):

- the concurrent dependence on different chemicals
- serious medical or psychiatric illness
- poor motivation for treatment
- heavy involvement in dealing drugs
- a past history of failure in outpatient treatment
- severe psychosocial problems
- a proven inability of the client to discontinue further drug use while in outpatient treatment

On the other hand, Miller and Foy (1981) believe that only three factors need to be considered by treatment professionals in working with the addicted person: (1) the client's physical condition, (2) the client's social support system, and (3) the client's expectations for treatment. The authors postulate that these factors are the most important in establishing a viable treatment plan with appropriate goals and are the factors to be evaluated when considering inpatient as opposed to outpatient treatment.

Turbo (1989), echoing Nace's (1987) work, mentions several criteria that seem to indicate when an inpatient treatment program might be better for the client than the outpatient setting. These criteria include (1) repeated failure to maintain sobriety in outpatient treatment, (2) an acutely suicidal state, (3) seriously disturbed home environment, (4) serious medical problems, and (5) serious psychiatric problems.

Allen and Phillips (1993) make an interesting suggestion, noting that the patient's legal status should also be one factor used to determine whether inpatient or outpatient treatment is best. Individuals who have been arrested for drug possession or for driving while under the influence of chemicals, might do better in an outpatient treatment program. Patients who have been able to achieve periods of sobriety but who then relapsed might be treated briefly on an inpatient basis. But, following a brief "stabilization" stay in the hospital, these patients could be switched to an outpatient treatment program.

As noted by Klar (1987), the final criterion to use to decide whether to suggest inpatient or outpatient treatment is, given the client's resources and needs, what is the *least restrictive treatment alternative*? The treatment referral criteria advanced by Miller and Foy (1981), Nace (1987), Turbo (1989), and Allen and Phillips (1993) are useful guides to the selection of the least restrictive alternative that will meet the client's needs.

Although some will argue that the inpatient treatment program sounds very much like a concentration camp, one must recall that the dysfunction caused by drug addiction often requires drastic forms of intervention. Just as drastic forms of intervention are often necessary in the practice of medicine, so is the step of inpatient treatment necessary in more advanced cases of addiction to chemicals.

Partial Hospitalization Options

In recent years, several new treatment formats that combine elements of inpatient and outpatient rehabilitation programs have been explored. Each has its advantages and disadvantages, yet all are viable treatment options for clients who present themselves for treatment. Depending on the client's needs, some of the new treatment formats could prove to be quite beneficial.

Two-by-Four Programs

One proposed solution to the dilemma of whether to utilize inpatient or outpatient treatment is the so-called two-by-four program. This program format borrows from both inpatient and outpatient treatment programs to establish a biphasic rehabilitation system that seems to have some promise.

The individual is first hospitalized for a short period of time, usually 2 weeks, to achieve total detoxification from chemicals. Depending on the individual's needs, the initial period of hospitalization might be somewhat shorter or longer than the 2-week time span. However, the goal is to help the client to reach a point where it is possible for him or her to participate in outpatient treatment as soon as possible. If, as will occasionally happen, the client is unable to function in the less restrictive outpatient rehabilitation program, he or she may be returned to the inpatient treatment format. Later, when additional progress has been made, the client can again return to an outpatient setting to complete his or her treatment program there.

Turbo (1989) discusses an interesting variation on the two-by-four program that is carried out through the Schick Shadel chain of hospitals in California, Texas, and Washington. These programs admit the individual for 10 days of inpatient treatment, followed by 2 additional inpatient "reinforcement" days 1 month after discharge, and another 2 days of inpatient treatment 2 months following the initial admission.

Berg and Dubin (1990), however, report that in their experience, admission to an inpatient treatment program for even short periods of time results in "a lower probability of complying with outpatient aftercare" by the client (p. 1177). The authors found a 60% dropout rate for those who were initially hospitalized and then referred to an intensive outpatient treatment program after the need for hospitalization had passed. It is not known at this time whether these results were specific only to the program with which Berg and Dubin (1990) are affiliated, or if this is a trend that exists in other partial hospitalization programs as well.

Day Hospitalization

The day hospitalization format is also known as partial day hospitalization. As Lewis, Dana, and Blevins (1988) point out, this type of rehabilitation program combines elements of inpatient treatment with the opportunities for growth that come from living at home. After detoxification has been achieved, the client is allowed to spend the evening hours at home, coming to the treatment center during normal working hours to participate in the rehabilitation program.

Although Klar (1987) explored the advantages and disadvantages of partial hospital programs for psychiatric patients, his insights into the advantages of day hospitalization for chemical dependency treatment are equally valid. Klar (1987) notes that, because the patients

> live at home, the acute partial hospital program is akin to a full-time job, and is consequently less disruptive to social and family roles and is less stigmatizing. Partial hospitalization is a less regressive treatment modality than inpatient care, asks more of the patient, and actively attempts to mobilize the patient's adaptive skills and support network in the treatment. (p. 338)

An essential element of day hospitalization is that the client has a supportive, stable family. Obviously, if the client's spouse (or other family member) also has a chemical abuse problem, day hospitalization will not be a viable treatment option. Similarly, if the client's spouse is severely codependent and continues to enable the client's continued chemical use, day hospitalization should not be the treatment of choice.

However, for the client with a stable home environment, day hospitalization offers the opportunity to combine the intensive programming possible through inpatient treatment programs with the opportunities for growth possible by having the client spend the evening hours at home. Such a program is of value for clients who need to rebuild family relationships after a protracted period of chemical use.

Halfway Houses

The halfway house concept emerged in the 1950s in response to the need for an intermediate step between the inpatient treatment format and independent living (Miller & Hester, 1980). For clients who lack a stable social support system, the period of time following treatment is often most difficult. Even if strongly motivated to remain sober, the client must struggle against the urge to return to chemical use without the social support necessary to aid in this struggle. The halfway house provides a transitional living facility for such a client.

Miller and Hester (1980) list several common characteristics of halfway houses: (1) small patient population (usually less than 25 individuals), (2) brief patient stay (less than a few months), (3) emphasis on Alcoholics Anonymous or similar twelve-step philosophy, (4) minimal rules, and (5) small number of professional staff members.

As noted, most halfway houses utilize a twelve-step philosophy, and many hold in-house self-help group meetings such as Alcoholics Anonymous. Other halfway houses require a specified number of community self-help group meetings a week. Each individual is expected to find work within a specified period of time (usually 2 to 3 weeks) or is assigned a job within the halfway house.

The degree of structure found in the traditional halfway house setting is somewhere between that of an inpatient treatment program setting and that of a traditional household. This structure provides the client with enough support to function during the transitional period between treatment and self-sufficiency, yet also allows the client to make choices about his or her life. As Miller and Hester (1980) point out, halfway houses usually have fewer rules than inpatient treatment centers. Halfway house participation is usually time-limited, generally from 3 to 6 months, after which clients are ready to assume their responsibilities again.

Surprisingly, there is little evidence to support effectiveness of the halfway house concept, according to Miller and Hester (1980). They report that research has failed to uncover significantly greater improvement from patients admitted to halfway houses following treatment than from patients who refused admission. Adelman and Weiss (1989) challenge this conclusion, however, observing that research has found an inverse relationship between length of stay and rehospitalization in the first 6 months following treatment. In other words, those patients who elected to enter a halfway house following inpatient treatment were less likely to be hospitalized for relapse than were those who did not. Finney, Moos, and Chan (1975) examined the relationship between length of stay in a halfway house setting following treatment and treatment outcome and concluded that, for some subgroups of patients, length of stay was correlated with successful treatment outcomes.

Summary

There is significant evidence that, at least for some addicted individuals, outpatient treatment is an option that should be considered by treatment professionals. For those with the proper social support and for whom there is no coexisting psychiatric illness or need for inpatient hospitalization, outpatient therapy for drug addiction may offer the individual the chance to participate in treatment while still living at home. This avoids the need for a reorientation period following treatment.

Outpatient treatment also allows for long-term therapeutic support that is often not available from inpatient programs. Within an outpatient drug addiction program, random urine toxicology screening can be utilized to check on medication compliance and identify those individuals who have engaged in illicit drug use. Research evidence suggests that, for many patients, outpatient drug addiction treatment is as effective as inpatient chemical dependency programs. There is a significant dropout rate from outpatient treatment programs, however, and there remains much to be learned about how to make outpatient addiction treatment more effective.

Inpatient treatment is often viewed as a drastic step. Yet, for a minority of those who are addicted to chemicals, such a drastic step is necessary if the client is ever to regain control of his or her life. The inpatient rehabilitation program offers many advantages over less restrictive treatment options, including a depth of support services unavailable in outpatient treatment. For many of those in the advanced stages of addiction, inpatient treatment offers the only realistic hope of recovery.

In recent years, questions have been raised concerning the need for inpatient treatment programs or halfway house placement following treatment. It has been suggested that inpatient treatment does not offer any advantage over outpatient treatment and that a longer length of stay is no more effective than short-term treatment. However, others have concluded that length of stay was inversely related to the probability of relapse following treatment.

Problems Encountered in the Treatment of Chemical Dependency

Research has consistently demonstrated that treatment is more effective than criminal justice sanctions as a way of dealing with the problem of drug abuse (Scheer, 1994b). But no matter which treatment approach the therapist chooses to utilize, there are a number of potential problems that he or she might experience in working with the recovering addict. In this chapter, we will examine some of the more common, and more serious, problems encountered by treatment professionals working with recovering addicts in different settings.

Limit Testing by Clients in Treatment

Clients in therapeutic relationships—including addicted clients in a treatment setting—often "test the limits" to determine whether or not the professional will be consistent in his or her treatment of the client. This limit-testing, done either consciously or unconsciously, might take on a number of different forms, from missed appointments to the use of chemicals while in treatment.

The chemical dependency professional should be aware that "dependability" and "consistency" also apply to the enforcement of the rules of the program. For example, to counter the problem of chemical use by patients in treatment, McCarthy and Borders (1985) told patients in a methadone maintenance program that their urine would be tested to detect continued chem-

ical abuse. The patients were told that if their urine tested positive for other drugs four times in the next year, they would be placed on a narcotics withdrawal program in place of the desired methadone maintenance. Patients in this structured program achieved significantly greater program compliance and were less likely to use drugs than were a matched control group of addicts who were not in such a structured program.

Treatment "Secrets"

A common scenario is for the client to ask for an individual conference with the staff member and then confess to a rules infraction. This admission of guilt is often made to a student or intern at the agency, rather than to a regular staff member. The confession might be an admission of having used chemicals while in treatment. After having made this admission, the client will ask that the staff member not tell the group, other staff members, or the program director about the rules violation for fear of being discharged from treatment.

For the chemical dependency professional to honor the request to not tell other staff members would constitute entering into a partnership with the addict. Such partnership, because it is set up by the addict, makes the professional an "enabler." In some situations, to not report a rules violation could make the professional vulnerable to later extortion by the client, who could threaten to report the professional to his or her superiors for not passing on the information to staff as he or she should have done.

The proper response to this situation is to properly document the material discussed *immediately*, in writing and through proper channels. This could be written as a memo or an entry into the client's progress notes and should also be discussed with the professional's immediate supervisor. This action is taken without malice to ensure both uniform enforcement of the rules for all clients and to protect the professional's reputation.

Relapse Prevention

One of the more frustrating facts about chemical addiction is that a significant percentage of those admitted to either inpatient or outpatient chemical dependency programs fail to "graduate" from treatment for one reason or another. Even of those who complete treatment, a large percentage relapse into the use of chemicals in the first months after discharge from the rehabilitation program. Thus, entry into treatment should not be taken as a guarantee that the person will actually complete the program or that he or she will benefit from treatment in any way.

In the past 20 years, the focus of treatment has shifted away from simply "getting them sober" to arming recovering addicts against the forces that may contribute to "relapse." Total abstinence from drugs of abuse is quite rare, even if the person has completed treatment. Instead, substance use patterns "are usually episodic, with alternating periods of abstinence and relapse" (DeJong, 1994, p. 682).

The first 90 days following discharge from treatment is a period of special vulnerability for relapse (DeJong, 1994). This does not mean that treatment is a waste of time; rather, it reflects the grim reality that the disease of addiction can be *arrested* but can never be *cured*. If the disease is only arrested, it can spring back into full bloom whenever conditions allow it to reassert itself.

The goal of relapse prevention, then, is to provide the individual with the tools that he or she might need to avoid returning to active drug use.

According to Chiauzzi (1990), there are four elements common to those who relapse. First, they often demonstrate *personality traits* that interfere with continued sobriety. For example, they may be compulsive, not adjusting well to even minor changes in routine. Often, they are dependent, having trouble asserting their wish to remain sober. Passive-aggressive personality traits also place the individual at risk for relapse because these personality types tend to blame others for their behavior. Narcissistic traits prevent many from admitting to the need for help during a weak moment, and antisocial personality traits underscore a tendency to be impulsive and a desire to "follow the road not taken" by others (Chiauzzi, 1990).

A second factor advanced by Chiauzzi as contributing to relapse is a tendency for the individual to *substitute addictions*. Recovering addicts often substitute work, a new relationship, or other chemicals for the drug they are no longer using. Caffeine or drug abuse, a dependent relationship, or an eating disorder could signal a high-risk situation for relapse.

Chiauzzi's third factor is a *narrow view of recovery*. All too often, the recovering addict equates abstinence or simple attendance at a self-help group with "recovery." This view of recovery places the individual at risk for relapse because he or she is not working to change the personality structure or work on the interpersonal problems that led to the addiction in the first place. Such individuals do not develop the self-awareness necessary to detect their drift toward relapse.

Finally, Chiauzzi found that what he calls *warning signals* of impending relapse were often overlooked by the individual. Chiauzzi's (1990) concept of warning signals is very similar to the concept of the mini-decisions first reported by Cummings, Gordon, and Marlatt (1980). They present a theoretical model in which relapse is viewed as evolving out of a series of "mini-decisions" (p. 297). According to this model, there is no major decision to return to drug use. Rather, the road to relapse is lined with smaller decisions that, added together, "begin a chain of behaviors which may set the stage for a relapse to occur" (p. 297).

Examples of such "mini-decisions" may be for the recovering addict to continue a friendship with an active addict or to go over to the local bar "just to play pool." Chiauzzi (1990) reports that individuals who relapse fail to notice negative thoughts; a desire to spend time with drug using friends or signs of a physical illness are dismissed by the recovering addict. Cummings, Gordon, and Marlatt (1980) point out that these seemingly innocent mini-decisions increase the chance that the recovering addict will encounter a situation in which he or she is likely to relapse.

Addicts have been known to "see if I could just walk down the same street, and not feel the urge to use anymore"; or they have only "stopped off to pay him some money that I owed him, and I found drugs all over the place!"—as if the friend's drug use were a revelation. This represents a decision point for the newly recovering addict. He or she must either reaffirm the commitment to sobriety or start back on the path to the active use of chemicals. If the individual has adequate coping skills, he or she will reaffirm the commitment to sobriety. However, if the individual's sobriety-based coping skills are inadequate, he or she might relapse. At best, the experience will be a frightening one that may make the individual question whether he or she is *ever* going to be capable of self-sustained sobriety.

Often, such a mini-decision is made to stop going to regular AA or NA meetings. The initial decision may be to cut back from five meetings a week to four meetings each week; then to cut back from four to perhaps only one or two meetings a week. Eventually, the decision might be to go to meetings only every other week, and then once a month, until the individual no longer has any contact with his or her sober support system.

It is virtually guaranteed that every recovering addict will encounter at least one high-risk situation; that is, a situation in which the possibility of drug use is high. Cummings, Gordon, and Marlatt (1980) group these high-risk situations into two categories. The first category consists of the acute period of drug withdrawal, when the individual is motivated to avoid further withdrawal discomfort through the ingestion of chemicals. The second group might be viewed as the social, environmental, and emotional states the individual perceives as stressful and for which drugs were previously used as a coping mechanism. In this second group of high-risk situations, cognitive evaluations of the social, environmental, or emotional stimuli mediate whether the individual considers the possibility of drug use or not. Such cognitive evaluations may then be interpreted by the individual as an urge or "craving" to use a substance.

Shiffman (1992) views the problem of relapse from the perspective of behavioral psychology, concluding that "stimulus factors" (p. 9) contribute to lapses in sobriety, in the sense that environmental stimuli might trigger craving for drug use. Research evidence now suggests that conditioned learning takes place during the individual's drug using period; when the individual is again exposed to the same (or similar) sights, sounds, or emotions, he or she may again feel a "craving" for chemicals. Recovering narcotics addicts have been known to suddenly experience craving for drugs when they return to the neighborhood where they once used chemicals, even if they had been abstinent for months or even years (Galanter, 1993).

To combat the influence of environmental triggers for chemical use, Shiffman advocates the use of behavioral rehearsals to help the client learn skills that enable him or her to avoid relapse. A second area of emphasis is the identification of the client's feelings of demoralization and self-blame during the early phases of recovery, according to Shiffman. Such "cognitive" intervention has been shown to be at least as effective as behavioral training for environmental triggers to relapse.

According to Lewis, Dana, and Blevins (1988), the first step in relapse prevention is the *identification of the high-risk situation* for each individual.

Self-monitoring and direct observation by treatment center staff are just two methods by which high-risk situations can be identified. The patient's history may also underscore high-risk situations of particular significance for that individual. Treatment staff should pay particular attention to the client's self-report to identify possible high-risk factors.

Once the high-risk factors have been identified, *specific coping responses* for each high-risk situation must be devised by the treatment center staff. Niaura, Rohsenow, Binkoff, Monti, Pedraza, and Abrams (1988) report that addicts are unlikely to relapse if they are armed with cognitive and behavioral coping mechanisms that counteract feelings of helplessness in the face of cognitive, social, or environmental cues for drug use. Lewis, Dana, and Blevins (1988) recommend that a reminder card be carried at all times, so that the individual who relapses will have written instructions on the steps to take to keep it within limits.

There are a number of situations that appear, either individually or in combination, to contribute to the addicted person's relapse. DeJong (1994) identified many of these "antecedents" of relapse: stress, negative emotional states, interpersonal conflict, social pressure, positive emotional states, use of other substances, and presence of drug-related cues.

The concept of relapse prevention has offered some insight into the forces that might undermine the initial success achieved in treatment. The theoretical models of relapse and its prevention offer some promise in the treatment of chemical dependency. In the next few years, research should disclose whether current models of relapse prevention are useful in the treatment of addiction or whether there is a need for further research in this area.

Controlled Drinking

The concept of helping the alcoholic return to "social" or "controlled" drinking has been a controversial one for many years (Helzer et al., 1985; Schuckit, 1989). Unfortunately, ever since the first preliminary reports that it *might* be possible to train a percentage of alcoholics to return to a state of "controlled" drinking, many alcoholics have seized on the concept as a justification for continued drinking.

Unfortunately, research (Helzer et al., 1985) suggests that less than 2% of alcoholics can return to a state of social drinking again. Although controlled drinking is a viable goal for individuals who are not clearly addicted and who have not experienced significant problems associated with addiction (Hester & Miller, 1989), it is not a goal for the alcoholic. In other words, it might be possible to teach a large percentage of those who *abuse* alcohol to control their drinking, but only about 2% of those who are clearly *addicted* can return to social drinking (Helzer et al., 1985).

Meyer (1989a) believes that individuals who are moderately to severely addicted to alcohol will quickly return to abusive drinking if they attempt to learn how to drink on a "social" basis. *Every* alcoholic, however, would like to believe that he or she is in the 1% to 2% of those who can be trained to return to "controlled" or "social" drinking.

Given that such a small percentage of alcoholics have been able to achieve a return to social drinking patterns, one must argue against the experiment of attempting to find out whether any given alcoholic is in this category. In a negative sense, Miller (1989) adopts the position of letting the alcoholic find out. If the individual maintains that he or she does not have an alcohol dependency problem, let the individual try to learn "controlled drinking," because "an unsuccessful trial at 'controlled drinking' may be a more persuasive confrontation of the need for abstinence than any amount of direct argumentation between therapist and client" (Miller, 1989, p. 77).

Thus, Miller believes that a trial of "controlled drinking" may prove of value in helping the individual realize the need for total abstinence. But the mental health or substance abuse professional needs to weigh the potential benefits of this trial against the potential risks. Confirmed alcoholics who believe that they can learn social drinking behaviors *and maintain* a pattern of social drinking for the rest of their lives are taking a chance where the odds are at best 49 to 1 against them.

Client Manipulation of Urine Toxicology Tests

When properly utilized, urine toxicology testing provides one of the most comprehensive means of monitoring patient compliance. But urine toxicology screens are not without their disadvantages. One drawback of urine toxicology screening is that the procedure involves an invasion of the patient's right to privacy (Cone, 1993). The staff of a treatment center must thus weigh the advantages of obtaining a urine sample for toxicology testing against the patient's right to privacy. Some treatment centers have clients sign a consent form stating that they are aware that one condition of treatment is that the staff might ask for a urine toxicology sample at any time. Such a statement provides a release clause, authorizing staff to collect a urine sample at its discretion. Another disadvantage is that some clients attempt to "fake" a urine sample, either by substituting another person's urine sample for their own or by other means.

One favorite trick is for the client to have a "clean" (drug-free) urine sample on hand, possibly hidden in a balloon or small bottle. When asked for a urine sample, the client may empty the container into the sample bottle, safe in the knowledge that the urine to be tested is "clean." Another trick is for the client to "accidentally" dip the bottle into the water in the toilet, diluting the urine so much that it is unlikely that the laboratory could detect any *urine*, never mind possible chemical traces! (One way to circumvent this action is to test the specific gravity and level of acidity of the urine sample, because water has a different specific gravity and acid level than urine.)

Many clients who are aware that they must provide a urine sample for toxicology testing will attempt to force-feed fluids, to dilute what-

ever traces of chemicals might be found in an unusually large volume of urine. "Street" addicts have long claimed that, if the individual can produce enough urine, it will dilute whatever metabolites of recreational chemicals exist to below the detection limits of most tests. The *Forensic Drug Abuse Advisor* (1994a) confirms that, if the addict ingests extra amounts of water, it is possible to dilute the metabolites of THC so much that the testing procedure is unable to detect the THC at a 50-ng/ml detection level. However, to accomplish this feat, the individual would have to ingest *a gallon* of water. Furthermore, the specific gravity and creatinine (a natural chemical found in urine) levels in the urine sample would drop so low as to alert staff that the urine sample had been altered in some way. Still, as a precaution against a diluted sample, many laboratories recommend that the urine sample submitted for testing be drawn from the client's first visit to the toilet in the morning, when urine is most concentrated.

Another way of defeating the urine toxicology screen is to substitute a small sample of a certain diet soda for the requested urine (*Playboy*, 1991). After being held under the arm for about an hour to simulate the body's warmth, 2 ounces of this unnamed diet soda would be accepted as a valid urine sample "98 percent of the time" (p. 56). Also, *Playboy* (1991) reports that adding a specific (unnamed) brand of eyedrops to a urine sample camouflages any evidence of marijuana use, and adding bleach to the urine sample camouflages traces of cocaine.

Thus, *extremely close supervision of the client must be the rule when using urine samples for detection of illicit drug use.* The person supervising the collection of the urine sample *must actually see the urine enter the bottle* and not just stand outside of the men's or women's room while the client is inside. Clients have been known to hide clean urine samples in the toilet area beforehand to substitute the urine sample for their own later that day.

Several techniques can be used to counter deception if the staff suspects that a client has substituted another person's urine for his or her own. First, because *urine is within 1 to 2 degrees of the core body temperature,* one can determine if the sample is a substitute by immediately testing its temperature. The client whose urine sample is 70°, for example, is likely to have substituted somebody else's and should be confronted with this fact.

Another technique is for a staff member to wait until the client is about to enter the lavatory before announcing that he or she has been selected for another urine sample for drug testing. It is unlikely that clients will carry around a bottle of substitute urine all the time, on the off chance that they will be asked for a urine sample. This procedure is likely to force clients to give a sample of their own urine, especially if care is taken to ensure that they provide a valid sample.

Still another technique is for the counselor to announce, at the beginning of a group session or other supervised activity, that the client will have to provide a supervised urine sample at the session's end. The client will be unable to retrieve a stored urine sample without staff being aware that he or she has left the group. The client should be given access to water, coffee, or soda to stimulate the production of urine and then be escorted to the bathroom for collection of the urine sample.

Test Results

Depending on the test method used, laboratories can detect either the drugs or the metabolites produced by the body as the liver breaks down the drugs for various periods of time. The chemical dependency professional should request a written summary from the laboratory that includes the following information:

- the *methods* used by the laboratory to detect illicit chemical use
- the *accuracy* of the methods
- the *specific chemicals that can be detected* by the laboratory
- the *duration of time over which the urine test will reveal such drug use*

- *other drugs* (including over-the-counter medications) that could yield false positive results

Ravel (1989) reports that a urine sample from a person who had smoked a *single* marijuana cigarette would be "positive" for 1 to 3 days at a cutoff level of 100 ng/ml, and if a lower cutoff level of 20 ng/ml were utilized, the same individual would test positive for THC for 5 to 8 days. Because the body stores THC and gradually releases it back into the blood, chronic marijuana users will test positive at the 20-ng/ml level for 30 to 40 days. Farrow (1990) gives an even higher estimate, stating that a daily marijuana user could continue to test positive for THC for between 6 and 81 days. Therefore, Ravel (1989) advocates testing new urine samples every 4 to 5 days for chronic users. If there has been no additional marijuana use, such serial urine samples should show "a progressive downward trend in the values" (p. 629).

Urine toxicology screening can detect other drugs of abuse besides marijuana. Depending on the route of administration and the amount of cocaine utilized, it is possible to detect metabolites of cocaine in urine samples for between 24 to 36 hours (House, 1990; Farrow, 1990; Schwartz, 1988) and 96 hours (Weddington, 1993) after the last drug use. Some of the factors that influence the time period in which cocaine can be detected in the urine depends on (1) the quantity ingested, (2) whether the individual had used cocaine once or several times, (3) individual variation in the period of time necessary for the body to metabolize cocaine, and (4) the sensitivity of the specific test for cocaine that is used (Ravel, 1989). However, as a general rule, a large dose of cocaine can be detected for 2 to 3 days using enzyme immunoassay techniques or for up to 7 days if the more sensitive radioimmunoassay techniques are utilized.

Ravel (1989) also states that PCP or its metabolites can be detected for up to one week following its use. As noted in the chapter on hallucinogens, however, the speed at which PCP is excreted from the body depends on the acidity of the urine, and thus there will be some variation in the speed at which PCP is eliminated from the body. Cone (1993) suggests that PCP might be detected in body fluids for up to 5 to 8 days in the casual user and for as long as 30 days in the chronic user.

The amphetamines, on the other hand, are eliminated more quickly. According to Cone (1993), they can be detected for only 24 to 48 hours after the last use. And Ravel (1989) reports that the narcotics can be detected for only 1 to 2 days following the last use of this class of drugs.

False Positive Test Results and Retesting

A number of chemicals can cause inaccurate test results. Poppy seeds, for example, often baked in bread products, might produce a "false positive" result on a urine toxicology screen for narcotics (Ravel, 1989). Over-the-counter medications such as pseudoephedrine hydrochloride (which is sold under a number of different brand names) may cause the urine sample to test positive for amphetamines (Schwartz, 1988).

Once illicit drug use is detected, the urine sample must be retested by another technique to rule out a false positive result. For example, Moyer and Ellefson (1987) report that, when a pure urine specimen is utilized, the enzyme-mediated immunotechnique (EMIT) is able to detect marijuana use with better than 95% accuracy. When combined with other tests such as gas chromatography/mass spectrometry (GC/MS), it is possible to obtain virtually 100% accuracy when testing urine specimens for evidence of marijuana use.

Given the fact that the EMIT procedure has a 3% false positive rate, testing with another technique such as GC/MS is essential to rule out any possibility of error. Ravel (1989) also advocates the use of additional testing such as mass spectrometry or gas chromatography to confirm or deny the original positive test results for all drugs of abuse. These are highly specialized test procedures that essentially separate the constituents of a urine sample for identification. Using multiple test procedures for all positive urine samples helps identify those individuals who

actually have used illicit chemicals and eliminates the danger of "false positive" test results (Schwartz, 1988).

Other Uses of Urine Toxicology Tests

A second use of urine toxicology testing is not to detect illicit drug use but to check medication compliance. In other words, urine toxicology screening can be used to help determine whether or not the client is taking the prescribed medications. Obviously, clients being detoxified from narcotics through methadone withdrawal should have methadone in their urine. Farrow (1990) reports that urine toxicology screening should be able to detect methadone for up to 56 hours after a dose of 40 mg. If the individual does not test positive for this drug, the staff should consider the possibility that this person has substituted another urine sample for his or her own.

Acquired Immune Deficiency Syndrome (AIDS)[1]

Both directly and indirectly, chronic chemical abuse contributes to the spread of a wide range of infectious diseases. In this section, we will discuss one of the most serious infections that can be transmitted by intravenous drug abuse: AIDS.

Addicts who inject drugs often fail to use proper "sterile technique" when injecting the chemicals into their bodies. In a hospital setting, the staff sterilizes the injection site either with alcohol or with an antiseptic solution. However, the addict usually just injects the drug into a vein without even attempting to wash the injection site first, thus allowing microorganisms at the injection site to gain direct admission to the blood-rich tissues below the skin of the addict and cause infection. Furthermore, the addict fre-

---

[1]The author would like to express appreciation to John P. Doweiko, M.D., for reviewing the next three sections of this chapter for technical accuracy.

quently uses chemical compounds that are contaminated with various microscopic pathogens.

These factors expose the addict to the risk of various localized, or systemic, infections. Some of the infections commonly found in intravenous drug addicts include peripheral cellulitis, skin abscesses, viral hepatitis (especially hepatitis B, which will be discussed later in this chapter), endocarditis (bacterial infection of the heart valves), pneumonia, lung abscesses, tetanus, and occasionally malaria (Cherubin & Sapira, 1993; Jenike, 1991).

Unfortunately, another common characteristic of intravenous drug addicts is that they often share needles with other addicts. This practice exposes each subsequent user to whatever infectious diseases previous users of that needle might have in their blood. One infection that can be transmitted through contaminated needles is caused by the human immunodeficiency virus (HIV) (King, 1994; Kruger & Jerrells, 1992), the virus that causes AIDS.

History of AIDS in the United States

In the early 1980s, it became clear to medical researchers that a previously unknown disease was spreading throughout the United States. Initially, the disease seemed to be isolated to the homosexual male population, but it was not immediately clear whether a new form of bacteria or a new virus was involved. All researchers knew was that the immune system in certain people would rapidly fail, leaving the victim open to any of a range of rare "opportunistic infections." Medical researchers termed this process the *acquired immune deficiency syndrome,* or AIDS.

Soon it was discovered that AIDS also developed in a number of intravenous drug addicts and in some patients whose only apparent "risk factor" for the infection was that they had received a blood transfusion in the past. These facts suggested to researchers that some kind of blood-borne infection was involved in the development of AIDS. Further studies quickly revealed that the infectious agent was most likely

a virus, rather than a new species of bacteria. Within a short period of time, researchers had isolated a virus that has since been called HIV (King, 1994; McCutchan, 1990).

What is AIDS?

It is surprising how many people speak of AIDS as if it were a disease in itself. AIDS is not a disease; it is a *syndrome,* or a specific pattern of symptoms. AIDS is the end stage of a viral infection in which HIV gains entry into the human body. For reasons that are still not understood, the individual's immune system is eventually overwhelmed and fails to function properly.

Since it was discovered, a number of theories have been advanced as to how HIV came into being, including theories that suggest that HIV was a "designer virus" made in a "germ warfare" laboratory (Weiss, 1994). Such stories are dismissed by most researchers, who view HIV as one of the multitude of viral infections that occasionally "jumps" from one species to another. Currently, researchers think that HIV evolved in Africa, possibly as a viral infection limited to a species of monkey. Sometime around the middle of the 20th century, the virus managed to shift from one "host" (monkeys) to another (humans), with devastating results (Weiss, 1994).

Another theory is that HIV was endemic to certain parts of Africa for perhaps the last 100 to 200 years (Anderson & May, 1992). Unfortunately, whereas geographic distance once provided an effective barrier to infectious diseases, modern travel has made it possible for numerous "new" forms of disease to move around the globe with surprising speed. This is how HIV is thought to have spread. First, as geographic barriers were removed, HIV traveled out of its region of origins in Africa, moving first to the major cities of Africa. Then, in a matter of a few months or years, it had traveled across the globe.

However, this is only a theory. Scientists have not discovered how HIV evolved into its present form or what its history was before it burst on the scene as a deadly viral infection. But there is little if any evidence to support the lurid reports passed from mouth to mouth that HIV is a "germ warfare" experiment that somehow escaped the laboratory or that it was intentionally released into the population to target homosexual males or other minority group members.

The process through which HIV is able to infect, and ultimately kill, the victim is based on a remarkable chain of events involving the individual's immune system.

In brief, every species of bacteria, virus, or fungus has a characteristic pattern of proteins within its cell walls. When the human body is invaded by a bacterium, fungus, or virus, the immune system learns to recognize these patterns and to distinguish between the protein pattern of an invading organism and that of the body's own cells. The body learns to protect itself from invading organisms by building "antibodies," the so-called white blood cells that recognize foreign cells and attack them.

The body "tailor makes" some antibodies for each species of bacteria, fungus, or virus that it encounters over the years. These pathogen-specific antibodies recognize specific protein patterns on the surface of the invader and protect the individual from further problems with that pathogen. This is why a person who once had an infection can become "immune" to that disease: a number of white blood cells that remain from the previous exposure to the invader can isolate and destroy others of the same species. When the body is exposed to a new organism, the process of producing the specific antibody necessary to fight it off can take hours, days, weeks, or sometimes years.

But the body also produces antibodies that are not pathogen-specific but that roam through the blood and seek out *any* invader with a foreign protein pattern in its cell wall. These antibodies are the ones that mount the initial attack against a new invader, before the body "learns" to produce pathogen-specific antibodies.

In the case of an HIV infection, it may require up to 9 months for the individual's body to begin to produce antibodies against the invading virus (McCutchan, 1990). This is one characteristic of the HIV disease process that has contributed to its rapid spread. Even before the body has started to produce antibodies against HIV, the infected person is capable of passing the virus on to others through blood or sexual contact. Thus, the person whose blood test is negative for HIV infection could still have the virus in his or her blood; the body just may not have had time to begin to manufacture antibodies that would be detected in a blood test.

Unfortunately, another characteristic of HIV infection is that it is able to work its way into different body tissues (Radetsky, 1990). This allows the virus to hide from the body's defenses while it reproduces. The AIDS virus infects various components of the immune system, especially the type of antibodies known as "T-helper" cells. Thus, in the infected individual, the virus often hides in the antibodies, many of which were produced by the body to attempt to fight off the HIV infection.

Ultimately, in the majority of individuals, HIV causes the destruction of the body's cellular immune system (Beardsley, 1994). The exact means by which HIV destroys the body's immune system is not clear at this time (King, 1994; Moore, 1993), but once the immune system is weakened, various "opportunistic infections" develop. These infections are usually caused by microorganisms that were once easily controlled by the immune system. In AIDS, the body's weakened defenses are overwhelmed by the invading microbes, and eventually the individual dies.

The Chain of HIV Infection

HIV is a fragile virus that is not easily transmitted from one person to another (Langone, 1989). The virus must be passed *directly* from individual to individual. The apparent modes of HIV transmission are limited to sexual intercourse with an infected person, direct mixing of one's blood with infected body fluids, the passage of the virus from the mother to the fetus, or transmission through the mother's milk to the nursing baby (King, 1994; Kruger & Jerrells, 1992; Glasner & Kaslow, 1990). Because it is a blood-borne infection, HIV can be transmitted through blood transfusions. New blood tests have been developed to screen out blood donors who might carry the virus. Currently the incidence of HIV infection through blood transfusions in the United States is estimated at between 1 case for every 45,000 to 225,000 units of blood transfused (Edelson, 1993).

One of the most common means by which HIV is transmitted from one person to another in the United States is the sharing of drug paraphernalia among intravenous drug addicts. Statistically, between 3 and 9% of intravenous drug addicts become infected with HIV each year. So common is this route of transmission that AIDS has become the leading cause of death for intravenous drug users (Pope & Morin, 1990). In some U.S. communities, blood tests show that between 60% (Glasner & Kaslow, 1990) and 80% (Michelson, Carroll, McLane, & Robin, 1988) of intravenous drug users tested are "seropositive," or that their blood samples contain antibodies against the HIV. This means they are infected with the virus.

The HIV virus is also found in the semen of all infected men and can be passed on to others through the semen. People involved in sexual relationships with those infected with the virus are themselves "at risk" for contracting HIV. It is for this reason that HIV is often classified as a sexually transmitted disease (STD). Promiscuous sexual activity increases the individual's risk of exposure to a wide range of STDs. The greater the number of sexual partners any one individual has, the greater are his or her chances of being exposed to HIV. Because of the high probability that drug addicts, promiscuous individuals, prostitutes, and bisexual or homosexual males are infected, sexual contact with people in these categories should be avoided.

In addition to the role that intravenous drug use plays in the transmission of HIV, recreational drug use may also *indirectly* contribute to HIV infection. For example, because alcohol is capable of lowering inhibitions, it may indirectly contribute to promiscuous behavior, exposing the individual to a partner who is infected with HIV. Furthermore, the use of alcohol by the individual who is infected with HIV might lower the individual's resistance, speeding up the progression of the viral infection (Kruger & Jerrells, 1992).

At one time, the two groups in the United States thought to have the greatest risk of contracting AIDS were homosexual males and intravenous drug users. These are still high-risk groups. Slightly over 52% of those people who are infected with HIV in the United States contracted the virus through homosexual or bisexual partners. Another 23% contracted the disease through the use of contaminated needles (Grigg, 1992). In the San Francisco area, perhaps as many as 50% of the homosexual or bisexual males are infected with HIV (Pope & Morin, 1990). Overall, homosexual and bisexual men form 60% to 70% of the U.S. population infected with HIV (Anderson, 1993).

Until recently, intravenous drug users formed the second-largest group of people infected with HIV. But the heterosexual transmission of the virus has now become the second most common means by which people become infected in the United States (Anderson, 1993). In other parts of the world, heterosexual transmission of HIV is *the* most common means of transmission. Globally, it is estimated that by the year 2000, 75% to 80% of those who have been infected with HIV will have acquired the infection through heterosexual intercourse with an infected partner.

To put the danger of the heterosexual transmission of HIV in a different perspective, Penney (1993) reports that a woman having a single sexual encounter with a new lover, without using appropriate precautions, has up to a 17.5% chance of contracting HIV. That is, statistically, a woman who spends a single night with a new male lover stands just under a *1 in 5* chance of having chosen a partner who is infected with HIV.

The Scope of the Problem

According to current theory, less than 20 years ago, HIV was an obscure virus found only in geographically isolated parts of Africa. In the span of a single generation, the disease has spread to the point where an estimated 20 million people around the world are currently infected with HIV (Greene, 1993). If the disease continues to spread at its present rate, 2% of the entire population of the world (or an estimated *120 million* people) will have been infected with HIV by the year 2000 (Greene, 1993).

It is estimated that two million people in the United States are currently infected with HIV (*Harvard Medical School Mental Health Letter*, 1994). Grigg (1992) breaks this estimate down by gender, stating that 1 in every 100 males and 1 in every 600 females is infected with HIV. The World Health Organization (WHO) gives an even higher estimate of 1 in 75 for males in North America, but a lower estimate of 1 in 700 women in North America being infected with HIV (CDC *AIDS Weekly*, 1992). In less than 20 years, AIDS went from a totally unknown disease in the United States to the second most common cause of death for men between the ages of 18 and 44 and the sixth most common cause of death for women 18 to 44 years old (Kelly, Murphy, Sikkema, & Kalicyhman, 1993).

At this time, AIDS is predominantly a male disease, at least in the United States. In more than 88% of the reported cases of AIDS in the United States, the victim is male (Dumas, 1992). For this reason, virtually all the research on the manifestations and treatment of AIDS has involved *male* victims (Squires, 1989). Very little is known about the evolution of AIDS in females or whether current treatment programs need to be modified for female victims.

As is the case with male AIDS victims, just over 50% of the cases of HIV infection in women involve intravenous drug users (Dumas, 1992). Approximately one-third of the infected women contracted AIDS through sexual contact with an infected man, and approximately 10% of the women who contracted HIV did so through con-taminated blood transfusions (*Medical Aspects of Human Sexuality*, 1990).[2] The homosexual transmission of AIDS between women is thought to be rare.

The Stages of AIDS

There is a long latency period between the initial exposure to the virus and the development of the full AIDS syndrome. During this time, HIV infection can be detected only through a series of blood tests. Pope and Morin (1990) outline the stages necessary to identify whether a person is (or is not) infected with HIV as follows.

> Generally, the initial tests screen blood samples of antibodies to the virus; such tests are termed ELISA (enzyme-linked immunosorbent assay). If the individual reacts positively to ELISA tests, a more difficult, expensive, and supposedly accurate test such as the Western Blot (which searches for antibodies against specific protein molecules) or radioimmunoprecipitation or radioimmunofluorescence assay [is carried out]. (p. 47)

The HIV infection progresses through three distinct stages, according to Atkinson and Grant (1994).

1. Seroconversion (the point where antibodies to HIV are detected in the individual's blood, indicating that he or she has been infected with the virus)
2. A period of time in which the individual is infected but is essentially asymptomatic
3. The period during which symptomatic disease and the progression to AIDS begins

The individual whose blood does not have antibodies for the AIDS virus and who does not test positive on the ELISA tests is classified as "seronegative." This means that either (1) the individual has never been exposed to the AIDS virus, or (2) the individual has not had sufficient time to develop antibodies to the AIDS virus. In

[2]The majority of these women received the blood transfusion *before* the current blood tests to detect HIV in the blood of donors were developed.

CD4$^+$ cell count (per cubic mm of blood)	A Asymptomatic	B Symptomatic but not full-blown AIDS	C Full-blown AIDS
500 or more cells	A1	B1	C1
200 to 499 cells	A2	B2	C2
Less than 200 cells	A3	B3	C3

→ Patients in column B would have developed infections—such as bacterial endocarditis, meningitis, pneumonia, or sepsis—that are not specific to AIDS patients alone. For example, it is not uncommon for individuals with normal immune systems to develop bacterial pneumonia. Contrast this with the defining criteria for column C.

→ Patients in column C have developed one or more infections rarely seen except in patients who have AIDS. For example, the patient might have a candidiasis infection of the esophagus, or AIDS-induced diarrhea that lasts longer than one month.

FIGURE 30.1 Modified Center for Disease Control HIV/AIDS classification chart

either case, the individual should be tested again at a later date, usually 6 to 10 months after the initial blood test or last "high risk" behavior, to rule out the second possibility.[3]

After the individual has contracted the virus, the person's body begins to develop antibodies over the next few months in an attempt to fight against the AIDS virus. This individual is classified as "seropositive." As noted earlier, an individual can be seropositive but essentially be asymptomatic for a number of years. During this time, the infection can be detected only through the use of appropriate blood tests for HIV infection.

[3]It should be noted that the blood test to detect exposure to HIV is not perfect. The most common blood test for HIV has a "false positive" rate of less than 1% and a "false negative" rate of about 3% (Rubin, 1993).

There are a number of other classification systems for the stages of the HIV infectious process. The system developed by the Centers for Disease Control (CDC) uses approximately the same three stages outlined by Atkinson and Grant combined with the number of certain specialized antibodies in the patient's blood. As researchers have come to understand more about the progression of the HIV infection in the body, they have discovered that the virus selectively destroys one component of the body's immune system, known as the CD4$^+$ lymphocyte cells (Hollander & Katz, 1993). The CD4$^+$ T-cell count is itself broken down into three levels by the CDC classification system (Rubin, 1993):

Category 1   500 or more cells per cubic mm of blood

Category 2   200–499 cells per cubic mm of blood

Category 3   fewer than 200 cells per cubic mm of blood

These two different criteria are then combined, providing a 3×3 classification table, as shown in Figure 30.1.

As HIV selectively destroys the individual's immune system, the CD4[+] T-cell count will fall. When the number of CD4[+] T-cells falls below 200 per mm of blood, the individual usually becomes vulnerable to any of a range of opportunistic infections rarely seen except in those patients whose immune system has been compromised in some manner. Such a disorder is *Pneumocystis carinii* (or *P. carinii*) pneumonia. Thus, if a physician encounters a patient whose pneumonia is caused by *P. carinii*, that physician would automatically suspect that the patient has AIDS.

Physicians once spoke of a stage of the HIV infection process known as "AIDS related complex," or ARC. During this phase, the individual was thought to have an impaired but still functional immune system. Also, the patient with ARC did not have the full spectrum of opportunistic infections seen in AIDS. In the past decade, this term has been replaced by the more accurate CD4[+] T-cell count method of determining the current stage of the HIV infectious process.

Over time, the infected individual's body becomes weakened by opportunistic infections that he or she could once easily control. Death is usually caused by one or more of these opportunistic infections. Thus, in a technical sense, AIDS is only one stage, in this case the final stage, of the infection caused by HIV (Glasner & Kaslow, 1990).

AIDS and Suicide

AIDS can kill indirectly through another mechanism. Pope and Morin (1990) conclude that individuals who knew they were infected with HIV had a suicide rate *more than 30 times higher* than for individuals who were not infected. However, with appropriate counseling, it is possible to reduce the risk of an individual committing suicide after learning that he or she has acquired the infection (*Harvard Medical School Mental Health Letter*, 1994).

AIDS and Kaposi's Sarcoma

There was a time when a rare form of cancer known as *Kaposi's sarcoma* was thought to be one of the opportunistic infections that indicated that an individual had AIDS. Recent research, however, suggests that Kaposi's sarcoma may be caused by a different infectious agent, possibly also a virus. Because of the similarities in the mode of transmission, both infections were commonly found in homosexual or bisexual males, which contributed to the mistaken conclusion that Kaposi's sarcoma was a manifestation of AIDS. Also, by coincidence, the virus seems to have been introduced into the United States at about the same time as the AIDS virus (Oliwenstein, 1990). By the early 1990s, researchers concluded that Kaposi's sarcoma is an entirely separate disease, and both Kaposi's sarcoma and HIV were classified as STDs.

The Treatment of AIDS

There is no cure for AIDS once HIV has been contracted, although researchers hope to develop treatment methods that will *arrest* the progression of the disease once the individual has been infected (Gallo & Montagnier, 1988; Heaton, 1990). If researchers are successful in finding a drug or drugs that arrest the progression of AIDS, it will be a significant step forward. However, at present, "Although antiviral and other medications may modestly prolong the lives of those infected, the great majority . . . will, barring some major advance, eventually die of an AIDS-related illness" (Greene, 1993, p. 99).

Once AIDS has developed, the average survival period is only 2 to 4 years (Hellinger, 1993). Furthermore, it is estimated that the lifetime cost of treating a person who has contracted the virus is $119,000. Considering that more than 2 million people in the United States are HIV positive, it is clear that the estimated cost of treating just those who are currently infected will eventually come to close to *$238 billion.*

If researchers are successful, they expect to develop a treatment program that will slow or completely arrest the progression of the disease. However, this will not be a cure for AIDS any more than insulin is a "cure" for diabetes mellitus. The injections of insulin serve as a substitute for the body's own insulin, slowing or even in some cases arresting the progression of the diabetes mellitus. But insulin is not a "cure" for the diabetes.

The ultimate "treatment" for AIDS at this time is prevention. Addicts, however, continue to share contaminated needles, syringes, or both, often simply because they do not want to wait until a clean needle or syringe is available. Although rinsing the needle and syringe with bleach often destroys the AIDS virus, many addicts do not engage in this practice simply because it takes too much time. Addicts have also been known to wait in line to use another person's needle and syringe—even though they have a new needle and syringe at home—because they do not want to wait to inject the drug.

There are people who continue to engage in high-risk behavior, although it is not known how representative this group is of national trends. People continue to engage in promiscuous sexual behavior, either heterosexual or homosexual, in spite of the known association between AIDS and sexual promiscuity. It is thus important for the chemical dependency professional to have a working knowledge of infections such as AIDS and other STDs to be better able to help their clients understand and come to terms with these diseases.

Tuberculosis

Both directly and indirectly, chronic chemical abuse contributes to the spread of a wide range of infectious diseases. Chronic substance abuse has indirectly contributed to the return of tuberculosis (TB) (Cherubin & Sapira, 1993). Because malnutrition is so frequently a side effect of chronic chemical abuse, alcoholics and drug addicts are at high risk for contracting TB. Furthermore, the typical addict's lifestyle makes treatment compliance difficult, a characteristic that has contributed to the rise of drug-resistant strains of the bacteria that cause TB. Finally, individuals whose immune system is compromised, such as individuals with HIV, are at risk for becoming infected with TB.

What Is Tuberculosis?

Tuberculosis is an infectious disease caused by the bacterium *Mycobacterium tuberculosis* (Boutotte, 1993). Although in the past the treatment of TB was a long, complicated affair with no guarantee of success, new medications were introduced in the 1950s that offered the hope of completely curing the patient of the disease in just a few months. For this reason, physicians thought that TB was no longer a major threat to the public. Unfortunately, new strains of TB are appearing that are resistant to many of the medications that were previously effective in treating it. Physicians have also discovered that many patients with HIV who were previously exposed to TB may develop TB as one of the "opportunistic infections" that develop when the individual's immune system is damaged.

TB usually invades the pulmonary system, although it is possible for TB to infect virtually every organ system in the body. The bacteria seem to prefer oxygen-rich body tissues, such as those found in the lungs, central nervous system, and kidneys (Boutotte, 1993). Because the most common site of infection in the United States is the lungs, we will focus our attention on this form of TB.

Tuberculosis is transmitted when the individual inhales a small droplet of body fluid that contains the bacteria. Whenever a person sings, talks, coughs, or sneezes, he or she releases microscopic droplets of moisture from the lungs that could remain suspended in the air for extended periods of time. If the person has active TB in the respiratory system, these moisture droplets will carry the bacteria into the surrounding air where another person might breathe them in (Boutotte, 1993).

Initially, once TB gains admission to the individual's body, the individual's immune system attacks the invading bacteria. The initial response by a part of the immune system known as *macrophages* is to engulf the invading bacteria, surround them, and wall them inside little pockets known as *granulomas*. This prevents the infection from proceeding further. However, *Mycobacterium tuberculosis* is difficult to destroy, and the bacteria could survive in a dormant stage within the granulomas for years or decades. If the immune system becomes weakened, perhaps by another infection or malnutrition, the body can no longer keep the bacteria isolated in the granulomas. Eventually, the TB bacteria can burst out and again invade the surrounding body tissue. This is known as "reactivation TB," which accounts for about 85% of all cases of TB in the United States (Boutotte, 1993).

At this point, the body tries a different approach to attacking the invading bacteria. Another part of the immune system, the *lymphocytes,* attempt to destroy the bacteria. Unfortunately, during this process, they release a toxin that also destroys surrounding lung tissue. Eventually, as less and less of the lung is able to function properly, the patient dies of pulmonary failure.

The Treatment of TB

Although a great deal has been written about "treatment resistant" TB in the past few years, physicians have access to a wide range of medications that they can call on to treat this infection. Unfortunately, the treatment process can take as long as 6 to 9 months, and the patient needs to take the proper medications on a daily basis for that period of time (Boutotte, 1993). Failure to follow the established treatment program allows some active TB germs to remain in the body. Because they have survived the patient's initial use of the medication, these germs would be more resistant to the same medications in the future.

Hepatitis B

One of the viral infections that is often transmitted between intravenous drug addicts is hepatitis B. Hepatitis B is one of four different viral diseases that infects the liver: hepatitis type A, B, C, and D. Each virus has a different mode of transmission and a different clinical course. In this section, we will focus our discussion on hepatitis type "B" (or HVB).

What Is Hepatitis B?

HVB is known to be *extremely* contagious, perhaps on the order of 100 times as contagious as HIV. The HIV virus is quite fragile and requires direct exposure to the infected individual's body fluids. But people have contracted HVB by sharing a toothbrush or a razor with an infected person or simply by kissing someone who is infected (Brody, 1991).

There are several mechanisms through which the hepatitis B virus can either directly or indirectly lead to death. First, the virus infects the liver, causing damage to that organ. If the liver damage is great enough, HVB might kill the individual through simple liver failure. This is a rare, but not unknown, result of hepatitis B infection. However, hepatitis B can kill in another way. For reasons that are not known at this time, a person who has been infected with the hepatitis B virus is *200 times as likely* to develop liver cancer as is a noninfected person (Brody, 1991). Liver cancer is quite difficult to detect or treat and is usually fatal. Thus, the hepatitis B virus can indirectly cause the death of the infected person by cancer of the liver.

The Route of Infection for Hepatitis B

Like HIV, hepatitis B can be transmitted through blood transfusions, which has led to the development of blood tests to screen out donors who might be carrying the virus. Two decades ago, the rate of infection with the hepatitis B virus was 1 per 100 units of blood transfused (Edelson, 1993). However, new blood tests for screening potential blood donors (and new ways of storing blood prior to use) have reduced the rate of hepatitis B infection to about 1 in 3,500 units of blood used.

In the United States, a common means by which hepatitis B is transmitted from one person to another is through the sharing of intravenous drug paraphernalia among addicts. Blood tests from intravenous drug users suggest that between 75 and 98% of intravenous drug users have been exposed to HVB virus at some time in their lives (Michelson et al., 1988).

HVB is also found in the semen of most infected men, and like HIV, can be passed on to another person through the semen. People involved in sexual relationships with infected partners are "at risk" for contracting HVB. For this reason, HVB could be classified as a sexually transmitted disease (STD). People involved in sexual relationships with homosexual or bisexual males are also considered to be "at risk" for HVB (and other STDs). Promiscuous sexual activity increases the individual's risk of exposure to a wide range of STDs. Because of the high probability that drug addicts, promiscuous individuals, prostitutes, and bisexual or homosexual males are infected, it is advised that sexual contact with people in these categories be avoided.

Scope of the Problem of HVB Infection

It is difficult to obtain a true picture of the hepatitis B infection pattern, if only because there are no symptoms of infection in up to half of those who are infected (Brody, 1991). But, to put the problem of HVB exposure into perspective, it was estimated in 1990 that there were 300,000 *new* cases of hepatitis B in the United States alone.

The Treatment of HVB

The most effective "treatment" for HVB is prevention. It is possible to immunize against HVB, and immunization is recommended for individuals who are likely to be exposed to the body fluids of an infected individual. For example, individuals who should be immunized against HVB include health care workers and the spouse of an infected individual.

Summary

It is impossible to identify in advance every potential complication that could arise during a substance abuse rehabilitation program. In this chapter, a few of the most common problems encountered by substance abuse treatment professionals were reviewed. Examples of such problems include the client who will "test the limits" of the treatment program and its staff, and the client who will attempt to control the process of treatment through the use of a "secret."

A major complication of treatment is the tendency for the client to relapse. The four elements that most commonly contribute to relapse were identified and discussed. The impact of infections such as that caused by HIV, TB, and hepatitis B were also discussed.

CHAPTER THIRTY-ONE

Pharmacological Intervention Tactics and Substance Abuse

In a very real sense, the pharmacological treatment of substance abuse is a logical extension of the medical model. It is based on the premise that the individual's substance use can be controlled or totally eliminated through various biochemical substances. The specific components of treatment may vary from one program to another. But, whether it is detoxification from alcohol, the prevention of relapse for the chronic drinker, or the control of the "craving" for cocaine, all forms of pharmacological interventions center on the use of selected chemicals to combat substance abuse.

The Pharmacological Treatment of Alcoholism

Frances and Miller (1991) struck a rather pessimistic note when they observed that, even after a century of searching for an antidipsotrophic medication, "at this writing there is no proven biological treatment for alcoholism. Each promising drug that has been tested in the hope it

The pharmacological support of alcohol or drug withdrawal, or as part of the treatment of an ongoing substance abuse problem, should be supervised by a licensed physician who is skilled and experienced in working with substance abuse cases. The information provided in this chapter is provided for educational purposes only. It is not intended to encourage self-treatment of substance abuse problems, nor should it be interpreted as a standard of care for patients who are addicted to chemicals.

would reduce relapse by intervening in the basic disease process has failed" (p. 13). However, the authors note, Antabuse (disulfiram) continues to provide one avenue for the symptomatic treatment of alcoholism.

Antabuse

For the past 40 years, the primary pharmacological agent that has been used in the fight against alcoholism is Antabuse (disulfiram). The theory behind the use of disulfiram is that, although the exact cause(s) of the individual's alcoholism may be unknown, it is still possible to utilize various chemical agents to interfere with the reward value of alcohol. Disulfiram is a potentially dangerous drug that should not be used with patients who have serious medical disorders (Schuckit, 1989), but it has been a useful tool in the fight against alcoholism.

For those patients who *can* use disulfiram, it often provides the time for a "second thought" desperately needed by the alcoholic who is tempted to drink. Disulfiram *does not decrease the alcoholic's desire to drink*, but it does interfere with the metabolism of alcohol after it enters the individual's body. The combination of alcohol with disulfiram causes a number of unpleasant—*and potentially fatal*—effects. This knowledge is then used to help the alcoholic who wants a "second chance" consider the consequences of even one drink in a new light.

The individual is warned about the effects of combining alcohol with disulfiram when the medication is started. Disulfiram allows acetaldehyde to build up in the blood. If the individual were to ingest even small amounts of alcohol, he or she would experience facial flushing, heart palpitations and a rapid heart rate, difficulty in breathing, nausea, vomiting, and possibly a serious drop in blood pressure (Schuckit, 1989).

The strength of these side effects depends on how much alcohol has been ingested, the amount of disulfiram being used each day, and how long it has been since the last dose of disulfiram was ingested. The period of time since the last dose of disulfiram is important because the body tends to metabolize the drug. Thus, over time, the effects of any given dose become less and less powerful. Although alcohol/disulfiram interactions have been reported for up to 2 weeks after the last dose was ingested, one cannot count on disulfiram reacting with alcohol for such an extended period of time. Usually, the individual will have to take the medication either daily or, at the very least, three times a week.

Another shortcoming of disulfiram is that it does not *immediately* interact with alcohol. Under normal conditions, it takes 3 to 12 hours after the first dose of disulfiram before it can begin to interfere with the metabolism of alcohol. After the individual has been using disulfiram for several days, however, he or she will experience the reaction within about 30 minutes of the time he or she ingests the first drink (Schuckit, 1989). Typically, the disulfiram/alcohol interaction lasts for 30 to 60 minutes, although there are reports of it lasting longer.

To make sure that the user understands the consequences of mixing alcohol with disulfiram, some treatment centers advocate a learning process in which the patient takes disulfiram for a short period of time (usually a few days) and then is allowed to drink a small amount of alcohol under controlled conditions. This is done so that the alcoholic can experience the negative consequences of mixing alcohol and disulfiram under supervision. When this technique is utilized, the treatment staff has access to the proper medications and respiratory support equipment to help the client recover from the alcohol/disulfiram interaction effects. The intention is that allowing alcoholics to experience the negative consequences after drinking only a small amount of alcohol will keep them from being tempted to drink a large amount of alcohol on their own, outside of the treatment center.

On occasion, treatment professionals have encountered the situation in which a codependent spouse inquires about obtaining disulfiram to "teach the alcoholic a lesson." The spouse usually wants a sample of disulfiram to place in the alcoholic's coffee or "eye opener." Then the next time the alcoholic drinks, he or she will experience the alcohol/disulfiram interaction without expecting it. Needless to say, *disulfiram should never be given to an individual without the user's knowledge and consent*. The interaction between disulfiram and alcohol is *potentially serious* and *may require emergency hospitalization for observation and treatment*. Death *is* possible from the mixture of alcohol and disulfiram.

A serious drawback of disulfiram is that the 30-minute delay between the individual's first drink and the development of the alcohol/disulfiram reaction makes disulfiram of little value in aversive conditioning programs. To be effective, aversive conditioning programs require *immediate* consequences paired to undesired behavior. Theoretically, an effective behavior modification program for alcoholism would involve the use of an immediate consequence. In this manner, the person learns to associate drinking behavior with a negative response and, in theory, will gradually discontinue the undesired behavior. The 30-minute delay between the ingestion of alcohol and the disulfiram/alcohol reaction is far too long for it to serve as an *immediate* consequence for the drinker, making it difficult for the person to associate the use of alcohol with the delayed discomfort caused by the alcohol/disulfiram reaction.

Another significant disadvantage of disulfiram is that its *full* effects last only about 24 to 48 hours. The individual needs to take the drug every day, or perhaps every other day, for optimal effectiveness. Between doses, the disulfiram is gradually eliminated from the body by the liver. Thus, it is up to the individual to take the medication according to the schedule worked out with a physician to ensure that there is an adequate supply of the drug in the body at all times. Obviously, medication compliance can be a serious problem for some alcoholics who use disulfiram.

Furthermore, disulfiram often reacts to the small amounts of alcohol found in many over-the-counter cough syrups, aftershaves, or any of a wide range of other products. The individual using disulfiram should be warned to avoid certain products to prevent an unintentional reaction. Most treatment centers or physicians who utilize disulfiram have lists of such products and foods that they provide to patients on disulfiram.

Research suggests that disulfiram interacts with the neurotransmitter serotonin, boosting brain levels of a byproduct of serotonin known as 5-hydroxytryptophol (5-HTOL) (Cowen, 1990). Animal research indicates that increased levels of 5-HTOL result in greater alcohol consumption. Although research with human subjects has yet to be completed, preliminary data suggests that there is a need for alcoholics to avoid "serotonin rich" foods, such as bananas and walnuts, to avoid increasing the craving for alcohol many recovering alcoholics experience.

Disulfiram is *not* recommended for individuals who have a history of cardiovascular disease, cerebrovascular disease, kidney failure, depression, seizure disorders, or liver disease or for those who might be pregnant (Fuller, 1989). Drug interactions have been reported between disulfiram and phenytoin (sold under the brand name of Dilantin), warfarin, isoniazid (used in the treatment of tuberculosis), diazepam (Valium), chlordiazepoxide (Librium), and several commonly used antidepressants (Fuller, 1989). Patients who are taking the antitubercular drug isoniazid (or "INH") should not take disulfiram. When used together, these drugs may bring on a

toxic psychosis or cause other neurological problems (Meyers, 1992).

Patients who use disulfiram should do so only under the supervision of a physician who has a *complete* medication use history on the patient. Because of the danger of disulfiram/medication interactions, the use of multiple prescriptions from different doctors should be strongly discouraged.

In spite of these disadvantages, research has demonstrated that alcoholism treatment programs that use disulfiram as a part of the overall treatment program have a lower relapse rate than programs that do not (Adelman & Weiss, 1989). What disulfiram does, once the person has taken the scheduled dose, is to provide the individual with the knowledge that he or she will be unable to drink for that day, or for perhaps as long as 2 weeks afterward—at least not without becoming very sick.

Disulfiram is not effective for everyone. Some alcoholics will drink in spite of the disulfiram in their system, which is known as trying to "drink through" the disulfiram. Many alcoholics stop taking the drug several days before a "spontaneous" relapse, and only about 20% of those individuals who start on the drug actually take it for a full year. Furthermore, many alcoholics believe that they know how to neutralize the drug while it is in their body. However, for the majority of those who use disulfiram as intended, the drug provides the individual an extra bit of support during a weak moment.

Lithium

Recently, there has been a great deal of attention devoted to the use of lithium in the treatment of alcoholism. Lithium is an element that has been useful in the treatment of bipolar affective disorders (formerly called the manic/depressive disorder). Surprisingly, lithium also apparently reduces the number of relapses that chronic alcoholics experience, reduces the apparent level of intoxication, and reduces the desire of chronic alcoholics to drink (Judd & Huey, 1984; Miller, Frances, & Holmes, 1989).

Unfortunately, research findings about the effectiveness of lithium in the treatment of chronic alcoholism are inconclusive, and there is no indication that lithium would be useful in the treatment of *every* chronic alcoholic (Miller, Frances, & Holmes, 1989). However, research into what subtypes of alcoholics might benefit from the use of lithium and under what circumstances lithium might be used continues at this time.

Naltrexone

In recent years, researchers have discovered that drugs that function as antagonists for the *mu* opioid receptor site in the brain—that is, those drugs that block the *mu* opioid receptor site— seem to reduce alcohol consumption in both animals and man (Swift, Whelihan, Kuznetsov, Buongiorno, & Hsuing, 1994). One such drug is naltrexone, a drug normally used in the treatment of narcotics addiction.

Volpicelli, Alterman, Hayashida, and O'Brien (1992) administered 50 mg/day of naltrexone to a sample of diagnosed alcoholics. The subjects received the naltrexone following detoxification from alcohol, and their relapse rate was contrasted with that of a matched group of alcoholics who received only a placebo. The authors found that the naltrexone treatment group reported significantly fewer "cravings" for alcohol than did those who received the placebo. Furthermore, the authors found that 54% of the alcoholics who received the placebo relapsed during the 12 weeks of the study, whereas only 23% of those who received naltrexone relapsed during the study.

The exact mechanism by which naltrexone may block the pleasurable effects of the alcohol is not known at this time. However, it does appear that naltrexone is able to reduce alcohol's reward value as a drug of abuse (Swift et al., 1994; Holloway, 1991). Further research suggests that naltrexone may offer other advan-

tages in the fight against alcohol dependence as well.

Other Pharmacological Treatments for Chronic Alcoholism

There are medications other than disulfiram that also cause discomfort when mixed with alcohol. Graedon (1980) reports that, when mixed with alcohol, Flagyl (metronidazole) causes nausea, vomiting, flushing, and headache. Researchers briefly experimented with metronidazole as a possible antidipsotrophic medication in the 1970s, but discontinued further research when they found little evidence to suggest it was effective (Holder et al., 1991).

However, one physician elected to use metronidazole as a short-term substitute for a patient who was allergic to Antabuse. This currently is not a recommended use of this medication by the Food and Drug Administration, but the physician was able to provide pharmacological support for an alcoholic who needed some external constraint during the initial period of sobriety, when most at risk of relapsing. This is not to say that metronidazole should be routinely administered to alcoholics who require pharmacological support. There is evidence that metronidazole has a significant potential for causing cancer (Graedon, 1980). The patient who uses metronidazole should do so only when the benefits clearly outweigh the risk.

In the 1980s, Blum and Trachtenberg (1988) proposed a different treatment approach to the rehabilitation of the alcoholic. They suggested that alcohol craving might be influenced by the neurochemicals available in the brain and that the use of a "neurotransmitter precursor loading" system (Blum & Trachtenberg, 1988, p. 5) may aid in the treatment of alcoholism. In theory, proper nutritional supplements will

> improve brain nutrition, improve the balance of the neurotransmitters, reduce the craving, and help the alcoholic respond more favorably to supportive treatment such as that provided by

treatment centers, counselors, and Alcoholics Anonymous. (Blum & Trachtenberg, 1988, p. 35)

This novel treatment approach was thought to show promise, according to the authors, who offer a patented combination of vitamins, amino acids, and minerals for use in the rehabilitation of alcoholics. This approach offered the advantage of using nonaddictive substances that the body could utilize to restore the balance of neurotransmitters found in the otherwise healthy brain. However, subsequent research has failed to find any positive effects from this approach (Peele, 1991).

The Pharmacological Treatment of Narcotics Addiction

Naltrexone hydrochloride (Trexan) is a new tool in the treatment of opioid abuse. This drug blocks the euphoric effects of injected opiates for up to 72 hours, depending on the dose used. The theory behind the use of the narcotics blocker is that, if the person taking it does not experience any feelings of euphoria from opiates, he or she is less likely to use opiates again.

Naltrexone *should be used only after the person is completely detoxified from opiates* to avoid bringing about an undesired withdrawal syndrome in an opiate addict. Callahan (1980) notes that few addicts attempt to use narcotics even once while on the blocker. However, when the medication is discontinued, the addict will again experience a craving for narcotics. Thus, there is no extinction of the craving for the drug during the period of time that the narcotics addict is being maintained on a narcotics blocker.

Jenike (1991) reports that a 50-mg dose of naltrexone will block the euphoria of an injection of narcotics for 24 hours, and a 100-mg dose will work for about 48 hours; a 150-mg dose of naltrexone will block the euphoria for 72 hours. According to Jenike, the usual dosage schedule is 3 times a week, with 100 mg being administered on Monday and Wednesday and 150 mg being administered on Friday to provide a longer term dose for the weekend.

To date, there is no research that demonstrates an *unequivocal* benefit from this medication in the treatment of narcotics addiction (Medical Economics Company, 1995). Indeed, research has discovered that a major drawback of naltrexone is that many addicts discontinue the drug on their own (Youngstrom, 1990a). In one study exploring the application of naltrexone in the treatment of narcotics addiction, *only 2%* of the original sample continued to take the drug for 9 months (Youngstrom, 1990a). Holloway (1991) suggests that naltrexone is most useful for the narcotics addict who is "motivated to stay drug free" (p. 100). Thus, although this drug does seem to offer pharmacological support during the initial period after detoxification when an addict is most vulnerable to relapse, its applicability in the long-term treatment of narcotics addiction is still unclear.

Narcotics Withdrawal

Programs that specialize in the treatment of narcotics addiction often offer controlled withdrawal from opiates. Occasionally, a hospital offers narcotics withdrawal programs even if that hospital does not attempt to provide long-term treatment for narcotics addicts. The detoxification component in each center is very much the same.

Methadone, which is taken orally, is the traditional drug of choice for narcotics withdrawal (Jenike, 1991). Methadone is a synthetic narcotic, first developed during World War II by German chemists as a substitute for morphine. Mirin, Weiss, and Greenfield (1991) point out that methadone has the additional advantage of a duration of action between 24 and 36 hours. They note that a daily dosage level of between 10 and 40 mg of methadone is usually sufficient to prevent withdrawal symptoms in narcotics addicts.

The individual is given an initial methadone dosage schedule of 10 mg/hour for the first day (Mirin, Weiss, & Greenfield, 1991), with an additional 10 mg of methadone administered each hour until the withdrawal symptoms are brought under control. Once the withdrawal symptoms have been controlled, the total dose of methadone administered becomes the starting dose for withdrawal. On the second day of withdrawal, the addict receives whatever dosage level terminated withdrawal symptoms on the first day, but the entire amount is administered in the morning in a single dose. Starting on the third day, the daily dose of methadone is reduced by 5 mg each day until the patient is completely detoxified from opiates (Mirin, Weiss, & Greenfield, 1991).

The usual detoxification program lasts between 3 and 21 days (Mirin, Weiss, & Greenfield, 1991), and if a detoxification program lasts longer, it must be licensed by the government as a methadone maintenance project (Jenike, 1991). Surprisingly, in spite of their length, detoxification programs have a significant dropout rate. For example, Mirin, Weiss, and Greenfield (1991) found that, as the daily dosage levels drop to the 15 or 20 mg/day range, the individual experiences a return of withdrawal symptoms. It is at this point that many individuals drop out of detoxification. Indeed, a timely reminder from the authors is that opiate addicts going through withdrawal should be warned that they should *not* expect a symptom-free withdrawal.

Other programs, however, operate on the philosophy that methadone withdrawal is inappropriate. Some narcotics addicts have reported that methadone withdrawal is, in their opinion, worse than going "cold turkey." However, as noted in the chapter on narcotics, withdrawal from opiates is not life-threatening, and many addicts have reported that, if the truth be told, withdrawal from narcotics is no worse than having a bad cold or the flu.

Some programs offer pharmacological support during the withdrawal phase, such as benzodiazepines to help the person relax and sleep, but they do not use narcotics. Other programs use a combination of nonnarcotic drugs to facilitate opiate withdrawal, such as the one outlined by Stein and Kosten (1992). They reviewed a treatment program in which two different drugs, an antihypertensive (clonidine hydrochloride) and an opiate blocker (naltrexone)

were used to bring about a 4- to 5-day opiate withdrawal. They concluded that, when used appropriately, the combination of clonidine and naltrexone was as effective as a 20-day methadone withdrawal program for opiate addicts. The interaction between the naltrexone and the clonidine allows for a rapid withdrawal from narcotics, and the clonidine hydrochloride also serves to control the individual's craving for narcotics.

Stein and Kosten found that over 95% of their sample were completely withdrawn from narcotics at the end of 5 days. Although there was some degree of discomfort, the addicts reported about the same level of discomfort from withdrawal using a combination of clonidine and naltrexone as they experienced during a methadone taper. Milhorn (1992) suggests that withdrawal discomfort might be further reduced through the use of transdermal clonidine patches, which provide a steady supply of the drug while the patch is in place. However, because of the delay in absorption, Milhorn advocates using an oral "loading" dose of 0.2 mg of clonidine at the beginning of the withdrawal cycle.

Although clonidine seems to be an effective tool to control the discomfort of narcotics withdrawal, some addicts have learned to combine clonidine with methadone, alcohol, benzodiazepines, or other drugs to produce a sense of euphoria (Jenike, 1991). Health care professionals must carefully monitor the patient's medication use to prevent abuse by the addict who is no longer able to use narcotics.

Methadone Maintenance Programs

The concept of methadone maintenance was first advanced by Dole and Nyswander (1965) and has since become the treatment of choice for narcotics addicts (especially those addicted to heroin). Estimates of the number of heroin addicts in the United States involved in a methadone maintenance program range from approximately 80,000 (Kanof, Aronson, & Ness, 1992) to 99,100 (Strain, Stritzer, Liebson, &

Bigelow, 1994). Of this number, perhaps 35,000 methadone maintenance patients are in New York City alone (Levy & Rutter, 1992).

The theory behind methadone maintenance is that the use of opiates in certain individuals causes permanent changes in brain function at the cellular level (Dole, 1988; Dole & Nyswander, 1965). Dole and Nyswander postulate that *even a single dose* of narcotics will bring about a change in the structure of the brain of the addict-to-be, forever altering the way his or her brain functions. According to this theory, when the narcotics are removed from the body, the individual will "crave" narcotics for months or even years afterward. This drug craving makes it more likely that the individual will ultimately return to the use of narcotics, if just to feel "normal" again.

This, according to Dole and Nyswander (1965), forms the basis of narcotics addiction. They knew that methadone, when administered orally in high dosage levels, would block the majority of the euphoric effects of injected narcotics. By substituting a sufficiently high dosage of oral methadone to "otherwise intractable" opioid addicts (Dole, 1989, p. 1880), they hoped to eliminate the individual's need for further illegal drug use to support the narcotics addiction. In theory, this was hoped to lead to an extinction of the intravenous narcotics use over time (National Academy of Sciences, 1990).

Dole (1988), who remains one of the major proponents of the methadone maintenance concept, refers to this treatment approach as "corrective, but not curative" (p. 3025) for the suspected (but as yet unproved) neurological dysfunction that brings about the compulsive use of narcotics. The usual dosage level, administered in a single dose is between 40 and 120 mg of methadone each day. It is usually administered in the morning in liquid form, often mixed with a fruit juice.

The initial results of the methadone maintenance concept were quite promising (Callahan, 1980). However, the original concept of methadone maintenance was that it would be a part of a larger rehabilitation program. Dole and Nyswander (1965) believed that when the suspected neurological dysfunction brought on by the use of narcotics "has been normalized, the ex-addict, supported by counseling and social services, can begin the long process of social rehabilitation" (Dole, 1988, p. 3025). Unfortunately, many methadone maintenance clinics became little more than drug distribution centers, with no effort being made at actual rehabilitation (Cohen & Levy, 1992; *The Addiction Letter*, 1989a).

McLellan, Arndt, Metzger, Woody, and O'Brien (1993) found that, when methadone maintenance was combined with a range of psychosocial support services (psychotherapy, vocational counseling, social services, and so on), significantly larger numbers of narcotics addicts were able to remain drug-free for longer periods of time than when such services were lacking. They conclude that providing such service was cost-effective for severely impaired addicts, and they recommend that methadone maintenance programs provide more than simply a steady supply of oral methadone.

Although these results are promising, the concept of methadone maintenance is still not without its critics. Some physicians challenge the concept of methadone maintenance on the grounds that it only replaces one addictive substance with another. A significant number of physicians also question the morality of physicians deliberately administering methadone, an addictive substance, to persons who are known to suffer from addictive disorders (Glass, 1993).

As many critics of methadone maintenance note, the assumption that narcotics use results in permanent neurological changes has never been proved. Furthermore, critics argue, although the person may not crave narcotics and may even be unable to experience the euphoria of injected narcotics while on methadone, this does not prevent him or her from abusing cocaine, alcohol, marijuana, benzodiazepines, or any other drug. Indeed, between 50 and 90% of the patients in methadone maintenance programs use other recreational drugs (Glantz & Woods, 1993). Even Dole (1989) acknowledges that methadone is "highly specific for the treatment of opiate addiction" (p. 1880), it will not block the euphoric effects of other drugs of abuse, and there is no similar pharmacological therapy for nonopiate addictions.

Methadone maintenance has always been a controversial concept. Yet, for a number of reasons, adequately staffed programs with appropriate psychosocial support do appear to be a viable treatment option for the treatment of opiate addicts. Yet in spite of the advantages supposedly offered by this treatment approach, methadone maintenance programs suffer from a significant dropout rate. This indicates that methadone maintenance programs are not the final answer to the problem of narcotics addiction.

Since methadone maintenance was first proposed as a "treatment" for narcotics addiction (some would say "substitute"), the program has been found to have other benefits beyond those suggested by Dole and Nyswander. First, and perhaps most important, methadone maintenance programs appear to slow the spread of HIV infection. Because methadone maintenance programs reduce the tendency for participants to use intravenously administered drugs, the chances that a given addict will be exposed to the virus through contaminated needles is reduced. One study in New York City found that less than 10% of those narcotics addicts who were admitted to methadone maintenance programs prior to 1978 were HIV positive, at a time when over 50% of the addicts who were still using narcotics were infected with this virus (Council on Addiction Psychiatry, 1994).

Second, the National Academy of Sciences (1990) concluded that by providing the addict with a supply of methadone so that he or she does not have to use "street" narcotics to avoid withdrawal symptoms, methadone maintenance programs reduce the level of criminal activity on the part of participants. This, in turn, makes methadone maintenance programs a cost-effective way of dealing with chronic narcotics addiction by offering a greater savings to society than the program costs. Thus, although there is little evidence to support the theory of Dole and Nyswander's (1965) original theory as to the *cause* of narcotics addiction, the concept of methadone maintenance does seem to have a role to play in the treatment of chronic narcotics addiction.

Recent Forms of Pharmacological Intervention in Narcotics Addiction

Recently, a synthetic narcotic agent developed in the 1960s, buprenorphine, was introduced as an alternative to methadone in the long-term maintenance of intravenous narcotics addicts. Researchers had discovered that buprenorphine binds to the same opiate receptor sites in the brain that are utilized by morphine.

As an analgesic, buprenorphine is thought to be between 25 and 40 times as potent as morphine (Singh, Mattoo, Malhotra, & Varma, 1992), making it of value in the control of high levels of pain. However, researchers also have discovered that orally administered doses of buprenorphine can actually block the euphoric effects of intravenously administered narcotics (Horgan, 1989; Rosen & Kosten, 1991). Indeed, low oral doses of buprenorphine are at least as effective as methadone in blocking the euphoria experienced when a narcotics addict injects an opiate-based drug (Strain, Stritzer, Liebson, & Bigelow, 1994). Furthermore, when used in a treatment program similar to methadone maintenance programs, buprenorphine can be administered just once a day. These features made buprenorphine an attractive alternative to methadone.

But buprenorphine offers other advantages over methadone. First, unlike methadone, there is little incentive for the individual to take more medication than is needed. High doses of buprenorphine actually act as a narcotic antagonist, producing effects similar to naltrexone. This means that the medication is, to a significant degree, self-limiting. At high doses, the antagonist effect actually blocks the respiratory depression and euphoria one might expect the user to experience from a narcotic analgesic that he or she has intentionally abused (Council on Addiction Psychiatry, 1994). Another advantage is that, whereas withdrawal from methadone can last up to 2 weeks, withdrawal from buprenorphine lasts only a few days (Horgan, 1989). And withdrawal from buprenorphine does not seem to make the individual as uncomfortable as happens during withdrawal from methadone (Council on Addiction Psychiatry, 1994; Rosen & Kosten, 1991).

However, buprenorphine is not a "magic bullet." Although *orally* administered buprenorphine has no euphoric value, *intravenously* administered buprenorphine has a significant abuse potential (Horgan, 1989). Intravenous buprenorphine, used either by itself or when mixed with diazepam, cyclizine, or temazepam, has been abused by narcotics addicts in New Zealand, Ireland, India (Singh et al., 1992), and the United States (Torrens, San, & Cami, 1993). Thus, although buprenorphine may prove to be a valuable tool in working with narcotics addicts, it is not the ultimate answer to the problem of how to treat intravenous opiate addicts.

Another chemical that has been approved as a possible agent in treating opiate addicts is L-alpha-acetylmethadol (LAAM). Like methadone, orally administered LAAM prevents the opiate addict from going into withdrawal. But the fact that LAAM has a biological half-life of in excess of 48 hours (as compared with methadone's half-life of 24 hours) means that the individual need only take the drug once every 2 to 3 days (*Alcoholism & Drug Abuse Week*, 1993). This virtually eliminates the need for the patient to take doses home, vastly reducing the problem of drug diversion to the illicit market.

Another advantage is that research suggests that withdrawal from LAAM may be easier than withdrawal from methadone (*Alcoholism & Drug Abuse Week*, 1993). However, at this point, it is too early to determine how effective LAAM may be in the treatment of narcotics addiction.

The Pharmacological Treatment of Cocaine Addiction

Since the last epidemic of cocaine abuse and addiction began, researchers have attempted to find an agent or agents that will control the "craving" or "hunger" for cocaine that many addicts experience in the earlier stages of recovery. Early reports suggest that antidepressant medications such as imipramine (Wilbur, 1986), or desipramine hydrochloride (Jenike, 1991; Gawin et al., 1989), when used at therapeutic dosage levels, are effective in curbing the postwithdrawal "craving" for cocaine.

Unfortunately, Meyer (1992) challenges the results of the study by Gawin et al. (1989) on methodological grounds, claiming that their study was flawed. Other researchers have also failed to replicate the results found by Gawin et al., according to Meyer. Thus, there is some doubt as to whether antidepressant medications such as desimipramine hydrochloride are actually effective in controlling the craving for cocaine that many addicts report.

Even if desimipramine hydrochloride is eventually found to be an effective agent in controlling the craving for cocaine, there is still some debate over whether or not it is *safe* to use antidepressants to curb postcocaine craving. Decker, Fins, and Frances (1987) note that "Little attention has been given to the possible cardiac risks of using antidepressants to prevent cocaine intoxication or to treat 'crashes' or withdrawal symptoms" (p. 465).

To avoid these possible cardiac complications, Margolin, Kosten, Petrakis, Avants, and Kosten (1991) used a "second generation" antidepressant, bupropion (Wellbutrin), to try to control postcocaine craving. The authors report that 5 of 6 subjects completed the experiment; 1 subject was dropped for medical reasons. Of the 5 remaining individuals, 4 subjects had stopped using cocaine after a period of 4 weeks and were still cocaine-free after 3 months. Unfortunately, their results are marred by the fact that the research sample was made up of only 6 subjects. Thus, further research into the applicability of bupropion and its effectiveness is needed before this medication is generally accepted as being of value in the treatment of cocaine abuse.

A significant problem with using tricyclic antidepressants to control the craving for cocaine that many addicts experience is that it typically takes 7 to 14 days for the antidepressant to *begin* to reduce the craving (Gawin, Allen, & Humblestone, 1989). It may take an additional 7 to 14 days before the medication reaches full effectiveness. Many addicts are unable or unwilling to tolerate the severe craving for cocaine they experience during this period, and so they drop out of treatment.

As a possible solution to this problem, Gawin, Allen, and Humblestone (1989) experimented with the drug flupenthixol as a means to control the craving for cocaine. Flupenthixol is currently available in Europe, the Far East, and the Caribbean but not the United States. This drug seems to be quite effective in the control of postcocaine craving, according to the authors, who call for further research into its use in the treatment of cocaine addicts. According to Holloway (1991), some cocaine addicts on flupenthixol report that their craving for cocaine is "manageable but is not eliminated" (p. 100). This suggests that flupenthixol shows some promise in the treatment of cocaine addiction, but other options still need to be explored.

Another drug that has demonstrated some promise in controlling cocaine craving, at least in experimental settings, is bromocriptine (sold in the United States under the brand name Parlodel) (DiGregorio, 1990). When administered in a single dose of 1.25 mg, bromocriptine was found to decrease cocaine withdrawal craving, according to DiGregorio (1990), and 0.625 mg given by mouth 4 times a day was found to reduce psychiatric symptoms associated with cocaine withdrawal.

Unfortunately, bromocriptine's side effects include headaches, sedation, muscle tremor, and dry mouth, which may make the user so uncomfortable as to discontinue use of this drug. Furthermore, the possibility that bromocriptine is itself addictive has been suggested. Holloway

(1991) reports that early clinical trials with bromocriptine have failed to yield any positive results, suggesting that this medication will ultimately prove of little value in the treatment of cocaine addiction.

Surprisingly, another agent that has shown promise in the treatment of cocaine withdrawal craving is buprenorphine. In addition to its effectiveness in laboratory studies with narcotics addicts, buprenorphine has also had an effect on the postcocaine craving (*The Economist*, 1989; Youngstrom, 1990a; Holloway, 1991; Rosen & Kosten, 1991). At low doses, oral buprenorphine seems to reduce the craving for cocaine, although the exact mechanism by which this is accomplished remains unknown (Holloway, 1991; Rosen & Kosten, 1991).

As Trachtenberg and Blum (1988) suggest, cocaine's effects may be brought about, at least in part, by activation of both dopamine and opioid peptide neurotransmitter systems. The authors point out, for example, that naloxone, which is normally used to block the effects of narcotics in the brain, actually potentiates the stimulation and euphoria of cocaine. If their theory is true, then the reward mechanisms for both cocaine and the narcotics seem to involve activation of the same neurotransmission systems. Thus, it seems to make sense that a drug such as buprenorphine might prove of value in controlling the craving for both narcotics and cocaine.

In 1988, a different treatment approach for cocaine addiction was suggested by Trachtenberg and Blum. They theorized that cocaine addiction may be influenced by neurochemicals naturally occurring in the brain. In an extension of the "neurotransmitter precursor loading" system used in their treatment of alcoholism, Blum and Trachtenberg advocate the use of a "nutritional neurochemical support" system (p. 326) to aid in the treatment of cocaine addiction. The authors suggest the use of a combination of amino acids and selected minerals and vitamins to try to stimulate the formation of the neurotransmitters depleted by chronic cocaine use. In one research study, the authors claimed a ninefold reduction in dropout rates for patients in an experimental group who received a patented formulation of "nutritional neurochemical support" over those who did not receive such support. But in the past few years, interest in the neuronutrient approach to the treatment of cocaine addiction has waned.

Surprisingly, after conducting an investigation into the cocaine withdrawal process, Satel et al. (1991) challenge the need for routine pharmacological support of recovering cocaine addicts. They concluded that their data "failed to demonstrate the emergence" (p. 1715) of severe withdrawal symptoms following the initiation of abstinence, and, although there were reports of craving for cocaine, their subjects experienced a marked decline in the strength and frequency of such craving over the first 3 weeks of recovery. For these reasons, Satel et al. conclude that there does not seem to be a need for routine pharma-

cological support during the early stages of recovery from cocaine addiction.

Summary

The pharmacological treatment of substance abuse involves the use of selected chemicals to aid the recovering addict in his or her attempt to maintain sobriety. To this end, a number of different chemicals have been utilized as experimental agents in the hopes that one or more would prove useful in controlling either the withdrawal symptoms experienced by a recovering addict in the early stages of sobriety or in controlling the craving that many addicts have reported they experience after they stop using chemicals.

CHAPTER THIRTY-TWO

Self-Help Groups

The Twelve Steps of Alcoholics Anonymous[1]

Step One: *We admitted we were powerless over alcohol—that our lives had become unmanageable.*

Step Two: *Came to believe that a Power greater than ourselves could restore us to sanity.*

Step Three: *Made a decision to turn our will and our lives over to the care of God* **as we understood Him.**

Step Four: *Made a searching and fearless moral inventory of ourselves.*

Step Five: *Admitted to God, to ourselves, and to another human being the exact nature of our wrongs.*

Step Six: *Were entirely ready to have God remove all these defects of character.*

Step Seven: *Humbly asked Him to remove our shortcomings.*

Step Eight: *Made a list of all persons we had harmed, and became willing to make amends to them all.*

Step Nine: *Made direct amends to such people wherever possible, except when to do so would injure them or others.*

Step Ten: *Continued to take personal inventory and when we were wrong promptly admitted it.*

Step Eleven: *Sought through prayer and meditation to improve our conscious contact with God* **as we understood Him,** *praying only for knowledge of His will for us and the power to carry that out.*

Step Twelve: *Having had a spiritual awakening as the result of these steps, we tried to carry this message to alcoholics, and to practice these principles in all our affairs.*

As we near the turn of the century, it is estimated that nearly 1 in 10 adults in the United States has attended at least one AA meeting (Miller & McCrady, 1993). Although AA is not the only treatment approach for alcoholism, it is the "most frequently consulted source of help for drinking problems" (Miller & McCrady, 1993, p. 3). Yet, in spite of its widespread acceptance, AA remains something of a mystery, not only to nonmembers but, all too often, even to those who profess to belong to one or more AA groups.

Although supporters of AA claim that it is the most effective means of treating alcoholism, it is

[1]The Twelve Steps are reprinted by permission of Alcoholics Anonymous World Services, Inc. Permission to reprint this material does not mean that AA has reviewed or approved the contents of this publication, nor that AA agrees with the views expressed herein. AA is a program of recovery from alcoholism—use of the Twelve Steps in connection with programs and activities which are patterned after AA, but which address other problems, does not imply otherwise.

not without its critics. In this chapter, we will look at AA and similar groups, what makes them work, and some of the criticism that has been aimed at this form of treatment.

A Brief History of Alcoholics Anonymous

The diverse forces that blended together to form Alcoholics Anonymous (AA) include the American temperance movement of the late 1800s (Peele, 1984, 1989); a nondenominational religious group known as the Oxford Group, which was popular in the 1930s (Nace, 1987); and the psychoanalysis of an American alcoholic by Carl Jung in the year 1931 (Edmeades, 1987). Over the years, many early members of Alcoholics Anonymous were hospitalized, mistakes were made, questions were asked, and the early pioneers of AA embarked on a struggle for sobriety that transcended individual members.

Historically, AA is thought to have been founded on June 10th, 1935, the day that an alcoholic physician, Dr. Robert Holbrook Smith, had his last drink (Nace, 1987). But the foundation of AA was set down earlier, during a meeting between Dr. Smith and William Griffith Wilson, an out-of-town stockbroker on a business trip, struggling to protect his new-found sobriety. After making several telephone calls to try to find support in his struggle, Wilson was asked to talk to Dr. Smith, who was drinking at the time that Wilson called. Rather than looking out for his own needs, Wilson chose a different approach. He carried a message of sobriety to another alcoholic.

The self-help philosophy of AA was born from this moment. In the half-century since then, it has grown to a fellowship of 87,000 "clubs," or AA groups, with chapters in 150 countries and a total membership estimated at more than 1.7 million people (Miller & McCrady, 1993).

During its early years, AA struggled to find a method that would support its members in their endeavor to both achieve and maintain sobriety. Within 3 years of its founding, three different AA groups were in existence, but even with three groups "it was hard to find twoscore of sure recoveries" (*Twelve Steps and Twelve Traditions*, 1981, p. 17). But the fledgling group continued to grow slowly, until, by the fourth year following its inception, there were about 100 members in isolated AA groups (Nace, 1987).

In spite of this rather limited beginning, the early members decided to write of their struggle to achieve sobriety to share their discoveries with others. The publication that was the result of this process was the first edition of the book *Alcoholics Anonymous* in 1939. The organization took its name from the title of this book (*Twelve Steps and Twelve Traditions*, 1981), which has since come to be known as the "Big Book" of AA.

Elements of Alcoholics Anonymous

Roots and Aanes (1992) identify several characteristics that seem to make some self-help groups so useful.

1. Members have *shared experience,* in this case their inability to control their drug or alcohol use.
2. *Education,* not psychotherapy, is the primary goal of AA membership.
3. Self-help groups are *self-governing.*
4. The group places emphasis on *accepting responsibility for one's behavior.*
5. There is but a *single purpose* to the group.
6. Membership is *voluntary.*
7. The individual member must make a *commitment to personal change.*
8. The group places emphasis on *anonymity and confidentiality.*

These are characteristics that apply to AA. As Peele (1984) notes, many of the features of AA are "peculiarly American" (p. 1338), including public confession, contrition, and salvation through spirituality. Furthermore, as the *Twelve Steps and Twelve Traditions* (1981) acknowledges, the early members of AA freely borrowed from the fields of medicine and religion to establish a program that worked for them. This program, embodied in the famous "Twelve Steps" of AA, serves as the core of the recovery program that AA offers.

A Breakdown of the Twelve Steps

The book *Al-Anon's Twelve Steps and Twelve Traditions,* which borrowed the Twelve Steps of AA for use with families, divides the steps into three groups. The first three steps are viewed as necessary for the acceptance of one's limitations. Through these first three steps, the individual is able to come to accept that his or her own resources are not sufficient to solve life's problems, especially the problems inherent in living with an addicted person. In the AA twelve-step program, these steps serve to help the individual accept that his or her resources are insufficient for dealing with the problems of life, especially the problem of addiction.

Steps four through nine are a series of change-oriented activities. These steps are designed to help the individual identify, confront, and ultimately overcome character shortcomings that were so much a part of the individual's addicted lifestyle. Through these steps, the individual can work through the guilt associated with past behaviors and learn to recognize the limits of personal responsibility. These steps allow the person to learn the tools of non-drug-centered living, something that at first is often alien to both the addict and his or her family.

Finally, steps ten through twelve challenge the individual to continue to build on the foundation established in steps four through nine. The individual is asked to continue to search out personal shortcomings and to confront them. The person is also challenged to continue the spiritual growth initiated during the earlier steps and to carry the message of hope to others.

It has been suggested that AA functions as a form of psychotherapy (Peck, 1993; Tobin, 1992; Alibrandi, 1978). As such, the AA program can be viewed as composed of five different phases as outlined by Alibrandi (1978). The first stage starts on the first day of membership in AA and lasts for the next week. During this phase, the individual's goal is simply to stay away from his or her first drink (or chemical use).

The second phase of recovery starts at the end of the first week and lasts until the end of the second month of AA membership. In this part of the recovery process, the recovering addict accepts the disease concept of addiction and learns to accept help with his or her addiction. During this phase, the individual struggles to replace old drug-centered behavioral habits with new, sobriety-oriented habits.

The third stage of recovery spans the interval from the second through the sixth month of sobriety. During this stage, the individual uses the Twelve Steps as a guide and tries to let go of old ideas. Guilt feelings about past chemical use are to be replaced with gratitude for sobriety, wherever possible, and the member is to stand available for service to other addicts.

The fourth stage begins at around the sixth month of sobriety and lasts until the first year of sobriety (Alibrandi, 1978). During the fourth stage, the addict is encouraged to take a searching and fearless moral inventory of "self" and to share this with another person. At the same time, if the individual is still "shaky," he or she is encouraged to work with another addict. Emphasis during this phase of recovery is on acceptance of responsibility and on the resolution of the anger and resentment on which addiction is so often established.

Finally, after the first year of sobriety, the recovery process has reached what Brown (1985) terms "ongoing sobriety." Alibrandi (1978) identifies the goal during this phase of recovery as the maintenance of a "spiritual condition." The person is warned to not dwell on the shortcomings of others, to suspend judgment of self and others, and to beware of the false pride that could lead to a return to chemical use.

The twelve-step program is essentially a program for spiritual growth (Peck, 1993). Although Dyer (1989) did not address AA specifically when he explored the issue of spiritual growth, his observations could also be applied to the process of spiritual growth that is a central component of the AA program:

> Once you start to make the transformational awakening journey, there is no going back. You develop a knowledge that is so powerful that you will wonder how you could have lived any other way. The awakened life begins to own you, and then you simply know within that you are on the right path. (p. 17)

In a very real sense, the Twelve Steps of AA is a program for living, a program for spiritual growth, and a series of 12 successive approximations toward a lifelong behavioral change: sobriety. What makes the Twelve Steps effective is often disputed, and there is a great deal of controversy over whether the twelve-step program is effective at all. But within the AA community, many believe that the Twelve Steps offer a program within which personality transformation can be accomplished (DiClemente, 1993). Others view them as a series of successive approximations toward the goal of sobriety.

In either case, although the steps are not required for AA membership, they are viewed within AA as a proven method of behavioral change that offers addicts a chance to rebuild their lives. There are many who believe that these steps were instrumental in saving their lives.

Alcoholics Anonymous and Religion

Alcoholics Anonymous distinguishes between spirituality and religion (Berenson, 1987). AA identifies with no single religious group or religious doctrine (*Twelve Steps and Twelve Traditions*, 1981), but it is a spiritual recovery program.

For example, Step Three of the program "doesn't demand an immediate conversion experience . . . but . . . does call for a decision" (Jensen, 1987b, p. 22). This decision is for addicts to make a conscious decision to turn their will over to their God. In addressing the issue of religion, Jensen (1987b) explains that "Step Three simply assumes that there is a God to understand

and that we each have a God of our own understanding" (p. 23).

In this manner, AA sidesteps the question of religion while addressing the spiritual disease that it views as existing within addiction. In turning their will over to another, addicts come to accept that their own will is not enough to maintain sobriety. Thus, AA offers a spiritual program that ties the individual's will to that of a "higher power" without offering a specific religious dogma that may offend some members.

One "A" Is for "Anonymous"

Anonymity is central to the AA and the NA programs (*Understanding Anonymity*, 1981). This is a major reason most meetings are "closed." During a "closed" meeting, which is limited to members only, members talk about "personal problems or interpretations of the Twelve Steps or the Twelve Traditions" (Lewis, Dana, & Blevins, 1988, p. 151). In an open meeting, which is open to any interested person, one or two volunteers speak and visitors are encouraged to ask questions about AA and how it works.

The anonymity that is central to AA protects the identities of members and ensures that no identified spokesperson emerges who "represents" AA (*Understanding Anonymity*, 1981). Through this policy, the members of AA strive for humility, each knowing that he or she is equal to the other members. The concept of anonymity is so important that it is said to serve "as the spiritual foundation of the Fellowship" of AA (*Understanding Anonymity*, 1981, p. 5).

The concept of equality of the members underlies the AA tradition that no "directors" are nominated or elected. Rather, "service boards" or special committees are created from the membership as needed. These boards always remain responsible to the group *as a whole* and must answer to the entire AA or NA group. As noted in Tradition Two of AA, "our leaders are but trusted servants; they do not govern" (*Twelve Steps and Twelve Traditions*, 1981, p. 10). Because of the emphasis on equality, the structure of AA has evolved into one in which "interpersonal conflicts and the petty jealousy, greed or self-importance that could create havoc among fellowship members" (DiClemente, 1993, p. 85) is minimized, if not totally avoided.

Alcoholics Anonymous and Outside Organizations

Alcoholics Anonymous is both a self-supporting and a nonprofit group. Each individual group is autonomous and must support itself only through the contributions of the members, each of whom is prohibited from contributing more than $1,000 per year. Outside donations are discouraged to avoid the problem of having to decide how to deal with these gifts. Outside commitments are also discouraged for AA groups. As is stated in the *Twelve Steps and Twelve Traditions* (1981), AA groups will not "endorse, finance, or lend the AA name to any related facility or outside enterprise, lest problems of money, property and prestige divert us from our primary purpose" (p. 11).

The relationship between different autonomous AA groups and that between different AA groups and other organizations are governed by the Twelve Traditions of AA. The Traditions are a set of guidelines for interactions among groups, and through which AA works as a whole. The Twelve Traditions will not be reviewed in this chapter, but interested readers may wish to read *Twelve Steps and Twelve Traditions* (1981) to learn more about the Traditions.

The Primary Purpose of Alcoholics Anonymous

This "primary purpose" of AA is actually twofold. First, the members of AA strive to "carry the message to the addict who still suffers" (*The Group*, 1976, p. 1). Second, AA seeks to provide for its members a program for living without chemicals. This is done not by preaching at the alcoholic or drug addict but by presenting to the addict a simple, truthful, realistic picture of the disease of addiction.

To accomplish this, it is necessary to confront the addict with the facts of his or her addiction in plain language that he or she can understand. The manner in which this confrontation is carried out is somewhat different than the usual methods of confrontation. In AA, speakers share their own life stories—a public confession, of sorts—where each individual tells of the lies, distortions, self-deceptions, and denial that supported his or her own chemical use. In so doing, the speaker hopes to break through the defensiveness of the addict by showing that others have walked the same road, yet found a way to sobriety. Helping others is a central theme of AA.

> Even the newest of newcomers finds undreamed rewards as he tries to help his brother alcoholic, the one who is even blinder than he.... And then he discovers that by the divine paradox of this kind of giving he has found his own reward, whether his brother has yet received anything or not. (*Twelve Steps and Twelve Traditions*, 1981, p. 109)

Yet here is a therapeutic paradox (not the only one!) in AA. For the speaker seeks first to help him- or herself through the public admission of powerlessness over chemicals. Through the public admission of weakness, the speaker seeks to gain strength. It is almost as if, by owning the reality of his or her own addiction, the speaker says "This is what *my* life was like, and by having shared it with you, I am reminded again of the reason I will not return to drugs again."

Through this process, the speaker uses the methods pioneered by Bill Wilson in his first meeting with Bob Smith. In that meeting, Bill Wilson spoke at length of his own addiction to alcohol and of the pain and suffering he had caused others and that he had suffered in the service of his addiction. He did not preach but simply shared with Dr. Smith the history of his own alcoholism. Bill Wilson concluded with the statement: "So thanks a lot for hearing me out. I know now that I'm not going to take a drink, and I'm grateful to you" (Kurtz, 1979, p. 29).

Earlier, it was noted that the methods of AA present a paradox—that by helping others, the speaker comes to receive help for his or her own addiction. At the same time, he or she confronts the new member by saying, in effect, "I am a mirror of yourself, and just as you cannot look into a mirror without seeing your own image, you cannot look at me without seeing yourself." In this way, the speaker seeks to carry the message to others.

As mentioned before, Alcoholics Anonymous is a spiritual program that is at the same time not religious. AA views alcoholism as a

> spiritual illness, and drinking as a symptom of that illness. The central spiritual "defect" of alcoholics is described as an excessive preoccupation with self.... Treatment of the preoccupation with self is at the core of A.A.'s approach. (McCrady & Irvine, 1989, p. 153)

In place of the disease of the spirit on which addiction rests, AA offers a program for living and a program for spiritual growth. Lewis, Dana, and Blevins (1988) point out that the Twelve Steps are usually introduced with the words, "Here are the steps we took, which are suggested as a program for recovery" (p. 149).

One is not *required* to follow the Twelve Steps to participate in AA. Jensen (1987a) observes that *"the program* does not issue orders; it merely *suggests* Twelve Steps to recovery" (p. 15, italics in original). Thus, the individual is offered a choice between the way of life that preceded AA or acceptance of a program that others have used to achieve and maintain their sobriety. However, the individual does not *passively* accept the Twelve Steps. Rather, the emphasis is on *working* the Twelve Steps, a process that requires "the active participation and intentional engagement of each individual who desires to change their drinking and become sober" (DiClemente, 1993, p. 80).

The Twelve Steps offer the promise and the tools necessary for daily sobriety. But the members of AA are encouraged not to look for the "cause" of their addiction but to accept their addiction as a given fact. "It is not so much *how*

you came to this place, as what you are going to do now that you are here," as one member said to a newcomer.

Neither is the member admonished for being unable to live without chemicals. Members of AA know from bitter experience that relapse is both possible and common (McCrady & Irvine, 1989). Chemical addiction is assumed in membership: "If chemicals were not a problem for you, you wouldn't be here!" In place of the chemical-centered lifestyle, new members are offered a step-by-step program for living that allows them to achieve and maintain sobriety.

To take advantage of this program, the member need only accept *the program.* Admittedly, in doing so the individual is asked to accept yet another therapeutic paradox—that of Step One. Step One of the program, the only step that specifically mentions alcohol by name, asks that the addict first accept that he or she is powerless over chemicals. The individual is asked to do so not on the most superficial of levels necessary to speak the words "I am powerless over chemicals" but on the deepest level of his or her being. Many addicts have found that conformity, at least to the point of saying the phrase "I am addicted to chemicals," is enough to help them escape from the consequences of their addiction. It is easy to say the words if one does not believe them to be true. To accept the *program,* members must look deep within themselves and completely accept that they are *addicted* and *totally powerless* over chemicals. William Springborn (1987) explains that when he confronts the rationalization that chemicals alone are the addict's bane and that the person is a helpless victim of the disease of addiction, he emphasizes "that it is we ourselves, not the pills or alcohol, who cause most of our problems. Chemicals will not bring destruction upon a person until that person learns how to justify continual use and abuse of those chemicals" (p. 8).

When addicts accept the painful, bitter, frightening reality that their lives are no longer their own but are spent in the service of their addiction, and when they come to understand that *nothing* they can do will allow them to control their chemical use, they have "hit bottom." It is at this point that the addict is able to turn to another person, and say: "My way does not work for me. I need help." At this moment, the person takes the First Step (the ultimate admission of powerlessness) and becomes receptive to learning another solution to addiction than to continue to use drugs.

Of Alcoholics Anonymous and Recovery

Alcoholics Anonymous does not refer to a "cure" for the disease of alcoholism, and the members of AA do not speak of themselves as having "recovered." Although members believe that addiction is a disease whose progress may be arrested, they acknowledge that alcoholism can never be cured. Thus, they speak of themselves as recovering, but never as having *recovered*.

Members of AA recognize that the recovering addict is only a moment away from the next "slip." The 25-year AA veteran may relapse in a weak moment. Simple affiliation with AA does not guarantee sobriety (McCrady & Irvine, 1989). No matter what a person's motivation is for sobriety, he or she can only strive to be sober for today. If "today" is too long a period to think about, the addict is encouraged to think about remaining sober for the next hour, the next minute, or just the next second.

Once addicts accept *the program*, they find a way of living that provides support for recovery 24 hours a day for the rest of their lives (DiClemente, 1993). In accepting the program, addicts may discover a second chance they thought was lost forever.

Sponsorship in Alcoholics Anonymous

To help each person on the spiritual odyssey that will hopefully result in their sobriety, new members of AA are encouraged to find a "sponsor."

Sponsors have worked their way through the twelve-step program and achieved a basic understanding of their own addiction. Sponsors act as spiritual (but not religious) guides, offering confrontation, insight, and support in equal amounts to the new member.

It is the duty of the sponsor to take an interest in the newcomer's progress but *not to take responsibility for it* (Alibrandi, 1978; McCrady & Irvine, 1989). The responsibility for recovery is placed on the individual. The sponsor is thus saying, "I can be concerned for you, but I am not responsible for you." In today's terminology, the sponsor is a living example of what might be called "tough love." In a sense, the sponsor's role is similar to that of a psychotherapist (Peck, 1993).

The sponsor should not try to control the newcomer's life and ideally should recognize his or her limitations. Many characteristics of the healthy human services professional identified by Rogers (1961) apply to the AA sponsor as well. Acting as an extension of AA, the sponsor is a tool, but it is up to the newcomer to use this tool to achieve sobriety. AA offers no guarantees, and the sponsor often struggles with many of the same issues that face the newcomer. The newcomer must assume the responsibility for reaching out and using the tools that are offered.

Sponsorship is essentially an expression of the second mission of AA, which is to "carry the message" to other addicts who are still actively using chemicals. This is a reflection of Step Twelve, and one often hears the sponsor speak of having participated in a twelfth-step visit or of having been involved in twelfth-step work. The sponsor is a guide, friend, peer-counselor, fellow traveler, conscience and devil's advocate, all rolled into one.

Alcoholics Anonymous and Psychological Theory

The psychiatrist and popular writer M. Scott Peck (1993) advanced the theory that AA offers a form of folk psychology. But the AA and NA step programs are different from other therapeutic programs that the addict may have been exposed to. The Twelve Steps are "reports of action taken rather than rules not to be broken" (Alibrandi, 1978, p. 166). Each step then is a public (or private) demonstration of action taken in the struggle to achieve and maintain sobriety, rather than a rule that may be broken.

Brown (1985) speaks of the Twelve Steps as serving to keep the recovering addict focused on his or her addiction. Just as alcohol was an "axis" around which the individual centered his or her life while drinking, through the Twelve Steps the addict continues to center his or her life around alcohol but in a different way: a way without chemicals. The Twelve Steps provide a structured program by which the individual can continue to relate to his or her addiction while drawing on the group for support and strength.

What Makes Alcoholics Anonymous Effective?

AA has been a social force in the United States for more than half a century, but there has been surprisingly little research into what elements of the program are effective (Emrick, Tonigan, Montgomery, & Little, 1993). Charles Bufe (1988) offers three reasons for AA's effectiveness, "at least for some people" (p. 55). First, AA provides a social outlet for its members. "Loneliness," Bufe observes, "is a terrible problem in our society, and people will flock to almost *anything* that relieves it—even AA meetings" (p. 55, italics in original).

Second, AA shows its members that their problems are not unique (Bufe, 1988; Alibrandi, 1978). Nace (1987) notes that, through AA participation, the individual member is able to restore identity and self-esteem through the unconditional acceptance of the members, all of whom suffer from the same disease. Thus, each member of AA feels a connection to the others.

Finally, AA offers a proven path to follow that can "look awfully attractive when your world has turned upside down and you no longer have

your best friend—alcohol—to lean on" (Bufe, 1988, p. 55). Thus, the AA program is able to offer the individual hope at a time when he or she feels that there is nobody to turn to (Bean-Bayog, 1993). Although hope is an essential part of recovery, it is doubtful that, as Bufe (1988) concludes, "These things, especially the first two, are all that is really needed" (p. 55). Bufe's view, although perhaps accurate, is also rather limited. AA seems to offer more than just a way to deal with loneliness or a way of relating to others.

Herman (1988) adds one more feature that twelve-step programs such as AA offer the recovering addict: predictability. Consistency is one of the characteristics Rogers (1961) identifies as being of value in the helping relationship. Predictability may be one of AA's curative forces. However, this remains only a hypothesis.

According to Berenson (1987), the AA twelve-step program provides a format for "a planned spontaneous remission" (p. 29) that is "designed so that a person can stop drinking by either education, therapeutic change, or transformation" (p. 30). As part of the therapeutic transformation inherent in AA participation, Berenson (1987) speculates that people "bond to the group and use it as a social support and as a refuge to explore and release their suppressed and repressed feelings" (p. 30).

Alcoholics Anonymous meetings "are generally characterized by warmth, openness, honesty, and humor" (Nace, 1987, p. 242), attributes that may promote personal growth. AA is thought to be "the treatment of choice" (Berenson, 1987, p. 27) for active alcoholics, although Brodsky (1993) challenges this claim. Indeed, Brodsky believes that the twelve-step program advocated by AA is potentially "damaging, violative and ineffective" (p. 21) for many individuals. Brodsky's criticism is that, although it may be a useful tool for some, it is based on "a 19th century fundamentalist tradition" (p. 21) that is essentially conservative Protestant in nature. In Brodsky's view, such a program might prove more destructive than helpful for many people.

Outcome Studies on the Effectiveness of Alcoholics Anonymous

As we have seen, even though AA is viewed by many treatment professionals as the single most important component of a person's recovery program, AA is not without its critics (Brodsky, 1993; Uva, 1991; Ogborne & Glaser, 1985). At best, it has been suggested that AA "should be used only as a supportive adjunct to treatment" (Lewis, Dana, & Blevins, 1988, p. 151), and not as a "treatment" of alcoholism by itself. This latter point was challenged by Tobin (1992), who suggests that the AA twelve-step program has many similarities to a therapeutic program of change and thus should be viewed as a form of treatment.

In light of the controversy that surrounds AA, it is surprising that there has been very little research into the subject of what factors may make AA effective or for what types of people it may be most useful (Ogborne & Glaser, 1985; Galanter, Castaneda, & Franco, 1991). Questions have even been raised as to whether AA is necessary for every addict's recovery (Peele, 1989; Peele, Brodsky, & Arnold, 1991). However, even critics of AA seem to accept the fact that it might be helpful at least to some—but not necessarily all—people who have a problem with chemicals (Brodsky, 1993; Ogborne & Glaser, 1985).

It has been pointed out that those people who join and who remain in AA are *not* a representative sample of alcoholics (Galanter, Castaneda, & Franco, 1991). Rather, the fact that these people have freely chosen to join and remain in AA distinguishes them from those alcoholics who choose not to join AA or those who join but do not remain active members.[2]

Contrary to popular belief, membership in AA is not a guarantee of sobriety. *At least half* of the newcomers to AA stop attending within 3 months, and at the end of 1 year, 90% of the new members will have dropped out (Miller & McCrady, 1993; *The Alcoholism Report*, 1991). Even of those who remain in AA, there is a significant relapse rate. Only 70% of those who stay sober for a year will still be sober at the end of the second year, and 90% of those who are sober at the end of their second year are still sober at the end of their third year of AA participation.

Only a limited number of research studies have attempted to measure the effectiveness of Alcoholics Anonymous (Emrick, Tonigan, Montgomery, & Little, 1993; McCrady & Irvine, 1989). Indeed, at present, there is insufficient evidence to conclude that AA is effective in the treatment of alcoholism (Hester, 1994; Holder et al., 1991). Rather, according to Ogborne and Glaser (1985), it appears that AA "is not effective for *all* kinds of persons with alcohol problems" (p. 188); indeed, the majority of alcoholics never attend AA (Bean-Bayog, 1993). At best, it seems that AA is most effective with a subset of problem drinkers: socially stable white males, over 40 years of age, who are physically dependent on alcohol, prone to guilt, and the firstborn or only child.

But this picture of the person who is most likely to benefit from AA membership is only a preliminary effort to identify the "typical" AA member. In reality, the research data "is not currently developed enough to provide us with a composite profile of the most likely AA affiliates" (Emrick et al., 1993, p. 53). Thus, the conclusions reached by Ogborne and Glaser (1985) should be viewed only as initial approximations until further research into this area is conducted.

Obviously, many members of Alcoholics Anonymous do not demonstrate the characteristics of a successful member outlined by Ogborne and Glaser (1985). For example, in 1991, it was estimated that fully 35% of the membership of AA was composed of women (*The Alcoholism Report*, 1991). This is in direct contrast to Ogborne and Glaser's conclusion that the person for whom AA is most effective is male.

[2]Yet, as the reader will recall, it was on data obtained from members of AA that Jellinek (1960) based his model of alcoholism.

AA certainly does *not* seem to be effective with those who are coerced into attending AA by the courts (Glaser & Ogborne, 1982; Peele, 1989; Peele, Brodsky, & Arnold, 1991), although there are those who would dispute this observation. Indeed, individuals who face legal consequences as a result of driving while intoxicated (were sent to jail or placed on probation) had better subsequent driving records than did those "sentenced" to treatment (Peele, 1989; Peele, Brodsky, & Arnold, 1991).

Peele (1989) is quite critical of AA as it exists today, in part because the current AA philosophy has been accepted as established fact without research support. He offers, as a basis for this criticism, the fallacy that alcoholism will *always* grow worse without treatment and that alcoholics cannot cut back or quit drinking on their own. Research (Vaillant, 1983; Peele, 1989) has shown just the opposite to be true. Alcoholics tend to only infrequently follow the downward spiral thought to be inescapable by AA, and they often control or discontinue drinking without formal intervention.

It has been suggested that the issue of whether or not AA is effective is far too complex to be measured by a single research study (Ogborne, 1993; Glaser & Ogborne, 1982). Indeed, the very nature of AA is that there are vast differences between AA groups. Although they all share the same name, different AA groups do not offer a fixed form of treatment (Ogborne, 1993). There is a need for a series of well-controlled research studies to identify all the variables that might influence the outcome of AA participation (McCrady & Irvine, 1989).

It could be that the very nature of the question, Is AA effective? makes it unanswerable. Would the chronic alcoholic who stopped continual drinking as a result of participation in AA but then entered into a pattern of binge drinking with month-long periods of sobriety in between be measured as a successful outcome? Would the chronic alcoholic who entered AA, stopped drinking, but died 6 weeks later from the accumulated effects of many years of chronic alcohol use be measured as an unsuccessful outcome?

The thrust of Ogborne and Glaser's (1985) work is that the simplistic question, Is AA effective? is unlikely to generate a meaningful answer. Rather, one must examine the factors that make or do not make AA effective to better understand the strengths and abilities of AA.

Narcotics Anonymous

In 1953, another self-help group patterned after AA was founded—Narcotics Anonymous (NA). Although NA honors its debt to Alcoholics Anonymous, the members of Narcotics Anonymous state:

> We follow the same path with only a single exception. Our identification as addicts is all-inclusive in respect to any mood-changing, mind-altering substance. "Alcoholism" is too limited a term for us; our problem is not a specific substance, it is a disease called "addiction." (*Narcotics Anonymous*, 1982, p. x)

To the members of NA, it is not the specific chemical that is the problem but the common disease of addiction. Narcotics Anonymous focuses on helping those whose only "common denominator is that we failed to come to terms with our addiction" (*Narcotics Anonymous*, 1982, p. x).

To many outsiders, the major difference between AA and NA seems to be one of scope. Alcoholics Anonymous addresses only alcoholism, whereas NA addresses addiction to chemicals as well as to alcohol. The growth of NA has been phenomenal, with a *600%* increase in the number of NA groups in the period from 1983 until 1988 (Coleman, 1989). Currently, more than 14,000 NA meetings are held in the United States each week (Coleman, 1989).

Although AA and NA are not affiliated with each other, there is an element of cooperation between them (M. Jordan, personal communication, 27 February 1989). Each follows essentially the same twelve-step program that offers the addict a day-by-day program for recovery. AA speaks about alcoholism; NA speaks of "addiction" or "chemicals." Each offers the same program, with minor variations, to help the addicted person in the struggle to achieve sobriety.

The important question is, Which group works best for the individual? Some people feel quite comfortable going to AA for their addiction to alcohol. Other people believe that NA offers them what they need to deal with their addiction. In the final analysis, the name of the group does not matter so much as the fact that it offers the recovering person the support and understanding that he or she needs to remain sober for today.

Al-Anon and Alateen

The book *Al-Anon's Twelve Steps and Twelve Traditions* provides a short history of Al-Anon in its introduction. According to this history, while their husbands were at the early AA meetings, the wives would often meet. As they waited for their husbands, they would often talk over their problems. At some point, they decided to try to apply the same twelve steps that their husbands had found so helpful, and the group known as *Al-Anon* was born.

In the beginning, each isolated group made whatever changes it felt necessary in the Twelve Steps. However, by 1948, the wife of one of the cofounders of AA became involved in the growing organization, and in time a uniform family support program emerged. This program, known as the Al-Anon Family Group, modified the AA Twelve Steps and Twelve Traditions to make them applicable to the needs of families of alcoholics.

By 1957, in response to the recognition that teenagers present special needs and concerns, Al-Anon itself gave birth to a modified Al-Anon group for teens known as *Alateen*. Alateen members follow the Twelve Steps outlined in the Al-Anon program. The goal of the Alateen program, however, is to provide the opportunity for teenagers to come together to share their experiences, discuss current problems, learn how to cope more effectively with their various con-

cerns, and provide encouragement to each other (*Facts about Alateen*, 1969).

Through Alateen, teenagers learn that alcoholism is a disease. They are helped to detach emotionally from the alcoholic's behavior, while still loving the individual. The goal of Alateen is also to help the individual learn that he or she did not "cause" the alcoholic to drink and to see that they can build a rewarding life in spite of the alcoholic's continued drinking (*Facts about Alateen*, 1969).

Other Support Groups

Criticism has been aimed against the AA program for its emphasis on spiritual growth, its failure to empower women, and its basic philosophy. Several new self-help groups have emerged since 1986 that offer alternatives to AA.

Rational Recovery (RR)

Rational Recovery was founded in 1986 (*Alcoholism & Drug Abuse Week*, 1991d). The program draws heavily on the cognitive-behavioral school of psychotherapy and views alcoholism as reflecting negative, self-defeating thought patterns. Groups are advised by mental health professionals, with the goal of helping the addict identify and correct self-defeating ways of viewing "self" and the world.

Gorski (1993) identifies two general irrational thought groups that contribute to the individual's substance use. The first is termed *addictive thinking* (p. 26), defined as the individual's use of irrational thoughts to support a claim that he or she has a "right" to use chemicals and that chemical use is not the cause of the person's problems. The second group of irrational thoughts are *relapse justifications* (p. 26). These are specific thoughts used by the individual to justify his or her return to chemical use: "I didn't have a choice—they made me do it!"

From a Rational Recovery perspective the task of the group and of the individuals is to learn more rational ways of looking at their behavior so they do not continue to support their substance use through such self-defeating thoughts.

Secular Organizations of Sobriety (SOS)

Also founded in 1986, SOS is a self-help group that does not place emphasis on spirituality (*Alcoholism & Drug Abuse Week*, 1991d). Because many potential members of AA have taken offense at its heavy emphasis on spirituality, SOS was formed as an alternative self-help group, placing heavy emphasis on personal responsibility and critical thinking. In meetings, members struggle to identify how their "cycle of addiction" might be broken. It is estimated that approximately 1,000 SOS groups meet each week in the United States.

Women for Sobriety (WFS)

Women for Sobriety was founded in 1975 (*Alcoholism & Drug Abuse Week*, 1991d). The organization is specifically for women and was founded on the theory that the AA program fails to address the very real differences in the meaning of addiction between men and women. There are 13 core statements, or beliefs, aimed at providing the member with a new perspective on herself. There is a great deal of emphasis on building the member's self-esteem. WFS is small, with approximately 450 groups across the United States.

Summary

The self-help group Alcoholics Anonymous (AA) has emerged as one of the predominant forces in the field of drug abuse treatment. Drawing on the experience and knowledge of its members, AA has developed a program for living that is spiritual without being religious and confrontational without being abusive. AA relies on no outside support, and many of its members believe it is effective in helping them stay sober on a daily basis.

The program for living established by AA is based on those factors that early members believed were important to their own sobriety. This program for living is known as the Twelve Steps. These steps are suggested as a guide to new members. Emphasis is placed on the equality of all members, and there is no board of directors within the AA group.

AA's effectiveness is still being questioned. Researchers agree that it seems to be effective for some people but not for all who join. The question of how to measure the effectiveness of AA is quite complex. It requires a series of well-designed research projects to identify the multitude of variables involved in making AA effective for some people.

In spite of these unanswered questions, AA has served as a model for many other self-help groups, including Narcotics Anonymous (NA). One of the central tenets of NA is that the alcohol focus of AA is too narrow for people who are addicted to other chemicals, either alone or in combination with alcohol. Narcotics Anonymous expounds the belief that addiction is a common disease that may express itself through many different forms of drug dependency. Its twelve-step program is based on the Twelve Steps of Alcoholics Anonymous, and draws heavily from the AA philosophy.

Other self-help groups that have emerged as a result of the AA experience include Al-Anon and Alateen. Al-Anon emerged from informal encounters between the spouses of early AA members, and it strives to provide an avenue for helping the families of those who are addicted to alcohol. Alateen emerged from Al-Anon in response to the recognition that adolescents have special needs. Both groups strive to help the member learn how to be supportive without being dependent on the alcoholic and to learn how to detach from the alcoholic and his or her behavior.

CHAPTER THIRTY-THREE

Crime and Drug Use

In the United States, the problems of illicit drug use and criminal activity are closely intertwined. Indeed, many people believe that these two social problems are essentially the same. From this perspective, illicit drug use is the major cause of criminal activity. Some people actually believe that if the problem of recreational drug use were to magically end tomorrow, the problem of criminal activity would also disappear.

This is a rather simplistic view of the relationship between illegal drug use and crime. In reality, they are two separate social problems. But in the past century or so, the social problems of illicit chemical abuse and criminal activity have come to be interrelated in a number of ways. In this chapter, we will explore some of the ways that drug abuse and crime are connected.

Problems with Identifying the Drugs/Crime Relationship

If the truth be told, researchers really do not have a clear picture of the full extent of drug-related criminal behavior (Bradford, Greenberg, & Motayne, 1992). It is known that recreational chemical use is one of the most significant factors associated with violent crime (Lewis, 1989). Furthermore, it is estimated that fully 25% of all property crimes (such as car theft and burglary) can also be traced to recreational drug use (National Academy of Sciences, 1990).

Although these statistics sound impressive, it is still quite difficult to determine the degree to which chemical abuse is a causal factor in the problem of criminal behavior. One problem is that social scientists who explore the interrelationship between criminal behavior and substance abuse often utilize police investigation reports as at least part of their database. Although police reports are useful, they do not provide a comprehensive overview of the role substance abuse might play in the commission of criminal activity.

For example, some crimes never are solved. Thus the possible impact of substance use in the commission of unsolved crimes can never be determined. Other crimes are solved only after extended periods of time. In such cases, it is not clear what role (if any) chemical use might have played in the commission of these crimes. How could researchers determine whether substance use or abuse was a factor in a crime that the criminal might not even remember committing? Still other crimes are ignored by law enforcement authorities for various reasons, such as lack of evidence, or poor witnesses (Bradford, Greenberg, & Motayne, 1992). Obviously the role of chemical use in the commission of these crimes will never be investigated.

Even when an arrest is made shortly after the commission of a crime, law enforcement officials rarely conduct urine or blood toxicology tests to determine whether the offender was under the influence of alcohol or drugs. In some cases, researchers have been reduced to simply asking the criminal whether he or she had been under the influence of chemicals at the time of committing the crime. Such a research technique obviously assumes that the respondent is going to tell the truth, a dubious assumption at best when dealing with a criminal population.

It is a little known fact that the theoretical bias of the researcher can influence the outcome of a study. Although one goal of scientific research is to control for the influence of the researcher's personal bias, this is not always possible. Indeed, the researcher's personal bias, expectations, and possibly political beliefs will shape the manner in which the research study is designed, what "facts" are considered in the formulation of the study, and what conclusions are reached when the data are evaluated.[1]

Many researchers assume that *any* crime committed under the influence of chemicals or in the service of one's addiction is automatically drug-related. An often-repeated example is that heroin addicts are forced to resort to crime to support their habit. The criminal activity of heroin addicts is thus assumed to be caused by their addiction to heroin. The theoretical bias of this research is evident when one considers that most studies that discuss the relationship between heroin addiction and criminal activity fail to report that *more than 50%* of heroin addicts in this country have a legal history *prior to their first use of narcotics* (Jaffe, 1989).

A different perspective is that individuals who are predisposed to crime might also be predisposed to the use of alcohol and/or drugs (Moore, 1991). From this perspective, it is possible to argue that drug abuse or addiction does not force the individual to resort to crime; rather, those people who engage in the abusive use of chemicals tend to be the kind of people who also engage in criminal activity. In other words drug users might "commit crimes more frequently

than non-users not because they use . . . but because they happen to be the kinds of people who would be expected to have a higher crime rate" (*National Commission on Marihuana and Drug Abuse,* 1972, p. 77). According to this line of reasoning, drugs do not so much *cause* criminal activity as *attract* those who are predisposed to commit crimes in the first place. The fact that the crimes may now be committed to support an addiction to chemicals only obscures the fact that these individuals often committed crimes *before* their addiction developed as well.

Elliott (1992) offers another perspective on the relationship between criminal activity and chemical abuse. Elliott suggests that chemical abuse and criminal activity both reflect the "decline in the power of cultural restraints" (p. 599) taking place in the United States. Thus, to Elliott, drug use and criminal activity are two expressions of a more pervasive sociological phenomenon: a breakdown of traditional restraints and guidelines.

Elliott supports his argument by noting that Europe has experienced "Tidal waves of crime" (Elliott, 1992, p. 599) every few decades since the 14th century, and a similar pattern has emerged in the United States over the past 200 years. A common thread connecting these waves of crime is that, in each successive period of social unrest, one could observe "an erosion of personal integrity, widespread dehumanization, a contempt for life, material greed, corruption in high places, sexual promiscuity, *and increased recourse to drugs and alcohol*" (p. 599, italics added for emphasis). Thus, it is Elliott's (1992) contention that the relationship between drug abuse and criminal activity can be found in the more general breakdown in cultural constraints against antisocial behavior. Rather than a simplistic "drug use causes crime" equation, the author offers a theory that suggests that *both* drug abuse and criminal activity are a reflection of, or perhaps even a reaction to, the more inclusive breakdown in existing social constraints and mores.

Thus, although there does seem to be an interrelationship between chemical use and crime, the exact nature of this relationship remains un-

[1]For a further discussion of this topic, the reader is referred to Stephen Jay Gould's *The Mismeasure of Man* (New York: Norton, 1981).

clear, even after more than a century of intense research. Ultimately, the determination of whether the substance use is the cause of a crime, one of a number of factors associated with a crime, or totally unrelated to a crime must be made on a case-by-case basis.

Criminal Activity and Personal Responsibility

The issue of the degree of personal responsibility in cases in which an individual may have been under the influence of chemicals when the offense was committed is a difficult one for society to address. In many cases, this issue is neatly sidestepped through the use of the social fiction that the drugs somehow interfered with the individual's ability to think coherently. Thus, any "perceived correlation between the use of a drug and the unwanted consequences is attributed to the drug, removing the individual from any and all responsibility" (National Commission on Marihuana and Drug Abuse, 1973, p. 4). This view is an extension of the "demon rum" philosophy of the late 1800s (Peele, 1989), according to which once a person ingests even one drink, the alcohol totally overwhelms his or her self-control. From that point on, the person is controlled by the demon within the bottle of alcohol. The modern version of this belief is that, when a crime is committed by a person who is under the influence of chemicals, the responsibility for that crime is attributed to the chemical used. The individual's role in the commission of the crime is overlooked, and the person is viewed as a helpless victim of the drug's effects. The outcome of this process is that, although drug use in itself is not an excuse for criminal behavior, *extreme* drug use often derails the legal system.

The criminal justice system is often unable to determine whether the individual actually intended to commit a crime while under the influence of chemicals. In such cases, the criminal justice system often simply accepts the compromise that the individual suffered a "diminished capacity" as a result of his or her use of chemi-

cals. So popular has this compromise become that, "as of 1986, 15 states had . . . created a 'diminished capacity' defense as a legal way station between innocence and full criminal responsibility" (Graham, 1989, p. 21). As a result of this social and legal fiction, it is not unusual for defense attorneys to negotiate a reduced sentence, based on the claim of diminished capacity (Graham, 1989).

Thus, the "demon rum" philosophy has actually influenced the workings of the criminal justice system. The diminished capacity defense is quite unlike the "insanity" defense, however, which is often viewed as an act of desperation on the part of the defense attorney. Because of the social fiction that the person is a helpless victim of the drug's effects, crimes committed "under the influence, are the only crimes we can generally elude punishment for by utilizing an escape into the recovery process established by our medical society" (Newland, 1989, p. 18). In other words, by invoking the "demon rum" defense, questions are raised as to the individual's responsibility for the commission of the crime, and substance abuse "treatment" might actually be substituted for the criminal sanctions that would normally be imposed.

The Drug Underworld and Crime

In a very real sense, the "problem" of organized crime could be viewed as a result of U.S. society's attempt to deal with the use of illicit chemicals through the criminal justice system. With the exception of alcohol and tobacco, drugs of abuse are not sold in a "free market" economy. Rather, because these substances are illegal, their production, distribution, and sale are carried out through illegal channels, or the "black market."

The black market generates a significant profit for those who are willing to run the risk of criminal prosecution. Currently, it is estimated that the traffic in illicit chemicals generates an estimated $50 to $60 billion a year in *profits* for those who supply the drugs to users (Nadelmann & Wenner, 1994). On an individual level, some "pushers" have been known to earn as much as $400 or $500 *a day*, or more than $180,000 a year (Collier, 1989).

Such profits have helped the drug distribution and sales infrastructure become quite resistant to law enforcement attempts to interdict illegal drugs (*The Lancet*, 1991b). There is always someone willing to risk arrest for the chance to participate in such a highly profitable trade. Thus, law enforcement attempts to control the distribution of illegal drugs may have contributed to the development of an industry so resilient that it is able to defeat any attempt to control it through legislation or criminal sanctions.

Because most recreational drugs are illegal, the price that is charged for these chemicals is not set by market demand but by those who control the distribution monopoly. The high cost of the drugs is justified by the fact that they are illegal, and thus the dealer runs a risk by providing the chemical to those who purchase it. The addict must then find some way to obtain the money necessary to buy the drugs at these inflated prices. All too often, the money to support the individual's chemical purchases is obtained through criminal activity. Addicts have been known to engage in burglary, armed robbery, prostitution (heterosexual and homosexual), car theft, forgery, and a range of other crimes to obtain the money needed to support the drug "habit." Engaging in drug sales (itself a criminal act) to support an addiction is also not uncommon.

Addicts who support their drug use through theft will receive only a fraction of the stolen material's worth. The result is that the addict must steal more and more so that the pittance received for the stolen property will meet his or her drug needs. It has been estimated that the typical heroin addict in an average city would need to steal some $200,000 worth of goods annually, to support a drug "habit" (Thomason & Dilts, 1991).

Some argue that it is not the drugs that bring about the criminal activity, it is the legal sanctions *against* drug use that have helped create the combination of a drug "underworld" and a high crime rate (Nadelmann & Wenner, 1994; McWilliams, 1993; Nadelmann, 1989). Proponents of this position argue that crime is not a natural consequence of drug use or abuse but an attempt to control access and distribution of chemicals through the legal justice system that breeds criminal behavior. By making chemical use and abuse a criminal justice matter, it is argued, society has in effect created a whole new group of criminals (Nadelmann & Wenner, 1994; Nadelmann, 1989). The criminal activities of the pre-Prohibition era need only be contrasted with the criminal activities of the Prohibition era to prove this point.[2] In discussing the relationship between narcotics abuse and crime, Jaffe (1989) concludes that

> The association between opioid use and crime emerges primarily in countries such as the United States, that have tried to restrict the use of opioids to legitimate medical indications, but have been unable to eliminate illicit opioid traffic. (p. 656)

The Illicit Drug Production and Distribution System

The manufacture and distribution network for illicit chemicals is not a free market economy. The price charged to the consumer is usually the result of an inflationary process where, at each step in the production and distribution system, every person involved makes a profit. For example, from $75 worth of chemicals, a street "chemist" could manufacture PCP that might ultimately sell for as much as $20,000 on the black market (Shepherd & Jagoda, 1990).

Amphetamine tablets are also relatively inexpensive to manufacture. A thousand tablets of amphetamine might cost a pharmaceutical company only about *seventy-five cents* to produce

---

[2]Although most people believe that the Prohibition era gang leader "Scarface" Al Capone made most of his money through the manufacture and distribution of illegal alcohol, historical evidence suggests that he actually made most of his money through illegal gambling and prostitution activities (Shenkman, 1991).

(Brecher, 1972). It only requires a minimal knowledge of chemistry to manufacture one of the amphetamines in an illicit laboratory, and the chemicals needed can be legally purchased at virtually any chemical supply store. But the same amphetamine that was manufactured by a pharmaceutical company for only a few pennies would cost thousands of dollars on the street. An investment of $1,000 to buy the necessary chemicals could eventually yield a return of as much as $40,000 for methamphetamine (*Playboy*, 1990; Peluso & Peluso, 1988). Nationally, the illicit manufacture of amphetamines is thought to be a *$3 billion a year* industry, mainly centered in Texas and California (Cho, 1990).

Street Drugs and Adulterants

Another method by which the price of "street" drugs is inflated is through the process of mixing the drug with an adulterant. Byrne (1989b) reports, for example, that raw cocaine leaves are sold by the farmer in South America for $2 a kilogram (2.4 pounds). The coca paste produced from the leaves is then sold for $200 a kilogram, and the cocaine base that is isolated from the coca paste sells for about $1,500 a kilogram. The cocaine hydrochloride obtained from the base is sold for up to $3,000 a kilogram, which then is sold at wholesale for upwards of $20,000 a kilogram. When packaged for sale on the streets in 1-gram lots, the same kilogram sells for between $80,000 and $192,000.

At each step in the distribution process, the cocaine is mixed with adulterants, reducing the purity of the resulting mixture while increasing the amount of the "drug" to be sold. Cocaine and narcotics are adulterated only to increase the profit from the sale of these drugs. The raw opium necessary to produce a kilogram (2.4 pounds) of heroin costs only a few hundred dollars. This same kilogram of heroin will ultimately sell on the street for between *$1 and $5 million* after it is "cut" repeatedly.

Between the time that the raw opium is harvested and the finished product is sold on the streets, heroin might be "cut" (adulterated) be-

tween four and seven times (Lingeman, 1974). At each stage, the potency of the heroin may be reduced by half or even more. When it is finally sold on the street, a single kilogram of heroin is sold in powder form in small "bags" (or, occasionally, condoms) selling for between $5 (a "nickel bag") and $10 (a "dime bag") each. At best, a typical "bag" of heroin contains just 73% "pure" heroin. Often, the purity of the heroin purchased on the street is much lower than this. The rest of the "bag" is composed of the various adulterants that have been added along the way.[3]

According to Scaros, Westra, and Barone (1990), the purity of cocaine purchased on the street ranges from just 14% to 75% with an average purity of 49%. This means that, on the average, *more than half of each gram of cocaine purchased* on the street is actually some other substance. These adulterants fall into one of five categories, according to the authors: (1) various forms of sugar, (2) stimulants, (3) local anesthetics, (4) toxins, and (5) any of a number of inert compounds.

Cocaine, according to the authors, is frequently adulterated with many different substances. The various forms of sugar are the most common adulterants. Then, the CNS stimulants as a group

> are the second most common adulterants, and include caffeine, ephedrine, phenylpropanolamine, amphetamine, or methamphetamine. . . . The local anesthetics are the third most frequent adulterants, and include lidocaine, benzocaine, procaine, and tetracaine. . . . The two most common [lethal toxins used as adulterants] are quinine and strychnine. (p. 24)

Many of the same compounds used to adulterate cocaine are also mixed with street narcot-

[3]The adulterants add additional health risks to the user. For example, the intravenous injection of quinine (frequently used as an adulterant in street heroin) may result in toxic reactions in the sensitive nerve tissues of the visual system (Michelson et al., 1988). Talcum powder, which is also a frequent adulterant for street heroin and cocaine, may cause retinopathy (damage to the retina of the eye).

ics. Other adulterants found in narcotics include food coloring, talcum powder, starch, powdered milk, baking soda, brown sugar, and, on occasion, even dog manure (Scaros, Westra, & Barone, 1990). Other compounds that have been either mixed with or substituted for heroin that was sold on the "street" include (but are not limited to) aspirin, amphetamine compounds, belladonna, caffeine, instant coffee, lactose, LSD, magnesium sulfate, meprobamate, pentobarbital, pepper, secobarbital, starch, and warfarin (used in rat poison) (Schauben, 1990).

It is not uncommon for up to half of the marijuana purchased on the street to be seeds and woody stems, which must be removed before the marijuana can be smoked. Furthermore, the marijuana can be laced with other compounds, ranging from PCP, cocaine paste, or opium on to toxic compounds such as "Raid" insect spray (Scaros, Westra, & Barone, 1990). Marijuana samples have also been found to have been adulterated with dried shredded cow manure (which may expose the user to salmonella bacteria), as well as herbicide sprays such as paraquat (Jenike, 1991). Schauben (1990) has compiled a long list of compounds that have either been mixed in with or substituted for marijuana, including alfalfa, apple leaves, catnip, cigarette tobacco, hay, licorice, mescaline, methamphetamine, opium, pipe tobacco, straw, wax, and wood shavings. All these compounds also gain admission into the user's body when the adulterated marijuana is smoked.

Unfortunately, medical researchers have little understanding of the effects on the body of these various compounds used to adulterate or substitute for illicit drugs. Once the adulterants gain admission to the body, medical research is hard-pressed to predict the impact these substances will have. In an emergency situation, such as when the user has had a toxic reaction to one or more chemicals, the physician must try to anticipate the effects not only of the drug(s) of abuse but of literally any of several score of possible adulterants.

One reason that "pharmaceuticals" (drugs produced by legal pharmaceutical manufacturers that have been diverted to the streets) are so highly prized among addicts is that they are of a known quality and potency. They are also unlikely to be contaminated. However, pharmaceuticals are difficult to obtain, and with rare exceptions, the majority of addicts use chemicals produced in illegal laboratories that have been adulterated time and time again.

Pharmaceuticals are not without their own dangers. Addicts often attempt to use a "pharmaceutical" in a way that was not intended by the manufacturer. For example, many addicts inject tablets or the contents of capsules that were intended for oral use. They often irritate the blood vessel walls or even totally block a blood vessel (Taylor, 1993). This can result in an infection, gangrene, blood clots, and strokes and in many cases the need to amputate the afflicted limb (Taylor, 1993).

The problem of chemical adulterants is one that has existed for generations. Indeed, it could be argued that the very fact that the drug "market" is illegal makes the use of chemical adulterants inevitable. In a later section of this chapter, we will look at another danger inherent in the drug world today: mistakes that are made in the manufacture of illicit chemicals that are sold to unsuspecting drug users.

Drug Use and Violence: The Unseen Connection

For a number of reasons, the recreational drug user is vulnerable to violent attacks. Drug pushers have been known to attack customers to steal their money, armed with the knowledge that drug users are unlikely to press charges. Drug pushers have been known to attack addicts in retaliation for unpaid drug debts. Indeed, it is not uncommon for addicts who fail to pay drug debts on time to be murdered. For example, Goldstein (1990) concluded that fully *18%* of the homicides committed in New York State in 1986 were the result of drug-related debts.

On occasion, drug pushers themselves are shot, dropped in front of the hospital emergency room, or simply left to die. Sometimes, the crime is committed by other drug pushers to scare off competition over "territory." On other occasions, the murder is carried out by others associated with the drug trade to avenge an unpaid drug debt or for other drug-related reasons.

Obviously, there is a relationship between recreational drug use and violence. Many recreational chemicals lower the individual's inhibitions, making it more likely that he or she will engage in violent acts. Jaffe (1989) reports that a study in St. Louis found that 35% of the addicts reported having been shot or wounded with a knife at some point during their drug using careers. Bays (1990) estimates that one in every five homicide victims in this country may have been using cocaine shortly before his or her death.

The lifestyle associated with narcotics addiction has long been known to expose the individual to threats or acts of violence. Indeed, estimates of the risk of premature death for a narcotics addict vary, but center around a 1% per year death rate for urban narcotics addicts. Lingeman (1974) describes how heroin addicts live on the fringes of the criminal underworld, often dying as a result of overdoses, infections brought on by unsterile needles, malnutrition, accidents, and violence.

The "War on Drugs": Is It Time to Declare a Winner?

For some time, questions have been raised as to whether the efforts of law enforcement agencies to interdict the flow of illegal chemicals has really been very effective. For example, the theory has been advanced that the interdiction efforts against marijuana in the early to mid-1970s may have caused international drug smugglers to switch from smuggling marijuana to smuggling cocaine into the United States (Scheer,

1994a). Pound for pound, cocaine is "less bulky, less smelly, more compact, and more lucrative" than marijuana (Nadelmann, Kleiman, & Earls, 1990, p. 45). If this theory is true, then the efforts of law enforcement officials to deal with the marijuana problem through interdiction may actually have contributed to the subsequent development of a wave of cocaine abuse in the United States.

Another consequence of the prohibition against chemical use is that addicts must utilize chemicals under hazardous conditions. For example, narcotics addicts inject the drugs only because that is the most efficient method of administering the limited amount of the drug available. When allowed access to unlimited supplies of relatively pure narcotics, the preferred method of administration is by smoking, as was found in the turn-of-the-century opium dens. It is only when supplies become scarce that addicts begin to inject the drug and to share needles. In a very real sense, the prohibition against narcotics use could be said to be one contributing factor to the spread of HIV in this country.

The twin policies of prohibition and interdiction of illicit chemicals have become watchwords in the United States for almost a century. In the past generation, *$100 billion* was spent waging a "war" on drugs (Scheer, 1994a; Ruby, 1993). Yet, in spite of all of the time, energy, and money invested in this war, there is strong evidence that "the past decade's 'War on Drugs' has failed as a strategy to decrease the level of drug use in the United States" (Selwyn, 1993, p. 1044). Indeed, there is evidence that there are *more* drugs on the street now—and in many cases of greater purity—than there were *before* the war on drugs began (Scheer, 1994a; Sabbag, 1994).

Still, one must wonder how committed the government was to winning this war. In spite of the financial investment and legal resources committed to this war, the Central Intelligence Agency (CIA) was busy *smuggling more than a ton of cocaine into the United States* for drug dealers ("60 Minutes," 1993). Is it any wonder that a small number of people are openly calling the war on drugs a failure and are looking for alternatives for this social policy?

Should Drugs Be Legalized?

In the early 1980s, the U.S. government initiated a "zero tolerance" program in its "war" against drug use. Legal sanctions and incarceration were immediately imposed on anyone convicted of a drug-related criminal offense through mandatory sentencing provisions in the law. Although political support for mandatory sentencing was almost universal in the early to mid-1980s, its success has been criticized by many social scientists.

A little known historical fact is that, in the 1950s, Congress passed a series of mandatory minimum-sentence laws in the fight against narcotics use and abuse in the United States (Schlosser, 1994). These laws were loosely termed the "Boggs Act," which defined minimum prison sentences that Congress thought should be imposed for the illicit use of narcotics. Although support for the Boggs Act was almost universal, the then director of the United States Bureau of Prisons, James V. Bennett, expressed strong reservations about its effectiveness. Although he had not personally broken any laws in doing so, Mr. Bennett was subsequently followed by agents of the Federal Bureau of Narcotics, who submitted reports on the content of speeches that he gave (Schlosser, 1994).

By the late 1960s, it was clear that Mr. Bennett was right: mandatory sentencing did little to reduce the scope of narcotics use or abuse in the United States. In 1970, the Boggs Act was replaced by a more appropriate series of sentencing guidelines, through which judges could assign appropriate sentences to defendants based on the merits of each case. However, in one of the great reversals of all time, just 14 years later Congress again imposed mandatory prison sentences for drug-related offenses. The lessons of past decades were forgotten. Through the Sentencing Reform Act of 1984, Congress took away

the judges' power to determine appropriate prison sentences through the application of mandated minimum prison terms. Even first-time offenders were sent to prison for extended periods of time without hope of parole.

One result of the Sentencing Reform Act of 1984 was that the prison system soon became filled with individuals serving lengthy mandatory sentences. Whereas only 16% of all federal prisoners were incarcerated because of drug-related convictions in 1970, 62% of those currently incarcerated in federal penitentiaries are there because of drug-related convictions (Nadelmann & Wenner, 1994; Schlosser, 1994). By the turn of the century, it is possible that more than 75% of all federal inmates may be incarcerated for drug-related mandatory minimum prison terms.

Currently, some 300,000 individuals are incarcerated for drug-related convictions (Nadelmann & Wenner, 1994). Assuming that it costs $35,000 *per inmate per year* to keep a person incarcerated in 1996, this means that more than *$10.5 billion a year* is being spent just to keep already convicted drug offenders incarcerated. A significant number of these prisoners are "first-time" offenders, who have never had a prior conviction for *any* offense. Yet, because of mandatory sentencing guidelines, they are sentenced to lengthy prison terms without hope of parole.

Some critics of mandatory sentencing claim that it results in prison terms that are not proportional to the offense. For example, although an offender convicted of intentional homicide is usually sentenced to life in prison, "The average sentence *served* for murder in the U.S. is six and a half years, while eight years with no possibility of parole is *mandatory* for the possession of 700 marijuana plants" (Potterton, 1992, p. 47, italics added for emphasis). A first-time offender convicted of stealing $80,000,000 would face a mandatory sentence of 4 years in a federal correctional facility, and he or she could apply for early release from prison under the parole provisions of the law. Yet a first-time offender convicted of possession of $1500 worth of LSD would be sentenced to a mandatory 10 years in prison under the Sentencing Reform Act of 1984, without benefit of parole (*Playboy*, 1993). In fact, habitual and violent prisoners are now being released from prison just to make room for *first-time* offenders convicted and sentenced under mandatory drug-enforcement laws (Asseo, 1993; Potterton, 1992).

Other critics of the mandatory sentencing laws for possession of illegal substances point out that the small-time user is usually the victim of lengthy mandatory prison terms (Steinberg, 1994). Steinberg points out that mid- and upper-level suppliers are frequently able to bargain their knowledge of who is buying drugs from them for lighter prison sentences. As a result of the plea bargains offered to these drug dealers in return for "cooperation,"

> The former hippie with 1,000 marijuana plants growing in his basement and no drug ring to rat on gets the full decade in prison, while the savvy dealer bringing in boatloads of pot from south of the border can finger a few friends and be out in half the time. (p. 33)

An excellent example of the unfair application of this principle is the case (reported in Schlosser, 1994) of a major drug dealer who was caught with 20,000 kilograms (44,092 pounds) of cocaine. He was able to trade his knowledge of the drug distribution system for a reduced sentence of less than 4 years in prison.

This is not to endorse the legalization of drugs. The question of whether drugs should be legalized has sparked fierce debate in this country. Advocates of drug legalization point out that through legalization an important source of revenue for what is loosely called "organized crime" would be removed. Currently, the illegal drug trade supports organized crime not only in the United States but around the world (*The Economist*, 1993a).

It has even been argued that personal, recreational drug use (as opposed to distribution of illicit chemicals to others) is essentially a consensual crime; the individual who is using the chem-

icals is making a choice to do so (McWilliams, 1993; Royko, 1990). Indeed, many people have demonstrated a remarkable persistence in obtaining illicit chemicals, in spite of all that society has done to block their use. If these drugs were legal, they would at least be more easily available to those who wished to "sniff away his nose or addle his brain" (Royko, 1990, p. 46). One advantage of this system, according to Royko, is that it would be possible to avoid the "gun battles, the corruption and the wasted money and effort trying to save the brains and noses of those who don't want them saved" (p. 46) to begin with. Through the legalization of drugs, Royko suggests that some measure of control could be gained over who has access to drugs and at what age they would be allowed to use them, much the same way that access to alcohol is restricted by law.

On the other hand, Frances (1991) argues against the legalization of drugs, in part because the increased availability of drugs would result in higher levels of chemical use. For example, Frances states that the number of cocaine users would triple if cocaine were legalized. Furthermore, Frances (1991) points out, when drugs were legal during the past century, society was swept by a wave of addiction the likes of which has never been seen before or since. If drugs were to be legalized now, the "black market" would be destroyed, but the price of chemicals of abuse would fall so drastically that prices would come "within reach of lunch money for elementary school children" (p. 120). This is a frightening prediction.

However, Lessard (1989) suggests an alternative to the free-market legalization program fearfully envisioned by Frances. Rather than have drugs freely available on the marketplace, Lessard (1989) proposes that drugs be made available through a physician's prescription. This is similar to the approach adopted in England, where physicians who hold a special license can prescribe drugs to proven addicts ("60 Minutes," 1992). In this way, access to the drugs could be limited, while the profit incentive for criminals would be removed. What Lessard (1989) suggests is that the problem of drug abuse be approached from a health perspective, as it is in Holland and England.

The Dutch Experience

The social experiment that has been underway in Holland for the last two decades has yielded conflicting evidence as to which approach to the problem of drug abuse might be the best one. In 1976, the Dutch revised their antidrug laws, making possession of less than 1 ounce of marijuana a misdemeanor offense. Further revisions of the antidrug statutes, or the ways that they were interpreted, resulted in a policy decision not to enforce the strict antidrug laws already on the books. To do so, government officials reasoned, would be to drive underground what was essentially a health problem, turning it into a legal problem.

In Holland, although the possession of heroin or cocaine for personal use was discouraged, it was tolerated by authorities as long as the individual did not engage in other illegal behaviors (R. Lewis, 1989; *The Economist*, 1990b). Small amounts of marijuana and hashish were sold openly in Dutch coffee houses, and users were allowed to purchase up to 13 grams of marijuana legally. The price of marijuana was quite low (approximately $1.50 per gram, according to *The Economist*, 1990b). Surprisingly, in spite of this open toleration for marijuana or drug use, the number of heroin addicts initially dropped by approximately one-third after this change in national philosophy took place (*The Lancet*, 1991b; Scheer, 1990; *The Economist*, 1990b).

But recently, substance abuse has become a serious problem in Holland. For example, Gay (1991) reported that only 5% of Dutch high school graduates admitted to experimenting with drugs, as compared to some 18% U.S. high school graduates. However, Schwartz challenged this figure in 1994, noting that the rate of marijuana use by teenagers in the Netherlands is now much higher than the 5% figure often cited in older studies.

However, Dutch authorities have started to clamp down on drug use in their country, in response to drug-related crime. Much of this crime is apparently committed by individuals who have moved to Holland just to take advantage of the permissive attitudes toward drugs there. At this point, it is not clear how the Dutch experiment will end or how the population will react to a wave of nonnative drug users moving to their country. But some Dutch officials have started to advocate mandatory treatment for drug addicts, in an attempt to deal with the problem of addiction (Kleber, 1994). This may signal a change in the "Dutch Experiment."

The English Experience

After following an American model of drug interdiction and incarceration for illegal drug users for some time, English policy makers found that drug addiction had tripled in England ("60 Minutes," 1992). The decision was made to return to the approach they had previously used, in which a limited number of physicians were given authority to prescribe the drugs addicts need to supply their "habit."

The physician who prescribes the drugs for the addict must hold a special license ("60 Minutes," 1992). At the same time, the addict must prove that he or she is unwilling or unable to give up drugs. The goal of this system is to help the addict avoid the dangers inherent in the drug using lifestyle, at least until he or she is able to "mature out" of the need to use drugs. One measure of the success of this approach is that whereas more than half of the addicts in cities like New York have been found to carry the virus that causes AIDS, only 1% of the addicts in Liverpool, England, have been found to have this virus in their blood ("60 Minutes," 1992).

It is too soon to determine whether this approach would work in the United States. However, both the Dutch and the English response to the drug "crisis" has been far different than the

U.S. approach. The success of each alternative approach suggests that there might be room for improvement in the traditional U.S. treatment of the problem of drug addiction.

Hidden Victims of Street Drugs

As we discussed earlier in this chapter, many of the drugs used in the United States are produced in illicit laboratories. Product reliability is hardly a strong component of clandestine, illegal drug laboratories, but this is not a new phenomenon. During the Prohibition era, a very real danger was that the "bathtub gin" or "homebrew" (beverages containing alcohol) might have accidentally included a form of alcohol that could blind or even kill the consumer. Indeed, Nadelmann, Kleiman, and Earls (1990) estimate that "tens of thousands" (p. 46) were blinded, or died, from illicitly produced alcohol during Prohibition. This was one reason smuggling alcohol was so popular during Prohibition: people could trust that a legitimate alcoholic beverage was safe.

Nor were the problems associated with illegally manufactured alcohol limited to the Prohibition era. Even today, whiskey produced by illegal "stills"—known in many parts of the country as "moonshine" (or "shine")—is frequently contaminated with high levels of lead (Pegues, Hughes, & Woernie, 1993). This contamination is caused by the tendency of many producers to filter the brew through old automobile radiators, according to the authors, where it comes into contact with lead from soldered joints. So common is this problem that the authors conclude that illegal whiskey is "an important and unappreciated source of lead poisoning" (p. 1501) in some parts of this country.

In today's world, contaminants are commonly found in the drugs sold on the street. If the drug was manufactured in an illegal laboratory, a simple mistake in the production process might produce a dangerous or even a lethal chemical combination. As often happened with alcohol during the Prohibition era, contaminated

or impure drugs are sold on the streets (Gallagher, 1986; Kirsch, 1986). Shafer (1985) explored the impact of many of these "mistakes" that were sold on California streets in the late 1970s under the guise of "new heroin." These drugs, produced in clandestine "laboratories," are reported to have included chemical impurities capable of literally "burning out" parts of the brain. Some addicts developed a drug-induced condition very similiar to advanced cases of Parkinson's disease after injecting what they were told was "synthetic heroin" (Kirsch, 1986). Chemists discovered that what had been mistakenly produced was not a synthetic narcotic known as MPPP but the chemical known as MPTP. Unfortunately, once in the body, an enzyme (monoamine oxidase) biotransforms MPTP into a neurotoxin known as MPP^+, which kills dopamine-using brain cells in the nigrostriatal region of the brain.

Subsequent research revealed that the loss of these neurons is also implicated in the development of Parkinson's disease. Thus, indirectly, this mistake in the manufacture of illicit narcotics allowed researchers to make an important medical discovery. Unfortunately, because MPTP was sold on the street, many addicts died and others developed lifelong drug-induced disorders that resemble Parkinson's disease.

There is no way to determine how many people have suffered or died because of impurities in illicit drugs. But it is known that addicts have been and still are being poisoned because of mistakes made in the production of street drugs. Parras, Patier, and Ezpeleta (1988), for example, relate the case of a heroin addict found to have developed lead poisoning as a result of lead-contaminated heroin. Cases have been reported of amphetamine users being exposed to toxic levels of lead or any of a number of possible carcinogenic compounds as a result of impure street drugs (Evanko, 1991; Centers for Disease Control, 1990).

Lombard, Levin, and Weiner (1989) describe a case in which a cocaine abuser was found to have had developed arsenic poisoning, a rather rare condition. Physicians concluded that the arsenic was contained in the cocaine the patient was using. When told that the cause of the nausea, vomiting, and diarrhea was a contaminant in the cocaine, the patient was reportedly quite unimpressed. The addict informed the physicians that it was "common knowledge" (p. 869) that cocaine might be mixed with compounds that contained arsenic. The authors warn that similar cases may occur as the cocaine epidemic spreads.

Nor is the problem of contaminated drugs limited to narcotics or cocaine. Most of the drugs

> intended for popular recreational use are most often produced in clandestine laboratories with little or no quality control, so generally speaking users cannot be sure of the purity of what they are ingesting. (Hayner & McKinney, 1986, p. 341)

Indeed, "Misrepresentation is the rule with illicit drugs" (Brown & Braden, 1987, p. 341). A capsule might be sold on the street as "THC" but actually contain PCP, a far different chemical. The buyer cannot, without a detailed chemical analysis, be sure what the substance purchased actually is, whether it is contaminated, or how potent it might be.

Near the end of the 1980s, one study found that only 60% of the samples of "amphetamines" purchased on the street actually contained amphetamines (Scaros, Westra, & Barone, 1990). It is not uncommon for "amphetamines" sold on the street to actually be nothing more than caffeine tablets or some other substance. In some cases, police chemists have found that what was sold as the hallucinogen MDMA might contain "anything from MDA, LSD and amphetamine to fish-tank oxygenating tablets and cold cure powders" (Abbott & Concar, 1992, p. 33).

Thus, one should not automatically assume that any illicit drug is actually what it is purported to be. Indeed, one should not even assume that the chemical is safe for human use, without a chemical analysis. In the world of illicit drug use, it is indeed a case of "let the buyer beware."

Drug Analogs: The "Designer" Drugs

The laws that identify a drug, be it legal or illegal, are highly specific. The drug's chemical structure is analyzed, and the exact location of each atom in relation to every other atom in the drug's chemical chain is identified and recorded. The specific chemical structure for a specific drug is then registered with the federal government, and its chemical structure is then used to identify the drug. This is true whether the chemical is legally copyrighted by a company or if the drug is an illegal substance.

The identification and regulation of new pharmaceuticals is a complex and difficult task that lies outside of the scope of this chapter. To simplify matters, our discussion will be limited to illegal drugs.

For the sake of discussion, let's say that the simplified drug molecule shown in Figure 33.1 has been outlawed as an illegal hallucinogen.[4] The exact location of every atom in this hypothetical drug molecule has been recorded, and the molecule has been described in specific detail to allow for its easy identification. However, a drug with the chemical structure shown in Figure 33.2 would technically be a "different" drug, since its molecular structure is not *exactly* the same as the first drug's. The molecule in Figure 33.2 is called a drug "analog" of the parent drug.

There is an obvious difference in the chemical structure of the drugs in Figures 33.1 and 33.2.

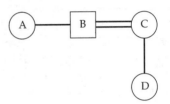

FIGURE 33.1

[4]The structures illustrated here are not actual drug molecules.

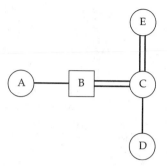

FIGURE 33.2

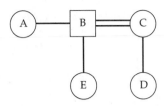

FIGURE 33.4

The new atom added in Figure 33.2 might not do *anything* to the potency of the drug, but it does change the chemical structure of the drug just enough that it is not covered by the law that made the parent drug illegal.

For this analog to be declared illegal, researchers would have to identify the location of every atom in the second drug and the nature of the chemical bond that held that atom in place. Then, law enforcement officials would have to present their findings to the appropriate agency for the drug analog to be outlawed. This is a process that could take months or even longer. When it is accomplished, though, it would be a simple matter to again change the chemical structure a little bit to build a new analog, as shown in Figure 33.3.

There is a very subtle difference in the chemical structure of the last two hypothetical drug molecules, but they are "different" drugs in the eyes of the law. Technically, this new "drug" is not covered by the law that prohibited the parent drug. If the drug molecule *were* to be outlawed, the "street" chemist could again change the drug, as shown in Figure 33.4.

The drug molecule used in this example was a very simple one, having only five atoms. However, even with this simple example, it was possible to produce several different analogs of the original molecule. When you consider that many psychoactive drugs have molecules that contain many hundreds or thousands of atoms, the number of potential combinations is impressive. For example, there are 184 known analogs of the hallucinogen MDMA, many of which have psychoactive properties and thus abuse potential (*The Economist*, 1993b).

Drug analogs vary in both potency and safety. When produced by underground laboratories, they are called "designer" drugs. Their regulation by the courts is extremely difficult, partly because it is so easy to alter the chemical structure to produce a "new" chemical and because it is so hard for chemists to identify the chemical structure of a drug.

Some Existing Drug Analogs

It should be no surprise that "street" chemists have been manipulating the chemical structure of known drugs of abuse for some time, hoping to come up with a new drug that has not yet been outlawed. Some analogs of the amphetamine family of drugs include the hallucinogen DOM (2,5-dimethoxy-4-methylamphetamine) (Scaros, Westra, & Barone, 1990). MDMA, also known as "ecstasy," is itself a drug analog of the amphetamine family of chemicals. As we noted in the chapter on the hallucinogens, research evidence suggests that MDMA is capable of selectively destroying certain neurons in the brain, indicating that this drug analog has some potential for harm to the human brain.

MDEA (3,4-methylenedioxyamphetamine) is another drug analog of the amphetamine family.

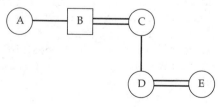

FIGURE 33.3

When the hallucinogen MDMA was classified as a controlled substance in 1985, many street chemists simply started to produce MDEA. The chemical structure of MDEA is very similar to that of MDMA, and its effects are reported to be very similar to those of MDMA (Mirin, Weiss, & Greenfield, 1991). This substance is often sold under the name of "Eve." There have been isolated reports of death associated with MDEA use, but it is not known what role, if any, MDEA had in these deaths. Furthermore, the long-term effects of MDEA are still unknown.

A recent addition to the illicit stimulants being produced by "street" chemists in the United States is methcathinone, or "cat." Easily manufactured from chemicals that can be purchased legally, in the United States, cat has long been used by addicts in the former Soviet Union (Goldstone, 1993). Chemically, 2-methylamino-1-phenylpropan-1-one is very similar to the amphetamines, although its effects are said to last up to 6 days, according to Goldstone. Tolerance to cat develops rapidly. Furthermore, as discussed in Chapter 7, cat has been identified as the cause of a drug-induced psychotic reaction and as a cause of death. Cat was classified as a controlled substance by the Drug Enforcement Administration in 1992. Although cat is not widespread at this time, it *has* been identified in "street" drug samples from both Wisconsin and Michigan, and it is expected to spread to other states (Goldstone, 1993).

Street chemists have also produced at least five drug analogs to the hallucinogen PCP, each of which has an effect similar to that of PCP (Scaros, Westra, & Barone, 1990). These are the drugs N-ethyl-1-phenylcyclohexylamine (also known as PCE), (1-(1-2-thienylcyclohexyl) piperidine) (or TCP), (1-(1-phenylcyclohexyl) pyrrolidine) (or PHP), (1-piperidinocyclohexanecarbonitrile) (or PCC), and Eu4ia (pronounced "euphoria"), an amphetamine-like drug synthesized from legally purchased, over-the-counter chemicals. Other street drugs that are occasionally produced by illicit laboratories include 2-(o-chlorophenyl)-2-(methylamino) cyclohexanone (or Ketamine).

Ketamine, surprisingly, is a legitimate pharmaceutical agent, which is used as a surgical anesthetic (Bushnell & Justins, 1993). When used as an anesthetic, Ketamine can be introduced into the body by intravenous injection, by intramuscular injection, or in oral form, according to the authors. Further, because Ketamine does not cause respiratory or cardiac depression, it is of value in situations where opioid-based anesthetics cannot be used. When it is abused, Ketamine is said to have effects similar to those of heroin (*The Economist*, 1989). In addition to causing a sense of euphoria, Ketamine can also bring about psychological dissociation, panic states, and hallucinations (Jansen, 1993). Long-term use, especially at high doses, may result in drug-induced memory problems.

A new entry into the world of drug analogs is 2-amino-4-methyl-5-phenyl-2-oxazoline, which is derived from a diet pill available in Europe known as "Aminorex" (Evanko, 1991). The effects of this drug, often sold on the street by the name of "U-4-E-UH" are not well known at this time, although there are reports that the drug has been sold on both the East and West coasts of the United States.

Obviously, these drugs are called a variety of other—easier—names on the street. There is no clinical research into their effects on the human body for the most part, and thus their potential for harm is unknown.

In the early 1980s, there was a series of fatal narcotic overdoses in California, as street chemists started to produce various "designer drugs" similar to the analgesic fentanyl (discussed in the chapter on narcotic analgesics) (Hibbs, Perper, & Winek, 1991). These new drug "analogs" could be more or less potent than the parent molecule. Kirsch (1986) identifies nine different drug analogs to fentanyl that are known or suspected to have been sold on the streets, ranging in potency from one-tenth that of morphine for the fentanyl analog benzylfentanyl, to between 1,000 times (Hibbs, Perper, & Winek, 1991) and 3,000 times (Kirsch, 1986) more potent than morphine for 3-methylfentanyl.

3-Methylfentanyl is also known to chemists as

"TMF." This analog of fentanyl has been identified as the cause of narcotics overdoses in the area around Pittsburgh, Pennsylvania (Hibbs, Perper, & Winek, 1991), and in New York City (*Newsweek,* 1991). Hibbs, Perper, and Winek (1991) conducted a retrospective analysis to determine how serious a problem TMF-induced overdoses were for the Allegheny County region, which surrounds Pittsburgh. Surprisingly, the authors found that, in 1988, fully 27% of the drug overdose deaths in Allegheny County were caused by TMF. This suggests that designer narcotics are a significant part of the narcotics problem in the United States.

Summary

The relationship between substance abuse and criminal activity is a very complex one. Although it appears on the surface that drug use *causes* crime, a deeper exploration reveals that this conclusion does not fit known facts. Indeed, an in-depth exploration of the relationship between chemical use and criminal activity reveals that these two social problems are so intertwined that it is difficult to determine how they contribute to one another. Even now, after a century of study, professionals are still unclear as to the true relationship between chemical use and crime.

The "U.S. model" of drug interdiction and criminal prosecution is not universally accepted. Indeed, the Dutch attempt to approach the problem differently has met with some success in both Holland and England. This social experiment casts doubt as to the utility of antidrug laws, which can be enforced only at a tremendous cost to society.

In the United States, the primary means by which the government has tried to deal with the drug use problem is through the judicial system. A number of laws have been passed in the hopes of controlling or eliminating recreational chemical use. One way that the manufacturers of illicit drugs try to circumvent these laws is by modifying the chemical structure of an existing drug, to produce a "new" substance that is not covered by any antidrug law. These new chemicals are called "analogs" of the parent drug, and they are becoming an increasingly common part of the drug use problem in this country.

Sample Assessment:
A Case of Alcohol Abuse

HISTORY AND IDENTIFYING INFORMATION

Mr John D. is a 35-year-old married white male from _____ County, Missouri. He is employed as an electrical engineer for the XYZ Company, where he has worked for the past 3 years. Prior to this, Mr. D. was in the United States Navy, where he served for 4 years. He was discharged under honorable conditions, and reported that he only had "a few" minor rules infractions. He was never brought before a court-martial.

CIRCUMSTANCES OF REFERRAL

Mr. D. was seen after having been arrested on the charge of driving while under the influence of alcohol. He reported that he had been drinking with co-workers to celebrate a promotion at work. His measured blood alcohol level (or BAL) was 0.150, well above the legal limit necessary for a charge of driving while under the influence. Mr. D. reported that he had had "seven or eight" mixed drinks in approximately a 2-hour time span. By his report, he had been arrested within 15 minutes after leaving the bar.

After his initial court appearance, Mr. D. was referred to this evaluator by the court, to determine whether he has a chemical dependency problem.

1

This case is entirely fictitious. Any similarity between the person in this report and any person, living or dead, is entirely coincidental.

DRUG AND ALCOHOL USE HISTORY

Mr. D. reported that he first began to drink at the age of 15, when he and a friend would steal beer from his father's supply in the basement. He would drink an occasional beer from time to time after that, and first became intoxicated when he was 17.

When he was eighteen, Mr. D. enlisted in the United States Navy, and after basic training he was stationed in the San Diego area. Mr. D. reported that he was first exposed to chemicals while he was stationed in San Diego, and that he tried both marijuana and cocaine while on weekend liberty. Mr. D. reported that he did not like the effects of cocaine and that he only used this chemical once or twice. He did like the effects of marijuana, and reported that he would smoke one or two marijuana cigarettes obtained from friends perhaps once a month.

Mr. D. reported that, during this portion of his life, he would drink about twice a weekend, when on liberty. The amount he would drink ranged from "one or two beers" up to 12 or 18 beers. Mr. D. reported that he first had an alcohol-related blackout while he was in the navy and that he "should have been arrested" for driving on base while under the influence of alcohol on several different occasions but was never stopped by the Shore Patrol.

Following his honorable discharge from the navy at the age of 22, Mr. D. enrolled in college. His chemical use declined to the weekend use of alcohol, usually in moderation, but Mr. D. reported that he did drink to the point of an alcohol-related blackout "once or twice" in the 4 years that he was in college. There was no other chemical use following his discharge from the navy, and Mr. D. reports that he has not used other chemicals since the age of 20 or 21.

Upon graduation, at the age of 26, Mr. D. began to work for the XYZ Company, where he is currently employed. He met his wife shortly after he began work, and they were married after a courtship of 1 year. Mr. D.'s wife, Pat, does not use chemicals other than an "occasional" social drink. On further questioning, it was revealed that Mrs. D. drinks a glass of wine with a meal about twice a month. She denied other chemical use.

Mrs. D. reported that her husband does not usually drink more than one or two beers, and that he will drink only on weekends. She reported that the night he was arrested was

2

"unusual" for him, in the sense that he is not a drinker. His employer was not contacted, but court records failed to reveal any other arrest records for Mr. D.

Mr. D. admitted to several alcohol-related blackouts, but none since he was in college. He denied seizures, DTs or alcohol-related tremor. There was no evidence of ulcers, gastritis, or cardiac problems. His last physical was "normal" according to information provided by his personal physician. There were no abnormal blood chemistry findings, nor did his physician find any evidence suggesting alcoholism. Mr. D. denied having ever been hospitalized for an alcohol-related injury, and there was no evidence suggesting that he has been involved in fights.

On the Michigan Alcoholism Screening Test, Mr. D.'s score of four (4) points would not suggest alcoholism. This information was reviewed in the presence of his wife, who did not suggest that there was any misrepresentation on his test scores. On this administration of the MMPI, there was no evidence of psychopathology noted. Mr. D.'s MacAndrew Alcoholism Scale score fell in the normal range, failing to suggest an addictive disorder at this time.

PSYCHIATRIC HISTORY

Mr. D. denied having had psychiatric treatment of any kind. He did admit to having seen a marriage counselor "once" shortly after he married, but reported that overall he and his wife are happy together. Apparently, they had a question about a marital communications issue that was cleared up after one visit, which took place after 3 or 4 years of marriage.

SUMMARY AND CONCLUSIONS

At this point, there is little evidence to suggest an ongoing alcohol problem. Mr. D. seems to be a well-adjusted young man who drank to the point of excess after having been offered a long-desired promotion at work. Excessive drinking seems to be unusual for Mr. D., who usually limits his drinking to one or two beers on the weekends. There was no evidence of alcohol-related injuries, accidents, or legal problems noted in Mr. D.'s record.

RECOMMENDATIONS

　　　Recommend light sentence, possibly a fine, limited probation, with no restrictions on license. It is also recommended that Mr. D. attend "DWI School" for 8 weeks to learn more about the effects of alcohol on driving.

Signed /s/

Sample Assessment:
A Case of Chemical Dependency

HISTORY AND IDENTIFYING FEATURES

Mr. Michael S. is a 35-year-old divorced white male who is self-employed. He has been a resident of ____ County, Kansas, for the past 3 months. Prior to this, he apparently was living in ____ County, New York, according to his account. On the night of June 6th of this year, Mr. S. was arrested on the charge of possession of a controlled substance. Specifically, Mr. S. was found to be in possession of 2 grams of cocaine, according to police records. This is his first arrest for a drug-related charge in Kansas, although he has been arrested on two other occasions for similar charges in New York State. A copy of his police record is attached to this report.

CIRCUMSTANCES OF REFERRAL

Mr. S. was referred to the undersigned for a chemical dependency evaluation, which will be part of his presentence investigation (PSI) for the charge of felony possession of a controlled substance, and the charge of sale of a controlled substance.

DRUG AND ALCOHOL USE HISTORY

Mr. S. reported that he began to use alcohol when he was

1

13 years of age, and that by the age of 14 he was drinking on a regular basis. Further questioning revealed that, by the time he was about to turn 15, Mr. S. was drinking on "weekends" with friends. He reported that he first became intoxicated on his 15th birthday, but projected responsibility for this onto his friends, who by his report "kept on pouring more and more into the glass until I was drunk."

By the age of 16, Mr. S. was using alcohol "four or five nights a week" and was also using marijuana and hallucinogenics perhaps two or three times a week. He projected responsibility for his expanded chemical use onto his environment, noting that "everybody was selling the stuff, you couldn't walk down the street without people stopping you to ask if you wanted to buy some."

Also, by the age of 16, Mr. S. was supporting his chemical use through burglaries, which he committed with his friends. He was never caught, but volunteered this information stating that since the statute of limitations has expired, he does not have to fear being charged for these crimes.

By the age of 21, Mr. S. was using cocaine "once or twice a week." He was arrested for the first time when he was about 22 for possession of cocaine. This was when he was living in the state of _____. After being tried in court, he was convicted of felony possession of cocaine and placed on probation for 5 years. When asked if he used chemicals while he was on probation, Mr. S. responded, "I don't have to answer that."

Mr. S. reported that he first entered treatment for chemical dependency when he was 27 years of age. At that time, he was found to be addicted to a number of drugs, including alcohol, cocaine, and "downers." Although in treatment for 2 months at the chemical dependency unit of _____ Hospital, Mr. S. stated that "I left as addicted as when I arrived." He reported with some degree of apparent pride that he had found a way to use chemicals even while in treatment. His chemical use apparently was the reason for his ultimate discharge from this program. Although Mr. S. was somewhat vague about the reasons for his discharge, he did report that the staff "did not like how I was doing" in treatment.

Since his discharge, Mr. S. has been using cocaine, alcohol, various drugs obtained from a series of physicians, and opiates. Mr. S. was quite vague as to how he supported his chemical use,

2

but noted that "there are ways of getting money if you really want some."

Mr. S. reported that, in the past year, he has been using cocaine "four or five times a week," although he did admit to having used cocaine on occasion "for a whole week straight." He admitted to sharing needles with other cocaine users from time to time but stated "I am careful." However, he did report that he was diagnosed as having hepatitis B in the past year. He also reported that he overdosed on cocaine "once or twice" but that he treated this overdose himself with benzodiazepines and alcohol.

In addition to the possible cocaine overdoses, Mr. S. admitted to having experienced chest pain while using cocaine on at least two occasions and that he regularly uses alcohol or tranquilizers to combat the side effects of cocaine. He admitted to frequently using tranquilizers or alcohol to help him sleep after using cocaine for extended periods of time. He also admitted to having spent money on drugs that was meant for other expenses (such as loan payments), and by his report he has had at least one automobile repossessed for failure to make payments on the loan.

Mr. S. has been unemployed for at least the past 2 years but is rather vague as to how he supports himself. He apparently was engaged in selling cocaine at the time of his arrest as this is one of the charges brought against him by the police.

Prior to this arrest, Mr. S. had not seen a physician for several years. During this interview, however, it was noted that he had scars strongly suggestive of intravenous needle use on both arms. When asked about these marks, he referred to them as "tracks," a street term for drug needle scars. This would suggest long-term intravenous drug use on Mr. S.'s part. He denied the intravenous use of opiates, but a urine toxicology screen detected narcotics. This suggests that Mr. S. has not been very open about his narcotic drug use.

On administration of the Michigan Alcoholism Screening Test (MAST) Mr. S. achieved a score of 17 points, a score that is strongly suggestive of alcoholism. He reported that the longest period that he has been able to go without using chemicals in the past 5 years was only "hours." His profile on the Minnesota Multiphasic Personality Inventory (MMPI) was suggestive of a very impulsive, immature individual who was likely to have a

3

chemical dependency problem.

PSYCHIATRIC HISTORY

Mr. S. reported that he has been hospitalized for psychiatric reasons only "once." This hospitalization took place several years ago, while Mr. S. was living in the state of _____. Apparently, he was hospitalized for observation following a suicide attempt in which he slit his wrists with a razor blade. Mr. S. was unable to recall whether he had been using cocaine prior to this suicide attempt, but he thought it was "quite possible" that he had experienced a cocaine-induced depression.

MEDICAL HISTORY

As noted above, Mr. S. had not seen a physician for several years prior to his arrest. Since the time of his arrest, however, he has been examined by a physician for a persistent, preexisting cough. The physician (report enclosed) concluded that Mr. S. is "seropositive" for HIV and classified him as falling into category CDC_1. Although it is not possible to determine whether Mr. S. contracted HIV through sharing needles, this is at least a possibility.

SUMMARY AND CONCLUSIONS

Overall, it is quite apparent that Mr. S. has a long-standing chemical dependency problem. In spite of his evasiveness and denial, there is strong evidence of significant chemical dependency problems. Mr. S. seems to support his drug and alcohol use through criminal activity, although he is rather vague about this. He has been convicted of drug-related charges in the state of _____ and was on probation following this conviction. Mr. S.'s motivation for treatment seems to be quite low at this time, as he has expressed the belief that his attorney will "make a deal for me" so he will not have to spend time in prison.

RECOMMENDATIONS

1. Given that Mr. S. has contracted HIV and hepatitis B, probably from infected needles, it is strongly recommended that he be referred to the appropriate medical facility for treatment.

2. It is the opinion of this reviewer that Mr. S.'s

4

motivation for treatment is low at this time. If he is referred
to treatment, it is recommended that this be made part of his
sentencing agreement with the court. If he is incarcerated,
chemical dependency treatment might be made part of his treatment
plan in prison.

    3. Referral to a therapeutic community should be considered
for Mr. S., for long-term residential treatment.

                                                      Signed /s/

References

AASE, J. M. (1994). Clinical recognition of FAS. *Alcohol Health & Research World, 18* (1), 5–9.

ABBOTT, A., & CONCAR, D. (1992). A trip into the unknown. *New Scientist, 135,* 30–34.

ABEL, E. L. (1982). *Drugs and behavior: A primer in neuropsychopharmacology.* Malabar, FL: Robert E. Krieger Publishing Co.

ABOOD, M. E., & MARTIN, B. R. (1992). Neurobiology of marijuana abuse. *Trends in Pharmacological Sciences, 13* (5), 201–206.

ABRAMS, R. C., & ALEXOPOULOS, G. (1987). Substance abuse in the elderly: Alcohol and prescription drugs. *Hospital and Community Psychiatry, 38,* 1285–1288.

ACKERMAN, R. J. (1983). *Children of alcoholics: A guidebook for educators, therapists, and parents.* Holmes Beach, FL: Learning Publications, Inc.

ADAMS, J. K. (1988). Setting free chemical dependency. *Alcoholism & Addiction, 8* (4), 20–21.

ADAMS, W. L., YUAN, Z., BARBORIAK, J. J., & RIMM, A. A. (1993). Alcohol-related hospitalizations of elderly people. *Journal of the American Medical Association, 270,* 1222–1225.

Addiction Letter, The. (1989a). Methadone centers ineffective in treating heroin addicts—GAO. *6* (5), 5.

Addiction Letter, The. (1989b). Therapeutic community research yields interesting results. *5* (1), 2.

Addiction Letter, The. (1993a). Blunts and crude: Two new marijuana products are on the streets. *9* (11), 1, 7.

Addiction Letter, The. (1993b). Dangerous inhalants are increasingly popular among adolescents. *9* (8), 1, 7.

ADELMAN, S. A., & WEISS, R. D. (1989). What is therapeutic about inpatient alcoholism treatment? *Hospital and Community Psychiatry, 40* (5), 515–519.

ADGER, H., & WERNER, M. J. (1994). The pediatrician. *Alcohol Health & Research World, 18,* 121–126.

AIDS Alert. (1989). Research on nitrites suggests drug plays role in AIDS epidemic. *4* (9), 153–156.

Al-Anon's Twelve Steps & Twelve Traditions. (1985). New York: Al-Anon Family Group Headquarters, Inc.

Alcohol Alert. (1993a). Alcohol and the liver. Washington, DC: National Institute on Alcohol Abuse and Alcoholism.

Alcohol Alert. (1993b). Alcohol and cancer. Washington, DC: National Institute on Alcohol Abuse and Alcoholism.

Alcohol Alert. (1993c). Alcohol and nutrition. Washington, DC: National Institute on Alcohol Abuse and Alcoholism.

Alcohol Alert. (1994). Alcohol-related impairment. Washington, DC: National Institute on Alcohol Abuse and Alcoholism.

Alcoholics Anonymous. (1976). New York: Alcoholics Anonymous World Services, Inc.

Alcoholism & Drug Abuse Week. (1990a). ONDCP gives rundown on treatment approaches. *2* (26), 3–5.

Alcoholism & Drug Abuse Week. (1990b). House panel considers impact of drugs on emergency rooms. *2* (38), 4–5.

Alcoholism & Drug Abuse Week. (1991a). DAWN: Emergency rooms seeing fewer drug cases. *3* (6), 1.

Alcoholism & Drug Abuse Week. (1991b). ONDCP says Americans spent $41 billion on drugs in 1990. *3* (24), 3.

Alcoholism & Drug Abuse Week. (1991c). Mixed signals on possible upsurge in heroin use. *3* (24), 4–5.

Alcoholism & Drug Abuse Week. (1991d). Groups offer self-help alternatives to AA. *3* (37), 6.

Alcoholism & Drug Abuse Week. (1993). Methadone alternative nears approval. *5* (22), 4.

Alcoholism & Drug Abuse Week. (1994a). Treating

women effectively doesn't mean simply treating women. *6* (17), 1–3.

Alcoholism & Drug Abuse Week. (1994b). Study: cocaine treatment more effective than supply control. *6* (24), 4.

The Alcoholism Report. (1991). AA survey findings released. *19* (7), 8–10.

ALEXANDER, B. (1991) Alcohol abuse in adolescents. *American Family Physician, 43* (2), 527–532.

ALIBRANDI, L. A. (1978). The folk psychotherapy of Alcoholics Anonymous. In S. Zimberg, J. Wallace, & S. Blume (Eds.), *Practical approaches to alcoholism psychotherapy.* New York: Plenum.

ALLEN, M. G., & PHILLIPS, K. L. (1993). Utilization review of treatment for chemical dependence. *Hospital and Community Psychiatry, 44,* 752–756.

ALLISON, M. C., HOWATSON, A. G., TORRANCE, C. J., LEE, F. D., & RUSSELL, R. I. (1992). Gastrointestinal damage associated with the use of nonsteroidal antiinflammatory drugs. *The New England Journal of Medicine, 327,* 749–754.

ALTERMAN, A. I., ERDLEN, D. I., LA PORTE, D. J., & ERDLEN, F. R. (1982). Effects of illicit drug use in an inpatient psychiatric population. *Addictive Behaviors, 7,* 231–242.

American Academy of Family Physicians. (1989). Screening for alcohol and other drug abuse. *American Family Physician, 40* (1), 137–147.

American Academy of Family Physicians. (1990a). Marijuana use and memory loss. *American Family Physician, 41* (3), 930–932.

American Academy of Family Physicians. (1990b). Effects of fetal exposure to cocaine and heroin. *American Family Physician, 41* (5), 1595–1597.

American Cancer Society. (1990). Data bank. *Breakthroughs, 1* (2), 12.

American Medical Association. (1992). Costs from drug abuse doubled since 1986. *American Medical News, 35* (30), 37.

American Medical Association. (1993a). Factors contributing to the health care cost problem. Chicago: American Medical Association.

American Medical Association. (1993b). Injury prevention must be part of nation's plan to reduce health costs, say control experts. *Journal of the American Medical Association, 270,* 19–20.

American Psychiatric Association. (1990). *Benzodiazepine dependence, toxicity, and abuse.* Washington, DC: American Psychiatric Association.

American Psychiatric Association. (1994). *Diagnostic and statistical manual of mental disorders (4th ed.).* Washington, DC: American Psychiatric Association.

American Society of Hospital Pharmacists. (1994). *AHFS drug information.* Bethesda, MD: Author.

AMES, D., WIRSHING, W. C., & FRIEDMAN, R. (1993).

Ecstasy, the serotonin syndrome, and neuroleptic malignant syndrome—a possible link? *Journal of the American Medical Association, 269,* 869–870.

ANAND, K. J. S., & ARNOLD, J. H. (1994). Opioid tolerance and dependence in infants and children. *Critical Care Medicine, 22,* 334–342.

ANANTH, J., VANDEWATER, S., KAMAL, M., BRODSKY, A., GAMAL, R., & MILLER, M. (1989). Missed diagnosis of substance abuse in psychiatric patients. *Hospital & Community Psychiatry, 40,* 297–299.

ANDERSON, D. J. (1989a). Inhalant abusers risk death, permanent injury. *Minneapolis Star-Tribune, VIII* (165), p. 4EX.

ANDERSON, D. J. (1989b). An alcoholic is never too old for treatment. *Minneapolis Star-Tribune, VIII* (200), p. 7EX.

ANDERSON, D. J. (1991). Alcohol abuse takes a toll in head injuries. *Minneapolis Star-Tribune, X* (152), p. 7E.

ANDERSON, D. J. (1993). Chemically dependent women still face barriers. *Minneapolis Star-Tribune, XII* (65), p. 8E.

ANDERSON, R. (1993). AIDS: Trends, predictions, controversy. *Nature, 363,* 393–394.

ANDERSON, R. M., & MAY, R. M. (1992). Understanding the AIDS pandemic. *Scientific American, 266* (5), pp. 58–66.

ANGELL, M., & KASSIFER, J. P. (1994). Alcohol and other drugs—toward a more rational and consistent policy. *The New England Journal of Medicine, 331,* 537–539

ANGIER, N. (1990). Storming the wall. *Discover, 11* (5), pp. 67–72.

ANKER, A. L., & SMILKSTEIN, M. J. (1994). Acetaminophen. *Emergency Medical Clinics of North America, 12,* 335–349.

ANSEVICS, N. L., & DOWEIKO, H. E. (1983). A conceptual framework for intervention with the antisocial personality. *Psychotherapy in Private Practice, 1* (3), 43–52.

APPELBAUM, P. S. (1992). Controlling prescription of benzodiazepines. *Hospital & Community Psychiatry, 43,* 12–13.

ARONOFF, G. M., WAGNER, J. M., & SPANGLER, A. S. (1986). Chemical interventions for pain. *Journal of Consulting and Clinical Psychology, 54,* 769–775.

ASHTON, H. (1992). *Brain Function and Psychotropic Drugs.* New York: Oxford University Press.

ASSEO, L. (1993). Drug war clogs system, ABA says. *St. Paul Pioneer Press, 144* (287), p. 2A.

Associated Press. (1992). Women smoker deaths are expected to double. *St. Paul Pioneer Press, 143* (341), p. 12A.

Associated Press. (1993). Drug dealers find new prey—the deaf. *San Francisco Examiner, 128* (21), p. B-7.

Associated Press. (1994a). About 2.2 million children smoke, heart group says. *Minneapolis Star-Tribune XII* (212), p. 2A.

Associated Press. (1994b). Spraying away the cigarette craving? *Minneapolis Star-Tribune, XIII* (120), pp. 5A, 6A.

ASTRACHAN, B. M., & TISCHLER, G. L. (1984). Normality from a health systems perspective. In D. Offer & M. Sabshin (Eds.), *Normality and the life cycle.* New York: Basic Books.

ATKINSON, I. H., & GRANT, I. (1994). Natural history of neuropsychiatric manifestations of HIV disease. *Psychiatric Clinics of North America, 17,* 17–33.

AUSABEL, D. P. (1983). Methadone maintenance treatment: The other side of the coin. *International Journal of the Addictions, 18,* 851–862.

AYD, F. J. (1994). Prescribing anxiolytics and hypnotics for the elderly. *Psychiatric Annals, 24* (2), 91–97.

AZUMA, S. D., & CHASNOFF, I. J. (1993). Outcome of children prenatally exposed to cocaine and other drugs: A path analysis of three-year data. *Pediatrics, 92,* 396–402.

BAHRKE, M. S. (1990). *Psychological research, methodological problems, and relevant issues.* Paper presented at the 1990 meeting of the American Psychological Association, Boston, MA.

BALES, J. (1988). Legalized drugs: Idea flawed, debate healthy. *APA Monitor, 19* (8), p. 22.

BANERJEE, S. (1990). Newest wrinkle for smokers is on their faces. *Minneapolis Star-Tribune, VIII* (341), pp. 1EX, 5EX.

BARDEN, J. C. (1991). In depth. *Minneapolis Star-Tribune, X* (153), pp. 4A, 6A.

BARNHILL, J. G., CIRAULO, A. M., CIRAULO, D. A. (1989). Interactions of importance in chemical dependence. In D. A. Ciraulo, R. I. Shader, D. J. Greenblatt, & W. Creelman (Eds.), *Drug interactions in psychiatry.* Baltimore: Williams & Wilkins.

BARR, W. G., & MERCHUT, M. P. (1992). Systemic lupus erythematosus with central nervous system involvement. *The Psychiatric Clinics of North America, 15,* 439–454.

BARTECCHI, C. E., MACKENZIE, T. D., & SCHRIER, R. W. (1994). The human costs of tobacco use. *The New England Journal of Medicine, 330,* 907–912.

BAUGHMAN, R. D. (1993). Psoriasis and cigarettes. *Archives of Dermatology, 129,* 1329–1330.

BAUMAN, J. L. (1988). Acute heroin withdrawal. *Hospital Therapy, 13,* 60–66.

BAUMAN, K. E., & ENNETT, S. T. (1994). Peer influence on adolescent drug use. *American Psychologist, 63,* 820–822.

BAYS, J. (1990). Substance abuse and child abuse. *Pediatric Clinics of North America, 37,* 881–903.

BAYS, J. (1992). The care of alcohol and drug-affected infants. *Pediatric Annals, 21* (8), 485–495.

BEAN-BAYOG, M. (1988). Alcohol and drug abuse: Alcoholism as a cause of psychopathology. *Hospital and Community Psychiatry, 39,* 352–354.

BEAN-BAYOG, M. (1993). AA processes and change: How does it work? In B. S. McCrady & W. R. Miller (Eds.), *Research on Alcoholics Anonymous.* New Brunswick, NJ: Rutgers Center of Alcohol Studies.

BEARDSLEY, T. (1994). The lucky ones. *Scientific American, 270* (5), pp. 20, 24, 28.

BEASLEY, J. D. (1987). *Wrong diagnosis, wrong treatment: The plight of the alcoholic in America.* New York: Creative Infomatics, Inc.

BEATTIE, M. (1987). *Codependent no more.* New York: Harper & Row.

BEATTIE, M. (1989). *Beyond codependency.* New York: Harper & Row.

BEAUVAIS, F., & OETTING, E. R. (1988). Inhalant abuse by young children. In *Epidemiology of inhalant abuse: An update.* Washington, DC: National Institute on Drug Abuse.

BECKMAN, L. J. (1993). Alcoholics Anonymous and gender issues. In B. S. McCrady & W. R. Miller (Eds.), *Research on Alcoholics Anonymous.* New Brunswick, NJ: Rutgers Center of Alcohol Studies.

BEEBE, D. K., & WALLEY, E. (1991). Substance abuse: The designer drugs. *American Family Physician, 43,* 1689–1698.

BEHNKE, M., & EYLER, F. D. (1993). The consequences of prenatal substance use for the developing fetus, newborn and young child. *International Journal of the Addictions, 28,* 1341–1391.

BEITNER-JOHNSON, D., & NESTLER, E. J. (1992). Basic neurobiology of cocaine: Actions within the mesolimbic dopamine system. In T. R. Kosten & H. D. Kleber (Eds.), *Clinician's guide to cocaine addiction.* New York: Guilford.

BENET, L. Z., MITCHELL, J. R., & SHEINER, L. B. (1991). Pharmacokinetics: The dynamics of drug absorption, distribution and elimination. In A. G. Gilman, T. W. Rall, A. S. Nies, & P. Taylor (Eds.), *The pharmacological basis of therapeutics* (8th ed.). New York: Pergamon.

BENOWITZ, N. L. (1992). Cigarette smoking and nicotine addiction. *Medical Clinics of North America, 76,* 415–437.

BENOWITZ, N. L., & HENNINGFIELD, J. E. (1994). Establishing a nicotine threshold for addiction. *New England Journal of Medicine, 331,* 123–126.

BENOWITZ, N. L., & JACOB, P. (1993). Nicotine and cotinine elimination pharmacokinetics in smokers and nonsmokers. *Clinical Pharmacology & Therapeutics, 53,* 316–323.

BERENSON, D. (1987). Alcoholics Anonymous: From surrender to transformation. *The Family Therapy Networker, 11* (4), 25–31.

BERG, B. J., & DUBIN, W. R. (1990). Economic grand

rounds: Why 28 days? An alternative approach to alcoholism treatment. *Hospital and Community Psychiatry, 41,* 1175–1178.

BERG, I. K., & MILLER, S. D. (1992). *Working with the problem drinker.* New York: Norton.

BERG, R., FRANZEN, M. M., & WEDDING, D. (1994). *Screening for brain impairment: A manual for mental health practice* (2nd ed.). New York: Springer.

BERGER, P. A., & DUNN, M. J. (1982). Substance induced and substance use disorders. In J. H. Griest, J. W. Jefferson, & R. L. Spitzer (Eds.), *Treatment of mental disorders.* New York: Oxford University Press.

BERKOWITZ, A., & PERKINS, H. W. (1988). Personality characteristics of children of alcoholics. *Journal of Consulting and Clinical Psychology, 56,* 206–209.

BLACK, C. (1982). *It will never happen to me.* Denver, CO: M.A.C. Printing and Publications.

BLACK, C. (1987). How different is recovery for a COA? *Alcoholism & Addiction, 8* (6), insert.

BLAKE, R. (1990). Mental health counseling and older problem drinkers. *Journal of Mental Health Counseling, 12* (3), 354–367.

BLANSJAAR, B. A., & ZWINDERMAN, A. H. (1992). The course of alcohol amnesic disorder: A three-year follow up study of clinical signs. *Acta Psychiatrica Scandinavica, 86,* 240–246.

BLAU, M. (1990). Toxic parents, perennial kids: Is it time for adult children to grow up? *Utne Reader, 42,* 60–65.

BLEIDT, B. A., & MOSS, J. T. (1989). Age-related changes in drug distribution. *U.S. Pharmacist, 14* (8), 24–32.

BLISS, R. E., GARVEY, A. J., HEINOLD, J. W., & HITCHCOCK, J. L. (1989). The influence of situation and coping on relapse crisis outcomes after smoking cessation. *Journal of Consulting and Clinical Psychology, 57,* 443–449.

BLOODWORTH, R. C. (1987). Major problems associated with marijuana abuse. *Psychiatric Medicine, 3* (3), 173–184.

BLOOMER, S. (1994). Caffeine abuse widespread, researchers show. *APA Monitor, 25* (2), 17.

BLUM, K. (1984). *Handbook of abusable drugs.* New York: Gardner.

BLUM, K. (1988). The disease process in alcoholism. *Alcoholism & Addiction, 8* (5), 5–8

BLUM, K., NOBLE, E. P., SHERIDAN, P. J., MONTGOMERY, A., RITCHIE, T., JAGADEESWARAN, P., NOGAMI, H., BRIGGS, A. H., & COHN, J. B. (1990). Allelic association of human dopamine D_2 receptor gene in alcoholism. *Journal of the American Medical Association, 263* (15), 2055–2060.

BLUM, K., & PAYNE, J. E. (1991). *Alcohol and the addictive brain.* New York: Free Press.

BLUM, K., & TRACHTENBERG, M. C. (1988). Neurochem-

istry and alcohol craving. *California Society for the Treatment of Alcoholism and Other Drug Dependencies News, 13* (2), 1–7.

BLUME, S. B. (1994). Gender differences in alcohol-related disorders. *Harvard Review of Psychiatry, 2,* 7–14.

Board of Trustees. (1991). Drug abuse in the United States. *Journal of the American Medical Association, 256,* 2102–2107.

BOHN, M. J. (1993). Alcoholism. *Psychiatric Clinics of North America, 16,* 679–692.

BOLOS, A. M., DEAN, M., LUCAS-DERSE, S., RAMSBURG, M., BROWN, G. L., & GOLDMAN, D. (1991). Population and pedigree studies reveal a lack of association between the dopamine D_2 receptor gene and alcoholism. *Journal of the American Medical Association, 264,* 3156–3160.

BOND, W. S. (1989). Smoking's effects on medications. *American Druggist, 200* (1), 24–25.

BONSTEDT, T., ULRICH, D. A., DOLINAR, L. J., & JOHNSON, J. J. (1984). When and where should we hospitalize alcoholics? *Hospital & Community Psychiatry, 35,* 1038–1040.

BOUTOTTE, J. (1993). T.B. The second time around . . . *Nursing 93, 23* (5), 42–49.

BOWEN, M. (1985). *Family therapy in clinical practice.* Northvale, NJ: Aronson.

BOWER, B. (1991). Pumped up and strung out. *Science News, 140* (2), 30–31.

BOYD, C. (1992). Self-help sickness? *St. Paul Pioneer Press, 143* (346), pp. 1C, 4C.

BRADFORD, J. M. W., GREENBERG, D. M., & MOTAYNE, G. G. (1992). Substance abuse and criminal behavior. *Psychiatric Clinics of North America, 15,* 605–622.

BRADLEY, B. P., GOSSOP, M., BREWIN, C. R., PHILLIPS, G., & GREEN, L. (1992). Attributions and relapse in opiate addicts. *Journal of Consulting and Clinical Psychology, 60,* 470–472.

BRADSHAW, J. (1988a). Compulsivity: The black plague of our day. *Lear's Magazine, 42,* pp. 89–90.

BRADSHAW, J. (1988b). *Bradshaw on: The family.* Deerfield Beach, FL: Health Communications, Inc.

BRADY, K. T., GRICE, D. E., DUSTAN, L., & RANDALL, C. (1993). Gender differences in substance use disorders. *American Journal of Psychiatry, 150,* 1707–1711.

BRANDT, J., & BUTTERS, N. (1986). The alcoholic Wernicke-Korsakoff syndrome and its relationship to long-term alcohol use. In I. Grant & K. M. Adams (Eds.), *Neuropsychological assessment of neuropsychiatric disorders.* New York: Oxford University Press.

BRECHER, E. M. (1972). *Licit and illicit drugs.* Boston: Little, Brown.

BRENNER, D. E., KUKULL, W. A., VAN BELLE, G., BOWEN, J. D., McCORMICK, W. C., TERI, L., & LARSON, E. B.

(1993). Relationship between cigarette smoking and Alzheimer's disease in a population-based case-control study. *Neurology, 43,* 293–300.

BRENT, D. A., KUPFER, D. J., BROMET, E. J., & DEW, M. A. (1988). The assessment and treatment of patients at risk for suicide. In A. J. Frances & R. E. Hales (Eds.), *American Psychiatric Association Annual Review: Vol. 7.* Washington, DC: American Psychiatric Association Press, Inc.

BREO, D. L. (1990). Of M.D.s and muscles—lessons from two "retired steroid doctors." *Journal of the American Medical Association, 263,* 1697–1705.

BRESLAU, N., KILBEY, M., & ANDRESKI, P. (1993). Vulnerability to psychopathology in nicotine-dependent smokers: An epidemiologic study of young adults. *American Journal of Psychiatry, 150,* 941–946.

BRESLIN, J. (1988). Crack. *Playboy, 35* (12), pp. 109–110, 210, 212–213, 215.

BRIGGS, G. G., FREEMAN, R. K., & YAFFE, S. J. (1986). *Drugs in pregnancy and lactation* (2nd ed.). Baltimore: Williams & Wilkins.

BRODSKY, A. (1993). The 12 Steps are not for everyone—Or even for most. *Addiction & Recovery, 13* (2), 21.

BRODY, J. (1991). Hepatitis B still spreading. *Minneapolis Star-Tribune, X* (269), p. 4E.

BRODY, J. (1993). To drink or not to drink? For women its benefit to heart vs. cancer risk. *Minneapolis Star-Tribune, XII* (168), p. 12EX.

BROOKOFF, D., COOK, C. S., WILLIAMS, C., & MANN, C. S. (1994). Testing reckless drivers for cocaine and marijuana. *The New England Journal of Medicine, 331,* 518–522.

BROPHY, J. J. (1993). Psychiatric disorders. In L. M. Tierney, S. J. McPhee, M. A. Papadakis, & S. A. Schroeder. (Eds.), *Current medical diagnosis and treatment.* Norwalk, CT: Appleton & Lange.

BROWER, K. J. (1993). Anabolic steroids. *Psychiatric Clinics of North America, 16,* 97–103.

BROWER, K. J., BLOW, F. C., YOUNG, J. P., & HILL, E. M. (1991). Symptoms and correlates of anabolic-androgenic steroid dependence. *British Journal of Addiction, 86,* 759–768.

BROWER, K. J., CATLIN, D. H., BLOW, F. C., ELIOPULOS, G. A., & BERESFORD, T. P. (1991). Clinical assessment and urine testing for anabolic-androgenic steroid abuse and dependence. *American Journal of Drug and Alcohol Abuse, 17* (2), 161–172.

BROWN, R. T., & BRADEN, N. J. (1987). Hallucinogens. *Pediatric Clinics of North America, 34* (2), 341–347.

BROWN, S. (1985). *Treating the alcoholic: A developmental model of recovery.* New York: Wiley.

BROWN, S. A. (1990). Adolescent alcohol expectancies and risk for alcohol abuse. *Addiction & Recovery, 10* (5/6), 16–19.

BROWN, S. A., CREAMER, V. A., & STETSON, B. A. (1987). Adolescent alcohol expectancies in relation to personal and parental drinking patterns. *Journal of Abnormal Psychology, 96,* 117–121.

BROWN, S. A., GOLDMAN, M. S., INN, A., & ANDERSON, L. R. (1980). Expectations of reinforcement from alcohol: Their domain and relation to drinking patterns. *Journal of Abnormal Psychology, 96,* 117–121.

Brown University Digest of Addiction Theory and Application. (1994). Whatever happened to ice? *13* (3), 6–8.

BROWN, V. B., RIDGELY, M. S., PEPPER, B., LEVINE, I. S., & RYGLEWICZ, H. (1989). The dual crisis: Mental illness and substance abuse. *American Psychologist, 44,* 565–569.

BROWNING, C., REYNOLDS, A. L., DWORKIN, S. H. (1991). Affirmative psychotherapy for lesbian women. *The Counseling Psychologist, 19,* 177–196.

BROWNING, M., HOFFER, B. J., & DUNWIDDIE, T. V. (1993). Alcohol, memory and molecules. *Alcohol Health & Research World, 16* (4), 280–284.

BROWNLEE, S., ROBERTS, S. V., COOPER, M., GOODE, E., HETTER, K., & WRIGHT, A. (1994). Should cigarettes be outlawed? *U.S. News & World Report, 116* (15), pp. 32–36, 38.

BROWNSON, R. C., NOVOTNY, T. E., & PERRY, M. C. (1993). Cigarette smoking and adult leukemia. *Archives of Internal Medicine, 153,* 469–475.

BRUNSWICK, M. (1989). More kids turning to inhalant abuse. *Minneapolis Star-Tribune, VII* (356), pp. 1A, 6A.

BRUNTON, S. A., HENNINGFIELD, J. E., & SOLBERG, L. I. (1994). Smoking cessation: What works best? *Patient Care, 25* (11), 89–115.

BRUST, J. C. M. (1992). Other agents: Phencyclidine, marijuana, hallucinogens, inhalants, and anticholinergics. *Neurologic Clinics, 11,* 555–561.

BUBER, M. (1970). *I and thou.* New York: Scribner's.

BUDIANSKY, S., GOODE, E. E., & GEST, T. (1994). The cold war experiments. *U.S. News & World Report, 116* (3), pp. 32–38.

BUFE, C. (1988). A. A.: Guilt and God for the gullible. *Utne Reader, 30,* 54–55.

BUKSTEIN, O. G., BRENT, D. A., PERPER, J. A., MORITZ, G., BAUGHER, M., SCHWEERS, J., ROTH, C., & BALACH, L. (1993). Risk factors for completed suicide among adolescents with a lifetime history of substance abuse: A case-controlled study. *Acta Psychiatrica Scandinavica, 88,* 403–408.

BURKE, J. D., BURKE, K. C., & RAE, D. S. (1994). Increased rates of drug abuse and dependence after onset of mood or anxiety disorders in adolescence. *Hospital and Community Psychiatry, 45,* 451–455.

BURNAM, M. A., STEIN, J. A., GOLDING, J. M., SIEGEL, J.

M., SORENSEN, S. B., FORSYTHE, A. B., & TELLES, C. A. (1989). Sexual assault and mental disorders in a community population. *Journal of Consulting and Clinical Psychology, 56* (6), 843–850.

BURNS, D. M. (1991). Cigarettes and cigarette smoking. *Clinics in Chest Medicine, 12,* 631–642.

BUSHNELL, T. G., & JUSTINS, D. M. (1993). Choosing the right analgesic. *Drugs, 46,* 394–408.

BUTCHER, J. N. (1988). Introduction to the special series. *Journal of Consulting and Clinical Psychology, 56,* 171.

BYCK, R. (1987). Cocaine use and research: Three histories. In S. Fisher, A. Rashkin, & E. H. Unlenhuth (Eds.), *Cocaine: clinical and behavioral aspects.* New York: Oxford University Press.

BYRNE, C. (1989a). Pregnancy and crack: Trying to heal horror. *Minneapolis Star-Tribune, VIII* (89), pp. 1, 4A.

BYRNE, C. (1989b). Cocaine alley. *Minneapolis Star-Tribune, VIII* (215), pp. 29A–32A.

CALABRESI, M., FOWLER, D., SCALA, T., THOMPSON, D., & WILLWERTH, J. (1994). The butt stops here. *Time, 143* (16), pp. 58–64.

CALLAHAN, E. J. (1980). Alternative strategies in the treatment of narcotic addiction: A review. In W. R. Miller (Ed.), *The addictive behaviors.* New York: Pergamon.

CALLAHAN, E. J., & PECSOK, E. H. (1988). Heroin addiction. In D. M. Donovan & G. A. Marlatt (Eds.), *Assessment of addictive behaviors.* New York: Guilford.

CALLAHAN, J. (1993). Blueprint for an adolescent suicidal crisis. *Psychiatric Annals, 23* (5), 263–270.

CALSYN, R. J., & MORSE, G. A. (1991). Correlates of problem drinking among homeless men. *Hospital and Community Psychiatry, 42,* 721–724.

CARDONI, A. A. (1990). Focus on adinazolam: A benzodiazepine with antidepressant activity. *Hospital Formulary, 25,* 155–158.

CAREY, K. B. (1989). Emerging treatment guidelines for mentally ill chemical abusers. *Hospital and Community Psychiatry, 40,* 341–342, 349.

CARLSON, J. L., STROM, B. L., MORSE, L., WEST, S. L., SOPER, K. A., STOLLEY, P. D., & Jones, J. K. (1987). The relative gastrointestinal toxicity of the nonsteroidal anti-inflammatory drugs. *Archives of Internal Medicine, 147,* 1054–1059.

CARROLL, K. M., & ROUNSAVILLE, B. J. (1992). Contrast of treatment-seeking and untreated cocaine abusers. *Archives of General Psychiatry, 49,* 464–471.

CASTLEMAN, M. (1994). Aspirin: Not just for your heart. *Reader's Digest, 144* (864), pp. 85–89.

CATON, C. L. M., GRALNICK, A., BENDER, S., & SIMON, R. (1989). Young chronic patients and substance abuse. *Hospitial and Community Psychiatry, 40,* 1037–1040.

CDC *AIDS Weekly.* (1992). Update on global AIDS situation. August 13, 1992, 2–4.

Centers for Disease Control. (1990). Lead poisoning associated with intravenous methamphetamine use—Oregon, 1988. *Journal of the American Medical Association, 263,* 797.

CHAN, P., CHEN, J. H., LEE, M. H., & DENG, J. F. (1994). Fatal and nonfatal methamphetamine intoxication in the intensive care unit. *Journal of Toxicology: Clinical Toxicology, 32,* 147–156.

CHARNESS, M. E., SIMON, R. P., & GREENBERG, D. A. (1989). Ethanol and the nervous system. *The New England Journal of Medicine, 321* (7), 442–454.

CHASNOFF, I. J. (1988). Drug use in pregnancy: Parameters of risk. *Pediatric Clinics of North America, 35* (6), 1403–1412.

CHASNOFF, I. J. (1991a). Drugs, alcohol, pregnancy, and the neonate. *Journal of the American Medical Association, 266,* 1567–1568.

CHASNOFF, I. J. (1991b). Cocaine and pregnancy: Clinical and methadologic issues. *Clinics in Perinatology, 18,* 113–123.

CHASNOFF, I. J., & SCHNOLL, S. H. (1987). Consequences of cocaine and other drug use in pregnancy. In A. M. Washton & M. S. Gold (Eds.), *Cocaine: A clinician's handbook.* New York: Guilford.

CHAVEZ, G. F., MULINARE, J., & CORDERO, J. F. (1989). Maternal cocaine use during early pregnancy as a risk factor for congenital urogenital anomalies. *Journal of the American Medical Association, 262* (6), 795–798.

CHERUBIN, C. E., & SAPIRA, J. D. (1993). The medical complications of drug addiction and the medical assessment of the intravenous drug user: 25 years later. *Annals of Internal Medicine, 119,* 1017–1028.

CHIAUZZI, E. (1990). Breaking the patterns that lead to relapse. *Psychology Today, 23* (12), pp. 18–19.

CHICK, J. (1993). Brief interventions for alcohol misuse. *British Medical Journal, 307,* 1374.

CHO, A. K. (1990). Ice: A new dosage form of an old drug. *Science, 249,* pp. 631–634.

CHRISTENSEN, W. G., MANSON, J. E., SEDDON, J. M., GLYNN, R. J., BURING, J. E., ROSNER, B., & HENNEKENS, C. H. (1992). A prospective study of cigarette smoking and risk of cataracts in men. *Journal of the American Medical Association, 268,* 989–993.

CIANCIO, S. G., & BOURGAULT, P. C. (1989). *Clinical pharmacology for dental professionals* (3rd ed.). Chicago: Year Book Medical Publishers, Inc.

CIRAULO, D. A., SHADER, R. I., CIRAULO, A., GREENBLATT, D. J., & VON MOLTKE, L. L. (1994a). Alcoholism and its treatment. In R. I. Shader (Ed.), *Manual of psychiatric therapeutics* (2nd ed.). Boston: Little, Brown.

CIRAULO, D. A., SHADER, R. I., CIRAULO, A.,

GREENBLATT, D. J., & VON MOLTKE, L. L. (1994b). Treatment of alcohol withdrawal. In R. I. Shader (Ed.), *Manual of psychiatric therapeutics* (2nd ed.). Boston: Little, Brown.

CIRAULO, D. A., SHADER, R. I., GREENBLATT, D. J., & BARNHILL, J. G. (1989). Basic concepts. In D. A. Ciraulo, R. I. Shader, D. J. Greenblatt, & W. Creelman (Eds.), *Drug interactions in psychiatry*. Baltimore: Williams & Wilkins.

CLARK, D. C., GIBBONS, R. D., HAVILAND, M. G., & HENDRYX, M. S. (1993). Assessing the severity of depressive states in recently detoxified alcoholics. *Journal of Studies on Alcohol, 54,* 107–114.

CLARK, R. E. (1994). Family costs associated with severe mental illness and substance abuse. *Hospital and Community Psychiatry, 45,* 808–813.

CLARK, W. G., BRATLER, D. C., & JOHNSON, A. R. (1991). *Goth's medical pharmacology* (13th ed.). Boston: Mosby.

CLAUNCH, L. (1994). Intervention can be used as a tool—or as a weapon against clients. *The Addiction Letter, 10* (4), 1–2.

CLIMKO, R. P., ROEHRICH, H., SWEENEY, D. R., & AL-RAZI, J. (1987). Ecstasy: A review of MDMA and MDA. *International Journal of Psychiatry in Medicine, 16* (4), 359–372.

CLONINGER, C. R., GOHMAN, M., & SIGVARDSSON, S. (1981). Inheritance of alcohol abuse: Cross-fostering analysis of adopted men. *Archives of General Psychiatry, 38,* 861–868.

COHEN, D. A., RICHARDSON, J., & LA BREE, L. (1994). Parenting behaviors and the onset of smoking and alcohol use: A longitudinal study. *Pediatrics, 94,* 368–375.

COHEN, J., & LEVY, S. J. (1992). *The mentally ill chemical abuser: Whose client.* New York: Lexington Books.

COHEN, L. S. (1989). Psychotropic drug use in pregnancy. *Hospital and Community Psychiatry, 40* (6), 566–567.

COHEN, N. L., & MARCOS, L. R. (1989). The bad-mad dilemma for public psychiatry. *Hospital and Community Psychiatry, 40,* 677.

COHEN, S. (1977). Inhalant abuse: An overview of the problem. In C. W. Sharp & M. L. Brehm (Eds.), *Review of inhalants: Euphoria to dysfunction*. Washington, DC: U.S. Government Printing Office.

COHEN, S., LICHTENSTEIN, E., PROCHASKA, J. O., ROSSI, J. S., GRITZ, E. R., CARR, C. R., ORLEANS, C.T., SCHOENBACH, V. J., BIENER, L., ABRAMS, D., DiCLEMENTE, C., CURRY, S., MARLATT, G. A., CUMMINGS, K. M., EMONT, S. L., GIOVINO, G., & OSSIP-KLEIN, D. (1989). Debunking myths about self-quitting. *American Psychologist, 44,* 1355–1365.

COHN, J. B., WILCOX, C. S., BOWDEN, C. L., FISHER, J. G., & RODOS, J. J. (1992). Double-blind clorazepate in anxious outpatients with and without depressive symptoms. *Psychopathology, 25* (Suppl. 1), 10–21.

COLBURN, N., MEYER, R. D., WRIGLEY, M., & BRADLEY, E. L. (1993). Should motorcycles be operated within the legal alcohol limits for automobiles? *The Journal of Trauma, 34* (1), 183–186.

COLE, J. O., & KANDO, J. C. (1993). Adverse behavioral events reported in patients taking alprazolam and other benzodiazepines. *Journal of Clinical Psychiatry, 54* (Suppl. 10), 49–61.

COLEMAN, E. (1988a). Chemical dependency and intimacy dysfunction: Inextricably bound. In E. Coleman (Ed.), *Chemical dependency and intimacy dysfunction*. New York: Haworth.

COLEMAN, E. (1988b). Child physical and sexual abuse among chemically dependent individuals. In E. Coleman (Ed.), *Chemical dependency and intimacy dysfunction*. New York: Haworth.

COLEMAN, P. (1989). Letter to the editor. *Journal of the American Medical Association, 261* (13), 1879–1880.

COLLETTE, L. (1988). Step by step: A skeptic's encounter. *Utne Reader, 30,* 69–76.

COLLETTE, L. (1990). After the anger, what then? *The Family Therapy Networker, 14* (1), 22–31.

COLLIER, A. (1989). To deal and die in L.A. *Ebony, 44* (10), pp. 106–108.

COLLINS, J. J., & ALLISON, M. (1983). Legal coercion and retention in drug abuse treatment. *Hospital and Community Psychiatry, 34,* 1145–1150.

COLLINS, J. J., & MESSERSCHMIDT, P. M. (1993). Epidemiology of alcohol-related violence. *Alcohol Health & Research World, 17* (2), 93–100.

Committee on Substance Abuse and Committee on Children With Disabilities. (1993). Fetal alcohol syndrome and fetal alcohol effects. *Pediatrics, 91,* 1004–1006.

CONE, E. J. (1993). Saliva testing for drugs of abuse. In D. Malamud & L. Tabak (Eds.), *Saliva as a diagnostic fluid*. New York: New York Academy of Sciences.

CONLAN, M. F. (1990). Research and development plan proposed for pharmacotherapy. *Drug Topics, 134* (1), 50.

CONRAD, S., HUGHES, P., BALDWIN, D. C., ACHENBACK, K. E., & SHEEHAN, D. V. (1989). Cocaine use by senior medical students. *American Journal of Psychiatry, 146,* 382–386.

COOPER, J. R., BLOOM, F. E., & ROTH, R. H. (1986). *The biochemical basis of neuropharmacology* (5th ed.). New York: Oxford University Press.

CORDERO, J. F. (1990). Effect of environmental agents on pregnancy outcomes: Disturbances of prenatal growth and development. *Medical Clinics of North America, 72* (2), 279–290.

CORWIN, J. (1994). Outlook. *U.S. News & World Report, 116* (23), pp. 15–16.

COTTON, P. (1990). Medium isn't accurate "ice age" message. *Journal of the American Medical Association, 263,* 2717.

COTTON, P. (1993). Low-tar cigarettes come under fire. *Journal of the American Medical Association, 270,* 1399.

COTTON, P. (1994). Smoking cigarettes may do developing fetus more harm than ingesting cocaine, some experts say. *Journal of the American Medical Association, 271,* 576–577.

Council on Addiction Psychiatry. (1994). Position statement on methadone maintenance treatment. *American Journal of Psychiatry, 151,* 792–794.

Council on Scientific Affairs. (1990a). The worldwide smoking epidemic. *Journal of the American Medical Association, 263,* 3312–3318.

Council on Scientific Affairs. (1990b). Medical and nonmedical uses of anabolic-androgenic steroids. *Journal of the American Medical Association, 264,* 2923–2927.

COUSINS, N. (1989). *Head first: The biology of hope.* New York: Dutton.

COVINGTON, S. S. (1987). Alcohol and female sexuality. *Alcoholism & Addiction, 7* (5), 21.

COWEN, R. (1990). Alcoholism treatment under scrutiny. *Science News, 137,* p. 254.

COWLEY, G. (1992). Halcion takes another hit. *Newsweek, CXIX* (7), p. 58.

CRABBE, J. C., & GOLDMAN, D. (1993). Alcoholism. *Alcohol Health & Research World, 16* (4), 297–303.

CREELMAN, W., CIRAULO, D. A, & SHADER, R. I. (1989). Lithium drug interactions. In D. A. Ciraulo, R. I. Shader, D. J. Greenblatt, & W. Creelman (Eds.), *Drug interactions in psychiatry.* Baltimore: Williams & Wilkins.

CREELMAN, W., SANDS, B. F., CIRAULO, D. A., GREENBLATT, D. J., & SHADER, R. I. (1989). Benzodiazepines. In D. A. Ciraulo, R. I. Shader, D. J. Greenblatt, & W. Creelman (Eds.), *Drug interactions in psychiatry.* Baltimore: Williams & Wilkins.

CREIGHTON, F. J., BLACK, D. L., & HYDE, C. E. (1991). "Ecstacy" psychosis and flashbacks. *British Journal of Psychiatry, 159,* 713–715.

CROWLEY, T. J. (1988). Substance abuse treatment and policy: Contributions of behavioral pharmacology. Paper presented at the 1988 meeting of the American Psychological Association, Atlanta, GA.

CUFFEL, B. J., HEITHOFF, K. A., & LAWSON, W. (1993). Correlates of patterns of substance abuse among patients with schizophrenia. *Hospital and Community Psychiatry, 44,* 247–251.

CUMMINGS, C., GORDON, J. R., & MARLATT, G. A. (1980). Relapse: Prevention and prediction. In W. R. Miller (Ed.), *The addictive behaviors.* New York: Pergamon.

CUNNIEN, A. J. (1988). Psychiatric and medical syndromes associated with deception. In R. Rogers (Ed.), *Clinical assessment of malingering and deception.* New York: Guilford.

CYR, M. G., & MOULTON, A. W. (1993). The physician's role in prevention, detection, and treatment of alcohol abuse in women. *Psychiatric Annals, 23,* 454–462.

DAGHESTANI, A. N., & SCHNOLL, S. H. (1994). Phencyclidine. In M. Galanter & H. D. Kleber (Eds.), *Textbook of substance abuse treatment.* Washington, DC: American Psychiatric Association Press, Inc.

DAIGLE, R. D. (1990). Anabolic steroids. *Journal of Psychoactive Drugs, 22* (1), 77–80.

D'ANDREA, L. M., FISHER, G. L., & HARRISON, T. C. (1994). Cluster analysis of adult children of alcoholics. *International Journal of the Addictions, 29,* 565–582.

DAVIS, J. M., & BRESNAHAN, D. B. (1987). Psychopharmacology in clinical psychiatry. In *American Psychiatric Association Annual Review: Vol. 6.* Washington, DC: American Psychiatric Association Press, Inc.

DAY, N. L., & RICHARDSON, G. A. (1991). Prenatal marijuana use: Epidemiology, methodologic issues, and infant outcome. *Clinics in Perinatology, 18,* 77–91.

DAY, N. L., & RICHARDSON, G. A. (1994). Comparative teratogenicity of alcohol and other drugs. *Alcohol Health & Research World, 18,* 42–48.

DEANGELIS, T. (1989). Behavior is included in report on smoking. *APA Monitor, 20* (3), 1, 4.

DEANGELIS, T. (1994). People's drug of choice offers potent side effects. *APA Monitor, 25* (2), 16.

DECKER, K. P., & RIES, R. K. (1993). Differential diagnosis and psychopharmacology of dual disorders. *Psychiatric Clinics of North America, 16,* 703–718.

DECKER, S., FINS, J., & FRANCES, R. (1987). Cocaine and chest pain. *Hospital & Community Psychiatry, 38,* 464–466.

DEJONG, W. (1994). Relapse prevention: An emerging technology for promoting long-term abstinence. *International Journal of the Addictions, 29,* 681–785.

DELEON, G. (1989). Psychopathology and substance abuse: What is being learned from research in therapeutic communities. *Journal of Psychoactive Drugs, 21* (2), 177–188.

DELEON, G. (1994). Therapeutic communities. In M. Galanter, & H. D. Kleber (Eds.), *Textbook of substance abuse treatment.* Washington, DC: American Psychiatric Association Press, Inc.

DERLET, R. W. (1989). Cocaine intoxication. *Postgraduate Medicine, 86* (5), 245–248, 253.

DERLET, R. W., & HEISCHOBER, B. (1990). Methamphetamine: Stimulant of the 1990s? *The Western Journal of Medicine, 153,* 625–629.

DEYKIN, E. Y., BUKA, D. P. H., & ZEENA, B. S. (1992).

Depressive illness among chemically dependent adolescents. *American Journal of Psychiatry, 149,* 1341–1347.

DiClemente, C. C. (1993). Alcoholics Anonymous and the structure of change. In B. S. McCrady & W. R. Miller (Eds.), *Research on Alcoholics Anonymous.* New Brunswick, NJ: Rutgers Center of Alcohol Studies.

Dietch, J. (1983). The nature and extent of benzodiazepine abuse: An overview of recent literature. *Hospital and Community Psychiatry, 34,* 1139–1144.

DiFranza, J. R., Richards, J. W., Paulman, P. M., Wolf-Gillespie, N., Fletcher, C., Jaffe, R. D., & Murray, D. (1991). RJR Nabisco's cartoon camel promotes Camel cigarettes to children. *Journal of the American Medical Association, 266,* 3149–3153.

DiFranza, J. R., & Tye, J. B. (1990). Who profits from tobacco sales to children? *Journal of the American Medical Association, 263,* 2784–2787.

DiGregorio, G. J. (1990). Cocaine update: Abuse and therapy. *American Family Physician, 41* (1), 247–251.

Dionne, R. A., & Gordon, S. M. (1994). Nonsteroidal antiinflammatory drugs for acute pain control. *Dental Clinics of North America, 38,* 645–667.

Discover. (1994). *Gallic hearts.* 15, (9), pp. 14–15.

Doghramji, K. (1989). Sleep disorders: A selective update. *Hospital and Community Psychiatry, 40,* 29–40.

Dole, V. P. (1988). Implications of methadone maintenance for theories of narcotic addiction. *Journal of the American Medical Association, 260,* 3025–3029.

Dole, V. P. (1989). Letter to the editor. *Journal of the American Medical Association, 261* (13), 1880.

Dole, V. P., & Nyswander, M. A. (1965). Medical treatment for diacetylmorphine (heroin) addiction. *Journal of the American Medical Association, 193,* 645–656.

Domenico, D., & Windle, M. (1993). Intrapersonal and interpersonal functioning among middle-aged female adult children of alcoholics. *Journal of Consulting and Clinical Psychology, 61,* 659–666.

Dominguez, R., Vila-Coro, A. A., Aguirre, V. C., Slipis, J. M., & Bohan, T. P. (1991). Brain and ocular abnormalities in infants in utero exposure to cocaine and other street drugs. *American Journal of Diseases of Children, 145,* 688–694.

Donovan, D. M. (1992). The assessment process in addictive behaviors. *The Behavior Therapist, 15* (1), 18.

Doria, J. (1990). Alcohol, women and heart disease. *Alcohol Health & Research World, 14* (4), 349–351.

Dorland's Illustrated Medical Dictionary (27th ed.). (1988). Philadelphia: Saunders.

Downing, C. (1990). The wounded healers. *Addiction & Recovery, 10* (3), 21–24.

Drake, R. E., Osher, F. C., & Wallach, M. A. (1989). Alcohol use and abuse in schizophrenia. *The Journal of Nervous and Mental Disease, 177,* 408–414.

Drake, R. E., & Wallach, M. A. (1989). Substance abuse among the chronic mentally ill. *Hospital and Community Psychiatry, 40,* 1041–1046.

Drake, R. E., & Wallach, M. A. (1993). Moderate drinking among people with severe mental illness. *Hospital and Community Psychiatry, 44,* 780–781.

Dreger, R. M. (1986). Does anyone really believe that alcoholism is a disease? *American Psychologist, 37,* 322.

Dreher, M. C., Nugent, K., & Hudgins, R. (1994). Prenatal marijuana exposure and neonatal outcomes in Jamaica: An ethnographic study. *Pediatrics, 93,* 254–260.

Drews, R. C. (1993). Alcohol and cataract. *Archives of Ophthalmology, 111,* 1312.

Dreyfuss, I. (1989). Federal agency to probe anabolic steroid abuse. *The Physician and Sports Medicine, 17* (7), 16.

Dube, C. E., & Lewis, D. C. (1994). Medical education in alcohol and other drugs: Curriculum development for primary care. *Alcohol Health & Research World, 18,* 146–155.

Dumas, L. (1992). Addicted women. *Nursing Clinics of North America, 27,* 901–915.

Dunlop, J., Manghelli, D., & Tolson, R. (1989). Senior alcohol and drug coalition statement of treatment philosophy for the elderly. *Professional Counselor, 4* (2), 39–42.

Dunn, G. E., Paolo, A. M., Ryan, J. J., & Van Fleet, J. (1993). Dissociative symptoms in a substance abuse population. *American Journal of Psychiatry, 150,* 1043–1047.

Dunne, F. J. (1994). Misuse of alcohol or drugs by elderly people. *British Medical Journal, 308,* 608–609.

DuRant, R. H., Rickert, V. I., Ashworth, C. S., Newman, C., & Slavens, G. (1993). Use of multiple drugs among adolescents who use anabolic steroids. *The New England Journal of Medicine, 328,* 922–926.

Durell, J., Lechtenberg, B., Corse, S., & Frances, R. J. (1993). Intensive case management of persons with chronic mental illness who abuse substances. *Hospital and Community Psychiatry, 44,* 415–416, 428.

Dyer, C. (1992). Upjohn claims exoneration after FDA's decision. *British Medical Journal, 305,* 1384.

Dyer, C. (1993). Halcion edges its way back into Britain in low doses. *British Medical Journal, 306,* 1085.

Dyer, W. W. (1989). *You'll see it when you believe it.* New York: William Morrow.

Dygert, S. L., & Minelli, M. J. (1993). Heroin abuse

progression chart. *Addiction & Recovery, 13* (1), 27–31.

ECCLES, J. S., MIDGLEY, C., WIGFIELD, A., BUCHANAN, C. M., REUMAN, D., FLANAGAN, C., & MacIVER, D. (1993). Development during adolescence. *American Psychologist, 48,* 90–101.

Economist, The. (1989). Ice overdose. *313* (7631), 29–31.

Economist, The. (1990a). Just say buprenorphine. *313* (7626), 95.

Economist, The. (1990b). War by other means. *314* (7641), 50.

Economist, The. (1993a). Bring drugs within the law. *327* (7811), 13–14.

Economist, The. (1993b). Market update. *329* (7830), 68.

EDELSON, E. (1993). Fear of blood. *Popular Science, 242* (6), pp. 108–111, 122.

EDMEADES, B. (1987). Alcoholics Anonymous celebrates its 50th year. In W. B. Rucker & M. E. Rucker (Eds.), *Drugs, society and behavior.* Guilford, CT: Dashkin Publishing Group, Inc.

EDWARDS, R. W. (1993). Drug use among 8th grade students is increasing. *International Journal of the Addictions, 28,* 1621–1623.

EFRAN, J. S., HEFFNER, K. P., & LUKENS, R. T. (1987). Alcoholism as an opinion. *The Family Therapy Networker, 11* (4), 43–46.

EHRENREICH, B. (1992). Stamping out a dread scourge. *Time, 139* (7), p. 88.

EISEN, S. A., LYONS, M. J., GOLDBERG, J., & TRUE, W. R. (1993). The impact of cigarette and alcohol consumption on weight and obesity. *Archives of Internal Medicine, 153,* 2457–2463.

EISENHANDLER, J., & DRUCKER, E. (1993). Opiate dependence among the subscribers of a New York area private insurance plan. *Journal of the American Medical Association, 269,* 2890–2891.

EISON, A. S., & TEMPLE, D. L. (1987). Buspirone: Review of its pharmacology and current perspectives on its mechanism of action. *The American Journal of Medicine, 80* (Suppl. 3B), 1–9.

ELLIOTT, F. A. (1992). Violence. *Archives of Neurology, 49,* 595–603.

ELLIS, A., McINERNEY, J. F., DiGIUSEPPE, R., & YEAGER, R. J. (1988). *Rational emotive therapy with alcoholics and substance abusers.* New York: Pergamon.

EMRICK, C. D., TONIGAN, S., MONTGOMERY, H., & LITTLE, L. (1993). Alcoholics Anonymous: What is currently known? In B. S. McCrady & W. R. Miller (Eds.), *Research on Alcoholics Anonymous.* New Brunswick, NJ: Rutgers Center of Alcohol Studies.

ENGELMAN, R. (1989). Researcher says quest for intoxication is common throughout animal kingdom. *Minneapolis Star-Tribune, VIII* (173), p. 12E.

ENGLISH, T. J. (1992). Hong Kong outlaws. *Playboy, 39* (6), pp. 94–96, 168–170.

ESMAIL, A., MEYER, L., POTTIER, A., & WRIGHT, S. (1993). Deaths from volatile substance abuse in those under 18 years: Results from a national epidemiological study. *Archives of Disease in Childhood, 69,* 356–360.

ESTROFF, T. W. (1987). Medical and biological consequences of cocaine abuse. In A. M. Washton & M. S. Gold (Eds.), *Cocaine: A clinician's handbook.* New York: Guilford.

EVANKO, D. (1991). Designer drugs. *Postgraduate Medicine, 89* (6), 67–71.

EVANS, G. D. (1993). Cigarette smoke = radiation hazard. *Pediatrics, 92,* 464.

EVANS, K., & SULLIVAN, J. M. (1990). *Dual diagnosis.* New York: Guilford.

EVANS, S. M., FUNDERBURK, F. R., & GRIFFITHS, R. R. (1990). Zolpidem and triazolam in humans: Behavioral and subjective effects and abuse liability. *Journal of Pharmacology and Experimental Therapeutics, 255,* 1246–1255.

EWING, J. A. (1984). Detecting alcoholism: The CAGE questionnaire. *Journal of the American Medical Association, 252,* 1905–1907.

Facts about Alateen. (1969). New York: Al-Anon Family Group Headquarters.

FALLS-STEWART, W., & LUCENTE, S. (1994). Treating obsessive-compulsive disorder among substance abusers: A guide. *Psychology of Addictive Behaviors, 8,* 14–23.

FARIELLO, D., & SCHEIDT, S. (1989). Clinical case management of the dually diagnosed patient. *Hospital and Community Psychiatry, 40,* 1065–1067.

FARROW, J. A. (1990). Adolescent chemical dependency. *Medical Clinics of North America, 74,* 1265–1274.

FASSINGER, R. E. (1991). The hidden minority: Issues and challenges in working with lesbian women and gay men. *The Counseling Psychologist, 19,* 157–176.

FEIGHNER, J. P. (1987). Impact of anxiety therapy on patients' quality of life. *The American Journal of Medicine, 82* (Suppl. A), 14–19.

FERNANDEZ-SOLA, J., ESTRUCH, R., GRAU, J. M., PARE, J. C., RUBIN, E., & URBANO-MARQUEZ, A. (1994). The relation of alcoholic myopathy to cardiomyopathy. *Annals of Internal Medicine, 120,* 529–536.

Fighting Drug Abuse: Tough Decisions for Our National Strategy. (1992). Majority staff of the United States Senate Judiciary Committee. Washington, DC.

FINGARETTE, H. (1988). Alcoholism: The mythical disease. *Utne Reader, 30,* 64–69.

FINNEY, J. W., MOOS, R. H., & CHAN, D. A. (1975). Length of stay and program component effects in the treatment of alcoholism. *Journal of Studies on Alcohol, 36,* 88–108.

FIORE, M. C. (1992). Trends in cigarette smoking in

the United States. *The Medical Clinics of North America, 76,* 289–303.

FIORE, M. C., EPPS, R. P., & MANLEY, M. W. (1994). A missed opportunity. *Journal of American Medical Association, 271,* 624–626.

FIORE, M. C., JORENBY, D. E., BAKER, T. B., & KENFORD, S. L. (1992). Tobacco dependence and the nicotine patch. *Journal of the American Medical Association, 268,* 2687–2694.

FIORE, M. C., NOVOTNY, T. E., PIERCE, J. P., GIOVINO, G. A., HATZIANDREU, E. J., NEWCOMB, P. A., SUR-AWICZ, T. S., & DAVIS, R. M. (1990). Methods used to quit smoking in the United States. *Journal of the American Medical Association, 263,* 2760–2765.

FIORE, M. C., SMITH, S. S., JORENBY, D. E., & BAKER, T. B. (1994). The effectiveness of the nicotine patch for smoking cessation. *Journal of the American Medical Association, 271,* 1940–1947.

FISCHBACH, G. D. (1992). Mind and brain. *Scientific American, 267* (3), pp. 48–57.

FISCHER, R. G. (1989). Clinical use of nonsteroidal anti-inflammatory drugs. *Pharmacy Times, 55* (8), 31–35.

FISHMAN, S. M., & CARR, D. B. (1992). Clinical issues in pain management. *Contemporary Medicine, 4* (10), 92–103.

FOA, P. P. (1989). Letters to the editor. *Smithsonian, 20* (6), p. 18.

FOLEY, K. M. (1993). Opioids. *Neurologic Clinics, 11,* 503–522.

FONTHAM, E. T. H., CORREA, P., REYNOLDS, P., WU-WILLIAMS, A., BUFFLER, P. A., GREENBERG, R. S., CHEN, V., ALTERMAN, T., BOYD, P., AUSTIN, D. F., & LIFF, J. (1994). Environmental tobacco smoke and lung cancer in nonsmoking women. *Journal of the American Medical Association, 271,* 1752–1759.

Forensic Drug Abuse Advisor. (1994a). Simple way to beat urine tests—Just drink water. *6* (3), 17–18.

Forensic Drug Abuse Advisor. (1994b). Take time to smell the fentanyl. *6* (5), 34–35.

Forensic Drug Abuse Advisor. (1994c). Feds say heroin use up, cocaine and heroin prices down, and cocaine snorting back in fashion. *6* (6), 41–43.

Forensic Drug Abuse Advisor. (1994d). Asiatic amphetamine abuse: Strokes, infarcts, agitated delirium, and postmortem levels. *6* (8), 60–62.

FORNAZZARI, L. (1988). Clinical recognition and management of solvent abusers. *Internal Medicine for the Specialist, 9* (6), 99–108.

FOSSUM, M. A., & MASON, M. J. (1986). *Facing shame: Families in recovery.* New York: Norton.

FRANCES, R. J. (1991). Should drugs be legalized? Implications of the debate for the mental health field. *Hospital and Community Psychiatry, 42,* 119–120, 125.

FRANCES, R. J., & MILLER, S. I. (1991). Addiction treatment: The widening scope. In R. J. Frances & S. I. Miller (Eds.), *Clinical textbook of addictive disorders.* New York: Guilford.

FRANK, D. A., BAUCHNER, H., ZUCKERMAN, B. S., & FRIED, L. (1992). Cocaine and marijuana use during pregnancy by women intending and not intending to breast-feed. *Journal of the American Dietetic Association, 92,* 215–217.

FRANKL, V. E. (1978). *The unheard cry for meaning.* New York: Touchstone Books.

FRANKLIN, J. (1987). *Molecules of the mind.* New York: Dell.

FRANKLIN, J. E. (1989). Alcoholism among blacks. *Hospital and Community Psychiatry, 40,* 1120–1122, 1127.

FRANKLIN, J. E. (1994). Addiction medicine. *Journal of the American Medical Association, 271,* 1650–1651.

FRANKS, P., HARP, J., & BELL, B. (1989). Randomized, controlled trial of clonidine for smoking cessation in a primary care setting. *The New England Journal of Medicine, 321,* 3011–3013.

FREDERICKSON, P. A., RICHARDSON, J. W., ESTHER, M. S., & LIN, S. (1990). Sleep disorders in psychiatric practice. *Mayo Clinic Procedures, 65,* 861–868.

FREIBERG, P. (1991). Panel hears of families victimized by alcoholism. *APA Monitor, 22* (4), 30.

FREZZA, M., DI PADOVA, C., POZZATO, G., TERPIN, M., BARAONA, E., & LIEBER, C. S. (1990). High blood alcohol levels in women. *The New England Journal of Medicine, 322,* 95–99.

FRIEDMAN, D. (1987). Toxic effects of marijuana. *Alcoholism & Addiction, 7* (6), 47.

FRIEDMAN, R. C., & DOWNEY, J. I. (1994). Homosexuality. *The New England Journal of Medicine, 331,* 923–930.

FROMM, E. (1956). *The art of loving.* New York: Harper & Row.

FROMM, E. (1968). *The revolution of hope.* New York: Harper & Row.

FULLER, R. K. (1989). Antidipsotropic medications. In R. K. Hester & W. R. Miller (Eds.), *Handbook of alcoholism treatment approaches.* New York: Pergamon.

FULTON, J. S., & JOHNSON, G. B. (1993). Using high-dose morphine to relieve cancer pain. *Nursing '93, 23* (2), 35–39.

FULTZ, O. (1991). 'Roid rage. *American Health, X* (4), 60–64.

FURSTENBERG, F. F. (1990). Coming of age in a changing family system. In S. S. Feldman & G. R. Elliott (Eds.), *At the threshold.* Cambridge, MA: Harvard University Press.

GABRIEL, T. (1994). Heroin finds a new market along cutting edge of style. *The New York Times, CXLIII* (49,690), pp. 1, 17.

GALANTER, M. (1993). Network therapy for addiction:

A model for office practice. *American Journal of Psychiatry, 150,* 28–36.

GALANTER, M., CASTANEDA, R., & FERMAN, J. (1988). Substance abuse among general psychiatric patients: Place of presentation, diagnosis, and treatment. *American Journal of Drug and Alcohol Abuse, 14* (2), 211–235.

GALANTER, M., CASTANEDA, R., & FRANCO, H. (1991). Group therapy and self-help groups. In R. J. Frances & S. I. Miller (Eds.), *Clinical textbook of addictive disorders.* New York: Guilford.

GALANTER, M., & FRANCES, R. (1992). Addiction psychiatry: Challenges for a new psychiatric subspecialty. *Hospital and Community Psychiatry, 43,* 1067–1068, 1072.

GALLAGHER, W. (1986). The looming menace of designer drugs. *Designer, 7* (8), 24–35.

GALLO, R. C., & MONTAGNIER, L. (1988). AIDS in 1988. *Scientific American, 259* (4), pp. 41–48.

GANNON, K. (1994). OTC naproxen sodium set to shake OTC analgesics. *Drug Topics, 138* (3), 34.

GARBARINO, J., DUBROW, N., KOSTELNY, K., & PARDO, C. (1992). *Children in danger.* San Francisco: Jossey-Bass.

GARRO, A. J., ESPINA, N., & LIEBER, C. S. (1992). Alcohol and cancer. *Alcohol Health & Research World, 16* (1), 81–85.

GAWIN, F. H., ALLEN, D., & HUMBLESTONE, B. (1989). Outpatient treatment of "crack" cocaine smoking with flupenthixol deconate: A preliminary report. *Archives of General Psychiatry, 46,* 122–126.

GAWIN, F. H., & ELLINWOOD, E. H. (1988). Cocaine and other stimulants: Actions, abuse, and treatment. *New England Journal of Medicine, 318,* 1173–1182.

GAWIN, F. H., KHALSA, M. E., & ELLINWOOD, E. (1994). Stimulants. In M. Galanter & H. D. Kleber (Eds.), *Textbook of substance abuse treatment.* Washington, DC: American Psychiatric Association Press, Inc.

GAWIN, F. H., & KLEBER, H. D. (1986). Abstinence symptomology and psychiatric diagnosis in cocaine abusers. *Archives of General Psychiatry, 43,* 107–113.

GAWIN, F. H., KLEBER, H. D., BYCK, R., ROUNSAVILLE, B. J., KOSTEN, T. R., JATLOW, P. I., & MORGAN, C. (1989). Desipramine facilitation of initial cocaine abstinence. *Archives of General Psychiatry, 46,* 117–121.

GAY, G. R. (1990). Another side effect of NSAIDs. *Journal of the American Medical Association, 164,* 2677–2678.

GAY, L. (1991). In Amsterdam, drug war is fought by example, not crackdowns. *Minneapolis Star-Tribune, IX* (285), p. 11A.

GAZZANIGA, M. S. (1988). *Mind matters.* Boston: Houghton-Mifflin.

GELERNTER, J., GOLDMAN, D., & RISCH, N. (1993). The A1 allele at the D_2 dopamine receptor gene and alcoholism. *Journal of the American Medical Association, 269,* 1673–1677.

GELLES, R. J., & STRAUS, M. A. (1988). *Intimate violence: The definitive study of the causes and consequences of abuse in the American family.* New York: Simon & Schuster.

GELMAN, D., UNDERWOOD, A., KING, P., HAGER, M., & GORDON, J. (1990). Some things work! *Newsweek, CXVI* (13), pp. 78–81.

GIACONA, N. S., DAHL, S. L., & HARE, B. D. (1987). The role of nonsteroidal antiinflammatory drugs and non-narcotics in analgesia. *Hospital Formulary, 22,* 723–733.

GILBERTSON, P. K., & WEINBERG, J. (1992). Fetal alcohol syndrome and functioning of the immune system. *Alcohol Health & Research World, 16* (1), 29–38.

GILLIN, J. C. (1991). The long and the short of sleeping pills. *The New England Journal of Medicine, 324,* 1735–1736.

GILMAN, S. (1992). Advances in neurology. *The New England Journal of Medicine, 326,* 1608–1616.

GIOVANNUCCI, E., RIMM, E. B., STAMPFER, M. J., COLDITZ, G. A., ASCHERIO, A., & WILLETT, W. C. (1994). Aspirin use and the risk of colorectal cancer and adenoma in male health professionals. *Annals of Internal Medicine, 121,* 241–245.

GIUNTA, C. T., & COMPAS, B. E. (1994). Adult daughters of alcoholics: Are they unique? *Journal of Studies on Alcohol, 55,* 600–606.

GLANTZ, J. C., & WOODS, J. R. (1993). Cocaine, heroin, and phencyclidine: Obstetric perspectives, *Clinical Obstetrics and Gynecology, 36,* 279–301.

GLASER, F. B., & OGBORNE, A. C. (1982). Does A. A. really work? *British Journal of the Addictions, 77,* 88–92.

GLASNER, P. D., & KASLOW, R. A. (1990). The epidemiology of human immunodeficiency virus infection. *Journal of Clinical and Consulting Psychology, 58,* 13–21.

GLASS, R. M. (1993). Methadone maintenance. *Journal of the American Medical Association, 269,* 1995–1996.

GLASSMAN, A. H. (1993). Cigarette smoking: Implications for psychiatric illness. *American Journal of Psychiatry, 150,* 546–553.

GLASSMAN, A. H., STETNER, F., WALSH, T., RAIZMAN, P. S., FLEISS, J. L., COOPER, T. B., & COVEY, L. S. (1988). Heavy smokers, smoking cessation and clonidine. *Journal of the American Medical Association, 259,* 2863–2866.

GLOWA, J. R. (1986). *Inhalants: The toxic fumes.* New York: Chelsea House Publishers.

GOLD, M. S. (1988). Alcohol, drugs, and sexual dysfunction. *Alcoholism & Addiction, 9* (2), 13.

GOLD, M. S. (1989a). Opiates. In A. J. Giannini & A.

E. Slaby (Eds.), *Drugs of abuse.* Oradell, NJ: Medical Economics Books.

GOLD, M. S. (1989b). Medical implications of cocaine intoxication. *Alcoholism & Addiction, 9* (3), 16.

GOLD, M. S. (1990a). Weekend warriors and addicts. *Alcoholism & Addiction, 10* (3), 12.

GOLD, M. S. (1990b). Another ice age? *Alcoholism & Addiction, 10* (2), 10.

GOLD, M. S. (1993). Opiate addiction and the locus coeruleus. *Psychiatric Clinics of North America, 16,* 61–73.

GOLD, M. S., & PALUMBO, J. M. (1991). The future treatment of cocaine addiction. *Alcohol & Addiction, 11* (3), 35–37.

GOLD, M. S., SCHUCHARD, K., & GLEATON, T. (1994). LSD use among U.S. high school students. *Journal of the American Medical Association, 271,* 426–427.

GOLD, M. S., & VEREBEY, K. (1984). The psychopharmacology of cocaine. *Psychiatric Annuals, 14,* 714–723.

GOLDMAN, B. (1991). How to thwart a drug seeker. *Emergency Medicine, 23* (6), 48–61.

GOLDSTEIN, P. (1990). Drugs and violence. Paper presented at the 1990 meeting of the American Psychological Association, Boston, MA.

GOLDSTONE, M. S. (1993). "Cat": Methcathinone, a new drug of abuse. *Journal of the American Medical Association, 269,* 2508.

GONDALF, E. W., & FOSTER, R. A. (1991). Wife assault among VA alcohol rehabilitation patients. *Hospital and Community Psychiatry, 42,* 74–79.

GONZALES, J. J., STERN, T. A., EMMERICH, A. D., & RAUCH, S. L. (1992). Recognition and management of benzodiazepine dependence. *American Family Physician, 45,* 2269–2276.

GOODWIN, D. W. (1989). Alcoholism. In H. I. Kaplan & B. J. Sadock (Eds.), *Comprehensive textbook of psychiatry/V.* Baltimore: Williams & Wilkins.

GOODWIN, D. W. (1991). Inpatient treatment of alcoholism—New life for the Minneapolis plan. *The New England Journal of Medicine, 325,* 804–806.

GOODWIN, D. W., & WARNOCK, J. K. (1991). Alcoholism: A family disease. In R. J. Frances & S. I. Miller (Eds.), *Clinical textbook of addictive disorders.* New York: Guilford.

GORSKI, T. T. (1992). Diagnosing codependence. *Addiction & Recovery, 12* (7), 14–16.

GORSKI, T. T. (1993). Relapse prevention. *Addiction & Recovery, 13* (2), 25–27.

GOSSOP, M., BATTERSBY, M., & STRANG, J. (1991). Self-detoxification by opiate addicts. *British Journal of Psychiatry, 159,* 208–212.

GOSSOP, M., GRIFFITHS, P., & STRANG, J. (1994). Sex differences in patterns of drug-taking behaviour. *British Journal of Psychiatry, 164,* 101–104.

GOTTESMAN, J. (1992). Little is known about effects of steroids on women. *Minneapolis Star-Tribune, XI* (211), p. 7C.

GOTTLIEB, A. M., KILLEN, J. D., MARLATT, G. A., & TAYLOR, C. B. (1987). Psychological and pharmacological influences in cigarette smoking withdrawal: Effects of nicotine gum and expectancy on smoking withdrawal symptoms and relapse. *Journal of Clinical and Consulting Psychology, 55,* 606–608.

GOTTLIEB, A., POPE, S., RICKERT, V. I., & HARDIN, B. H. (1993). Patterns of smokeless tobacco use by young adolescents. *Pediatrics, 91,* 75–78.

GOTTLIEB, M. I. (1994). Alcohol and pregnancy: A potential for disaster. *Emergency Medicine, 26* (1), 73–79.

GRAEDON, J. (1980). *The people's pharmacy—2.* New York: Avon Books.

GRAEDON, J., & FERGUSON, T. (1993). *The aspirin handbook.* New York: Bantam Books.

GRAEDON, J., & GRAEDON, T. (1991). *Graedons' best medicine.* New York: Bantam Books.

GRAHAM, B. (1988). The abuse of alcohol: Disease or disgrace? *Alcoholism & Addiction, 8* (4), 14–15.

GRAHAM, J. R. (1990). *MMPI-2 Assessing Personality and Psychopathology.* New York: Oxford University Press.

GRAHAM, M. (1989). One toke over the line. *The New Republic, 200* (16), 20–22.

GRANT, I. (1987). Alcohol and the brain: Neuropsychological correlates. *Journal of Clinical and Consulting Psychology, 55,* 310–324.

GRANT, P. D., & HEATON, R. K. (1990). Human immunodeficiency virus-type 1 (HIV-1) and the brain. *Journal of Clinical and Consulting Psychology, 58,* 22–30.

GREDEN, J. F., & WALTERS, A. (1992). Caffeine. In J. H. Lowinson, P. Ruiz, R. Millman, & J. G. Langrod (Eds.), *Substance abuse: A comprehensive textbook* (2nd ed.). New York: Williams & Wilkins.

GREENBERG, D. A. (1993). Ethanol and sedatives. *Neurologic Clinics, 11,* 523–534.

GREENBLATT, D. J., & SHADER, R. I. (1975). Treatment of the alcohol withdrawal syndrome. In R. I. Shader (Ed.), *Manual of psychiatric therapeutics.* Boston: Little, Brown.

GREENE, W. C. (1993). AIDS and the immune system. *Scientific American, 269* (3), 99–105.

GRIFFIN, M. L., WEISS, R. D., MIRIN, S. M., & LANG, U. (1989). A comparison of male and female cocaine abusers. *Archives of General Psychiatry, 46,* 122–126.

GRIFFITHS, H. J., PARANTAINEN, H., & OLSON, P. (1994). Alcohol and bone disorders. *Alcohol Health & Research World, 17,* 299–304.

GRIGG, W. (1992). Don't bet your life on statistics. *Minneapolis Star-Tribune, XI* (106), p. 23A.

GRINSPOON, L., & BAKALAR, J. B. (1990). What is

phencyclidine? *The Harvard Medical School Mental Health Letter, 6* (7), 8.

GRINSPOON, L., & BAKALAR, J. B. (1992). Marijuana. In J. H. Lowinson, P. Ruiz, R. B. Millman, & J. G. Langrod (Eds.), *Substance abuse: A comprehensive textbook* (2nd ed.). New York: Williams & Wilkins.

GROB, L. H., BRAVO, G., & WALSH, R. (1990). Second thoughts on 3, 4–methylenedioxymethamphetamine (MDMA) neurotoxicity. *Archives of General Psychiatry, 47,* 288.

Group for the Advancement of Psychiatry. (1990). Substance abuse disorders: A psychiatric priority. *American Journal of Psychiatry, 148,* 1291–1300.

Group, The. (1976). Narcotics Anonymous World Service Office, Inc.

GROVER, S. A., GRAY-DONALD, K., JOSEPH, L., ABRAHAMOWICZ, M., & COUPAL, L. (1994). Life expectancy following dietary modification or smoking cessation. *Archives of Internal Medicine, 154,* 1697–1704.

HALL, S. M., HAVASSY, B. E., & WASSERMAN, D. A. (1991). Effects of commitment to abstinence, positive moods, stress and coping on relapse to cocaine use. *Journal of Consulting and Clinical Psychology, 59,* 526–532.

HALL, W. C., TALBERT, R. L., & ERESHEFSKY, L. (1990). Cocaine abuse and its treatment. *Pharmacotherapy, 10* (1), 47–65.

HAMMER, S., & HAZELTON, L. (1984). Cocaine and the chemical brain. *Science Digest, 92* (10), pp. 58–62, 100–103.

HAMNER, M. B. (1993). PTSD and cocaine abuse. *Hospital and Community Psychiatry, 44,* 591–592.

HAND, R. P. (1989). Taking another look at triazolam—Is this drug safe? *Focus on Pharmacology: Theory and practice, 11* (6), 1–3.

HANDELSMAN, L., ARONSON, M. J., NESS, R., COCHRANE, K. J., & KANOF, P. D. (1992). The dysphoria of heroin addiction. *American Journal of Drug and Alcohol Abuse, 18* (3), 275–287.

HANKINSON, S. E., WILLETT, W. C., COLDITZ, G. A., SEDDON, J. M., ROSNER, B., SPEIZER, F. E., & STAMPFER, M. J. (1992). A prospective study of cigarette smoking and risk of cataract surgery in women. *Journal of the American Medical Association, 268,* 994–998.

HARRIS, M., & BACHRACH, L. L. (1990). Perspectives on homeless mentally ill women. *Hospital & Community Psychiatry, 41,* 253–254.

Harvard Medical School Mental Health Letter. (1988). Sleeping pills and antianxiety drugs. *5* (6), 1–4.

Harvard Medical School Mental Health Letter. (1990). Amphetamines. *6* (10), 1–4.

Harvard Medical School Mental Health Letter. (1992a). Addiction—Part I. *9* (4), 1–4.

Harvard Medical School Mental Health Letter (1992b). Addiction—Part II. *9* (5), 1–4.

Harvard Medical School Mental Health Letter (1994). AIDS and mental health—Part I. *10* (7), 1–4.

HATFIELD, A. B. (1989). Patients' accounts of stress and coping in schizophrenia. *Hospital and Community Psychiatry, 40,* 1141–1145.

HAUPT, H. A. (1993). Anabolic steroids and growth hormone (somatotropin). *The American Journal of Sports Medicine, 21* (3), 468–475.

HAWKES, C. H. (1992). Endorphins: The basis of pleasure? *Journal of Neurology, Neurosurgery and Psychiatry, 55,* 247–250.

HAYNER, G. N., & MCKINNEY, H. (1986). MDMA: The dark side of Ecstasy. *Journal of Psychoactive Drugs, 18* (4), 341–347.

Health Facts. (1991). Medical benefits of marijuana. *XVI* (147), 1, 4.

Health News. (1990). Drug problems in perspective. *8* (3), 1–10.

HEATH, D. B. (1994). Inhalant abuse. *Behavioral Health Management, 14* (3), 47–48.

HEATON, R. K. (1990). Introduction to the special series on acquired immune deficiency syndrome (AIDS). *Journal of Consulting and Clinical Psychology, 58,* 3–4.

HEEREMA, D. L. (1990). Drug use in the 1990s. *Business Horizons, 33* (1), 127–132.

HEIMEL, C. (1990). It's now, it's trendy, it's codependency. *Playboy, 37* (5), p. 43.

HEIMEL, C. (1991). Sickos "R" us. *Playboy, 38* (9), p. 42.

HELLINGER, F. J. (1993). The lifetime cost of treating a person with HIV. *Journal of the American Medical Association, 270,* 474–478.

HELLMAN, R. E., STANTON, M., LEE, J., TYTUN, A., & VACHON, R. (1989). Treatment of homosexual alcoholics in government-funded agencies: Provider training and attitudes. *Hospital and Community Psychiatry, 40,* 1163–1168.

HELZER, J. E., ROBINS, L. N., TAYLOR, J. R., CAREY, K., MILLER, R. H., COMBS-ORME, T., & FARMER, A. (1985). The extent of long-term moderate drinking among alcoholics discharged from medical and psychiatric treatment facilities. *The New England Journal of Medicine, 312,* 1678–1682.

HENDERSON, L. A. (1994a). About LSD. In L. A. Henderson & W. J. Glass (Eds.), *LSD: Still with us after all these years.* New York: Lexington Books.

HENDERSON, L. A. (1994b). Adverse reactions. In L. A. Henderson & W. J. Glass (Eds.), *LSD: Still with us after all these years.* New York: Lexington Books.

HENNEKENS, C. H., JONAS, M. A., & BURING, J. E. (1994). The benefits of aspirin in acute myocardial infarction. *Archives of Internal Medicine, 154,* 37–39.

HENNESSEY, M. B. (1992). Identifying the woman with

alcohol problems. *Nursing Clinics of North America,*
27, 917–924.

HENNINGFIELD, J. E., & NEMETH-COSLETT, R. (1988).
Nicotine dependence. *Chest, 93* (2), 37s–55s.

HENRY, J. A., JEFFREYS, J. A., & DAWLING, S. (1992).
Toxicity and deaths from 3,4–methylenedioxymethamphetamine ("Ecstasy"). *The Lancet, 340,*
384–387.

HERMAN, E. (1988). The twelve step program: Cure or
cover? *Utne Reader, 30,* 52–53.

HERMAN, R. (1993). Alcohol debate may drive you to
drink. *St. Paul Pioneer Press, 144* (356), p. 11G.

HESTER, R. K. (1994). Outcome research: Alcoholism.
In M. Galanter & H. D. Kleber (Eds.), *Textbook of
substance abuse treatment.* Washington, DC: American Psychiatric Association Press, Inc.

HESTER, R. K., & MILLER, W. R. (1989). Self-control
training. In R. K. Hester & W. R. Miller (Eds.),
Handbook of alcoholism treatment approaches. New
York: Pergamon.

HIBBS, J., PERPER, J., & WINEK, C. L. (1991). An outbreak of designer drug-related deaths in Pennsylvania. *Journal of the American Medical Association,
265,* 1011–1013.

HILTS, P. J. (1994). Labeling on cigarettes called a
smoke screen. *St. Paul Pioneer Press, 146* (5), pp.
1A, 6A.

HIRSCHFIELD, R. M. A., & DAVIDSON, L. (1988). Risk
factors for suicide. In A. J. Frances & R. E. Hales
(Eds.), *Review of Psychiatry, Vol. 7.* Washington,
DC: American Psychiatric Association Press, Inc.

HOBSON, J. A. (1989). Dream theory: A new view of
the brain-mind. *The Harvard Medical School Mental
Health Letter, 5* (8), 3–5.

HOCHBERG, M. C. (1992). NSAIDs: Mechanisms and
pathways of actions. *Hospital Practice, 24* (3), 185–
198.

HOEGERMAN, G., & SCHNOLL, S. (1991). Narcotic use
in pregnancy. *Clinics in Perinatology, 18,* 52–76.

HOEKSEMA, H. L., & DE BOCK, G. H. (1993). The value
of laboratory tests for the screening and recognition of alcohol abuse in primary care patients. *The
Journal of Family Practice, 37,* 268–276.

HOFFMAN, H., LOPER, R. G., & KAMMEIER, M. L. (1974).
Identifying future alcoholics with MMPI alcohol
scales. *Quarterly Journal of Studies on Alcohol, 35,*
490–498.

HOFFMANN, N. G., BELILLE, C. A., & HARRISON, P. A.
(1987). Adequate resources for a complex population? *Alcoholism & Addiction, 7* (5), 17.

HOLDER, H., LONGABAUGH, R., MILLER, W. R., &
RUBONIS, A. V. (1991). The cost effectiveness of
treatment for alcoholism: A first approximation.
Journal of Studies on Alcohol, 52, 517–540.

HOLLAND, W. W., & FITZSIMONS, B. (1991). Smoking

in children. *Archives of Disease in Childhood, 66,*
1269–1270.

HOLLANDER, H., & KATZ, M. H. (1993). HIV infection.
In L. M. Tierney, S. J. McPhee, M. A. Papadakis, &
S. A. Schroeder (Eds.), *Current medical diagnosis &
treatment.* Norwalk, CT: Appleton & Lange.

HOLLOWAY, M. (1991). Rx for addiction. *Scientific
American, 264* (3), pp. 94–103.

HONG, R., MATSUYAMA, E., & NUR, K. (1991). Cardiomyopathy associated with smoking of crystal
methamphetamine. *Journal of the American Medical
Association, 265,* 1152–1154.

HOPPER, J. L., & SEEMAN, E. (1994). The bone density
of female twins discordant for tobacco use. *The
New England Journal of Medicine, 330,* 387–392.

HORGAN, J. (1989). Lukewarm turkey: Drug firms balk
at pursuing a heroin-addiction treatment. *Scientific
American, 260* (3), p. 32.

HORNEY, K. (1964). *The neurotic personality of our time.*
New York: Norton.

Hospital and Community Psychiatry. (1994). Report to
Congress on alcohol and health paints comprehensive picture of alcoholism's impact. *45* (1),
86.

HOUGH, D. O., & KOVAN, J. R. (1990). Is your patient
a steroid abuser? *Medical Aspects of Human Sexuality, 24* (11), 24–32.

HOUSE, M. A. (1990). Cocaine. *American Journal of
Nursing, 90* (4), 40–45.

HOWLAND, R. H. (1990). Barriers to community treatment of patients with dual diagnoses. *Hospital &
Community Psychiatry, 41,* 1136–1138.

HSER, Y., ANGLIN, D., & POWERS, K. (1993). A 24-year
follow-up of California narcotics addicts. *Archives
of General Psychiatry, 50,* 577–584.

HUGHES, J. R. (1992). Tobacco withdrawal in self-quit-
ters. *Journal of Consulting and Clinical Psychology,
60,* 689–697.

HUGHES, J. R., GUST, S. W., SKOOG, K., KEENAN, R. M.,
& FENWICK, J. W. (1991). Symptoms of tobacco
withdrawal. *Archives of General Psychiatry, 48,* 52–
59.

HUGHES, R. (1993). Bitch, bitch, bitch . . . *Psychology
Today, 26* (5), pp. 28–30.

HUMPHREYS, K., & RAPPAPORT, J. (1993). From the
community mental health movement to the war
on drugs. *American Psychologist, 48,* 892–901.

HUNTER, M., & KELLOGG, T. (1989). Redefining ACA
characteristics. *Alcoholism & Addiction, 9* (3), 28–29.

HURT, R. D., FINLAYSON, R. E., MORSE, R. M., & DAVIS,
L. J. (1988). Alcoholism in elderly persons: Medical
aspects and prognosis of 216 inpatients. *Mayo
Clinic Proceedings, 63,* 753–760.

HUSSAR, D. A. (1990). Update 90: New drugs. *Nursing
90,* 20 (12), 41–51.

HUTCHINSON, B. M., & HOOK, E. W. (1990). Syphilis in adults. *Medical Clinics of North America, 74,* 1389–1416.

HYDE, G. L. (1989). Management of the impaired person in the O.R. *Bulletin of the American College of Surgeons, 74* (11), 6–9.

HYMOWITZ, N., FEUERMAN, M., HOLLANDER, M., & FRANCES, R. J. (1993). Smoking deterence using silver acetate. *Hospital and Community Psychiatry, 44,* 113–114, 116.

IGGERS, J. (1990). The addiction industry. *Minneapolis Star-Tribune, IX* (102), pp. 1E, 4E, 10EX.

Internal Medicine Alert. (1989). Aspirin reduces the risk of heart attack—The physician's health study data. *11* (15), 57–58.

ISNER, J. M., & CHOKSHI, S. K. (1989). Cocaine and vasospasm. *The New England Journal of Medicine, 321,* 1604–1606.

JACOBSON, J. M. (1992). Alcoholism and tuberculosis. *Alcohol Health & Research World, 16* (1), 39–45.

JAFFE, J. H. (1986). Opioids. In *American Psychiatric Association Annual Review. Vol. 5.* Washington, DC: American Psychiatric Association.

JAFFE, J. H. (1989). Drug dependence: Opioids, non-narcotics, nicotine (tobacco) and caffeine. In H. I. Kaplan & B. J. Sadock (Eds.), *Comprehensive textbook of psychiatry/V.* Baltimore: Williams & Wilkins.

JAFFE, J. H. (1990). Drug addiction and drug abuse. In A. G. Gilman, T. W. Rall, A. S. Nies, & P. Taylor (Eds.), *The pharmacological basis of therapeutics* (8th ed.). New York: Macmillan.

JAFFE, J. H. (1992). Opiates: Clinical aspects. In J. H. Lowinson, P. Ruiz, R. B. Millman, & J. G. Langrod (Eds.), *Substance abuse: A comprehensive textbook* (2nd ed.). New York: Williams & Wilkins.

JAFFE, J. H., & MARTIN, W. R. (1990). Opioid analgesics and antagonists. In A. G. Gilman, T. W. Rall, A. S. Nies, & P. Taylor (Eds.), *The pharmacological basis of therapeutics* (8th ed.). New York: Macmillan.

JANSEN, K. L. R. (1993). Non-medical use of ketamine. *The Lancet, 306,* 601–602.

JAPENGA, A. (1991). You're tougher than you think! *Self, 13* (4), pp. 174–175, 187.

JARVIK, M. E., & SCHNEIDER, N. G. (1992). Nicotine. In J. H. Lowinson, P. Ruiz, R. B. Millman, & J. G. Langrod (Eds.), *Substance abuse: A comprehensive textbook* (2nd ed.). New York: Williams & Wilkins.

JAY, S. M., ELLIOTT, C., & VARNI, J. W. (1986). Acute and chronic pain in adults and children with cancer. *Journal of Consulting and Clinical Psychology, 54,* 601–607.

JELLINEK, E. M. (1952). Phases of alcohol addiction. *Quarterly Journal of Studies on Alcohol, 13,* 673–674.

JELLINEK, E. M. (1960). *The disease concept of alcoholism.* New Haven, CT: College and University Press.

JENIKE, M. A. (1991). Drug abuse. In E. Rubenstein & D. D. Federman (Eds.), *Scientific American medicine.* New York: Scientific American Press, Inc.

JENSEN, G. B., & PAKKENBERG, B. (1993). Do alcoholics drink their neurons away? *The Lancet, 342,* 1201–1204.

JENSEN, J. G. (1987a). Step Two: A promise of hope. In *The Twelve Steps of Alcoholics Anonymous.* New York: Harper & Row.

JENSEN, J. G. (1987b). Step Three: Turning it over. In *The Twelve Steps of Alcoholics Anonymous.* New York: Harper & Row.

Johnson Institute. (1987). *The family enablers.* Minneapolis: The Johnson Institute.

JOHNSON, M. D. (1990). Anabolic steroid use in adolescent athletes. *The Pediatric Clinics of North America, 37,* 1111–1123.

JOHNSON, V. E. (1980). *I'll quit tomorrow.* San Francisco: Harper & Row.

JOHNSTON, L. D., O'MALLEY, P. M., & BACHMAN, J. G. (1993). *National survey results on drug use from the Monitoring the Future Study, 1975–1992.* Rockville, MD: U.S. Department of Health and Human Services.

JOHNSTON, L. D., O'MALLEY, P. M., & BACHMAN, J. G. (1994). *Monitoring the future study, 1993.* Rockville, MD: U.S. Department of Health and Human Services.

JONES, R. L. (1990). Evaluation of drug use in the adolescent. In L. M. Haddad & J. F. Winchester (Eds.), *Clinical management of poisoning and drug overdoses* (2nd ed.). New York: W. B. Saunders.

JONES, R. T. (1987). Psychopharmacology of cocaine. In A. G. Washton & M. S. Gold (Eds.), *Cocaine: A clinician's handbook.* New York: Guilford.

JOSHI, N. P., & SCOTT, M. (1988). Drug use, depression, and adolescents. *The Pediatric Clinics of North America, 35* (6), 1349–1364.

JOYCE, C. (1989). The woman alcoholic. *American Journal of Nursing, 89,* 1314–1316.

JUDD, L. L., & HUEY, L. Y. (1984). Lithium antagonizes ethanol intoxication in alcoholics. *The American Journal of Psychiatry, 141,* 1517–1521.

JUERGENS, S. M. (1993). Benzodiazepines and addiction. *Psychiatric Clinics of North America, 16,* 75–86.

JUERGENS, S. M., & MORSE, R. M. (1988). Alprazolam dependence in seven patients. *The American Journal of Psychiatry, 145,* 625–627.

JULIEN, R. M. (1992). *A primer of drug action* (6th ed.). New York: W. H. Freeman.

KACSO, G., & TEREZHALMY, G. T. (1994). Acetylsalicylic acid and acetaminophen. *Dental Clinics of North America, 38,* 633–644.

KAMBACK, M. C. (1978). Animal models of addictive

behavior. In G. U. Balis (Ed.), *Basic Psychopathology. Vol. III.* Boston: Butterworth Publishers, Inc.

KAMINER, W. (1992). *I'm dysfunctional, you're dysfunctional.* New York: Addison-Wesley.

KAMINER, Y. (1991). Adolescent substance abuse. In R. J. Frances & S. I. Miller (Eds.), *Clinical textbook of addictive disorders.* New York: Guilford.

KAMINER, Y. (1994). Adolescent substance abuse. In M. Galanter & H. D. Kleber (Eds.), *Textbook of substance abuse treatment.* Washington, DC: American Psychiatric Association Press, Inc.

KAMINER, Y., & FRANCES, R. J. (1991). Inpatient treatment of adolescents with psychiatric and substance abuse disorders. *Hospital and Community Psychiatry, 42,* 894–896.

KAMINSKI, A. (1992). *Mind-altering drugs.* Madison, WI: Wisconsin Clearinghouse, Board of Regents, University of Wisconsin System.

KANDALL, S. R., GAINES, J., HABEL, L., DAVIDSON, G., & JESSOP, D. (1993). The relationship of maternal substance abuse to subsequent sudden infant death syndrome in offspring. *The Journal of Pediatrics, 123,* 120–126.

KANDEL, D. B., & RAVEIS, V. H. (1989). Cessation of illicit drug use in young adulthood. *Archives of General Psychiatry, 46,* 109–116.

KANDEL, D. B., YAMAGUCHI, K., & CHEN, K. (1992). Stages of progression in drug involvement from adolescence to adulthood: Further evidence for the gateway theory. *Journal of Studies on Alcohol, 53* (5), 447–458.

KANOF, P. D., ARONSON, M. J., & NESS, R. (1992). Organic mood syndrome associated with detoxification from methadone maintenance. *American Journal of Psychiatry, 150,* 423–428.

KANWISCHER, R. W., & HUNDLEY, J. (1990). Screening for substance abuse in hospitalized psychiatric patients. *Hospital & Community Psychiatry, 41,* 795–797.

KAPLAN, H. I., & SADOCK, B. J. (1990). *Pocket handbook of clinical psychiatry.* Baltimore: Williams & Wilkins.

KAPLAN, H. I., SADOCK, B. J., & GREBB, J. A. (1994). *Synopsis of psychiatry* (7th ed.). Baltimore: Williams & Wilkins.

KASHKIN, K. B. (1992). Anabolic steroids. In J. H. Lowinson, P. Ruiz, R. B. Millman, & J. G. Langrod (Eds.), *Substance abuse: A comprehensive textbook* (2nd ed.). New York: Williams & Wilkins.

KASHKIN, K. B., & KLEBER, H. D. (1989). Hooked on hormones? An anabolic steroid addiction hypothesis. *Journal of the American Medical Association, 262,* 3166–3173.

KATZ, S. J., & LIU, A. E. (1991). *The codependency conspiracy.* New York: Warner Books.

KAUFMAN, E., & MCNAUL, J. P. (1992). Recent developments in understanding and treating drug abuse and dependence. *Hospital and Community Psychiatry, 43,* 223–236.

KAUFMAN, G. (1989). *The psychology of shame.* New York: Springer.

KAY, S. R., KALATHARA, M., & MEINZER, A. E. (1989). Diagnostic and behavioral characteristics of psychiatric patients who abuse substances. *Hospital and Community Psychiatry, 40,* 1062–1065.

KELLY, J. A., MURPHY, D. A., SIKKEMA, K. J., & KALICYHMAN, S. C. (1993). Psychological interventions to prevent HIV infection are urgently needed. *American Psychologist, 48,* 1023–1034.

KEMM, J. (1993). Alcohol and heart disease: The implications of the U-shaped curve. *British Medical Journal, 307,* 1373–1374.

KENDER, K. S., HEATH, A. C., NEALE, M. C., KESSLER, R. C., & EVES, J. (1992). A population-based twin study of alcoholism in women. *Journal of the American Medical Association, 268,* 1877–1882.

KENFORD, S. L., FIORE, M. C., JORENBY, D. E., SMITH, S. S., WETTER, D., & BAKER, T. B. (1994). Predicting smoking cessation. *Journal of the American Medical Association, 271,* 589–594.

KESSLER, R. C., MCGONAGLE, K. A., ZHAO, S., NELSON, C. B., HUGHES, M., ESHLEMAN, S., HANS-ULRICH, W., & KENDLER, K. S. (1994). Lifetime and 12-month prevalence of *DSM-III-R* psychiatric disorders in the United States. *Archives of General Psychiatry, 51,* 8–19.

KHANTZIAN, E. J. (1985). The self-medication hypothesis of addictive disorders: Focus on heroin and cocaine dependence. *American Journal of Psychiatry, 142,* 1259–1274.

KHURI, E. T. (1989). Narcotic poisoning. In R. E. Rakel (Ed.), *Conn's current therapy.* Philadelphia: W. B. Saunders.

KILPATRICK, C. (1990). Violence as a precursor of women's substance abuse: The rest of the drugs–violence story. Paper presented at the 1990 meeting of the American Psychological Association, Boston, MA.

KING, G. R., & ELLINWOOD, E. H. (1992). Amphetamines and other stimulants. In J. H. Lowinson, P. Ruiz, R. B. Millman, & J. G. Langrod (Eds.), *Substance abuse: A comprehensive textbook* (2nd ed.). New York: Williams & Wilkins.

KING, S. R. (1994). HIV: Virology and mechanisms of disease. *Annals of Emergency Medicine, 24,* 443–449.

KIRN, T. F. (1989). Studies of adolescents indicate just how complex the situation is for this age group. *Journal of the American Medical Association, 261,* 3362.

KIRSCH, M. M. (1986). *Designer drugs.* Minneapolis: CompCare Publications.

KITRIDOU, R. C. (1993). The efficacy and safety of oxaproxin versus aspirin: Pooled results of double-blind trials in rheumatoid arthritis. *Drug Therapy, 23* (Suppl.), 21–25.

KIVLAHAN, D. R., HEIMAN, J. R., WRIGHT, R. C., MUNDT, J. W., & SHUPE, J. A. (1991). Treatment cost and rehospitalization rate in schizophrenic outpatients with a history of substance abuse. *Hospital and Community Psychiatry, 42,* 609–614.

KLAG, M. J., & WHELTON, P. K. (1987). Risk of stroke in male cigarette smokers. *The New England Journal of Medicine, 316,* 628.

KLAR, H. (1987). The setting for psychiatric treatment. In *American Psychiatric Association Annual Review. Vol. 6.* Washington, DC: American Psychiatric Association Press, Inc.

KLASS, P. (1989). Vital signs. *Discover, 10* (1), pp. 12–14.

KLATSKY, A. L. (1990). Alcohol and coronary artery disease. *Alcohol Health & Research World, 14* (4), 289–300.

KLEBER, H. D. (1991). Tracking the cocaine epidemic. *Journal of the American Medical Association, 266,* 2272–2273.

KLEBER, H. D. (1994). Letter to the editor. *New England Journal of Medicine, 331,* 129.

KLEIN, M. The emperor's new addiction. *Playboy, 37* (3), p. 41.

KLEIN, J. M., & MILLER, S. I. (1986). Three approaches to the treatment of drug addiction. *Hospital and Community Psychiatry, 37,* 1083–1085.

KLINGER, R. L., & CABAJ, R. P. (1993). Characteristics of gay and lesbian relationships. In J. M. Oldham, M. B. Riba, & A. Tasman (Eds.), *Review of psychiatry. Vol. 12.* Washington, DC: American Psychiatric Association.

KOFOED, L., KANIA, J., WALSH, T., & ATKINSON, R. M. (1986). Outpatient treatment of patients with substance abuse and coexisting psychiatric disorders. *The American Journal of Psychiatry, 143,* 867–872.

KOFOED, L., & KEYS, A. (1988). Using group therapy to persuade dual-diagnosis patients to seek substance abuse treatment. *Hospital & Community Psychiatry, 39,* 1209–1211.

KOLODNER, G., & FRANCES, R. (1993). Recognizing dissociative disorders in patients with chemical dependency. *Hospital and Community Psychiatry, 44,* 1041–1044.

KOLODNY, R. C. (1985). The clinical management of sexual problems in substance abusers. In T. E. Bratter & G. G. Forrest (Eds.), *Alcoholism and substance abuse: Strategies for clinical intervention.* New York: Free Press.

KONSTAN, M. W., HOPPEL, C. L., CHAI, B., DAVIS, P. B. (1991). Ibuprofen in children with cystic fibrosis: Pharmacokinetics and adverse effects. *Journal of Pediatrics, 118,* 956–965.

KOTTLER, J. A. (1992). *Compassionate therapy.* San Francisco: Jossey-Bass.

KOTULAK, R. (1992). Recent discoveries about cocaine may help unlock secrets of brain. *St. Paul Pioneer Press, 143* (345), p. 4C.

KOVASZNAY, B., BROMET, E., SCHWARTZ, J. E., RANGANATHAN, R., LAVELLE, J., & BRANDON, L. (1993). Substance abuse and onset of psychotic illness. *Hospital and Community Psychiatry, 44,* 567–571.

KOZLOWSKI, L. T., WILKINSON, A., SKINNER, W., KENT, W., FRANKLIN, T., & POPE, M. (1989). Comparing tobacco cigarette dependence with other drug dependencies. *Journal of the American Medical Association, 261,* 898–901.

KRUGER, T. E., & JERRELLS, T. R. (1992). Potential role of alcohol in human immunodeficiency virus infection. *Alcohol Health & Research World, 16* (1), 57–63.

KRUZICKI, J. (1987). Dispelling a myth: The facts about female alcoholics. *Corrections Today, 49,* 110–115.

KRYGER, M. H., STELJES, D., POULIOT, Z., NEUFELD, H., & ODYNSKI, T. (1991). Subjective versus objective evaluation of hypnotic efficacy: Experience with Zolpidem. *Sleep, 14* (5), 399–407.

KUNITZ, S. J., & LEVY, J. E. (1974). Changing ideas of alcohol use among Navaho Indians. *Quarterly Journal of Studies on Alcohol, 46,* 953–960.

KURTZ, E. (1979). *Not God: A history of Alcoholics Anonymous.* Center City, MN: Hazelden.

KUSHNER, M. G., SHER, K. J., & BEITMAN, B. D. (1990). The relation between alcohol problems and the anxiety disorders. *American Journal of Psychiatry, 147,* 685–695.

LACKS, P., & MORIN, C. M. (1992). Recent advances in the assessment and treatment of insomnia. *Journal of Consulting and Clinical Psychology, 60,* 586–594.

LADER, M. (1987). Assessing the potential for buspirone dependence or abuse and effects of its withdrawal. *The American Journal of Medicine, 82* (Suppl. 5A), 20–26.

LAEGREID, L., RAGNAR, O., NILS, C., HAGBERG, G., WAHLSTROM, J., & ABRAHAMSSON, L. (1990). Congenital malformations and maternal consumption of benzodiazepines: A case control study. *Developmental Medicine and Child Neurology, 32,* 432–442.

LAMAR, J. V., RILEY, M., SAMGHABADI, R. (1986). Crack: A cheap and deadly cocaine is spreading menace. *Time, 128,* pp. 16–18.

The Lancet. (1991a). The smoking epidemic. *338,* 1387.

The Lancet. (1991b). Your heroin, sir. *337,* 402.

The Lancet. (1993). Controlling the weed in public. *341,* 525–526.

LAND, W., PINSKY, D., & SALZMAN, C. (1991). Abuse

and misuse of anticholinergic medications. *Hospital and Community Psychiatry, 42,* 580–581.

LANDRY, G. L., & PRIMOS, W. A. (1990). Anabolic steroid abuse. *Advances in Pediatrics, 37,* 185–205.

LANGE, R. A., CIGARROA, R. G., YANCY, C. W., WILLARD, J. E., POPMA, J. J., SILLS, M. N., MCBRIDE, W., KIM, A. S., & HOLLIS, L. D. (1989). Cocaine induced coronary artery vasoconstriction. *The New England Journal of Medicine, 321,* 1557–1562.

LANGE, W. R., WHITE, N., & ROBINSON, N. (1992). Medical complications of substance abuse. *Postgraduate Medicine, 92,* 205–214.

LANGONE, J. (1989). Hot to block a killer's path. *Time, 133* (5), pp. 60–62.

LARSON, K. K. (1982). Birthplace of "The Minnesota Model." *Alcoholism, 3* (2), 34–35.

LAURENCE, D. R., & BENNETT, P. N. (1992). *Clinical pharmacology* (7th ed.). New York: Churchill Livingstone.

LAWSON, C. (1994). Flirting with tragedy: Women who say yes to drugs. *Cosmopolitan, 217* (1), pp. 138–141.

LAYNE, G. S. (1990). Schizophrenia and substance abuse. In D. F. O'Connell (Ed.), *Managing the dually diagnosed patient.* New York: Haworth.

LEDERBERG, M. S., & HOLLAND, J. C. (1989). Psychooncology. In H. I. Kaplan & B. J. Sadock (Eds.), *Comprehensive textbook of psychiatry/V.* Baltimore: Williams & Wilkins.

LEE, E. W., & D'ALONZO, G. E. (1993). Cigarette smoking, nicotine addiction, and its pharmacologic treatment. *Archives of Internal Medicine, 153,* 34–48.

LEHMAN, A. F., MYERS, C. P., & CORTY, E. (1989). Assessment and classification of patients with psychiatric and substance abuse syndromes. *Hospital and Community Psychiatry, 40,* 1019–1025.

LEHMAN, L. B., PILICH, A., & ANDREWS, N. (1994). Neurological disorders resulting from alcoholism. *Alcohol Health & Research World, 17,* 305–309.

LEIGH, G. (1985). Psychosocial factors in the etiology of substance abuse. In T. E. Bratter & G. G. Forrest (Eds.), *Alcoholism and substance abuse: Strategies for clinical intervention.* New York: Free Press.

LENDER, M. E. (1981). The disease concept of alcoholism in the United States: Was Jellinek first? *Digest of Alcoholism Theory and Application, 1* (1), 25–31.

LEO, J. (1990). The it's-not-my-fault syndrome. *U.S. News & World Report, 109* (12), p. 16.

LESSARD, S. (1989). Busting our mental blocks on drugs and crime. *Washington Monthly, 21* (1), 70.

LEVERS, L. L., & HAWES, A. R. (1990). Drugs and gender: A woman's recovery program. *Journal of Mental Health Counseling, 12,* 527–531.

LEVY, S. J., & RUTTER, E. (1992). *Children of drug abusers.* New York: Lexington Books.

LEWIS, D. O. (1989). Adult antisocial behavior and criminality. In H. I. Kaplan & B. J. Sadock (Eds.), *Comprehensive textbook of psychiatry/V.* New York: Williams & Wilkins.

LEWIS, J. A., DANA, R. Q., & BLEVINS, G. A. (1988). *Substance abuse counseling.* Pacific Grove, CA: Brooks/Cole.

LEWIS, R. (1989). Drug tolerance apparently works in Holland. *Minneapolis Star-Tribune, VIII* (173), p. 15A.

LIBERTO, J. G., OSLIN, D. W., & RUSKIN, P. E. (1992). Alcoholism in older persons: A review of the literature. *Hospital and Community Psychiatry, 43,* 975–984.

LICHTENSTEIN, E., & GLASGOW, R. E. (1992). Smoking cessation: What we have learned over the past decade. *Journal of Consulting and Clinical Psychology, 60,* 518–526.

LIEBERMAN, M. L. (1988). *The sexual pharmacy.* New York: New American Library.

LIEVELD, P. E., & ARUNA, A. (1991). Diagnosis and management of the alcohol withdrawal syndrome. *U.S. Pharmacist, 16* (1), H1–H11.

LINGEMAN, R. R. (1974). *Drugs from A to Z: A dictionary.* New York: McGraw-Hill.

LINNOILA, M., DEJONG, J., & VIRKKUNEN, M. (1989). Family history of alcoholism in violent offenders and impulsive fire setters. *Archives of General Psychiatry, 46,* 613–616.

LINSZEN, D. H., DINGEMANS, P. M., & LENIOR, M. E. (1994). Cannabis abuse and the course of recent-onset schizophrenic disorders. *Archives of General Psychiatry, 51,* 273–279.

LIPKIN, M. (1989). Psychiatry and medicine. In H. I. Kaplan & B. J. Sadock (Eds.), *Comprehensive textbook of psychiatry/V.* Baltimore: Williams & Wilkins.

LIPSCOMB, J. W. (1989). What pharmacists should know about home poisonings. *Drug Topics, 133* (15), 72–80.

LITTLE, R. E., ANDERSON, K. W., ERVIN, C. H., WORTHINGTON-ROBERTS, B., & CLARREN, S. K. (1989). Maternal alcohol use during breast-feeding and infant mental and motor development at one year. *The New England Journal of Medicine, 321,* 425–430.

LØBERG, T. (1986). Neuropsychological findings in the early and middle phases of alcoholism. In I. Grant & K. M. Adams (Eds.), *Neuropsychological assessment of neuropsychiatric disorders.* New York: Oxford University Press.

LOEBL, S., SPRATTO, G. R., & WOODS, A. L. (1994). *The nurse's drug handbook* (7th ed.). New York: Delmar.

LOMBARD, J., LEVIN, I. H., & WEINER, W. J. (1989).

Arsenic intoxication in a cocaine abuser. *The New England Journal of Medicine, 320,* 869.

LOPER, R. G., KAMMEIER, M. L., & HOFFMAN, H. (1973). MMPI characteristics of college freshman males who later become alcoholics. *Journal of Abnormal Psychology, 82,* 159–162.

LOUIE, A. K. (1990). Panic attacks—When cocaine is the cause. *Medical Aspects of Human Sexuality, 24* (12), 44–46.

LOURWOOD, D. L., & RIEDLINGER, J. E. (1989). The use of drugs in the breast-feeding mother. *Drug Topics, 133* (21), 77–85.

LOVETT, A. R. (1994, May 5). Wired in California. *Rolling Stone,* pp. 39–40.

LYONS, J. S., & McGOVERN, M. P. (1989). Use of mental health services by dually diagnosed persons. *Hospital & Community Psychiatry, 40,* 1067–1069.

MAAS, E. F., ASHE, J., SPIEGEL, P., ZEE, D. S., & LEIGH, R. J. (1991). Acquired pendular nystagmus in toluene addiction. *Neurology, 41,* 282–286.

MacKENZIE, T. D., BARTECCHI, C. E., & SCHRIER, R. W. (1994a). The human costs of tobacco use. *The New England Journal of Medicine (First of Two Parts), 330,* 907–912.

MacKENZIE, T. D., BARTECCHI, C. E., & SCHRIER, R. W. (1994b). The human costs of tobacco use. *The New England Journal of Medicine (Second of Two Parts), 330,* 975–980.

MADDUX, J. F., DESMOND, D. P., & COSTELLO, R. (1987). Depression in opioid users varies with substance use status. *American Journal of Drug & Alcohol Abuse, 13* (4), 375–378.

MAGUIRE, J. (1990). *Care and feeding of the brain.* New York: Doubleday.

MAISTO, S. A., & CONNORS, G. J. (1988). Assessment of treatment outcome. In D. M. Donovan & G. A. Marlatt (Eds.), *Assessment of addictive disorders.* New York: Guilford.

MALES, M. (1992). Tobacco: Promotion and smoking. *Journal of the American Medical Association, 267,* 3282.

MANFREDI, R. L., KALES, A., VGONTZAS, A. N., BIXLER, E. O., ISAAC, M. A., & FALCONE, C. M. (1991). Buspirone: Sedative or stimulant effect? *American Journal of Psychiatry, 148,* 1213–1217.

MANN, C. C., & PLUMMER, M. L. (1991). *The aspirin wars.* New York: Knopf.

MANN, J. (1994). *Murder, magic and medicine.* New York: Oxford University Press.

MARANTO, G. (1985). Coke: The random killer. *Discover, 12* (3), pp. 16–21.

MARGOLIN, A., KOSTEN, T., PETRAKIS, I., AVANTS, S. K., & KOSTEN, T. (1991). Bupropion reduces cocaine abuse in methadone-maintained patients. *Archives of General Psychiatry, 48,* 87.

MARLATT, G. A. (1994). Harm reduction: A public health approach to addictive behavior. *Division on Addictions Newsletter, 2* (1), 1, 3.

MARSANO, L. (1994). Alcohol and malnutrition. *Alcohol Health & Research World, 17,* 284–291.

MARSHALL, J. R. (1994). The diagnosis and treatment of social phobia and alcohol abuse. *Bulletin of the Menninger Clinic, 58,* A58–A66.

MARZUK, P. M., TARDIFF, K., LEON, A. C., STAJIC, M., MORGAN, E. B., & MANN, J. J. (1992). Prevalence of cocaine use among residents of New York City who committed suicide during a one-year period. *American Journal of Psychiatry, 149,* 371–375.

MASSING, M. (1992). Mixed messages. *Modern Maturity, 35* (1), 38–41, 93.

MATHERS, D. C., & GHODSE, A. D. (1992). Cannabis and psychotic illness. *British Journal of Psychiatry, 161,* 648–653.

MATHEW, R. D., WILSON, W. H., BLAZER, D. G., & GEORGE, L. K. (1993). Psychiatric disorders in adult children of alcoholics: Data from the epidemiologic catchment area project. *American Journal of Psychiatry, 150,* 793–800.

MATSUDA, L. A., LOLAIT, S. J., BROWNSTEIN, M. J., YOUNG, A. C., & BONNER, T. I. (1990). Structure of a cannabinoid receptor and functional expression of the cloned cDNA. *Nature, 346,* 561–564.

MATUSCHKA, E. (1985). Treatment, outcomes and clinical evaluation. In T. E. Bratter & G. G. Forrest (Eds.), *Alcoholism and substance abuse: Strategies for clinical intervention.* New York: Free Press.

MATUSCHKA, P. R. (1985). The psychopharmacology of addiction. In T. E. Bratter & G. G. Forrest (Eds.), *Alcoholism and substance abuse: Strategies for clinical intervention.* New York: Free Press.

MAY, G. G. (1988). *Addiction & grace.* New York: Harper & Row.

MAY, G. G. (1991). *The awakened heart.* New York: Harper & Row.

MAYES, L. C., GRANGER, R. H., BORNSTEIN, M. H., & ZUCKERMAN, B. (1992). The problem of prenatal cocaine exposure. *Journal of the American Medical Association, 267,* 406–408.

MAYES, L. C., GRANGER, R. H., FRANK, M. A., SCHOTTENFELD, R., & BORNSTEIN, M. H. (1993). Neurobehavioral profiles of neonates exposed to cocaine prenatally. *Pediatrics, 91,* 778–783.

Mayo Clinic Health Letter. (1989). America's drug crisis. Rochester, MN: Mayo Foundation for Medical Education and Research.

McCAFFERY, M., & FERRELL, B. R. (1994). Understanding opioids and addiction. *Nursing 94, 24* (8), 56–59.

McCARTHY, J. J., & BORDERS, O. T. (1985). Limit setting on drug abuse in methadone maintenance patients. *American Journal of Psychiatry, 142,* 1419–1423.

McCarty, D., Argeriou, M., Huebner, R. B., & Lubran, B. (1991). Alcoholism, drug abuse, and the homeless. *American Psychologist, 46,* 1139–1148.

McCrady, B. S., & Irvine, S. (1989). Self-help groups. In R. K. Hester & W. R. Miller (Eds.), *Handbook of alcoholism treatment approaches.* New York: Pergamon.

McCutchan, J. A. (1990). Virology, immunology, and clinical course of HIV infection. *Journal of Clinical and Consulting Psychology, 58,* 5–12.

McEnroe, P. (1990). Hawaii is fighting losing battle against the popularity of drug "ice." *Minneapolis Star-Tribune, IX* (44), pp. 1, 20A.

McGinnis, J. M., & Foege, W. H. (1993). Actual causes of death in the United States. *Journal of the American Medical Association, 270,* 2207–2212.

McGuire, L. (1990). The power of non-narcotic pain relievers. *RN, 53* (4), 28–35.

McGuire, P., & Fahy, T. (1991). Chronic paranoid psychosis after misuse of MDMA ("Ecstasy"). *British Medical Journal, 302,* 697.

McHugh, M. J. (1987). The abuse of volatile substances. *The Pediatric Clinics of North America, 34* (2), 333–340.

McLellan, A. T., Arndt, I. O., Metzger, D. S., Woody, G. E., & O'Brien, C. P. (1993). The effects of psychosocial services in substance abuse treatment. *Journal of the American Medical Association, 269,* 1953–1959.

McMicken, D. B. (1990). Alcohol withdrawal syndromes. *Emergency Medicine Clinics of North America, 8,* 805–819.

McWilliams, P. (1993). Ain't nobody's business. *Playboy, 40* (9), pp. 49–52.

Mead, R. (1993). Teen access to cigarettes in Green Bay, Wisconsin. *Wisconsin Medical Journal, 92,* 23–25.

Medical Aspects of Human Sexuality. (1990). Women with AIDS: The growing threat. *24* (10), 68–69.

Medical Economics Company. (1989). Anabolic steroid abuse and primary care. *Patient Care, 23* (8), 12.

Medical Economics Company. (1995). *1995 Physician's desk reference* (47th ed.). Oradell, NJ: Author.

Medical Letter, The. (1989). Aspirin for prevention of myocardial infarction and stroke. *31* (799), 77–79.

Medical Update. (1994). The agony of "Ecstasy." *17* (11), 5–6.

Meer, J. (1986). Marijuana in the air: Delayed buzz bomb. *Psychology Today, 20,* p. 68.

Melzack, R. (1990). The tragedy of needless pain. *Scientific American, 262* (2), pp. 27–33.

Mendelson, W. B., & Rich, C. L. (1993). Sedatives and suicide: The San Diego study. *Acta Psychiatrica Scandinavica, 88,* 337–341.

Mendoza, R., & Miller, B. L. (1992). Neuropsychiatric disorders associated with cocaine use. *Hospital and Community Psychiatry, 43,* 677–678.

Merlotti, L., Roehrs, T., Koshorek, G., Zorick, F., Lamphere, J., & Roth, T. (1989). The dose effects of zolpidem on the sleep of healthy normals. *Journal of Clinical Psychopharmacology, 9* (1), 9–14.

Merton, T. (1961). *New seeds of contemplation.* New York: New Directions Publishing.

Merton, T. (1978). *No man is an island.* New York: New Directions Publishing.

Meyer, R. (1988). Intervention: Opportunity for healing. *Alcoholism & Addiction, 9* (1), 7.

Meyer, R. E. (1989a). Who can say no to illicit drug use? *Archives of General Psychiatry, 46,* 189–190.

Meyer, R. E. (1989b). What characterizes addiction? *Alcohol Health & Research World, 13* (4), 316–321.

Meyer, R. E. (1992). New pharmacotherapies for cocaine dependence. . . revisited. *Archives of General Psychiatry, 49,* 900–904.

Meyer, R. E. (1994). What for, alcohol research? *American Journal of Psychiatry, 151,* 165–168.

Meyers, B. R. (1992). *Antimicrobial therapy guide.* Newtown, PA: Antimicrobial Prescribing, Inc.

Michelson, J. B., Carroll, D., McLane, N. J., & Robin, H. S. (1988). Drug abuse and ocular disease. In J. B. Michelson & R. A. Nozik (Eds.), *Surgical treatment of ocular inflammatory disease.* New York: Lippincott.

Mikkelsen, E. (1985). Substance abuse in adolescents and children. In R. Michels, J. O. Cavenar, H. K. H. Brodie, A. M. Cooper, S. B. Guze, S. B. Judd, G. Klerman, & A. J. Solnit (Eds.), *Psychiatry.* New York: Basic Books.

Milby, J. B., Hohmann, A. A., Gentile, M., Huggins, N., Sims, M. K., McLellan, T., Woody, G., & Haas, N. (1994). Methadone maintenance outcome as a function of detoxification phobia. *American Journal of Psychiatry, 151,* 1031–1037.

Milhorn, H. T. (1991). Diagnosis and management of phenocyclidine intoxication. *American Family Physician, 43,* 1293–1302.

Milhorn, H. T. (1992). Pharmacologic management of acute abstinence syndromes. *American Family Physician, 45,* 231–239.

Miller, A. (1988). *The enabler.* Claremont, CA: Hunter House.

Miller, F. T., & Tanenbaum, J. H. (1989). Drug abuse in schizophrenia. *Hospital and Community Psychiatry, 40,* 847–849.

Miller, L. J. (1994). Psychiatric medication during pregnancy: Understanding and minimizing risks. *Psychiatric Annals, 24* (2), 69–75.

Miller, N. S., & Gold, M. S. (1991a). Dual diagnosis: Psychiatric syndromes in alcoholism and drug addiction. *American Family Physician, 43,* 2071–2076.

MILLER, N. S., & GOLD, M. S. (1991b). Organic solvent and aerosol abuse. *American Family Physician, 44,* 183–190.

MILLER, N. S., & GOLD, M. S. (1991c). Abuse, addiction, tolerance, and dependence to benzodiazepines in medical and nonmedical populations. *American Journal of Drug and Alcohol Abuse, 17* (1), 27–37.

MILLER, N. S., & GOLD, M. S. (1993). A hypothesis for a common neurochemical basis for alcohol and drug disorders. *Psychiatric Clinics of North America, 16,* 105–117.

MILLER, P. M., & FOY, D. W. (1981). Substance abuse. In S. M. Turner, K. S. Calhoun, & H. E. Adams (Eds.), *Handbook of clinical behavior therapy.* New York: Wiley.

MILLER, R. R. (1990). Athletes and steroids: Playing a deadly game. *Journal of Chiropractic, 27* (2), 35–38.

MILLER, S. I., FRANCES, R. J., & HOLMES, D. J. (1988). Use of psychotropic drugs in alcoholism treatment: A summary. *Hospital & Community Psychiatry, 39,* 1251–1252.

MILLER, S. I., FRANCES, R. J., & HOLMES, D. J. (1989). Psychotropic medications. In R. K. Hester & W. R. Miller (Eds.), *Handbook of alcoholism treatment approaches.* New York: Pergamon.

MILLER, W. R. (1976). Alcoholism scales and objective measures. *Psychological Bulletin, 83,* 649–674.

MILLER, W. R. (1989). Increasing motivation for change. In R. K. Hester & W. R. Miller (Eds.), *Handbook of alcoholism treatment approaches.* New York: Pergamon.

MILLER, W. R. (1992). Client/treatment matching in addictive behaviors. *The Behavior Therapist, 15* (1), 7–8.

MILLER, W. R., GENEFIELD, G., & TONIGAN, J. S. (1993). Enhancing motivation for change in problem drinking: A controlled comparison of two therapist styles. *Journal of Consulting and Clinical Psychology, 61,* 455–462.

MILLER, W. R., & HESTER, R. K. (1980). Treating the problem drinker: Modern approaches. In W. R. Miller (Ed.), *The addictive behaviors.* New York: Pergamon.

MILLER, W. R., & HESTER, R. K. (1986). Inpatient alcoholism treatment. *American Psychologist, 41* (7), 794–806.

MILLER, W. R., & HESTER, R. K. (1989). Treating alcohol problems: Toward an informed eclecticism. In R. K. Hester, & W. R. Miller, (Eds.), *Handbook of alcoholism treatment approaches.* New York: Pergamon.

MILLER, W. R., & KURTZ, E. (1994). Models of alcoholism used in treatment: Contrasting AA and other perspectives with which it is often confused. *Journal of Studies on Alcohol, 55,* 159–166.

MILLER, W. R., & McCRADY, B. S. (1993). The importance of research on Alcoholics Anonymous. In B. S. McCrady & W. R. Miller (Eds.), *Research on Alcoholics Anonymous.* New Brunswick, NJ: Rutgers Center of Alcohol Studies.

MILLER, W. R., & ROLLNICK, S. (1991). *Motivational interviewing.* New York: Guilford.

MILLMAN, R. B., & BEEDER, A. B. (1994). Cannabis. In M. Galanter & H. D. Kleber (Eds.), *Textbook of substance abuse treatment.* Washington, DC: American Psychiatric Association Press, Inc.

MILLON, T. (1981). *Disorders of personality.* New York: Wiley.

MILZMAN, D. P., & SODERSTROM, C. A. (1994). Substance use disorders in trauma patients. *Critical Care Clinics, 10,* 595–612.

MINKOFF, K. (1989). An integrated treatment model for dual diagnosis of psychosis and addiction. *Hospital and Community Psychiatry, 40,* 1031–1036.

Minneapolis Star-Tribune. (1989). New drug "ice" grips Hawaii, threatens mainland. *VIII* (150), p. 12a.

Minneapolis Star-Tribune. (1994). Study: Drug treatment makes cents. *XIII* (71), p. 8A.

MIRIN, S. M., WEISS, R. D., & GREENFIELD, S. F. (1991). Psychoactive substance use disorders. In A. J. Galenberg, E. L. Bassuk, & S. C. Schoonover (Eds.), *The practitioner's guide to psychoactive drugs* (3rd ed.). New York: Plenum.

MITCHELL, J. R. (1988). Acetaminophen toxicity. *The New England Journal of Medicine, 319,* 1601–1602.

MOLITERNO, D. J., WILLARD, J. E., LANGE, R. A., NEGUS, B. H., BOEHRER, J. D., GLAMANN, B., LANDAU, C., ROSSEN, J. D., WINNIFORD, M. D., & HOLLIS, L. D. (1994). Coronary-artery vasoconstriction induced by cocaine, cigarette smoking, or both. *The New England Journal of Medicine, 330,* 454–459.

MONCHER, M. S., HOLDEN, G. W., & TRIMBLE, J. E. (1990). Substance abuse among native-American youth. *Journal of Consulting and Clinical Psychology, 58,* 408–415.

MONDI, L., HOOTEN, J., & PETERZELL, J. (1994). Are smokers junkies? *Time, 143* (12), p. 62.

MOORE, J. (1993). AIDS: Striking the happy media. *Nature, 363,* pp. 391–392.

MOORE, M. H. (1991). Drugs, the criminal law, and the administration of justice. *The Milbank Quarterly, 69* (4), 529–560.

MORGENROTH, L. (1989). High-risk pain pills. *The Atlantic, 264* (6), pp. 36–42.

MORRISON, M. A. (1990). Addiction in adolescents. *The Western Journal of Medicine, 152,* 543–547.

MORSE, R. M., & FLAVIN, D. K. (1992). The definition of alcoholism. *Journal of the American Medical Association, 268,* 1012–1014.

MORTENSEN, M. E., & RENNEBOHM, R. M. (1989). Clinical pharmacology and use of nonsteroidal anti-inflammatory drugs. *Pediatric Clinics of North America, 36,* 1113–1139.

MORTON, H. G. (1987). Occurrence and treatment of solvent abuse in children and adolescents. *Pharmacological Therapy, 33,* 449–469.

MORTON, W. A., & SANTOS, A. (1989). New indications for benzodiazepines in the treatment of major psychiatric disorders. *Hospital Formulary, 24,* 274–278.

MOTT, S. H., PACKER, R. J., & SOLDIN, S. J. (1994). Neurologic manifestations of cocaine exposure in childhood. *Pediatrics, 93,* 557–560.

MOYER, T. P., & ELLEFSON, P. J. (1987). Marijuana testing—How good is it? *Mayo Clinic Procedures, 62,* 413–417.

MOYLAN, D. W. (1990). Court intervention. *Adolescent Counselor, 2* (5), 23–27.

MUESER, K. T., BELLACK, A. S. & BLANCHARD, J. J. (1992). Comorbidity of schizophrenia and substance abuse: Implications for treatment. *Journal of Counseling and Clinical Psychology, 60,* 845–856.

MUESER, K. T., YARNOLD, P. R., & BELLACK, A. S. (1992). Diagnostic and demographic correlates of substance abuse in schizophrenia and major affective disorder. *Acta Psychiatrica Scandinavica, 85,* 48–55.

MURPHY, D. F. (1993). NSAIDs and postoperative pain. *British Medical Journal, 306,* 1493.

MURPHY, G. E., WETZEL, R. D., ROBINS, E., & McEVOY, L. (1992). Multiple risk factors predict suicide in alcoholism. *Archives of General Psychiatry, 49,* 459–463.

MURPHY, S. M., OWEN, R., & TYRER, P. (1989). Comparative assessment of efficacy and withdrawal symptoms after 6 and 12 weeks' treatment with diazepam or buspirone. *British Journal of Psychiatry, 154,* 529–534.

MURRAY, R. M., CLIFFORD, C. A., & GURLING, H. M. D. (1983). Twin and adoption studies: How good is the evidence for a genetic role? In M. Galanter (Ed.), *Recent Developments in Alcoholism. Vol. 1.* New York: Plenum.

MUSTO, D. F. (1991). Opium, cocaine and marijuana in American history. *Scientific American, 265* (1), pp. 40–47.

MYERS, M. G., & BROWN, S. A. (1994). Smoking and health in substance-abusing adolescents: A two year follow-up. *Pediatrics, 93,* 561–566.

NACE, E. P. (1987). *The treatment of alcoholism.* New York: Brunner/Mazel.

NACE, E. P., & ISBELL, P. G. (1991). Alcohol. In R. J. Frances & S. I. Miller (Eds.), *Clinical textbook of addictive disorders.* New York: Guilford.

NADELMANN, E. A. (1989). Drug prohibition in the United States: Costs, consequences, and alternatives. *Science, 245,* pp. 939–946.

NADELMANN, E. A., KLEIMAN, M. A. R., & EARLS, F. J. (1990). Should some illegal drugs be legalized? *Issues in Science and Technology, VI* (4), 43–49.

NADELMANN, E., & WENNER, J. S. (1994, May 5). Towards a sane national drug policy. *Rolling Stone,* pp. 24–26.

NAHAS, G. G. (1986). Cannabis: Toxicological properties and epidemiological aspects. *The Medical Journal of Australia, 145,* 82–87.

Narcotics Anonymous. (1982). Van Nuys, CA: Narcotics Anonymous World Service Office, Inc.

NATHAN, P. E. (1980). Etiology and process in the addictive behaviors. In W. R. Miller (Ed.), *The addictive behaviors.* New York: Pergamon.

NATHAN, P. E. (1988). The addictive personality *is* the behavior of the addict. *Journal of Consulting and Clinical Psychology, 56,* 183–188.

NATHAN, P. E. (1991). Substance use disorders in the DSM-IV. *Journal of Abnormal Psychology, 100,* 356–361.

National Academy of Sciences. (1990). *Treating drug problems. Vol. 1.* Washington, DC: National Academy Press.

National Commission on Marihuana and Drug Abuse. (1972). *Marihuana: A signal of misunderstanding.* Washington, DC: U.S. Government Printing Office.

National Commission on Marihuana and Drug Abuse. (1973). *Drug use in America: Problem in perspective.* Washington, DC: U.S. Government Printing Office.

National Foundation for Brain Research. (1992). *The Cost of Disorders of the Brain.* Washington, DC: Author.

National Institute on Alcohol Abuse and Alcoholism. (1989). Relapse and craving. *Alcohol Alert (#6).* Washington, DC: U.S. Dept. of Health and Human Services.

National Institute on Drug Abuse. (1991). *National household survey on drug abuse: Population estimates 1990.* Rockville, MD: U.S. Government Printing Office.

Nation's Health, The. (1990). Sex-for-drugs pushes U.S. syphilis rates up. *20* (1), p. 17.

NELIPOVICH, M., & BUSS, E. (1991). Investigating alcohol abuse among persons who are blind. *Journal of Visual Impairment & Blindness, 85,* 343–345.

NEWCOMB, M. D., & BENTLER, P. M. (1989). Substance use and abuse among children and teenagers. *American Psychologist, 44,* 242–248.

NEWELL, T., & COSGROVE, J. (1988). Recovery of neuropsychological functions during reduction of PCP use. Paper presented at the 1988 annual meeting of the American Psychological Association, Atlanta, GA.

NEWELL, T., & COSGROVE, J. (1994). Paper presented

at the 1994 annual meeting of the American Psychological Association, Los Angeles, CA.

NEWLAND, D. (1989). Alcohol and drug addiction—A disease or a crime? *Supervision, 50* (6), 16–19.

Newsweek. (1991). A new market for a lethal drug. *CXVII* (7), p. 58.

NEWTON, R. E., MARUNYCZ, J. D., ALDERDICE, M. C., & NAPOLIELLO, M. J. (1986). Review of the side effects of buspirone. *The American Journal of Medicine, 80* (Suppl. 3B).

NEY, J. A., DOOLEY, S. L., KEITH, L. G., CHASNOFF, I. J., & SOCOL, M. L. (1990). The prevalence of substance abuse in patients with suspected preterm labor. *American Journal of Obstetrics and Gynecology, 162,* 1562–1568.

NIAURA, R. S., ROHSENOW, D. J., BINKOFF, J. A., MONTI, P. M., PEDRAZA, M., & ABRAMS, D. B. (1988). Relevance of cue reactivity to understanding alcohol and smoking relapse. *Journal of Abnormal Psychology, 97* (2), 133–153.

NICASTRO, N. (1989). Visual disturbances associated with over-the-counter ibuprofen in three patients. *Annals of Ophthalmology, 21,* 447–450.

NOBLE, E. P., BLUM, K., RITCHIE, T., MONTGOMERY, A., & SHERIDAN, P. F. (1991). Allelic association of the D2 dopamine receptor gene with receptor-binding characteristics in alcoholism. *Archives of General Psychiatry, 48,* 648–654.

NORRIS, D. (1994). War's "wonder" drugs. *America's Civil War, 7* (2), 50–57.

NOVELLO, A. C., & SHOSKY, J. (1992). From the Surgeon General, U.S. Public Health Service. *Journal of the American Medical Association, 268,* 961.

O'BRIEN, P. E., & GABORIT, M. (1992). Codependency: A disorder separate from chemical dependency. *Journal of Clinical Psychology, 48* (1), 129–136.

OCHS, L. (1992). EEG treatment of addictions. *Biofeedback, 20* (1), 8–16.

O'CONNOR, P. G., CHANG, G., & SHI, J. (1992). Medical complications of cocaine use. In T. R. Kosten & H. D. Kleber (Eds.), *Clinician's guide to cocaine addiction.* New York: Guilford.

O'DONNELL, M. (1986). The executive ailment: "Curable only by death." *International Management, 41* (7), 64.

O'DONOVAN, M. C., & McGUFFIN, P. (1993). Short-acting benzodiazepines. *British Medical Journal, 306,* 182–183.

OETTING, E. R., & BEAUVAIS, F. (1990). Adolescent drug use: Findings of national and local surveys. *Journal of Consulting and Clinical Psychology, 58,* 385–394.

OGBORNE, A. C. (1993). Assessing the effectiveness of Alcoholics Anonymous in the community: Meeting the challenges. In B. S. McCrady & W. R. Miller (Eds.), *Research on Alcoholics Anonymous.* New Brunswick, NJ: Rutgers Center of Alcohol Studies.

OGBORNE, A. C., & GLASER, F. B. (1985). Evaluating Alcoholics Anonymous. In T. E. Bratter & G. G. Forrest (Eds.), *Alcoholism and substance abuse: Strategies for clinical intervention.* New York: Free Press.

OLDS, D. L., HENDERSON, C. R., & TATELBAUM, R. (1994). Intellectual impairment in children of women who smoke cigarettes during pregnancy. *Pediatrics, 93,* 221–227.

OLIWENSTEIN, L. (1988). The perils of pot. *Discover, 9* (6), p. 18.

OLIWENSTEIN, L. (1990). The Kaposi's connection. *Discover, 11* (8), p. 28.

OLSON, J. (1992). *Clinical pharmacology made ridiculously simple.* Miami, FL: MedMaster, Inc.

O'MALLEY, S., ADAMSE, M., HEATON, R. K., & GAWIN, F. G. (1992). Neuropsychological impairment in chronic cocaine abusers. *American Journal of Drug and Alcohol Abuse, 18* (2), 131–144.

OSHER, F. C., DRAKE, R. E., NOORDSY, D. L., TEAGUE, G. B., HURLBUT, S. C., BIESANZ, J. C., & BEAUDETT, M. S. (1994). Correlates and outcomes of alcohol use disorder among rural outpatients with schizophrenia. *Journal of Clinical Psychiatry, 55,* 109–113.

OSHER, F. C., & KOFOED, L. L. (1989). Treating patients with psychiatric and psychoactive substance abuse disorders. *Hospital and Community Psychiatry, 40,* 1025–1030.

OTTO, R. K., LANG, A. R., MEGARGEE, E. I., & ROSENBLATT, A. I. (1989). Ability of alcoholics to escape detection by the MMPI. *Critical Items, 4* (2), 2, 7–8.

OWINGS-WEST, M., & PRINZ, R. J. (1987). Parental alcoholism and child psychopathology. *Psychological Bulletin, 102* (2), 204–281.

PACKE, G. E., GARTON, M. J., & JENNINGS, K. (1990). Acute myocardial infarction caused by intravenous amphetamine abuse. *British Heart Journal, 64,* 23–24.

PAPE, P. A. (1988). EAPs and chemically dependent women. *Alcoholism & Addiction, 8* (6), 43–44.

PAPPAS, N. (1990). Dangerous liaisons: When food and drugs don't mix. *In Health, 4* (4), 22–24.

PARKER, G. B., BARRETT, E. A., & HICKIE, I. B. (1992). From nurture to network: Examining links between perceptions of parenting received in childhood and social bonds in adulthood. *American Journal of Psychiatry, 149,* 877–885.

PARKER, R. N. (1993). The effects of context on alcohol and violence. *Alcohol Health & Research World, 17* (2), 117–122.

PARRAS, F., PATIER, J. L., & EZPELETA, C. (1988). Lead contaminated heroin as a source of inorganic lead intoxication. *The Staff, 316,* 755.

PARRY, A. (1992). Taking heroin maintenance seriously: The politics of tolerance. *The Lancet, 339,* 350–351.

PARSIAN, A., & CLONINGER, C. R. (1991). Genetics of high-risk populations. *Addiction & Recovery, 11* (6), 9–11.

PARSIAN, A., TODD, R. D., DEVOR, E. J., O'MALLEY, K. L., SUAREZ, B. K., REICH, T., & CLONINGER, C. R. (1991). Alcoholism and alleles of the human D_2 dopamine receptor locus: Studies of association and linkage. *Archives of General Psychiatry, 48,* 655–663.

PARSONS, O. A., & NIXON, S. J. (1993). Neurobehavioral sequelae of alcoholism. *Behavioral Neurology, 11,* 205–218.

PATLAK, M. (1989). The fickle virus. *Discover, 10* (2), pp. 24–25.

PATRONO, C. (1994). Aspirin as an antiplatelet drug. *New England Journal of Medicine, 330,* 1287–1294.

PAUL, J. P., STALL, R., & BLOOMFIELD, K. A. (1991). Gay and alcoholic. *Alcoholic Health & Research World, 15,* 151–160.

PAULOS, J. A. (1994). Counting on dyscalculia. *Discover, 15* (3), pp. 30, 34–36.

PEARLSON, G. D., JEFFERY, P. J., HARRIS, G. J., ROSS, C. A., FISCHMAN, M. W., & CAMARGO, E. E. (1993). Correlation of acute cocaine-induced changes in local cerebral blood flow with subjective effects. *American Journal of Psychiatry, 150,* 495–497.

PEARSON, M. A., HOYME, E., SEAVER, L. H., & RIMSZA, M. E. (1994). Toluene embryopathy: Delineation of the phenotype and comparison with fetal alcohol syndrome. *Pediatrics, 93,* 211–215.

PECK, M. S. (1978). *The road less traveled.* New York: Simon & Schuster.

PECK, M. S. (1993). *Further along the road less traveled.* New York: Simon & Schuster.

Pediatrics for Parents. (1990). Marijuana and breast-feeding. *11* (10), 1.

PEELE, S. (1984). The cultural context of psychological approaches to alcoholism. *American Psychologist, 39,* 1337–1351.

PEELE, S. (1985). *The Meaning of Addiction.* Lexington, MA: D. C. Heath.

PEELE, S. (1988). On the diseasing of America. *Utne Reader, 30,* 67.

PEELE, S. (1989). *Diseasing of America.* Lexington, MA: D. C. Heath.

PEELE, S. (1991). What we now know about treating alcoholism and other addictions. *The Harvard Medical School Mental Health Letter, 8* (6), 5–7.

PEELE, S., BRODSKY, A., & ARNOLD, M. (1991). *The truth about addiction and recovery.* New York: Simon & Schuster.

PEGUES, D. A., HUGHES, B. J., & WOERNIE, C. H. (1993). Elevated blood lead levels associated with illegally distilled alcohol. *Archives of Internal Medicine, 153,* 1501–1504.

PELUSO, E., & PELUSO, L. S. (1988). *Women & Drugs.* Minneapolis: CompCare Publishers.

PELUSO, E., & PELUSO, L. S. (1989). Alcohol and the elderly. *Professional Counselor, 4* (2), 44–46.

PENICK, E. C., NICKEL, E. J., CANTRELL, P. F., POWELL, B. J., READ, M. R., & THOMAS, M. M. (1990). The emerging concept of dual diagnosis: An overview and implications. In D. F. O'Connell (Ed.), *Managing the dually diagnosed patient.* New York: Haworth.

PENISTON, E. G., & KULKOSKY, P. J. (1990). Alcoholic personality and alpha-theta brainwave training. *Medical Psychotherapy, 3,* 37–55.

PENNEY, A. (1993). *How to make love to a man (safely).* New York: Crown Publishers.

PENTZ, M. A., DWYER, J. H., MACKINNON, D. P., FLAY, B. R., HANDEN, W. B., WANG, E. Y. I., & JOHNSON, A. (1989). A multicommunity trial for primary prevention of adolescent drug abuse. *Journal of the American Medical Association, 261* (2), 3259–3266.

PEROUTKA, S. J. (1989). "Ecstasy": A human neurotoxin? *Archives of General Psychiatry, 46,* 191.

PERRY, J. C., & COOPER, S. H. (1989). An empirical study of defense mechanisms. *Archives of General Psychiatry, 46,* 444–452.

PETERS, H., & THEORELL, C. J. (1991). Fetal and neonatal effects of maternal cocaine use. *Journal of Obstetric, Gynecologic, and Neonatal Nursing, 20* (2), 121–126.

PETO, R., LOPEZ, A. D., BOREHAM, J., THUN, M., & HEATH, C. (1992). Mortality from tobacco in developed countries: Indirect estimation from national vital statistics. *The Lancet, 339,* 1268–1278.

PETTINE, K. A. (1991). Association of anabolic steroids and avascular necrosis of femoral heads. *The American Journal of Sports Medicine, 19* (1), 96–98.

PEYSER, H. S. (l989). Alcohol and drug abuse: Underrecognized and untreated. *Hospital and Community Psychiatry, 40* (3), 221.

PICKENS, R. W., SVIKIS, D. S., MCGUE, M., LYKKEN, D. T., HESTON, L. L., & CLAYTON, P. J. (1991). Heterogeneity in the inheritance of alcoholism: A study of male and female twins. *Archives of General Psychiatry, 48,* 19–28.

PIERCE, J. P., GILPIN, E., BURNS, D. M., WHALEN, E., ROSBROOK, B., SHOPLAND, D., & JOHNSON, M. (1991). Does tobacco advertising target young people to start smoking? *Journal of the American Medical Association, 266,* 3154–3158.

PIHL, R. O., & PETERSON, J. B. (1993). Alcohol, serotonin, and aggression. *Alcohol Health & Research World, 17,* 113–116.

PINKNEY, D. S. (1990). Substance abusers seen shifting to "kitchen lab" drugs. *American Medical News, 33* (16), 5–7.

PLASKY, P., MARCUS, L., & SALZMAN, C. (1988). Effects

of psychotropic drugs on memory: Part 2. *Hospital & Community Psychiatry, 39,* 501–502.

Playboy. (1990). Raw data. *37* (1), 16.

Playboy. (1991). Forum. *38* (1), 52.

Playboy. (1992). Raw data. *39* (8), 14.

Playboy. (1993). Raw data. *40* (12), 22.

PLESSINGER, M. A., & WOODS, J. R. (1993). Maternal, placental, and fetal pathophysiology of cocaine exposure during pregnancy. *Clinical Obstetrics and Gynecology, 36,* 267–278.

POLEN, M. R., SIDNEY, S., TEKAWA, I. S., SADLER, M., & FRIEDMAN, G. D. (1993). Health care use by frequent marijuana smokers who do not smoke tobacco. *Western Journal of Medicine, 158,* 596–601.

POMERLEAU, O. D., COLLINS, A. C., SHIFFMAN, S., & POMERLEAU, C. S. (1993). Why some people smoke and others do not: New perspectives. *Journal of Clinical and Consulting Psychology, 61,* 723–731.

POPE, H. G., & KATZ, D. L. (1987). Bodybuilder's psychosis. *The Lancet, 334,* 863.

POPE, H. G., & KATZ, D. L. (1988). Affective and psychotic symptoms associated with anabolic steroid use. *American Journal of Psychiatry, 145,* 487–490.

POPE, H. G., & KATZ, D. L. (1990). Homicide and near-homicide by anabolic steroid users. *Journal of Clinical Psychiatry, 51* (1), 28–31.

POPE, H. G., & KATZ, D. L. (1991). What are the psychiatric risks of anabolic steroids? *The Harvard Medical School Mental Health Letter, 7* (10), 8.

POPE, H. G., & KATZ, D. L. (1994). Psychiatric and medical effects of anabolic-androgenic steroid use. *Archives of General Psychiatry, 51,* 375–382.

POPE, H. G., KATZ, D. L., & CHAMPOUX, R. (1986). Anabolic-androgenic steroid use among 1,010 college men. *The Physician and Sports Medicine, 17* (7), 75–81.

POPE, K. S., & MORIN, S. F. (1990). AIDS and HIV infection update: New research, ethical responsibilities, evolving legal frameworks, and published sources. *The Independent Practitioner, 10* (4), 43–53.

PORTERFIELD, L. M. (1991). Steroid abuse. *Advancing Clinical Care, 6* (2), 44.

POST, R. M., WEISS, S. R. B., PERT, A., & UHDE, T. W. (1987). Chronic cocaine administration: Sensitization and kindling effects. In S. Fisher, A. Rashkin, & E. H. Unlenhuth (Eds.), *Cocaine: Clinical and behavioral aspects.* New York: Oxford University Press.

POTTER, W. Z., RUDORFER, M. V., & GOODWIN, F. K. (1987). Biological findings in bipolar disorders. In *American Psychiatric Association Annual Review. Vol. 6.* Washington, DC: American Psychiatric Association Press, Inc.

POTTERTON, R. (1992). A criminal system of justice. *Playboy, 39* (9), pp. 46–47.

POWELL, B. J., READ, M. R., PENICK, E. C., MILLER, N. S., & BINGHAM, S. F. (1987). Primary and secondary depression in alcoholic men: An important distinction. *Journal of Clinical Psychiatry, 48,* 98–101.

PRATT, C. T. (1990). Addiction treatment for health care professionals. *Addiction & Recovery, 10* (3), 17–19, 38–41.

PRICE, L. H., RICAURTE, G. A., KRYSTAL, J. H., & HENINGER, G. R. (1989). Neuroendocrine and mood responses to intravenous L-tryptophan in 3, 4–Methylenedioxymethamphetamine (MDMA) users. *Archives of General Psychiatry, 46,* 20–22.

PRICE, L. H., RICAURTE, G. A., KRYSTAL, J. H., & HENINGER, G. R. (1990). In reply. *Archives of General Psychiatry, 47,* 289.

PRISTACH, C. A., & SMITH, C. M. (1990). Medication compliance and substance abuse among schizophrenic patients. *Hospital and Community Psychiatry, 41,* 1345–1348.

PROCHASKA, J. O., DICLEMENTE, C. C., & NORCROSS, J. C. (1992). In search of how people change. *American Psychologist, 47,* 1102–1114.

PRUMMEL, M. F., & WIERSINGA, W. M. (1993). Smoking and the risk of Graves' disease. *Journal of the American Medical Association, 269,* 479–482.

Psychiatry Drug Alerts. (1989). Aspirin in the prevention of cardiovascular disease. *III* (8), 64.

Psychology Today. (1992). Pot shot. *25* (3), p. 8.

PUIG-ANTICH, J., GOETS, D., DAVIES, M., KAPLAN, T., DAVIES, S., OSTROW, L., ASNIS, L., TOWMEY, J., IYENGAR, S., & RYAN, N. D. (1989). A controlled family history of prepubertal major depressive disorder. *Archives of General Psychiatry, 46,* 406–418.

PURSCH, J. A. (1987). Mental illness and addiction. *Alcoholism & Addiction, 7* (6), 42.

PUTNAM, F. W. (1989). *Diagnosis and treatment of multiple personality disorder.* New York: Guilford.

RACINE, A., JOYCE, T., & ANDERSON, R. (1993). The association between prenatal care and birth weight among women exposed to cocaine in New York City. *Journal of the American Medical Association, 270,* 1581–1586.

RADETSKY, P. (1990). Closing in on an AIDS vaccine. *Discover, 11* (9), pp. 71–77.

RADO, T. (1988). The client with a dual diagnosis—A personal perspective. *The Alcohol Quarterly, 1* (1), 5–7.

RAINS, V. S. (1990). Alcoholism in the elderly—The hidden addiction. *Medical Aspects of Human Sexuality, 24* (10), 40–42, 43.

RALL, T. W. (1990). Hypnotics and sedatives. In A. G. Gilman, T. W. Rall, A. S. Nies, & P. Taylor (Eds.), *The Pharmacological Basis of Therapeutics* (8th ed.). New York: Pergamon.

RANDALL, T. (1992). Medical news and perspectives.

Journal of the American Medical Association, 268, 1505–1506.

RAPOPORT, R. J. (1993). The efficacy and safety of oxaproxin versus aspirin: Pooled results of double-blind trials in osteoarthritis. *Drug Therapy, 23* (Suppl.), 3–8.

RAPPORT, D. J., & COVINGTON, E. D. (1989). Motor phenomena in benzodiazepine withdrawal. *Hospital and Community Psychiatry, 40,* 1277–1280.

RASKIN, V. D. (1994). Psychiatric aspects of substance use disorders in childbearing populations. *Psychiatric Clinics of North America, 16,* 157–165.

RASYMAS, A. (1992). Basic pharmacology and pharmacokinetics. *Clinics in Pediatric Medicine and Surgery, 9,* 211–221.

RAVEL, R. (1989). *Clinical laboratory medicine: Clinical application of laboratory data* (5th ed.). Chicago: Year Book Medical Publishers, Inc.

RAY, O. S., & KSIR, C. (1993). *Drugs, society and human behavior* (6th ed.). St. Louis: C. V. Mosby.

REDMAN, G. L. (1990). Adolescents and anabolics. *American Fitness, 8* (3), 30–33.

REGIER, D. A., FARMER, M. E., RAE, D. S., LOCKE, B. Z., KIETH, S. J., JUDD, L. L., & GOODWIN, F. K. (1990). Comorbidity of mental disorders with alcohol and other drug abuse. *Journal of the American Medical Association, 264,* 2511–2518.

REISER, M. F. (1984). *Mind, brain, body.* New York: Basic Books.

RENAUD, S., & DELORGERIL, M. (1992). Wine, alcohol, and the French paradox for coronary heart disease. *The Lancet, 339,* 1523–1526.

RESTAK, R. (1984). *The brain.* New York: Bantam Books.

RESTAK, R. (1991). *The brain has a mind of its own.* New York: Harmony Books.

RESTAK, R. (1993). Brain by design. *The Sciences, 33* (5), 27–33.

RESTAK, R. (1994). *Receptors.* New York: Bantam Books.

REULER, J. B., GIRARD, D. E., & COONEY, T. G. (1985). Wernicke's encephalopathy. *New England Journal of Medicine, 316,* 1035–1039.

REVKIN, A. C. (1989). Crack in the cradle. *Discover, 10* (9), pp. 63–69.

RHODES, J. E., & JASON, L. A. (1990). A social stress model of substance abuse. *Journal of Consulting and Clinical Psychology, 58,* 395–401.

RICE, D. P. (1993). The economic cost of alcohol abuse and alcohol dependence: 1990. *Alcohol Health & Research World, 17* (1), 10–11.

RICKELS, L. K., GIESECKE, M. A., & GELLER, A. (1987). Differential effects of the anxiolytic drugs, diazepam and buspirone on memory function. *British Journal of Clinical Pharmacology, 23,* 207–211.

RICKELS, K., SCHWEIZER, E., CASE, W. G., &

GREENBLATT, D. J. (1990). Long-term therapeutic use of benzodiazepines: I. Effects of abrupt discontinuation. *Archives of General Psychiatry, 47,* 899–907.

RICKELS, K., SCHWEIZER, E., CSANALOSI, I., CASE, W. G., & CHUNG, H. (1988). Long-term treatment of anxiety and risk of withdrawal. *Archives of General Psychiatry, 45,* 444–450.

RICKELS, K., SCHWEIZER, E., & LUCKI, I. (1987). Benzodiazepine side effects. In R. E. Hales & A. J. Frances (Eds.), *American Psychiatric Association Annual Review. Vol. 6.* Washington, DC: American Psychiatric Association Press, Inc.

RIES, R. K., & ELLINGSON, T. (1990). A pilot assessment at one month of 17 dual diagnosis patients. *Hospital and Community Psychiatry, 41,* 1230–1233.

RILEY, J. A. (1994). Dual diagnosis. *Nursing Clinics of North America, 29,* 29–34.

ROBBINS, A. S., MANSON, J. E., LEE, I., SATTERFIELD, S., & HENNEKENS, C. H. (1994). Cigarette smoking and stroke in a cohort of U.S. male physicians. *Annals of Internal Medicine, 120,* 458–462.

ROBERTS, J. R., & TAFURE, J. A. (1990). Benzodiazepines. In L. Haddad & J. F. Winchester (Eds.), *Clinical management of poisoning and drug overdose* (2nd ed.). Philadelphia: W. B. Saunders.

ROBERTS, M. (1986). MDMA: "Madness, not ecstasy." *Psychology Today, 20,* pp. 14–16.

ROBERTS, S. V., & WATSON, T. (1994). Teens on tobacco. *U.S. News & World Report, 116* (15), pp. 38, 43.

ROBERTSON, J. R., & RONALD, P. J. M. (1992). Prescribing benzodiazepines to drug misusers. *The Lancet, 339,* 1169–1170.

RODGERS, J. E. (1994). Addiction—A whole new view. *Psychology Today, 27* (5), pp. 32–38, 72, 74, 76, 79.

RODMAN, M. J. (1993). OCT interactions. *RN, 56* (1), 54–60.

RODRIGUES, C. (1990). Drug market runs on a cycle of poverty and greed. *Minneapolis Star-Tribune, IX* (155), p. 21A.

ROEHLING, P., KOELBEL, N., & RUTGERS, C. (1994). Codependence—pathologizing femininity? Paper presented at the 1994 annual meeting of the American Psychological Association, Los Angeles, CA.

ROFFMAN, R. A., & GEORGE, W. H. (1988). Cannabis abuse. In D. M. Donovan & G. A. Marlatt (Eds.), *Assessment of addictive behaviors.* New York: Guilford.

ROGERS, C. R. (1961). *On becoming a person.* Boston: Houghton-Mifflin.

ROGERS, P. D., HARRIS, J., & JARMUSKEWICZ, J. (1987). Alcohol and adolescence. *The Pediatric Clinics of North America, 34* (2), 289–303.

ROHSENOW, D. J., & BACHOROWSKI, J. (1984). Effects of alcohol and expectancies on verbal aggression in men and women. *Journal of Abnormal Psychology, 93,* 418–432.

ROINE, R., GENTRY, T., HERNANDEZ-MUNOZ, R., BARAONA, E., & LIEBER, C. S. (1990). Aspirin increases blood alcohol concentrations in humans after ingestion of alcohol. *Journal of the American Medical Association, 264,* 2406–2408.

ROLD, J. F. (1993). Mushroom madness. *Postgraduate Medicine, 78* (5), 217–218.

ROME, H. P. (1984). Psychobotanica revisited. *Psychiatric Annals, 14,* 711–712.

ROOTS, L. E., & AANES, D. L. (1992). A conceptual framework for understanding self-help groups. *Hospital and Community Psychiatry, 43,* 379–381.

ROSE, K. J. (1988). *The body in time.* New York: Wiley.

ROSEN, M. I., & KOSTEN, T. R. (1991). Buprenorphine: Beyond methadone? *Hospital and Community Psychiatry, 42,* 347–349.

ROSENBAUM, J. F. (1990). Switching patients from alprazolam to clonazepam. *Hospital and Community Psychiatry, 41,* 1302.

ROSENBAUM, J. F., & GELENBERG, A. J. (1991). Anxiety. In A. J. Gelenberg, E. L. Bassuk, & S. C. Schoonover (Eds.), *The practitioner's guide to psychoactive drugs* (3rd ed.). New York: Plenum.

ROSENBERG, N. (1989). Nervous systems effects of toluene and other organic solvents. *The Western Journal of Medicine, 150,* 571–573.

ROSENBLUM, M. (1992). Ibuprofen provides longer lasting analgesia than fentanyl after laparoscopic surgery. *Journal of the American Medical Association, 267,* 219.

ROSENTHAL, E. (1992). Bad fix. *Discover, 13* (2), pp. 82–84.

ROSS, A. (1991). Poland's dark harvest. *In Health, 5* (4), 66–70.

ROSSE, R. B., COLLINS, J. P., FAY-McCARTHY, M., ALIM, T. N., WYATT, R. J., & DEUTSCH, S. I. (1994). Phenomenologic comparison of the idiopathic psychosis of schizophrenia and drug-induced cocaine and phencyclidine psychosis: A retrospective study. *Clinical Neuropharmacology, 17,* 359–369.

ROTHENBERG, L. (1988). The ethics of intervention. *Alcoholism & Addiction, 9* (1), 22–24.

ROTHWELL, P. M., & GRANT, R. (1993). Cerebral venous sinus thrombosis induced by "Ecstasy." *Journal of Neurology, Neurosurgery and Psychiatry, 56,* 1035.

ROUNSAVILLE, B. J., ANTON, S. F., CARROLL, K., BUDDE, D., PRUSOFF, B. A., & GAWIN, F. (1991). Psychiatric diagnoses of treatment-seeking cocaine abusers. *Archives of General Psychiatry, 48,* 43–51.

ROY, A. (1993). Risk factors for suicide among adult alcoholics. *Alcohol Health & Research World, 17,* 133–136.

ROYKO, M. (1990). Drug war's over: Guess who won. *Playboy, 37* (1), p. 46.

RUBIN, E., & DORIA, J. (1990). Alcoholic cardiomyopathy. *Alcohol Health & Research World, 14* (4), 277–284.

RUBIN, R. H. (1993). Acquired immunodeficiency syndrome. In E. Rubenstein & D. D. Federman (Eds.), *Scientific American Medicine.* New York: Scientific American Press, Inc.

RUBINO, F. A. (1992). Neurologic complications of alcoholism. *Psychiatric Clinics of North America, 15,* 359–372.

RUBINSTEIN, L., CAMPBELL, F., & DALEY, D. (1990). Four perspectives on dual diagnosis: Overview of treatment issues. In D. F. O'Connell (Ed.), *Managing the dually diagnosed patient.* New York: Haworth.

RUBY, M. (1993). Should drugs be legalized? *U.S. News & World Report, 115* (24), p. 80.

RUSSELL, J. M., NEWMAN, S. C., & BLAND, R. C. (1994). Drug abuse and dependence. *Acta Psychiatrica Scandinavica* (Suppl. 376), 54–62.

RUSTIN, T. (1988). Treating nicotine addiction. *Alcoholism & Addiction, 9* (2), 18–19.

RUSTIN, T. (1992, August). Review of nicotine dependence and its treatment. *Consultation to La Crosse addiction treatment programs: Lutheran Hospital and St. Francis Hospital.* Symposium conducted for staff, Lutheran Hospital, La Crosse, WI.

RYDON, P., REDMAN, S., SANSON-FISHER, R. W., & REID, A. L. A. (1992). Detection of alcohol-related problems in general practice. *Journal of Studies on Alcohol, 53* (3), 197–202.

SABBAG, R. (1994, May 5). The cartels would like a second chance. *Rolling Stone,* pp. 35–37, 43.

SACKS, O. (1970). *The man who mistook his wife for a hat.* New York: Harper & Row.

SAGAR, S. M. (1991). Toxic and metabolic disorders. In M. A. Samuels (Ed.), *Manual of Neurology.* Boston: Little, Brown.

SAGAR, S. M., & McGUIRE, D. (1991). Infectious diseases. In M. A. Samuels (Ed.), *Manual of Neurology.* Boston: Little, Brown.

SAITZ, R., MAYO-SMITH, M. F., ROBERTS, M. S., REDMOND, H. A., BERNARD, D. R., & CALKINS, D. R. (1994). Individualized treatment for alcohol withdrawal. *Journal of the American Medical Association, 272,* 519–523.

SALLOWAY, S., SOUTHWICK, S., & SADOWSKY, M. (1990). Opiate withdrawal presenting as posttraumatic stress disorder. *Hospital & Community Psychiatry, 41,* 666–667.

SALZMAN, C. (1990). What are the uses and dangers of the controversial drug Halcion? *The Harvard Medical School Mental Health Letter, 6* (9), 8.

SANDERS, S. R. (1990). Under the influence. *The Family Therapy Networker, 14* (1), 32–37.

SANDS, B. F., KNAPP, C. M., & CIRAULO, D. A. (1993). Medical consequences of alcohol–drug interactions. *Alcohol Health & Research World, 17*, 316–320.

SATEL, S. L. (1992). "Craving for and fear of cocaine": A phenomenologic update on cocaine craving and paranoia. In T. R. Kosten & H. D. Kleber (Eds.), *Clinician's guide to cocaine addiction*. New York: Guilford.

SATEL, S. L., & EDELL, W. S. (1991). Cocaine-induced paranoia and psychosis proneness. *American Journal of Psychiatry, 148*, 1708–1711.

SATEL, S. L., KOSTEN, T. R., SCHUCKIT, M. A., & FISCHMAN, M. W. (1993). Should protracted withdrawal from drugs be included in DSM-IV? *American Journal of Psychiatry, 150*, 695–704.

SATEL, S. L., PRICE, L. H., PALUMBO, J. M., MCDOUGLE, C. J., KRYSTAL, J. H., GAWIN, F., CHARNEY, D. S., HENINGER, G. R., & KLEBER, H. D. (1991). Clinical phenomenology and neurobiology of cocaine abstinence: A prospective inpatient study. *American Journal of Psychiatry, 148*, 1712–1716.

SAVAGE, S. R. (1993). Opium: The gift and its shadow. *Addiction & Recovery, 13* (1), 38–39.

SBRIGLIO, R., & MILLMAN, R. B. (1987). Emergency treatment of acute cocaine reactions. In A. M. Washton & M. S. Gold (Eds.), *Cocaine: A clinician's handbook*. New York: Guilford.

SCARF, M. (1980). *Unfinished business*. New York: Ballantine.

SCAROS, L. P., WESTRA, S., & BARONE, J. A. (1990). Illegal use of drugs: A current review. *U. S. Pharmacist, 15* (5), 17–39.

SCHAFER, J., & BROWN, S. A. (1991). Marijuana and cocaine effect expectancies and drug use patterns. *Journal of Consulting and Clinical Psychology, 59*, 558–565.

SCHAUBEN, J. L. (1990). Adulterants and substitutes. *Emergency Medicine Clinics of North America, 8*, 595–611.

SCHEER, R. (1990). Drugs: Another wrong war. *Playboy, 37* (1), pp. 51–52.

SCHEER, R. (1994a). The drug war's a bust. *Playboy, 41* (2), p. 49.

SCHEER, R. (1994b). Fighting the wrong war. *Playboy, 41* (10), p. 49.

SCHENKER, S., & SPEEG, K. V. (1990). The risk of alcohol intake in men and women. *The New England Journal of Medicine, 322*, 127–129.

SCHLOSSER, E. (1994). Marijuana and the law. *The Atlantic Monthly, 274* (3), pp. 84–86, 89–90, 92–94.

SCHNEIDERMAN, H. (1990). What's your diagnosis? *Consultant, 30* (7), 61–65.

SCHROF, J. M. (1992). Pumped up. *U.S. News & World Report, 112* (21), pp. 54–63.

SCHUCKIT, M. A. (1986). Primary men alcoholics with histories of suicide attempts. *Journal of Studies on Alcohol, 47*, 78–81.

SCHUCKIT, M. A. (1987). Biological vulnerability to alcoholism. *Journal of Consulting and Clinical Psychology, 55*, 301–309.

SCHUCKIT, M. A. (1989). *Drug and alcohol abuse: A clinical guide to diagnosis and treatment* (3rd ed.). New York: Plenum.

SCHUCKIT, M. A. (1994). Low level of response to alcohol as a predictor of future alcoholism. *American Journal of Psychiatry, 151*, 184–189.

SCHUCKIT, M. A., KLEIN, J., TWITCHELL, G., & SMITH, T. (1994). Personality test scores as predictors of alcoholism almost a decade later. *American Journal of Psychiatry, 151*, 1038–1042.

SCHUCKIT, M. A., SMITH, T. L., ANTHENELLI, R., & IRWIN, M. (1993). Clinical course of alcoholism in 636 male inpatients. *American Journal of Psychiatry, 150*, 786–792.

SCHUCKIT, M. A., ZISOOK, S., & MORTOLA, J. (1985). Clinical implications of DSM-III diagnoses of alcohol abuse and alcohol dependence. *American Journal of Psychiatry, 142*, 1403–1408.

SCHUSTER, C. R. (1990). The National Institute on Drug Abuse in the decade of the brain. *Neuropsychopharmacology, 3*, 315–318.

SCHWARTZ, R. H. (1987). Marijuana: An overview. *The Pediatric Clinics of North America, 34* (2), 305–317.

SCHWARTZ, R. H. (1988). Urine testing in the detection of drugs of abuse. *Archives of Internal Medicine, 148*, 2407–2412.

SCHWARTZ, R. H. (1989). When to suspect inhalant abuse. *Patient Care, 23* (10), 39–50.

SCHWARTZ, R. H. (1994). Letter to the editor. *New England Journal of Medicine, 331*, 126–127.

SCHWEIZER, E., & RICKELS, K. (1994). New and emerging clinical uses of buspirone. *Journal of Clinical Psychiatry, 55* (Suppl. 5), 46–54.

SCHWEIZER, E., RICKELS, K., CASE, W. G., & GREENBLATT, D. J. (1990). Long term therapeutic use of benzodiazepines: II. Effects of gradual taper. *Archives of General Psychiatry, 47*, 908–916.

SCHWERTZ, D. W. (1991). Basic principles of pharmacologic action. *Nursing Clinics of North America, 26*, 245–262.

Science Digest. (1989). Nightcap dangers. 2 (5), p. 90.

SCOTT, M. J., & SCOTT, M. J. (1989). HIV infection associated with injections of anabolic steroids. *Journal of the American Medical Association, 262* (2), 207–208.

SEGAL, R., & SISSON, B. V. (1985). Medical complications associated with alcohol use and the assessment of risk of physical damage. In T. E. Bratter & G. G. Forrest (Eds.), *Alcoholism and substance abuse: Strategies for clinical intervention*. New York: Free Press.

SEIDMAN, S. N., & RIEDER, R. O. (1994). A review of sexual behavior in the United States. *American Journal of Psychiatry, 151,* 330–341.

SEILHAMER, R. A., JACOB, T., & DUNN, N. J. (1993). The impact of alcohol consumption on parent–child relationships in families of alcoholics. *Journal of Studies on Alcohol, 54* (2), 189–198.

SELLERS, E. M., CIRAULO, D. A., DUPONT, R. L., GRIFFITHS, R. R., KOSTEN, T. R., ROMACH, M. K., & WOODY, G. E. (1993). Alprazolam and benzodiazepine dependence. *Journal of Clinical Psychiatry, 54* (Suppl. 10), 64–74.

SELWYN, P. A. (1993). Illicit drug use revisited: What a long, strange trip it's been. *Annals of Internal Medicine, 119,* 1044–1046.

SELZER, M. (1971). The Michigan Alcoholism Screening Test: The quest for a new diagnostic instrument. *American Journal of Psychiatry, 127,* 1653–1658.

SERFATY, M., & MASTERTON, G. (1993). Fatal poisonings attributed to benzodiazepines in Britain during the 1980s. *British Journal of Psychiatry, 163,* 386–393.

SEXSON, W. R. (1994). Cocaine: A neonatal perspective. *International Journal of the Addictions, 28,* 585–598.

SHADER, R. I. (1994). A perspective on contemporary psychiatry. In *Manual of psychiatric therapeutics* (2nd ed.). Boston: Little, Brown.

SHADER, R. I., & GREENBLATT, D. J. (1993). Use of benzodiazepines in anxiety disorders. *The New England Journal of Medicine, 328,* 1398–1405.

SHADER, R. I., GREENBLATT, D. J., & CIRAULO, D. A. (1994). Treatment of physical dependence on barbiturates, benzodiazepines, and other sedative-hypnotics. In *Manual of psychiatric therapeutics* (2nd ed.). Boston: Little, Brown.

SHAFER, J. (1985). Designer drugs. *Science '85, 12* (3), pp. 60–67.

SHANER, A., KHALSA, E., ROBERTS, L., WILKINS, J., ANGLIN, D., & HSIECH, S. C. (1993). Unrecognized cocaine use among schizophrenic patients. *American Journal of Psychiatry, 150,* 758–762.

SHANNON, M. T., WILSON, B. A., & STANG, C. L. (1992). *Drugs and nursing implications* (7th ed.). Norwalk, CT: Appleton & Lange.

SHAPIRO, D. (1981). *Autonomy and rigid character.* New York: Basic Books.

SHARP, C. W., & BREHM, M. L. (1977). Review of inhalants: Euphoria to dysfunction. *NIDA Research Monograph, 15.* Washington, DC: U.S. Government Printing Office.

SHEDLER, J., & BLOCK, J. (1990). Adolescent drug use and psychological health. *American Psychologist, 45,* 612–630.

SHENKMAN, R. (1991). *I love Paul Revere, whether he rode or not.* New York: Harper Collins.

SHEPHERD, S. M., & JAGODA, A. S. (1990). PCP. In L. D. Haddad & J. F. Winchester (Eds.), *Clinical management of poisoning and drug overdose* (2nd ed.). Philadelphia: W. B. Saunders.

SHER, K. J. (1991). *Children of alcoholics.* Chicago: University of Chicago Press.

SHER, K. J., WALITZER, K. S., WOOD, P. K., & BRENT, E. E. (1991). Characteristics of children of alcoholics: Putative risk factors, substance use and abuse, and psychopathology. *Journal of Abnormal Psychology, 100,* 427–448.

SHERIDAN, E., PATTERSON, H. R., & GUSTAFSON, E. A. (1982). *Falconer's The drug, the nurse, the patient* (7th ed.). Philadelphia: W. B. Saunders.

SHERMAN, C. (1994). Kicking butts. *Psychology Today, 27* (5), pp. 40–45.

SHERMAN, C. B. (1991). Health effects of cigarette smoking. *Clinics in Chest Medicine, 12,* 643–658.

SHERMAN, D. I. N., WARD, R. J., WARREN-PERRY, M., WILLIAMS, R., & PETERS, T. J. (1993). Association of restriction fragment length polymorphism in alcohol dehydrogenase 2 gene with alcohol induced liver damage. *British Medical Journal, 307,* 1388–1390.

SHIELDS, R. O. (1990). Amphetamines. In L. M. Haddad & J. F. Winchester (Eds.), *Clinical management of poisoning and drug overdose* (2nd ed.). Philadelphia: W. B. Saunders.

SHIFFMAN, L. B., FISCHER, L. B., ZETTLER-SEGAL, M., & BENOWITZ, N. L. (1990). Nicotine exposure among nondependent smokers. *Archives of General Psychiatry, 47,* 333–340.

SHIFFMAN, S. (1992). Relapse process and relapse prevention in addictive behaviors. *The Behavior Therapist, 15* (1), 99–110.

SHINTON, R., SAGAR, G., & BEEVERS, G. (1993). The relation of alcohol consumption to cardiovascular risk factors and stroke. The West Birmingham stroke project. *Journal of Neurology, Neurosurgery and Psychiatry, 56,* 458–462.

SICHERMAN, A. (1992). Two fingers of Tagamet. *Minneapolis Star-Tribune, X* (342), p. 1T.

SIEGEL, B. S. (1986). *Love, medicine & miracles.* New York: Harper & Row.

SIEGEL, B. S. (1989). *Peace, love & healing.* New York: Harper & Row.

SIEGEL, L. (1989). Want to take the risks? It should be your choice. *Playboy, 36* (1), p. 59.

SIEGEL, R. K. (1982). Cocaine smoking disorders: Diagnosis and treatment. *Psychiatric Annals, 14,* 728–732.

SIEGEL, R. K. (1991). Crystal meth or speed or crank. *Lear's, 3* (1), pp. 72–73.

SIEGEL, R. L. (1986). Jungle revelers: When beasts take drugs to race or relax, things get zooey. *Omni, 8* (6), pp. 70–74, 100.

SIERLES, F. S. (1984). Correlates of malingering. *Behavioral Sciences and the Law, 2* (1), 113–118.

SILAGY, C. A., McNEIL, J. J., DONNAN, G. A., TONKIN, A. M., WORSAM, B., & CAMPION, K. (1993). Adverse effects of low-dose aspirin in a healthy elderly population. *Clinical Pharmacology Therapeutics, 54,* 84–89.

SILVERMAN, M. M. (1989). Children of psychiatrically ill parents: A prevention perspective. *Hospital & Community Psychiatry, 40,* 1257–1265.

SILVERS, J. (1990). Wounded country. *Playboy, 37* (8), pp. 76–77, 80, 147–150.

SIMMONS, A. L. (1991). A peculiar dialect in the land of 10,000 treatment centers. *Minneapolis Star-Tribune, X* (24), p. 23A.

SIMON, E. J. (1992). Opiates: Neurobiology. In J. H. Lowinson, P. Ruiz, R. B. Millman, & J. G. Langrod (Eds.), *Substance abuse: A comprehensive textbook* (2nd ed.). New York: Williams & Wilkins.

SIMONS, A. M., PHILLIPS, D. H., & COLEMAN, D. V. (1993). Damage to DNA in cervical epithelium related to smoking tobacco. *British Medical Journal, 306,* 1444–1448.

SIMPSON, D. D., CRANDALL, R. L., SAVAGE, J., & PAVA-KRUEGER, E. (1981). Leisure of opiate addicts at posttreatment follow-up. *Journal of Counseling Psychology, 28,* 36–39.

SINGH, R. A., MATTOO, S. K., MALHOTRA, A., & VARMA, V. K. (1992). Cases of buprenorphine abuse in India. *Acta Psychiatrica Scandinavica, 86,* 46–48.

"60 Minutes." (1992). RX drugs. *XXV* (15).

"60 Minutes." (1993). The CIA's cocaine. *XXVI* (10).

"60 Minutes." (1994). Halcion. *XXVI* (42).

SKOG, O. J., & DUCKERT, F. (1993). The development of alcoholics' and heavy drinkers' consumption: A longitudinal study. *Journal of Studies on Alcohol, 54,* 178–188.

SKOLNICK, A. A. (1993). Injury prevention must be part of nation's plan to reduce health care costs, say control experts. *Journal of the American Medical Association, 270,* 19–21.

SLABY, A. E., LIEB, J., & TANCREDI, L. R. (1981). *Handbook of psychiatric emergencies* (2nd ed.). Garden City, NY: Medical Examination Publishing Co., Inc.

SLOVUT, G. (1992). Sports medicine. *Minneapolis Star-Tribune, X* (353), p. 20C.

SMITH, B. D., & SALZMAN, C. (1991). Do benzodiazepines cause depression? *Hospital and Community Psychiatry, 42,* 1101–1102.

SMITH, G. T. (1994). Psychological expectancy as mediator of vulnerability to alcoholism. In T. F. Babor, V. Hesselbrock, R. E. Meyer, & W. Shoemaker (Eds.), *Types of alcoholics.* New York: New York Academy of Sciences.

SMITH, R. (1990). Psychopathology and substance abuse: A psychoanalytic perspective. In D. F. O'Connell (Ed.), *Managing the dually diagnosed patient.* New York: Haworth.

SMITH, T. (1994). How dangerous is heroin? *British Medical Journal, 307,* 807.

Smithsonian. (1989). Letters to the editor. *20* (6), p. 18.

SMOLOWE, J. (1993). Choose your poison. *Time, 142* (4), pp. 56–57.

SNYDER, S. H. (1977). Opiate receptors and internal opiates. *Scientific American, 260* (3), pp. 44–56.

SNYDER, S. H. (1986). *Drugs and the brain.* New York: Scientific American Books, Inc.

SPARADEO, F. R., & GILL, D. (1989). Effects of prior alcohol use on head injury recovery. *Journal of Head Trauma Rehabilitation, 4* (1), 75–82.

SPOHR, H. L., WILLMS, J., & STEINHAUSEN, H. C. (1993). Prenatal alcohol exposure and long-term consequences. *The Lancet, 341,* 907–910.

SPRINGBORN, W. (1987). Step One: The foundation of recovery. In *The twelve steps of Alcoholics Anonymous.* New York: Harper & Row.

SQUIRES, S. (1989). Studies slight women's medical problems. *Minneapolis Star-Tribune, VIII* (257), p. 6Ex.

SQUIRES, S. (1990). Popular painkiller ibuprofen is linked to kidney damage. *Minneapolis Star-Tribune, VIII* (315), pp. 1E, 4E.

STEELE, T. E., & MORTON, W. A. (1986). Salicylate-induced delirium. *Psychosomatics, 27* (6), 455–456.

STEIN, J. A., NEWCOMB, M. D., & BENTLER, P. M. (1993). Differential effects of parent and grandparent drug use on behavior problems of male and female children. *Developmental Psychology, 29,* 31–43.

STEIN, S. M., & KOSTEN, T. R. (1992). Use of drug combinations in treatment of opioid withdrawal. *Journal of Clinical Psychopharmacology, 12* (3), 203–209.

STEINBERG, A. D. (1993). Should chloral hydrate be banned? *Pediatrics, 92,* 442–446.

STEINBERG, L. (1991). Adolescent transitions and alcohol and other drug use prevention. In *Preventing adolescent drug use: From theory to practice.* Rockville, MD: U.S. Dept. of Health and Human Services.

STEINBERG, N. (1994, May 5). The cartels would like a second chance. *Rolling Stone,* pp. 33–34.

STEINBERG, W., & TENNER, S. (1994). Acute pancreatitis. *New England Journal of Medicine, 330,* 1198–1210.

STERNBACH, G. L., & VARON, J. (1992). "Designer drugs." *Postgraduate Medicine, 91,* 169–176.

STEPHENS, R. S., ROFFMAN, R. A., & SIMPSON, E. E. (1994). Treating adult marijuana dependence: A test of the relapse prevention model. *Journal of Consulting and Clinical Psychology, 62,* 92–99.

STEVENS, V. J., & HOLLIS, J. F. (1989). Preventing smoking relapse, using an individually tailored skills-training technique. *Journal of Consulting and Clinical Psychology, 57,* 420–424.

STINCHFIELD, R. D., NIFOROPULOS, L., & FEDER, S. H. (1994). Follow-up contact bias in adolescent substance abuse treatment research. *Journal of Studies on Alcohol, 55* (3), 285–270.

STIX, G. (1994). Lollipop, lollipop. *Scientific American, 270* (5), p. 113.

STOCKWELL, T., & TOWN, C. (1989). Anxiety and stress management. In H. K. Hester & W. R. Miller (Eds.), *Handbook of alcoholism treatment approaches.* New York: Pergamon.

STOFFELMAYR, B. E., BENISHEK, L. A., HUMPHREYS, K., LEE, J. A., & MAVIS, B. E. (1989). Substance abuse prognosis with an additional psychiatric diagnosis: Understanding the relationship. *Journal of Psychoactive Drugs, 21* (2), 145–152.

STOLBERG, S. (1994). Aspirin isn't just for headaches. *Minneapolis Star-Tribune, XIII* (179), p. 4A.

STONE, J. (1991). Light elements. *Discover, 12* (1), pp. 12–16.

STRAIN, E. C., STRITZER, M. L., LIEBSON, I. A., & BIGELOW, G. E. (1994). Comparison of buprenorphine and methadone in the treatment of opioid dependence. *American Journal of Psychiatry, 151,* 1025–1030.

STRANG, J., GRIFFITHS, P., POWIS, B., & GOSSOP, M. (1992). First use of heroin: Changes in route of administration over time. *British Medical Journal, 304,* 1222–1223.

STRANG, J., JOHNS, A., & CAAN, W. (1993). Cocaine in the UK—1991. *British Journal of Psychiatry, 162,* 1–13.

STREISSGUTH, A. P., AASE, J. M., CLARREN, S. K., RANDELS, S. P., LADUE, R. A., & SMITH, D. F. (1991). Fetal alcohol syndrome in adolescents and adults. *Journal of the American Medical Association, 265,* 1961–1967.

STUART, R. B. (1980). *Helping couples change.* New York: Guilford.

SUPERNAW, R. B. (1991). Pharmacotherapeutic management of acute pain. *U.S. Pharmacist, 16* (2), H1–H14.

SUSSMAN, N. (1988). Diagnosis and drug treatment of anxiety in the elderly. *Geriatric Medicine Today, 7* (10), 1–8.

SUSSMAN, N. (1994). The uses of buspirone in psychiatry. *Journal of Clinical Psychiatry, 55* (5), (Suppl.), 3–19.

SUTER, P. M., SCHULTZ, Y., & JEQUIER, E. (1992). The effect of ethanol on fat storage in healthy subjects. *The New England Journal of Medicine, 326,* 983–987.

SUTHERLAND, G., STAPLETON, J. A., RUSSELL, M. A. H., JARVIS, M. J., HAJEK, P., BELCHER, M., & FEYERABEND, C. (1992). Randomised controlled trial of nasal nicotine spray in smoking cessation. *The Lancet, 340,* 324–329.

SVANUM, S., & MCADOO, W. G. (1989). Predicting rapid relapse following treatment for chemical dependence: A matched-subjects design. *Journal of Consulting and Clinical Psychology, 34,* 1027–1030.

SWADI, H. (1993). Alcohol abuse in adolescence: An update. *Archives of Disease in Childhood, 68,* 341–343.

SWAIM, R. C., OETTING, R. W., EDWARDS, R. W., & BEAUVAIS, F. (1989). Links from emotional distress to adolescent drug use: A path model. *Journal of Consulting and Clinical Psychology, 57,* 227–231.

SWIFT, R. M., WHELIHAN, W., KUZNETSOV, O., BUONGIORNO, G., & HSUING, H. (1994). Naltrexone-induced alterations in human ethanol intoxication. *American Journal of Psychiatry, 151,* 1463–1467.

SZASZ, T. S. (1972). Bad habits are not diseases: A refutation of the claim that alcoholism is a disease. *The Lancet, 319,* 83–84.

SZASZ, T. S. (1988). A plea for the cessation of the longest war of the twentieth century—The war on drugs. *The Humanistic Psychologist, 16* (2), 314–322.

SZASZ, T. S. (1991). Diagnoses are not diseases. *The Lancet, 338,* 1574–1576.

SZASZ, T. S. (1994). Mental illness is still a myth. *Transaction Social Science and Modern Society, 31* (4), 34–39.

SZUSTER, R. R., SCHANBACHER, B. L., & MCCANN, S. C. (1990). Characteristics of psychiatric emergency room patients with alcohol- or drug-induced disorders. *Hospital and Community Psychiatry, 41,* 1342–1345.

SZWABO, P. A. (1993). Substance abuse in older women. *Clinics in Geriatric Medicine, 9,* 197–208.

TABAKOFF, B., & HOFFMAN, P. L. (1992). Alcohol: Neurobiology. In J. H. Lowinson, P. Ruiz, R. B. Millman, & J. G. Langrod (Eds.), *Substance abuse: A comprehensive textbook* (2nd ed.). New York: Williams & Wilkins.

TAHA, A. S., DAHILL, S., STURROCK, R. D., LEE, F. D., & RUSSELL, R. I. (1994). Predicting NSAID related ulcers—Assessment of clinical and pathological risk factors and importance of differences in NSAID. *Gut, 35,* 891–895.

TAKANISHI, R. (1993). The opportunities of adolescence—Research, interventions, and policy. *American Psychologist, 48,* 85–87.

TALLEY, N. J. (1993). The effects of NSAIDs on the gut. *Contemporary Internal Medicine, 5* (2), 14–28.

TARTER, R. E. (1988). Are there inherited behavioral traits that predispose to substance abuse? *Journal of Consulting and Clinical Psychology, 56,* 189–197.

TARTER, R. E., OTT, P. J., & MEZZICH, A. C. (1991). Psychometric assessment. In R. J. Frances & S. I. Miller (Eds.), *Clinical textbook of addictive disorders.* New York: Guilford.

TASHKIN, D. P. (1990). Pulmonary complications of smoked substance abuse. *The Western Journal of Medicine, 152,* 525–531.

TASHKIN, D. P. (1993). Is frequent marijuana smoking harmful to health? The Western Journal of Medicine, *158,* 635–637.

TATE, C. (1989). In the 1800s, antismoking was a burning issue. *Smithsonian, 20* (4), pp. 107–117.

TATE, J. C., STANTON, A. L., GREEN, S. B., SCHMITZ, J. M., LE, T., & MARSHALL, B. (1994). Experimental analysis of the role of expectancy in nicotine withdrawal. *Psychology of Addictive Behaviors, 8,* 169–178.

TAVRIS, C. (1990). One more guilt trip for women. *Minneapolis Star-Tribune, VIII* (341), p. 21A.

TAVRIS, C. (1992). *The mismeasure of woman.* New York: Simon & Schuster.

TAYLOR, D. (1993). Addicts' abuse of sleeping pills brings call for tough curbs. *The Observer, No. 10531,* p. 6.

TAYLOR, W. A., & GOLD, M. S. (1990). Pharmacologic approaches to the treatment of cocaine dependence. *Western Journal of Medicine, 152,* 573–578.

TEST, M. A., WALLISCH, L. S., ALLNESS, D. J., & RIPP, K. (1990). Substance use in young adults with schizophrenic disorders. *Schizophrenia Bulletin, 15,* 465–476.

THACKER, W., & TREMAINE, L. (1989). Systems issues in serving the mentally ill substance abuser: Virginia's experience. *Hospital and Community Psychiatry, 40,* 1046–1049.

THOMASON, H. H., & DILTS, S. L. (1991). Opioids. In R. J. Frances & S. I. Miller (Eds.), *Clinical textbook of addictive disorders.* New York: Guilford.

THOMSON, A. D. (1994). Alcoholic hepatitis. *The Lancet, 343,* 810.

THORNTON, J. (1990). Pharm aid: 10 new medicines you should know about. *Men's Health, 5* (4), 73–78.

THUN, M. J., NAMBOODIRI, M. M., & HEATH, C. W. (1991). Aspirin use and reduced risk of fatal colon cancer. *The New England Journal of Medicine, 325,* 1593–1596.

TOBIN, J. W. (1992). Is A.A. "treatment"? You bet. *Addiction & Recovery, 12* (3), 40.

TONEATTO, T., SOBELL, L. C., SOBELL, M. B., & LEO, G. I. (1991). Psychoactive substance use disorder (alcohol). In M. Hersen & S. M. Turner (Eds.), *Adult Psychopathology & Diagnosis* (2nd ed.). New York: Wiley.

TORRENS, M., SAN, L., & CAMI, J. (1993). Buprenorphine versus heroin dependence: Comparison of toxicologic and psychopathologic characteristics. *American Journal of Psychiatry, 150,* 822–824.

TRABERT, W., CASPARI, D., BERNHARD, P., & BIRO, G. (1992). Inappropriate vasopressin secretion in severe alcohol withdrawal. *Acta Psychiatrica Scandinavica, 85,* 376–379.

TRACHTENBERG, M. C., & BLUM, K. (1987). Alcohol and opioid peptides: Neuropharmacological rationale for physical craving of alcohol. *American Journal of Drug and Alcohol Abuse, 13* (3), 365–372.

TRACHTENBERG, M. C., & BLUM, K. (1988). Improvement of cocaine-induced neuromodulator deficits by the neuronutrient Tropamine. *Journal of Psychoactive Drugs, 20* (3), 315–331.

TRAYNOR, M. P., BEGAY, M. E., & GLANTZ, S. A. (1993). New tobacco industry strategy to prevent local tobacco control. *Journal of the American Medical Association, 270,* 479–486.

TREADWAY, D. (1987). The ties that bind. *The Family Therapy Networker, 11* (4), 17–23.

TREADWAY, D. (1990). Codependency: Disease, metaphor, or fad? *The Family Therapy Networker, 14* (1), 39–43.

Triangle of Self-Obsession, The. (1983). New York: Narcotics Anonymous World Service Office.

TRICHOPOULOS, D., MOLLO, F., TOMATIS, L., AGAPITOS, E., DELSEDIME, L., ZAVITSANOS, X., KALANDIDI, A., KATSOUYANNI, K., RIBOLI, E., & SARACCI, R. (1992). Active and passive smoking and pathological indicators of lung cancer risk in an autopsy study. *Journal of the American Medical Association, 268,* 1697–1701.

TRUOG, R. D., BERDE, C. B., MITCHELL, C., & GRIER, H. E. (1992). Barbiturates in the care of the terminally ill. *The New England Journal of Medicine, 327,* 1678–1682.

TUCKER, J. A., & SOBELL, L. C. (1992). Influences on help-seeking for drinking problems and on natural recovery without treatment. *The Behavior Therapist, 15* (1), 12–14.

TURBO, R. (1989). Drying out is just a start: Alcoholism. *Medical World News, 30* (3), 56–63.

TURKINGTON, C. (1994). Study of xanthines could lead to drug discoveries. *APA Monitor, 25* (2), 18.

TWEED, S. H., & RYFF, C. D. (1991). Profiles of wellness amidst distress. *Journal of Studies on Alcohol, 52,* 133–141.

Twelve Steps and Twelve Traditions. (1981). New York: Alcoholics Anonymous World Services, Inc.

TWERSKI, A. J., (1983). Early intervention in alcoholism: Confrontational techniques. *Hospital & Community Psychiatry, 34,* 1027–1030.

TWERSKI, A. J. (1989). Diagnosing and treating dual disorders. *Alcoholism & Addiction, 9* (3), 37–40.

TYAS, S., & RUSH, B. (1993). The treatment of disabled persons with alcohol and drug problems: Results of a survey of addiction services. *Journal of Studies on Alcohol, 54,* 275–282.

TYLER, D. C. (1994). Pharmacology of pain management. *Pediatric Clinics of North America, 41,* 59–71.

TYRER, P. (1993). Withdrawal from hypnotic drugs. *British Medical Journal, 306,* 706–708.

UHL, G. R., PERSICO, A. M., & SMITH, S. S. (1992). Current excitement with D$_2$ dopamine receptor gene alleles in substance abuse. *Archives of General Psychiatry, 49,* 157–160.

Understanding Anonymity. (1981). New York: Alcoholics Anonymous World Services, Inc.

United States Pharmacopeial Convention, Inc. (1990). *Advice for the patient* (10th ed.). Rockville, MD: USPC Board of Trustees.

University of California, Berkeley. (1990a). Codependency. *The Wellness Letter 7* (1), 7.

University of California, Berkeley. (1990b). Marijuana: What we know. *The Wellness Letter, 6* (6), 2–4.

University of California, Berkeley. (1990c). Women's magazines: Whose side are they on? *The Wellness Letter, 7* (3), 7.

University of California, Berkeley. (1990d). Is there an addictive personality? *The Wellness Letter, 6* (9), 1–2.

University of California, Berkeley. (1991). The changing face of AIDS. *The Wellness Letter, 7* (8), 6.

Upjohn Company. (1989). Anxiety center. *Science Digest, 2* (1), pp. 69–70.

USA Today. (1994). *Cocaine use . . . by the ton. 12* (235), p. 1A.

U.S. News & World Report. (1991). The men who created crack. *111* (8), pp. 44–53.

U.S. News & World Report. (1993). A call for new curbs on teens. *114* (10), p. 15.

U.S. News & World Report. (1994). Take 2 aspirins and come back in 76 years. *117* (12), p. 24.

UVA, J. L. (1991). Alcoholics Anonymous: Medical recovery through a higher power. *Journal of the American Medical Association, 266,* 3065–3068.

VAILLANT, G. E. (1983). *The natural history of alcoholism.* Cambridge, MA: Harvard University Press.

VAILLANT, G. E. (1990). We should retain the disease concept of alcoholism. *The Harvard Medical School Mental Health Letter, 9* (6), 4–6.

VANDEPUTTE, C. (1989). Why bother to treat older adults? The answer is compelling. *Professional Counselor, 4* (2), 34–38.

VEREBEY, K., & TURNER, C. E. (1991). Laboratory testing. In R. J. Frances & S. I. Miller (Eds.), *Clinical textbook of addictive disorders.* New York: Guilford.

VICTOR, M. (1993). Persistent altered mentation due to ethanol. *Neurologic Clinics, 11,* 639–661.

VOELKER, R. (1994). Medical marijuana: A trial of science and politics. *Journal of the American Medical Association, 271,* 1645–1648.

VOLKOW, N. D., HITZEMANN, R., WANG, G. J., FOWLER, J. S., BURR, G., PASCANI, K., DEWEY, S. L., & WOLF, A. P. (1992). Decreased brain metabolism in neurologically intact healthy alcoholics. *American Journal of Psychiatry, 149,* 1016–1022.

VOLPE, J. J. (1995). *Neurology of the newborn* (3rd ed.). Philadelphia: W. B. Saunders.

VOLPICELLI, J. R., ALTERMAN, A. I., HAYASHIDA, M., & O'BRIEN, C. P. (1992). Naltrexone in the treatment of alcohol dependence. *Archives of General Psychiatry, 49,* 876–880.

WADLER, G. I. (1994). Drug use update. *Medical Clinics of North America, 78,* 439–455.

WALKER, C. E., BONNER, B. L., & KAUFMAN, K. I. (1988). *The physically and sexually abused child.* New York: Pergamon.

WALKER, J. D. (1993). The tobacco epidemic: How far have we come? *Canadian Medical Association Journal, 148,* 145–147.

WALLACE, J. M., OISHI, J. S., BARBERS, R. G., SIMMONS, M. S., & TASHKIN, D. P. (1994). Lymphocytic subpopulation profiles in bronchoalveolar lavage fluid and peripheral blood from tobacco and marijuana smokers. *Chest, 105,* 847–852.

WALLEN, M. C., & WEINER, H. D. (1989). Impediments to effective treatment of the dually diagnosed patient. *Journal of Psychoactive Drugs, 21,* 161–168.

WALSH, D. C., HINGSON, R. W., MERRIGAN, D. M., LEVENSON, S. M., CUPPLES, L. A., HEEREN, T., COFFMAN, G. A., BECKER, C. A., BARKER, T. A., HAMILTON, S. A., MCGUIRE, T. G., & KELLY, C. A. (1991). A randomized trial of treatment options for alcohol-abusing workers. *The New England Journal of Medicine, 325,* 775–782.

WALTERS, G. D. (1994). The drug lifestyle: One pattern or several? *Psychology of Addictive Behaviors, 8,* 8–13.

WASHTON, A. M. (1990). Crack and other substance abuse in the suburbs. *Medical Aspects of Human Sexuality, 24* (5), 54–58.

WASHTON, A. M., STONE, N. S., & HENDRICKSON, E. C. (1988). Cocaine abuse. In D. M. Donovan & G. A. Marlatt (Eds.), *Assessment of addictive behaviors.* New York: Guilford Press.

WASMAN, H. (1991). Tobacco marketing. *Journal of the American Medical Association, 266,* 3186–3188.

WATSON, J. M. (1984). Solvent abuse and adolescents. *The Practitioner, 228,* 487–490.

WEATHERS, W. T., CRANE, M. M., SAUVAIN, K. J., & BLACKHURST, D. W. (1993). Cocaine use in women from a defined population: Prevalence at delivery and effects on growth in infants. *Pediatrics, 91,* 350–354.

WEBB, S. T. (1989). Some developmental issues of adolescent children of alcoholics. *Adolescent Counselor, 1* (6), 47–48, 67.

WEDDINGTON, W. W. (1993). Cocaine. *Psychiatric Clinics of North America, 16,* 87–95.

WEGSCHEIDER-CRUSE, S. (1985). *Choice-making.* Pompano Beach, FL: Health Communications.

WEGSCHEIDER-CRUSE, S., & CRUSE, J. R. (1990). *Understanding co-dependency.* Pompano Beach, FL: Health Communications.

WEIL, A. (1986). *The natural mind.* Boston: Houghton-Mifflin.

WEINER, N. (1985). Norepinephrine, epinephrine and the sympathomimetic amines. In A. G. Gilman, L. S. Goodman, T. W. Rall, & F. Murad (Eds.), *The pharmacological basis of therapeutics* (7th ed.). New York: Houghton-Mifflin.

WEINRIEB, R. M., & O' BRIEN, C. P. (1993). Persistent cognitive deficits attributed to substance abuse. *Neurologic Clinics, 11,* 663–691.

WEISNER, C., & SCHMIDT, L. (1992). Gender disparities in treatment for alcohol problems. *Journal of the American Medical Association, 268,* 1872–1876.

WEISS, R. (1994). Of myths and mischief. *Discover, 15* (10), pp. 36–42.

WEISS, R. D., & MIRIN, S. M. (1988). Intoxication and withdrawal syndromes. In S. E. Hyman (Ed.), *Handbook of psychiatric emergencies* (2nd ed.). Boston: Little, Brown.

WEISS, R. D., MIRIN, S. M., & FRANCES, R. J. (1992). The myth of the typical dual diagnosis patient. *Hospital and Community Psychiatry, 43,* 107–108.

WEISS, R. D., MIRIN, S. M., GRIFFIN, M. L., & MICHAEL, J. L. (1988). Psychopathology in cocaine users: Changing trends. *Journal of Nervous and Mental Disease, 176,* 719–725.

WERNER, E. E. (1989). Children of the garden island. *Scientific American, 260* (4), pp. 106–111.

WESTERMEYER, J. (1987). The psychiatrist and solvent-inhalant abuse: Recognition, assessment and treatment. *American Journal of Psychiatry, 144,* 903–907.

WETLI, C. V. (1987). Fatal reactions to cocaine. In A. M. Washton & M. S. Gold (Eds.), *Cocaine: A clinician's handbook.* New York: Guilford.

WETTER, D. W., YOUNG, T. B., BIDWELL, T. R., BADR, M. S., & PALTA, M. (1994). Smoking as a risk factor for sleep-disordered breathing. *Archives of Internal Medicine, 154,* 2219–2224.

WHEELER, K., & MALMQUIST, J. (1987). Treatment approaches in adolescent chemical dependency. *The Pediatric Clinics of North America, 34* (2), 437–447.

WHITE, P. T. (1989). Coca. *National Geographic, 175* (1), pp. 3–47.

WHITE, R. J. (1993). Washington figuring out it has fought drug war on wrong fronts. *Minneapolis Star-Tribune, XI* (351), p. 23A.

WHITEHEAD, R., CHILLAG, S., & ELLIOTT, D. (1992). Anabolic steroid use among adolescents in a rural state. *Journal of Family Practice, 35,* 401–405.

WHITMAN, D., FRIEDMAN, D., & THOMAS, L. (1990). The return of skid row. *U.S. News & World Report, 108* (2), pp. 27–30.

WILBUR, R. (1986). A drug to fight cocaine. *Science '86, 7* (2), pp. 42–46.

WILCOX, C. M., SHALEK, K. A., & COTSONIS, G. (1994). Striking prevalence of over-the-counter nonsteroidal anti-inflammatory drug use in patients with upper gastrointestinal hemorrhage. *Archives of Internal Medicine, 154,* 42–46.

WILEY, J. P. (1993). Phenomena, comment and notes. *Smithsonian, 24* (6), pp. 21–25.

WILFORD, J. N. (1991). 3500 B.C.: They have served no wine before this time. *Minneapolis Star-Tribune, X* (26), p. 7A.

WILL, G. F. (1993). U.S. drug policy sets off slew of unintended consequences. *Minneapolis Star-Tribune, XII* (84), p. 21A.

WILLIAMS, B. R., & BAER, C. L. (1994). *Essentials of clinical pharmacology in nursing* (2nd ed.). Springhouse, PA: Springhouse Corp.

WILLIAMS, E. (1989). Strategies for intervention. *The Nursing Clinics of North America, 24* (1), 95–107.

WILLIAMSON, D. F., MADANS, J., ANDA, R., KLEINMAN, J. C., GIOVINO, G. A., & BYERS, T. (1991). Smoking cessation and severity of weight gain in a national cohort. *The New England Journal of Medicine, 324,* 739–745.

WILLOUGHBY, A. (1984). *The alcohol-troubled person: Known and unknown.* Chicago: Nelson-Hall.

WILSNACK, S. C. (1991). Barriers to treatment for alcoholic women. *Addiction & Recovery, 11* (4), 10–12.

WINCHESTER, J. F. (1990). Barbiturates, methaqualone and primidone. In L. M. Haddad & J. F. Winchester (Eds.), *Clinical management of poisoning and drug overdose* (2nd ed.). Philadelphia: W. B. Saunders.

WISNEIWSKI, L. (1994). Use of household products as inhalants rising among young teens. *Minneapolis Star-Tribune, XIII* (9), p. 8Ex.

WITKIN, G., & GRIFFIN, J. (1994). The new opium wars. *U.S. News & World Report, 117* (114), pp. 39–44.

WOITITZ, J. G. (1983). *Adult children of alcoholics.* Pompano Beach, FL: Health Communications.

WOLF-REEVE, B. S. (1990). A guide to the assessment of psychiatric symptoms in the addictions treatment setting. In D. F. O'Connell (Ed.), *Managing the dually diagnosed patient.* New York: Haworth.

WOLIN, S. J., & WOLIN, S. (1993). *The resilient self.* New York: Villard Books.

WOLKOWITZ, O. M. (1990). Long-lasting behavioral

changes following prednisone withdrawal. *Journal of the American Medical Association, 261,* 1731.

WOLKOWITZ, O. M., RUBINOW, D., DORAN, A. R., BREIER, A., BERRETTINI, W. H., KLING, M. A., & PICKAR, D. (1990). Prednisone effects on neurochemistry and behavior: Preliminary findings. *Archives of General Psychiatry, 47,* 963–968.

WOODS, J. H., KATZ, J. L., & WINGER, G. (1988). Use and abuse of benzodiazepines. *Journal of the American Medical Association, 260* (23), 3476–3480.

WOODS, J. H., WINGER, G. D., & FRANCE, C. P. (1987). Reinforcing and discriminative stimulus effects of cocaine: Analysis of pharmacological mechanisms. In S. Fisher, A. Raskin, & E. H. Unlenhuth (Eds.), *Cocaine: Clinical and behavioral aspects.* New York: Oxford University Press.

WORMSLEY, K. G. (1993). Safety profile of ranitidine. *Drugs, 46,* 976–985.

WRAY, S. R., & MURTHY, N. V. A. (1987). Review of the effects of cannabis on mental and physiological functions. *West Indian Medical Journal, 36* (4), 197–201.

YABLONSKY, L. (1967). *Synanon: The tunnel back.* Baltimore: Penguin.

YALOM, I. D. (1985). *The theory and practice of group psychotherapy* (3rd ed.). New York: Basic Books.

YESALIS, C. E., KENNEDY, N. J., KOPSTEIN, A. N., & BAHRKE, M. S. (1993). Anabolic-androgenic steroid use in the United States. *Journal of the American Medical Association, 270,* 1217–1221.

YIP, L., DART, R. C., & GABOW, P. A. (1994). Concepts and controversies in salicylate toxicity. *Emergency Medical Clinics of North America, 12,* 351–364.

YOUCHA, G. A. (1978). *A dangerous pleasure.* New York: Hawthorn Books.

YOUNGSTROM, N. (1990a). The drugs used to treat drug abuse. *APA Monitor, 21* (10), 19.

YOUNGSTROM, N. (1990b). Debate rages on: In- or outpatient? *APA Monitor, 21* (10), 19.

YOUNGSTROM, N. (1991). Field, APA address drug abuse in society. *APA Monitor, 22* (1), 14.

YOUNGSTROM, N. (1992). Fetal alcohol syndrome carries severe deficits. *APA Monitor, 23* (4), 32.

ZAREK, D., HAWKINS, D., & ROGERS, P. D. (1987). Risk factors for adolescent substance abuse. *The Pediatric Clinics of North America, 34* (2), 481–493.

ZERWEKH, J., & MICHAELS, B. (1989). Co-dependency. *The Nursing Clinics of North America, 24* (1), 109–120.

ZIMBERG, S. (1978). Psychosocial treatment of elderly alcoholics. In S. Zimberg, J. Wallace, & S. B. Blume (Eds.), *Practical approaches to alcoholism psychotherapy.* New York: Plenum.

ZISOOK, S., HEATON, R., MORANVILLE, J., KUCK, J., JERNIGAN, T., & BRAFF, D. (1992). Past substance abuse and clinical course of schizophrenia. *American Journal of Psychiatry, 149,* 552–553.

ZITO, J. M. (1994). *Psychotherapeutic drug manual* (3rd ed.). New York: Wiley.

ZUCKER, R. A., & GOMBERG, E. S. L. (1986). Etiology of alcoholism reconsidered: The case for a biopsychosocial process. *American Psychologist, 41,* 783–794.

ZUCKERMAN, B., & BRESNAHAN, K. (1991). Developmental and behavioral consequences of prenatal drug and alcohol exposure. *Pediatric Clinics of North America, 38,* 1387–1406.

ZUGER, A. (1994). Meningitis mystery. *Discover, 15* (3), pp. 40–43.

ZUKIN, S. R., & ZUKIN, R. S. (1992). Phencyclidine. In J. H. Lowinson, P. Ruiz, R. B. Millman, & J. G. Langrod (Eds.), *Substance abuse: A comprehensive textbook* (2nd ed.). New York: Williams & Wilkins.

Index

TO THE OWNER OF THIS BOOK:

I hope that you have enjoyed *Concepts of Chemical Dependency,* Third Edition, as much as I've enjoyed writing it. I'd like to know as much about your experiences with the book as you care to offer. Only through your comments and comments of others can I learn how to make a better book for future readers.

School and address: _____

Your instructor's name: _____

1. For what course was this book assigned? _____

2. What did you like most about the book? _____

_____

_____

3. What did you like least about the book? _____

_____

_____

4. Were all of the chapters of the book assigned for you to read? _____

    If not, which ones weren't? _____

_____

5. In the space below, or on a separate sheet of paper, please let me know what other comments about the book you'd like to make. (For example, were any chapters or concepts particularly difficult?) I'd be delighted to hear from you.

_____

_____

_____

_____

_____

_____

Optional:

Your name: _____ Date: _____

May Brooks/Cole quote you, either in promotion for *Concepts of Chemical Dependency,*
Third Edition, or in future publishing ventures?

Yes: _____ No: _____

Sincerely,

Harold Doweiko

FOLD HERE

BUSINESS REPLY MAIL

FIRST CLASS   PERMIT NO. 358   PACIFIC GROVE, CA

POSTAGE WILL BE PAID BY ADDRESSEE

ATT: *Harold Doweiko* _____

Brooks/Cole Publishing Company
511 Forest Lodge Road
Pacific Grove, California 93950-9968

FOLD HERE

Brooks/Cole is dedicated to publishing quality books for the helping professions. If you would like to learn more about our publications, please use this mailer to request our catalogue.

Name: ————————————————————————————

Street Address: ————————————————————————

City, State, and Zip: ————————————————————